Nutrition and feeding of the broodmare

The EAAP series is published under the direction of Dr. P. Rafai

EAAP – European Federation of Animal Science

Molise University

EWEN – European Workshop on Equine Nutrition

The organisation acknowledges the following organisations for their finacial support:

FISE – Federazione Italiana Sport Equestri

Regione Molise

The European Association for Animal Production wishes to express its appreciation to the *Ministero per le Politiche Agricole e Forestali* and the *Associazione Italiana Allevatori* for their valuable support of its activities

Nutrition and feeding of the broodmare

EAAP publication No. 120

Editors:

N. Miraglia and W. Martin-Rosset

Wageningen Academic
Publishers

ISBN-10: 90-8686-014-1
ISBN-13: 978-90-8686-014-2

ISSN 0071-2477

First published, 2006

Wageningen Academic Publishers
The Netherlands, 2006

Table of contents

Foreword 11
Nicoletta Miraglia William Martin-Rosset

Part A – Pregnancy

Energy and protein requirements and recommended allowances in pregnant mares 15
W. Martin-Rosset, I. Vervuert and D. Austbo

Apparent digestibility of two diets in the Amiata breed of donkey in late pregnancy 41
L. Casini, M. Sgorbini, L. Magni, M. Corazza and D. Gatta

Part B – Lactation

Physiology of lactation in the mare 49
G.R. Starbuck

Milk yield of nursing and dairy mares 57
M. Doreau and F. Martuzzi

Mare milk composition: recent findings about protein fractions and mineral content 65
F. Martuzzi and M. Doreau

Fat content and composition of mare's milk 77
M. Doreau and F. Martuzzi

Energy and protein requirements and recommended allowances in lactating mares 89
W. Martin-Rosset, D. Austbo and M. Coenen

Asses: milk yield and composition 117
E. Salimei and B. Chiofalo

Other utilisation of mare's and ass's milk 133
B. Chiofalo, C. Drogoul and E. Salimei

The lactation curve in Lusitano mares - a preliminary study 149
A.S. Santos and A.M. Silvestre

A novel restrictive grazing approach to enhance leptin sensitivity in obese pony mares* 155
P.R. Buff, D.H. Keisler, P.J. Johnson, N.T. Messer IV and V.K. Ganjam

A weigh-suckle-weigh approach for estimating milk yield in the Arabian mare 163
N.L. Trottier, T. Stamper, J. Moore, J. Liesman and B.D. Nielsen

Different fibre sources in dairy ass's diet: effects on body condition and plasma leptin level 167
C. Maglieri, F. Rosi, D. Magistrelli, M. Polidori, F. Fantuz and E. Salimei

Nutritional status of lactating asses fed two different dietary fibre sources 169
C. Maglieri, M. Palazzo, D. Casamassima, P. Polidori and E. Salimei

Values on serum metabolites in lactating jennies of Martina Franca breed 171
A.G. D'Alessandro, G. Martemucci, M. Palazzo, N. Simone, G.E. Colella, R. Pizzo and D. Casamassima

Different fibre sources in dairy ass's diet. I. Effects on milk fatty acid composition 175
B. Chiofalo, D. Piccolo, E.B. Riolo, C. Maglieri and E. Salimei

Different fibre sources in dairy ass's diet. II. Effects on plasma fatty acid profile 177
B. Chiofalo, D. Piccolo, E.B. Riolo, C. Maglieri and E. Salimei

Ass' s milk nitrogen distribution: effects of different dietary fibre source 179
F. Fantuz, P. Polidori, C. Maglieri, G. Varisco, S. Vincenzetti and E. Salimei

Machine milking of dairy asses as related to milk production and body condition 181
E. Salimei, C. Maglieri, M. Polidori, R. Socci, B. Chiofalo, M. Gambacorta and G. Varisco

Behaviour and milk yield of Murgese mares subjected to machine or hand milking 183
M. Caroprese, M. Albenzio, A. Santillo, R. Marino, S.Pelosi and F. D'Emilio

Part C – The foal

Physiology and metabolism in the newborn foal with reference to orphaned or sick foals 187
J.C. Ousey

Equine colostrum production and utilisation: basic and applied aspects 203
C. Drogoul, F. Clément, M. Ventorp and M. Orlandi

Energy and protein requirements and feeding of the suckling foal 221
W. Martin-Rosset and B. Younge

Body weight and condition of Kentucky Thoroughbred mares and their foals as influenced by month of foaling, season, and gender 245
J.D. Pagan, C.G. Brown-Douglas and S. Caddel

The utilisation of morphometric measurements to estimate horse body weight: Application to the Lusitano breed 253
A.S. Santos, B.C. Sousa, L.C. Leitão and V.C. Alves

Passive immunity transfer forecast in different horse breeds 257
M. Orlandi and M.C. Curadi

TAHITIAN NONI™ Equine Essentials™ Regulates LPS-Induced COX-2 and cytokine expression in equine neonatal monocytes: A preliminary study 259
J. Xu, J. Cai, R.G. Godbee, S.F. Peek and B.J. Darien

Part D – Feeding practices and pastures management

Overview practices in the field in Europe: rationing and prevention of nutritional related problems in the mares 263
D. Bergero, M. Ventorp, I. Vervuert, N. Miraglia, C. Trillaud-Geyl and E. Valle

Role of pasture in mares and foals management in Europe 279
N. Miraglia, M. Saastamoinen and W. Martin-Rosset

Relationships between the management and health of pastures and mares and foals: A U.S. perspective 299
W. Burton Staniar

Part E – Nutrition and reproductive performances

Effects of nutrition level in mares' ovarian activity and in equines' puberty 315
D. Guillaume, J. Salazar-Ortiz and W. Martin-Rosset

Nutrition and equine fertility 341
A.D. Ellis, M. Boekhoff, L. Bailoni and R. Mantovani

Intrauterine nutrition: Effect on subsequent health 367
A.H. Tauson, P. Harris and M. Coenen

Part F - Advances in reproductive biotechnologies

The new biotechnologies of reproduction in horses: recent progresses and applications 389
F. Camillo, C. Galli and E. Palmer

Management strategy of the broodmare: The case of trotter mares in Italy 403
A. Falaschini and F. Cappelli

Author index 415

Foreword

This proceedings provide a compilation of the abstracts of papers presented at the 3rd European Workshop on Equine Nutrition (EWEN) held at the University of Molise in Campobasso, Italy, June 20-22 June, 2006.

The meeting is placed under the umbrella of the Horse commission of the European association for Animal Production (EAAP) as a satellite of the annual meeting of EAAP. Yearly, the Horse commission sets up, in the scope of the EAAP meeting, six scientific sessions devoted either to disciplinary areas (genetics, physiology, nutrition, behaviour, etc.) to initiate discussion between scientists, advisers officers, or to multidisciplinary approaches to answer to rising multi factorial questions raised by equine industry. But no enough time and space are left in each discipline and related sessions to extend oral presentation and large discussion. Hence, European working groups (EWG) have been set up at the initiative of Horse commission to improve the situation. The EWG Nutrition decided years ago to perform biannual workshops to give the opportunity to deepen more extensively three key points:
The evaluation and prediction of nutrients requirements.
The means to overcome the limiting factors met in the application of the different nutritional systems for rationing horses, comparing the feeding practices throughout Europe.
The increases interaction between health and nutrition, which limits the performance and welfare of horses.

The workshop held in 2006 dealt with the broodmare which is the key animal in the Equine chain. In the new competitive context of Equine Industry, the mare should foal yearly a healthy offspring at an optimum cost. The foal should be born and weaned at the accurate months of the year to fit the goals of production: races, sports or leisure horses. So far the improvement of the knowledge of biology of pregnancy and lactation, of nutrition and the interaction between nutrition and physiology of reproduction is of major concern to outline and disseminate relevant husbandry and feeding systems to the Equine industry.

An International Scientific Committee (ISC) determined the scientific programme: Dag Austbo* (N), Domenico Bergero* (I), Manfred Coenen* (D), Carole Drogoul*(F), Andrea Ellis* (UK), Anders Herlin (SW), Jan Eric Lindberg* (SW), William Martin-Rosset* (EAAP, President of the ISC), Nicoletta Miraglia* (I), Markku Saastamoinen* (Fin), Pat Harris** (UK)
* Members of EWG Nutrition at EAAP
** Member of EWG Nutrition at EAAP and a representative of Equine industry (Feed company)

The meeting was organised by a National Committee (NC): Lucia Bailoni (University of Padova); Sandro Barbacini (Studio Cristella), Domenico Bergero (University of Torino), Francesco Camillo (University of Pisa), Antonio Lucio Catalano (University of Parma), Biagina Chiofalo (University of Messina), Adalberto Falaschini (University of Bologna), Domenico Gatta (University of Pisa), Roberto Mantovani (University of Padova), Francesca Martuzzi (University of Parma), Elisabetta Salimei (University of Molise), Nicoletta Miraglia (University of Molise, President of NC), Maurizzio Silvestrelli (University of Perugia), Maria Federica Trombetta (University of Ancona)

The meeting was placed under the patronage of the University of Molise in Campobasso, located in Molise county in the South of Italy. The scientific secretariat was carried out by Nicoletta Miraglia assisted by Marco Costantini and Mimmo Polidori whereas Rosalba Albanese, Incoronata Cavaliere and Fiore Carpenito achieved the administrative secretariat. Mimmo Polidori was in charge of all the technical assistance too.

The scientific programme was focused around 4 main topics designed in four main sessions with main reports given by invited speakers, and communications and posters. A round table was organised with invited speakers.

Session 1: Pregnancy
Session 2: Lactation
Session 3: The foal (3a) – Pasture management (3b)
Session 4:Nutrition and reproductive performances
Round table: Advances in reproductive biotechnologies
Scientific tour:

- Visit at the breeding area of wild Pentro horses
- Visit of the experimental farm of "La Torre Feudozzo";

The sessions were chaired by:

- Session 1: Main reports: Jan Eric Lindberg (Sweden)
- Session 2: Main reports: John Burton (Canada); Communications and posters: Michel Doreau (France)
- Session 3: Main reports 3a: Joe D Pagan (US); Communications and posters: Manfred Coenen (Germany); Main reports 3b: Dag Austbo (Norway)
- Session 4: Main reports: Markku Saastamoinen (Finland)
- Round table: Sandro Barbacini (Italy)
- Scientific tour: Nicoletta Miraglia (Italy)

The workshop was under the patronage of Italian Scientific Organisations: ASPA – Scientific Association for Animal Productions; SIDI - Italian Society of Equine Practitioners; SISVet - Italian Society of Veterinary Sciences; SIVE – Italian Society of Equine Veterinarians. It was financially supported by:

- The University of Molise
- The Department of Animals, Vegetables and Environmental Sciences of the University of Molise
- The European Association for Animal Production: EAAP
- The Italian Equestrian Federation (FISE)
- The County of Molise (Assessorato Regionale Agricoltura, Foreste e Pesca Produttiva)
- The Equine industry: ACME (Italy); ALLTECH (US); CAVALOR (Belgium); WALTHAM (UK); IMV technologies Italia; PEGUS Horse feeds (Italy)
- The Scuderia Orsi Mangelli

Nicoletta Miraglia
President of the National committee
Vice- President of EAAP Horse commission

William Martin-Rosset
President of the International committee
President of EAAP Horse commission

Part A – Pregnancy

Energy and protein requirements and recommended allowances in pregnant mares

W. Martin-Rosset[1], I. Vervuert[2] and D. Austbo[3]
[1]INRA-Department of Animal Science, Research Center of Clermont-Ferrand/Theix, 63122 St Genès Champanelle, France
[2]University of Leipzig, Institute of Animal Nutrition Nutritional Diseases and Dietetics, Leipzig, Germany
[3]University of Norway, Department of Animal and Aquacultural Science, Norwegian University of Life Sciences, Box 5003, N-1432 Aas, Norway

Abstract

Original feeding standards/systems were proposed in the US (1978-1989) and in France (1984-1990). Several feeding standards were derived in Germany (GEH, 1994), in the Netherlands (CVB, 1996-2005) and in Scandinavia (SCAND; 2002-2004). In all the feeding standards/systems total energy requirements are broken down in maintenance and pregnancy requirements. Maintenance requirements are estimated from body weight (BW) (NRC) or BW^{75} (all the others). Pregnancy requirements are estimated from the accretion of energy in the conceptus using the efficiency rates of energy for pregnancy (CVB, GEH, INRA). Or the requirements are expressed as an increase of the maintenance requirement based on the accretion of energy in the conceptus (NRC, SCAND). The nutritional models performed by INRA and NRC were based or/and validated with feeding trials. In all the feeding standards/systems total protein requirements are broken down in maintenance or pregnancy requirements for CVB, GEH and INRA. Pregnancy requirements are estimated from the accretion of protein in the conceptus using the efficiency rates of energy for pregnancy. For the expression of the requirements NRC is using a N/E ratio and SCAND expresses the requirements as an increase of maintenance. The protein requirements have not been extensively validated with feeding experiments. Difference in energy or protein requirements are discussed. The harmonisation of the estimation of energy or protein requirements could be easily carried out between European Countries if a common model of the foetus growth curve could be designed. Recommended allowances related to body weight, body condition score, intake capacity are proposed by INRA. Other proposals could be elaborated in other European countries using feeding trials carried out to take care of breeds diversity and local conditions.

Keywords: mare, pregnancy, energy, protein, requirements, allowances

Introduction

Pregnancy is of high concern in the breeding cycle of the mare. The pregnant mare should deliver a healthy foal at the right month of year appropriate to the goal of production: race, sport, leisure or horse for meat. The mare should be in good condition at foaling too for rebreeding within the month following delivery.

Requirements are mainly related to physiological expenditure due to tissue accretion in the conceptus. Foetal development and metabolism have been studied to some extend. Energy and protein requirements have been estimated in different systems (CVB, GEH, INRA, NRC, SCAND). Comparison of those estimations are relevant to improve our knowledge and to suggest some harmonisation. Nutrients and feed allowances depend on intake capacity, body reserves of the mares throughout, the breeding cycle, namely the period of pregnancy. The effects of these characteristics should be determined to perform allowances which should be well adapted to the mares devoted to produce either race, sport or leisure horses, or horses meat in the conditions of the different countries.

This chapter is focused on energy and protein requirements and allowances only as there are enough data to discuss the recommendations proposed in the different countries. Minerals and vitamins requirements are of high concern as well, but most the recommendations proposed are based on the same data used by NRC, 1978, 1989 and there are not a lot of new experiments carried out at present in the world to argue new figures. (see the reviews published in the proceedings of Ker 2001)

Conceptus development and metabolism

Conceptus development

Foetus growth was determined in ponies, sports and heavy breeds from the data of Dusek, 1966[1], den Engelsen, 1966[2], Meyer and Alshwede, 1976[3] (Figure 1a). The gain is very low until the 7th month of pregnancy. But the increase is nearly linear during the last months. The development of the placenta, the amnios, the uterus and the udder take place earlier than the foetus during the pregnancy (Figure 1b). All these maternal tissues account for 70 percent of foetus body weight at mid-pregnancy and then 45 percent at foaling. The placenta weight would be about 4 kg for a 500 kg mare (Allen *et al.*, 2002). The udders and uterus weight is twice or twenty times higher respectively at the end of pregnancy (Barone and Monnet, 1955; Douglas and Ginther, 1975). The weight of foetal liquids is drawn from Arthur, 1969.

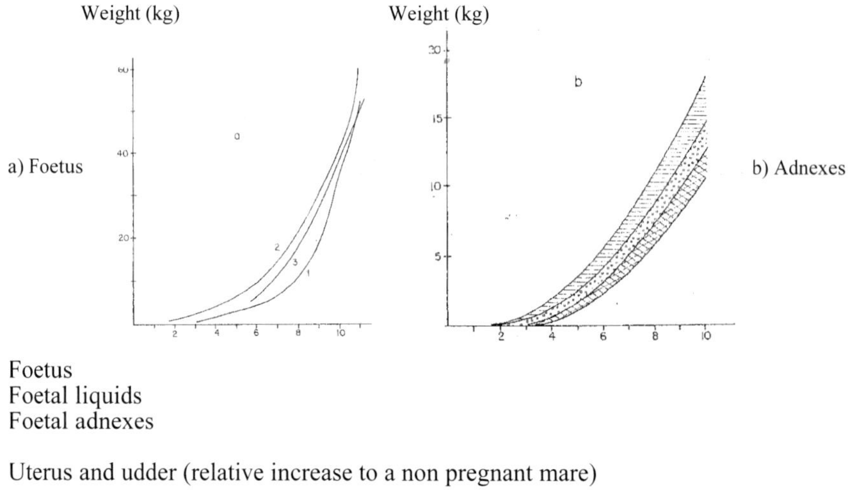

Figure 1. Variation of the weight of the foetus (a) and the foetus components (b).

Amount of nutrients fixed in the conceptus

The chemical composition of the foetus was determined (Table 1).

The accretion of the nutrients can be estimated from the chemical composition of the foetus and the daily gain using an appropriate model. The accretion of the nutrients in the placenta, amnios, uterus and udder can be estimated if we assumed that their chemical composition is similar to that of the cows. Using the weight of these tissues determined by Douglas and Ginther (1975), the accretion of energy and protein in these tissues would account for 20 percent of the daily gain of these nutrients

Table 1. Chemical composition of the foetus at birth (per kg) (from Meyer and Ahlswede, 1976).

Energy	5.48 MJ	Calcium	18.2 g
Protein	171 g	Phosphorus	9.7 g
Lipids	26 g	Magnesium	0.38 g
Ash	56 g	Potassium	1.9 g
		Chloridee	1.2 g
		Iron	120 mg
		Copper	5.0 mg

in the foetus. As a result the accretion of nutrients in the conceptus would be estimated from that in the foetus multiplied by 1.20.

Metabolism of the foetus and adnexes

During the last four month of pregnancy, weight, energy and protein gain of the foetus would account for 80, 90 and 90 percent of total gain respectively (Meyer and Ahlswede, 1976). So far oxygen and substrates needs of the foetus are very high (Fowden and Silver, 1995a). The placenta and the uterus grow and change in chemical composition too (Douglas and Ginther, 1975, Baur, 1977). Those tissues are metabolically very active as they are implemented into the transfer of substances to the foetus and the synthesis of nutrients, hormones and growth factors (Hay, 1977). Hence oxygen and substrates demand and subsequent requirement for these tissues are of high concern too (Fowden and Silver, 1995a).

In the last 5 months of pregnancy absolute uptake and utilization of glucose rise until 9-10th months then plateaued (Figure 2). But the weight specific rates of umbilical uptake and utilisation decrease simultaneously as far as the weight of the foetus increases (Figure 3).

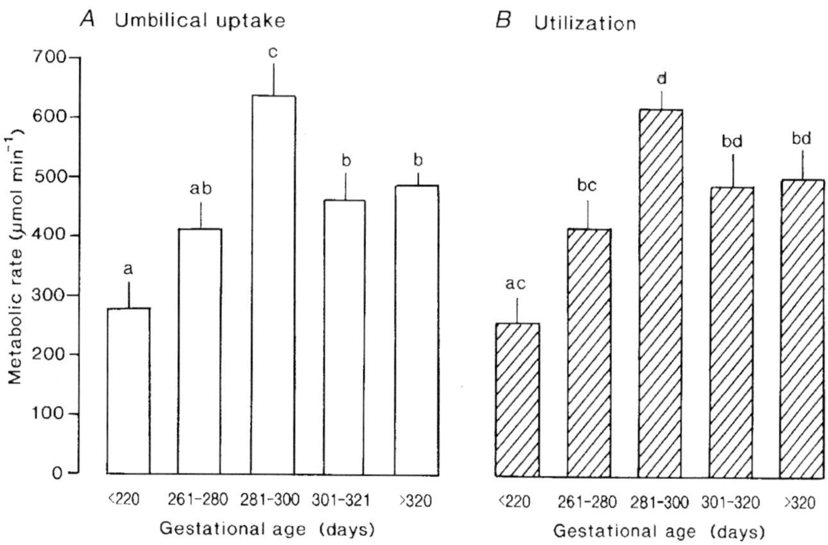

Figure 2. Absolute rates of umbilical uptake and utilization of glucose (from Fowden et al., 2000a).

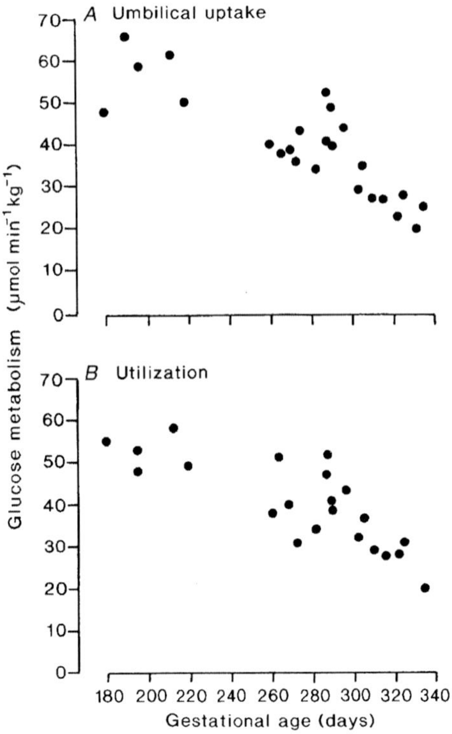

Figure 3. Weight specific rates of umbilical uptake and utilization of glucose (from Fowden et al., 2000a).

Absolute and weight specific rate of lactate uptake peak at 9-10th months then plateaued too. Urea clearance does not change during late pregnancy either in absolute terms or on weight specific bases.

Oxygen uptake is 3.5 times higher at the last month than at the 7th month of pregnancy. But weight specific rates oxygen uptake is not significant during late pregnancy. It results that the requirements of the foetus are highly dependant of glucose supply (85 percent) and to a lesser extend to lactate supply (15 percent) when the mares are fed adequately (Fowden *et al.*, 2000a). There is no endogenous production of glucose by the foetus. The glycogenic activity is low as the hepatic glycogen content and glycogenic enzymes activities are low (Fowden *et al.*, 1991). But the rise in carbohydrate and oxygen delivery reaches at the beginning of the 11th month a maximum of about 90 percent of the total requirements requested in the late pregnancy whereas the growth of the foetus is still very high: 23 percent of foal birth weight (Meyer and Ahlswede, 1976).

When the mare is experimentally fasted proportionately more glucose is oxidized by the foetus eventhough less glucose is utilised in total. But other substrates are likely oxidised as glucose carbon account only for 30 to 40 percent of total oxygen by the foetus. Lactate uptake is unaffected by maternal fasting. Amino acid oxidation could account for 10-15 percent as indicated in the rate of urea production. Lipids are the most likely supplementary energy source in response to the restriction of the mares (Stammers *et al.*, 1995). It would result in the last months of pregnancy that the weight specific rate of glucose decrease (60 percent), the lactate uptake increases whereas lipids are likely increasingly mobilised. Amino acids are likely oxidised in drastic conditions.

In late gestation, the relative weight of total adnexes (uterus and uteral placental tissue) in the conceptus decrease from 70 percent to 45 percent at birth (Douglas and Ginther, 1975). Glucose uptake of the foetus decrease from 73 to 61 percent and the weight specific rate of glucose is lower too. But the proportion of glucose intake of the foetus in the total intake of the conceptus, increases at the expenses of the uteroplacental tissue in late pregnancy. The oxygen uptake of the uteroplacental tissues is 2-3 times higher but the weight specific rates do not change in late gestation (Fowden *et al.*, 2000d). There is no change in the distribution of uterine oxygen uptake between the foetus and uteroplacental tissue with increasing gestational age conversely to sheep (Figure 4). The uteroplacental tissue account for about 50 percent of the uterine oxygen uptake at all gestational ages.

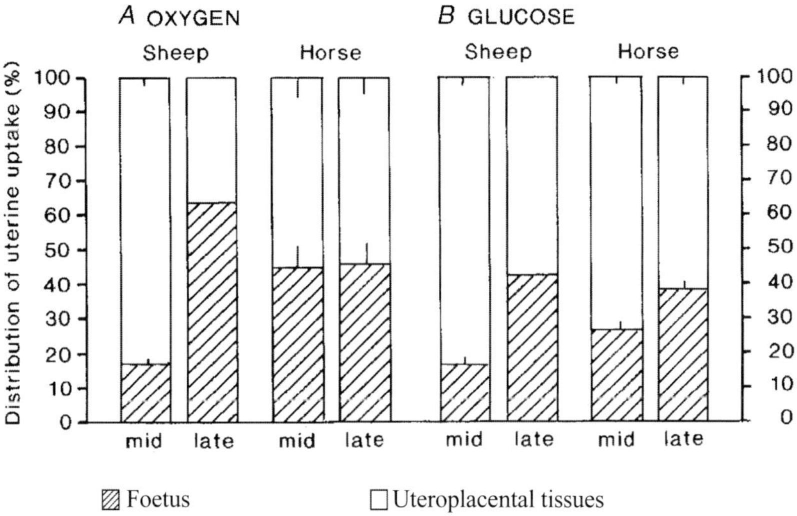

Figure 4. Distribution of the uterine oxygen and glucose uptakes.(from Fowden et al 2000b) The percentage distribution of the uterine uptake of oxygen (A) and glucose (B) in pregnant horses and sheep at mid- (50-60% gestation) and late gestation (> 90% gestation). Data for horses from this study and for sheep from Bell et al.,1986; Molina et al., 1991 and Fowden and Silver, 1995b.

Methods for evaluating nutrients requirements and recommended allowances

Definitions

Requirements and recommended allowances have to be clearly distinguished. The requirements stand for estimated or measured physiological expenditure of energy and protein in horses during different physiological situations. Allowances stand for the amount of nutrients, which are provided by the appropriate ration to meet the requirement of horses, and thus include estimation of energy and protein provided by feed and intake capacity horses. Recommended allowances stand for the amount of nutrients provided by the ration optimised for meeting the goal of production and utilisation of horses – these link the breeders' goal, the physiological requirements of the horse and feed allowances. It means that the amount of nutrients required for pregnancy of the same mare, can be lower, equal or higher than the nutritional requirements depending on husbandry or/and economical aims.

Methods for determination

Requirements are basically determined by factorial method. For maintenance, requirements are determined using balance experiments and then appropriate nutrients conversion rates for calculation. For pregnancy, requirements are determined using weight gain and accretion of nutrients, estimated with the appropriate method and then nutrients conversion rates if these are known. Allowances are determined by global method e.g. feeding experiments carried out with a high number of animals during long period corresponding to husbandry system to include the effect of individual animal variation, breeds, environmental factors as far as animals are expected to be in good health and well managed. In these experiments energy and nitrogen intakes are related to the true performances.

Evaluation of energy requirements

Calculation of energy requirements in different countries: data base – methodology – requirements

US

In US according to NRC (1989) (National Research Council) daily energy requirements for maintenance and pregnancy are calculated by using the following model:

DE = (Maintenance) + (Pregnancy) for mares which weight 200 to 900 kg BW

- 200 – 600 kg BW

$$DE = (1.4 + 0.03\ BW) + (maintenance \times F)$$

- 900 kg BW

$$DE = (1.82 + 0.0383\ BW - 0.000015\ BW^2) + (maintenance \times F)$$

Where

DE = Digestible Energy (MJ)
BW = Body weight (kg)
F = 1.11 (9 months) – 1.13 (10 months) – 1.20 (11 months)

These models are based on the data of Meyer and Ahlswede (1976); Platt (1984). The daily requirements calculated using this model are given in Table 2

Table2. Daily energy requirement (MJ DE) for pregnant mares (500 kg BW) according to NRC (1989).

Maintenance	Maintenance + Pregnancy		
	9 months	10 Months	11 months
68.6	76.1	77.3	82.4

Germany

In Germany, according to GEH (1994) (Gesellschaft für Ernärhungsphysiologie) daily requirements for maintenance and pregnancy are calculated by using the following equation

DE = (Maintenance) + (Pregnancy) for mares which weight 100 to 800 kg BW.
Daily maintenance requirement is calculated using this relationship:
$DE_m = 0.6$ MJ/kg BW^{75}
based on Hoffman *et al.* (1967), Knox *et al.* (1970), Wooden *et al.* (1970), Argenzio and Hintz (1971), Barth *et al.* (1977).
Daily pregnancy requirement is calculated using this relationship.
$DEp = (0.004851 * a * BW^{75})\ 1.20$
Total daily energy requirement is calculated using the following model
$DE = (0.6\ \text{MJ/kg}\ BW^{75}) + (0.004851 * a * BW^{75})\ 1.20$

Where

a = chemical composition of foetus (Table 3 – 4)
BW^{75} = metabolic body weight of the mare
1.20 = include extra requirement for adnexes (20 percent)

Table 3. Chemical composition of the foetus at birth (from Meyer and Ahlswede, 1976).

Energy (MJ)	Protein (%)	Ash (%)	Water (%)
5.48	17.1	5.6	72.7

Table 4. Body weight and nutrients gain of the foetus (from Meyer and Ahlswede, 1976). BW of the foetus at birth = (0.45 x BW^{75} of mare).

Months	Weight gain in p. 100 of birth weight	Gross Energy gain in p. 100 of total birth content	Protein gain
7	17	10.5	10.5
8	18	14.0	14.0
9	19	21.5	21.5
10	23	23.0	23.0
11	23	31.0	31.0

Efficiency of energy for pregnancy is assumed to be 20 percent. As a result the daily requirement calculated using this model is given in the Table 5.

Table 5. Daily energy requirement (MJ/DE) of pregnant mares (500 kg BW) according to GEH (1994).

Maintenance	Maintenance + Pregnancy		
	8 Months	9 – 10 Months	11 Months
69.7	79.0	83.0	88.0

France

In France according to INRA (1984-1990) (Institut National Recherche Agronomique) daily requirement are calculated by using the following model:

NE = (Maintenance) + (Pregnancy)

NE (MJ) = (0.351 MJ/Kg BW^{75}) + (Y * a * GE * kp)
UFC = (0.038 UFC/kg BW^{75}) + (Y * a * GE * km/kp)/9.2

Where

NE = Net Energy expressed either in MJ or UFC
(NE_m) = 9.2 MJ of 1 kg of Barley at maintenance in UFC system
BW^{75} = Metabolic body weight
GE = Gross Energy (MJ/kg BW foetus)
km = Efficiency rate of energy for maintenance (= 0.785)
Kp = Efficiency rate of energy for pregnancy (= 0.25)
Y = Body weight of foetus estimated using the following equation
a = Chemical composition of the foetus (Table 6)

Table 6. Weight gain and chemical composition of the foetus (from Martin-Rosset et al., 1994)

Month of pregnancy	Weight gain (in p. 100 of birth weight)	Gross Energy (MJ/kg)	Protein content (%)
8	19	4.18	11.5
9		4.60	13.0
10	30	4.93	15.3
11	31	5.35	17.1

A model based on data obtained in ponies (Douglas and Ginther, 1975); in light breeds (Meyer and Ahlswede, 1976) and in heavy breeds (Martin-Rosset, unpublished) was performed by INRA (1984) (see Martin-Rosset and Doreau, 1984a) to predict body weight of foetus along the pregnancy.

$$Y = - 1.99 + 13.67 X – 37.38 X^2 + 45.51 X^3 – 18.32 X^4$$

Where

Y = Body weight of foetus / Body weight of foal at birth

and BW = 19 kg for pony
BW = 53 kg for light breed
BW = 67 kg for heavy breed
} at birth

X = days from fecundation / days of pregnancy (= 340 d)

The daily requirement calculated using the model is given in Table 7.

Table 7. Daily energy requirements (NE) of pregnant mares (500 kg BW) according to INRA (1990).

Unit	Maintenance	Maintenance + Pregnancy		
		8 Months	9 – 10 Months	11 Months
UFC	4.2	4.6	5.2	5.3
MJ	38.6	42.3	47.8	48.7

The Netherlands

In the Netherlands, according to CVB (1996-2005) (Central Veevorde Bureau) daily requirements for maintenance and pregnancy are calculated by using the following equation:

NE = (Maintenance) + (Pregnancy)

$NE (MJ) = (0.378 * BW^{75}) + (G_f * GE_f * K_p)]$
$NE (EWpa) = [(0.0390 * BW^{75}) + (G_f * GE_f * Km/K_p)]\ 8.93$

Where

BW^{75} = Metabolic Body weight (*0.0390 for Underbred * 0.0411 for Thoroughbred)
G_f = Growth of the foetus = $(BW_{t=0} + 0.02\ BW\ mare) * (PG/100)\ 30.5$

BWto: birth weight of the foal
PG = Growth of the foetus per month in percent of birth weight

BW adult (kg)	100	200	400	800
BW_t = birth weight of foal (percent of adult weight)	14.2	12.0	10.0	8.5

GE_f: Gross energy of the foetus (MJ/kg)

km = Efficiency rate for maintenance = 0.779
K_p = efficiency rate for pregnancy = 0.25
} km/kp = 3

In CVB, 2005 system, energy requirements are evaluated in NE for maintenance. Hence NE requirements calculated should be multiplied by the ratio km/k_p. And NE is expressed in EWpa: a Dutch unit (Energie Worden Paard) and 1 EWpa = 8.93 MJ NEm/kgDM.

The daily requirement calculated using this model and GEf, PG value are given in the Tables 8 and 9

Table 8. Gain (PG) and Gross Energy (GE) content of gain of the foetus according to CVB, 2005.

Month	GE (MJ/kg)	Protein deposition (g/kg gain)	PG (p. 100 of birth weight)
8	4.184	148	10
9	4.602	192	18
10	4.937	168	23
11	5.355	213	30

Table 9. Daily energy requirements (EN) of pregnant mares (500 kg BW) according to CVB (2005).

Unit	Maintenance	Maintenance + Pregnancy		
		8 Months	9 – 10 Months	11 Months
EWpa	4.1	4.3	4.5	4.7
MJ	36.8	38.2	40.0	42.1

Scandinavia

In Scandinavia according to Austbo (2004) daily energy requirements are calculated by using the following model:

NE = (Maintenance) ∗ (Pregnancy: F)

Maintenance requirements are:

Maintenance requirement (NE) = 0.351 MJ/kg BW^{75} referring to INRA

DK, N, IS Maintenance requirement (NE) = (0.351/9.414) = 0.0373 UFC/kg BW^{75}

Sweden Maintenance requirement (ME) = (0.351/0.7) = 0.51 MJ/kg BW^{75}

Finland Maintenance requirement (ME) = [(0.351/0.7)]/ 11.7 = 0.0429 ME/kg BW^{75}

F: expressed in percent of maintenance

The basis for calculation of the requirements are:
weight of foals at birth is set to be 10 percent of the body weight of the mare
the growth of the foetus (as percent of birth weight has been calculated according to Meyer and Stadermann (1991) (Table 10)

Table 10. Growth and protein retention by the foetus according to SCAND (2004) (Austbo, 2004).

Months of pregnancy	Growth of foetus (p. 100 of birth weight)	GE (MJ/kg)	Protein retention (g/kg growth)
Total for 1 to 7 months	19		101
8	10	?	148
9	18		192
10	23		168
11	30		213

These basis are implemented for calculating the energy requirements for pregnancy expressed in proportion of the maintenance requirements depending of the month of pregnancy (Table 11).

Table 11. Energy requirement for pregnancy: F in percentage of maintenance requirement (Austbo, 2004).

Body weight of mares (kg)		Months of pregnancy			
		8	9	10	11
200	F =	5	11	15	21
500		7	13	18	25
700		7	14	20	28

The daily energy requirements calculated using the general model are given in Table 12.

Table 12. Daily requirements of pregnant mares (500 kg BW) according to SCAND (2004) (Austbo, 2004).

Country	Unit	Maintenance	Maintenance + Pregnancy			
			8th Month	9th Month	10th Month	11th Month
DK, N, IS	NE	3.94	4.22	4.45	4.65	4.93
SW[1]	ME	52.85	56.55	59.72	62.36	66.06
Fin[2]	Fu (ME)	4.54	4.86	5.13	5.36	5.68

[1]SLU, 2004; [2]MTT, 2004

Comparison of energy requirements in the different countries

In US and Scandinavia the energy requirements are given as an increase of maintenance for the last four months of pregnancy.

In France, Germany and the Netherlands the energy requirements for pregnancy are calculated from the variation in daily accretion of nutrients in the foals and in the uteroplacental tissues, using efficiency rates which range from 20 to 25 percent. The countries use different models to estimate the growth of the foetus but the same chemical composition of the foetus published by Meyer and Ahlswede (1976).

As a result the requirement can be compared only referring to maintenance (Table 13).

Table 13. Comparison of the energy requirements for pregnancy in the different countries.

<table>
<tr><th></th><th></th><th>NRC
1989</th><th>GEH
1994</th><th>INRA
1990</th><th>CVB
2005</th><th>SCAND
2004</th></tr>
<tr><td>Maintenance</td><td></td><td>100</td><td>100</td><td>100</td><td>100</td><td>100</td></tr>
<tr><td>Pregnancy Months</td><td>8</td><td>-</td><td>113</td><td rowspan="2">110</td><td>105</td><td>107</td></tr>
<tr><td></td><td>9</td><td>111</td><td rowspan="2">119</td><td rowspan="2">110</td><td>113</td></tr>
<tr><td></td><td>10</td><td>113</td><td>124</td><td>118</td></tr>
<tr><td></td><td>11</td><td>120</td><td>126</td><td>126</td><td>115</td><td>125</td></tr>
</table>

Energy requirements calculated in European Countries except in the Netherlands are higher than those proposed in US, whatever the months of pregnancy. An agreement for the last month of pregnancy between European Countries would arise. Compromise might be met for the other months if an agreement might be stated about the model of the foetus growth and the use of the chemical composition of the foetus published by Meyer and Ahlswede (1976). The efficiency rate used for energy is very close 20 – 25 percent.

Evaluation of protein requirements

Calculation of protein requirements in different countries: data - base – methodology – requirements

US

In US, according to NRC (1989). Daily protein requirement for maintenance and pregnancy are calculated by using the following model

gCP/d = (Maintenance) + (Pregnancy) for mares which weight 200 to 900 kg BW.

For maintenance DP requirements is estimated to be 0.6 g DP/kg BW (Teeter *et al.*, 1967; Slade *et al.*, 1970; Hintz and Schryver, 1972; Quinn, 1975; Meyer *et al.*, 1985). Assuming that digestibility of forage diet consumes by horses is 46 percent, the requirements would be 1.3 g CP/kg BW. Dividing the CP requirements by DE requirements results in value of 40 g CP/Mcal.DE (e.g. 10 g CP/MJDE).

A 500 kg pregnant mare requires for the 9th, 10th and 11th months: 127, 130 and 178 g/d for foetal deposition respectively based on the foetal composition (Meyer and Ahlswede, 1976) and an efficiency rate of 60 percent for protein. The total DCP requirements for pregnant mare would be 427, 430, 478 g. If 55 percent protein digestibility is assumed the total CP requirement is 776, 782 and 869 g/d for 9th – 10th and 11th months. Dividing these CP requirements by DE requirements results in a 44 gCP/Mcal of DE (e.g. 11 g CP/MJ). As a result daily protein requirement for pregnant mare is estimated using the following model:

gCP = (10 g CP/MJ of DE) + (11 g CP/MJ of DE)
the daily requirement calculated using this equation is given in the Table 14.

Table 14. Daily protein requirement (gCP) for a pregnant mare (500 kg BW) according to NRC (1989).

Maintenance	Maintenance + Pregnancy		
	9 Months	10 Months	11 Months
656	801	815	866

Germany

In Germany according to GEH (1994), requirements for maintenance and pregnancy are calculated by using the following model:

gDCP = (Maintenance) + (Pregnancy) for mares which weight 100 to 800 kg BW.

Daily maintenance requirement is calculated using the following relationship based on Olsson and Ruudvere (1955); Teeter *et al.* (1967); Slade *et al.* (1970)

$gDCP_m - 3 \text{ g/kg } BW^{75}$

Daily requirement for pregnancy is calculated using the following relationship assuming an efficiency rate for protein of 50 percent.

$gDCP/d = 0.06055 * a * BW^{75}$

Where:

BW^{75} Metabolic Body Weight of the mare
a = Chemical composition and gain of foetus (Tables 3 – 4)
The calculation includes extra requirements for adnexes (+ 20 percent)

The daily requirements of pregnant can be calculated using the following equation is given Table 15.
$gDCP = 3g/BW^{75} + 0.06055 * a * BW^{75}$

The daily requirement of a pregnant mare using this model is given in Table 15.

Table 15. Daily protein requirement (gDCP) for pregnant mare (500 kg BW) according to GEH (1994).

Maintenance	Maintenance + Pregnancy		
	8 Months	9 – 10 Months	11 Months
450	450	505	580

France

In France according to INRA (1984-1990) requirements are calculated by using the following model:

gMADC/d = (Maintenance) + (Pregnancy)

$gMADC/d = (2.8\ g/kgBW^{75}) + [(Y * a) / 0.55)] * 1.20$

Where:

MADC: Matières Azotées Digestibles Cheval or Horse Digestible Crude Protein
BW^{75} = Metabolic weight of the mare
Y = Protein gain of the foetus estimated using
Growth curve and protein content of the foetus (Table 6)
Growth curve using the equation described for calculating energy requirement

a = Chemical composition of the foetus (Table 6)
0.55 = Efficiency rate of the utilization of DCP for pregnancy (55 percent)
1.20 = Additional requirement for adnexes (+ 20 percent)

The daily requirement of a pregnant mare calculated using this equation is given in the Table 16.

Table 16. Daily requirement (gMADC) of pregnant mare according to INRA (1990) (500 kg BW).

Maintenance	Maintenance + Pregnancy		
	8 - 9 Months	10 Months	11 Months
295	340	460	485

The Netherlands

In the Netherlands, according to CVB (2005) the requirements are calculated using the following model:

gDCP/d (VRE/d) = (Maintenance) + (Pregnancy)
VRE: Dutch unit which means DCP

Maintenance is estimated using this relationship
$gDCP/d = 3.0\ g\ DCP \times BW^{75}$

Extra DCP requirement for pregnancy is estimated to be: 296 – 360 – 360 – 426 g for 8 – 9 – 10 – 11 months using growth and protein disposition in the foetus given Table 8.

As a result the total daily requirement of a pregnant mare (Table 17) is calculated using the following equation.

$gDCP = (3.0\ g\ DCP/BW^{75})$ + (296 to 426 g/kg gain of foetus according to the months of pregnancy)

Table 17. Daily protein requirement (gDCP) of pregnant mare (500 kg BW) according to CVB (2005).

Maintenance	Maintenance + Pregnancy		
	8 Months	9 – 10 Months	11 Months
317	369	446	541

Scandinavia

In Scandinavia, according to Austbo (2004). The total protein requirement is estimated using the following model:

gDCP/d = (Maintenance) ∗ (Pregancy: F)

Where:

Maintenance = 3 g DCP/BW^{75}
BW^{75}: metabolic body weight
F expressed in percent of maintenance
F is a factor which has been performed from the growth of the foetus and the protein per kg of growth, assuming the efficiency rate of protein for pregnancy to be = 50 percent

The daily requirement is calculated using the following equation
gDCP/d = 3 g DCP/BW^{75} ∗ (F = 1.12 to 1.50% BW see Table 18)

Where:

BW^{75} is the metabolic weight of the mare
BW is the body weight of the mare

Table 18. F: performed for the last 4 months of pregnancy according to SCAND (2004), Austbo (2004).

Month of pregnancy	DCP requirement	F
8	12% BW	1.12
9	25% BW	1.25
10	33% BW	1.33
11	50% BW	1.50

The total daily requirements of a pregnant mare an given in the Table 19.

Table 19. Daily requirements (gDCP/d) of pregnant mares (500 kg BW) for SCAND (2004) according to Austbo (2004).

Maintenance	Maintenance + Pregnancy			
	8 Months	9 Months	10 Months	11 Months
317	377	442	482	567

Comparison of requirements between the Countries

NRC and GEH requirements are very close but much lower than those of INRA, CVB and SCAND, namely during the last 3 months of pregnancy (Table 20). European countries are using the same chemical composition of the foetus (Meyer and Alshwede, 1976) directly or indirectly and efficiency rate for protein disposition, of 50 percent. As a result the main discrepancy is the curve of foal growth.

Table 20. Comparison of the requirement for pregnancy between the countries.

<table>
<tr><td>Maintenance
Pregnancy (Months)</td><td>NRC
1989
100</td><td>GEH
1994
1000</td><td>INRA
1990
100</td><td>CVB
2005
100</td><td>SCAND
2004
100</td></tr>
<tr><td>8</td><td>-</td><td>100</td><td rowspan="2">115</td><td>116</td><td>119</td></tr>
<tr><td>9</td><td>122</td><td rowspan="2">118</td><td rowspan="2">141</td><td>139</td></tr>
<tr><td>10</td><td>124</td><td>156</td><td>152</td></tr>
<tr><td>11</td><td>132</td><td>128</td><td>164</td><td>171</td><td>179</td></tr>
</table>

Recommended allowances for energy and protein

A recommended allowances is the amount of nutrients which should be supplied to horses to achieve a desirable level of performance consistent with their potential: genotype, stage of pregnancy. The horses are assumed to be in good health, well managed and housed during the winter period. These should be as optimum allowances which cover the physiological expenditure of horses so called net requirements. Exceptions are mares of heavy breeds or light breed devoted to horse meat production or leisure horse production respectively, where a moderate and controlled use of body reserves is assumed during the winter period to reduce the feed costs. In all the situations: optimum, restricted or maximum allowances according to the types of horse production: race or sport horses, leisure horses, horses for meat production, energy and protein allowances are related to the intake capacity and to the amount and ability of body reserves to be mobilised throughout the pregnancy period to meet at foaling a nutritional balance compatible with normal milk yield, and reproductive performances.

Intake capacity

Dry matter intake is proposed by INRA and NRC to cover the requirements in late pregnancy. (Table 21). INRA proposals come from feeding trials carried out in heavy breed and light breed (INRA, 1984; INRA, 1990). NRC proposals are drawn to some extend from feeding experiments in light breeds (NRC, 1989).

Table 21. Dry matter intake in late pregnancy (kg DM/100 kg BW).

	8th Month	9th Month	10th Month	11th month	Concentrate p. 100 BW
NRC, 1989	<------------------------1.5 – 2.0 ---------------------->				35 - 40
INRA, 1990	<------ 1.8 – 2.2 ------>		1.6 – 2.1	1.4 – 1.8	20 - 25

The range of variation of dry matter intake is rather closed between NRC and INRA but the proportion of concentrate in the diet to meet the requirements is much higher in NRC than in INRA recommendations. Voluntary intake is related to the animal: stage of pregnancy and the feeds: quality of forage (Figure 5).

Voluntary feed intake regularly decreased on average by 20 percent between 5 and 1 weeks before foaling (9 to 30 percent according to mares (Martin-Rosset and Doreau, 1984; Doreau, Boulot, 1986; Doreau *et al.*, 1990). Comparing with non lactating (and non pregnant) mares fed the same hay based diet (F./C: 85/15) dry matter intake of pregnant mares is 13 percent lower during late pregnancy due to the increase of the foetus weight which rises by 80 percent in the last four months according to the equation set up by INRA, 1984. Elevated oestrogen's levels are believed to depress intake in late pregnancy in ruminants (Forbes, 1971). However in mares, oestrogen's secretion is not enhanced in late pregnancy (Nett *et al.*, 1973). The mean retention time of digesta passage is faster in pregnant (21.7 hours) than in non pregnant mares (32.2 hours) fed the same hay based diet (F/C

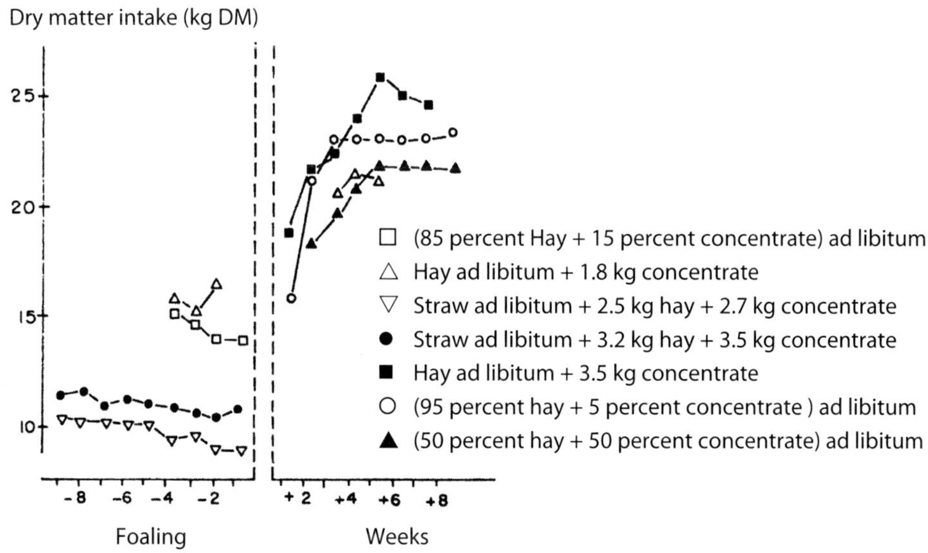

Figure 5. Dry matter intake of mare (heavy breed: 700 kg BW at foaling) in late pregnancy and early lactation (Martin-Rosset and Doreau, 1984b).

= 85/15) (Miraglia *et al.*, 1992). As a result dry matter intake ranges from 1.4 to 2.2 kg DM/100 kg BW during the late pregnancy (Table 21). And the digestibility of the diet (dOM) is 5 point lower in pregnant mares than in non pregnant mares fed the same previous diet (Martin-Rosset *et al.*, 1990). Individual differences of intake is rather high: variation coefficient = 16 percent with standard deviation in total dry matter intake of 2.0 to 2.5 kg DM (Doreau and Boulot, 1986).

Such level of intake allow small increase in the body weight of the mare: 2 percent on average over the last month. According to Martin-Rosset *et al.*, 1986a, well fed mares should increase their body weight on average by 8 percent over the last 3 months; however the main part of the gain takes place before one month delivery and a slight decrease may even occur during the last 2 weeks. After corrections for digestive content variations (Martin-Rosset *et al.*, 1986b) and for conceptus growth (Martin-Rosset and Doreau, 1984a) it appears that energy and nitrogen balances of mares fed *ad libitum* a hay based diet (F/C = 85.15) are positive (20 to 25 percent) (Table 22).

But intake depends also on quality of forage. Comparing two groups of mares of light breed fed *ad libitum* two hay-based diets (F: C = 90: 10) composed of high (HQ) or low (LQ) quality hay during the last month of pregnancy, daily intake was on average 11 percent higher for HQ diet than for LQ diet (Table 22). Energy requirements were met in both groups whereas protein requirements were cowered only in HQ groups (Table 22). Intake might be likely related to the proportion of concentrate in the diet but no data are available as proportion of concentrate is routinely rather restricted due the limited requirement to be covered and the intake capacity of forage by pregnant does not seem to be a limiting factor, except with very poor hay or straw fed in high proportion as exhibited by the trial 3 vs trial 1 (Table 22).

Table 22. Effect of diet composition and quality of hay on intake and nutritional balance of mare in late pregnancy.

Trials no.	1[1]	2[2]a	2[2]b	3[3]a	3[3]b
Number of mares	11*	7**	7**	14*	14*
Body weight (kg)	784	612	612	795	793
Length of experimental period	5 weeks	5 weeks	5 weeks	8 weeks	12 weeks
Forage: concentrate	85:15	90:10		76:34 52 p. 100 straw	78:32 60 p. 100 straw
Chemical composition of hay %					
Crude fibre	31.9	38.2	29.0	29.5	29.5
Crude Protein	11.3	5.7	11.7	12.3	12.3
Dry matter intake (kg/d) (average)	15.5	11.2	12.4	12.0	12.6
Body weight gain (% initial BW)	2.0	1.6	2.0	0.8	1.0
Balance (intake/requirements)					
Energy	125	100	151	104	101
Nitrogen	120	65	165	88	93
Body conditions score[4]	-	1.9	3.0	2.3	2.5

[1]Doreau and Boulot, 1986; [2]Doreau *et al.*, 1990; [3]Martin-Rosset *et al.*, unpublished; *Heavy breeds; **Light breeds; [4]INRA-HN-IE Method, 1997

Variation in body weight

Throughout the year, the live weight of mares can vary by 15 – 20 percent with normal management practices (Figure 6). Body weight is maximum and minimum before and after foaling respectively. The body weight in the last four months of pregnancy would increase by 2 to 15 p. 100 or decrease depending on body condition and feeding level (Martin-Rosset and Doreau, 1980; Henneke *et al.*, 1984; Martin-Rosset *et al.*, 1986a; Hines *et al.*, 1987; Lawrence *et al.*, 1992).

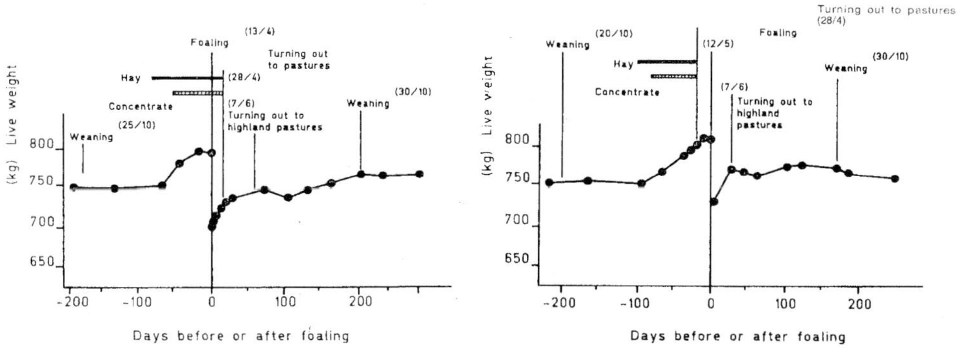

a b

a : Mares foaling during the winter (n = 13) b : Mares foaling during the grazing season (n = 6)

Figure 6. Variation in the body weight of mare depending on foaling time (Martin-Rosset et al., 1986a).

The greatest variation would result in a loss of weight at foaling which represents 11 to 15 percent of the body weight of the mare that is 1.3 – 1.5 times of the foal birth weight depending on foal and fluids that are delivered at foaling; and from changes in total gut content. The conceptus represents 85 – 90 percent of this variation for mare in moderate body condition. That is 9 to 13 percent of mare body weight at foaling. The total gut content ranges from 8 to 10 percent of horses'body weight (Martin-Rosset *et al.*, 1983) and the large intestine account for 70 percent of total gut content, that is 7 percent of body weight of horses. Body weight variation is strongly related to dry matter intake. The body weight of dry mare changes significantly at last 24 – 48 hours later on a variation in dry matter intake of forage or concentrate because the mean retention time of digesta in the total tract is only 25 to 30 hours. It can be slightly reduced in pregnant mares fed the same diet as the non pregnant mares (Miraglia *et al.*, 1995). The variation of body weight (Y) is fairly well related to the variation in dry matter intake of forage (X_1) and concentrate (X_2) (Martin-Rosset *et al.*, 1986b).

$$Y = 1.636 + 3.48\, X_1 + 3.45\, X_2 \qquad n = 29 \qquad R^2 = 0.77$$

It results that body weight of the mare can vary by 3.48 ± 1.40 kg and 3.45 ± 0.95 kg when there is 1 kg change in dry matter intake of forage or concentrate respectively. This relationship is very useful to explain in the late pregnancy the simultaneous variations in body weight and the decrease in dry matter intake.

In conclusion the conceptus and the variation in digesta content would represent 85-90 and 10-15 percent of the loss of body weight of mare in good conditions at foaling. If the body condition score is poor, additional variation is related to the mobilisation of the body reserves, which is of high concern to calculate total energy balance and resulting energy allowances to be fed.

Role of body reserves

The proportion of adipose tissues in horses range between 8 to 12 percent of body weight (Martin-Rosset *et al.*, 1983; Robelin *et al.*, 1984) in horses fed to meet the requirements. This large reserve in energy is highly related to the feeding level of the mare. Variation in body reserves can be estimated using a scoring method. INRA has proposed a method (INRA-HN-IE, 1997) based on simultaneous scoring of the horses before slaughtering and the weight of adipose tissue (and energy content) determined after total anatomical dissection of the tissues and analysis for GE determination (Figure 7).

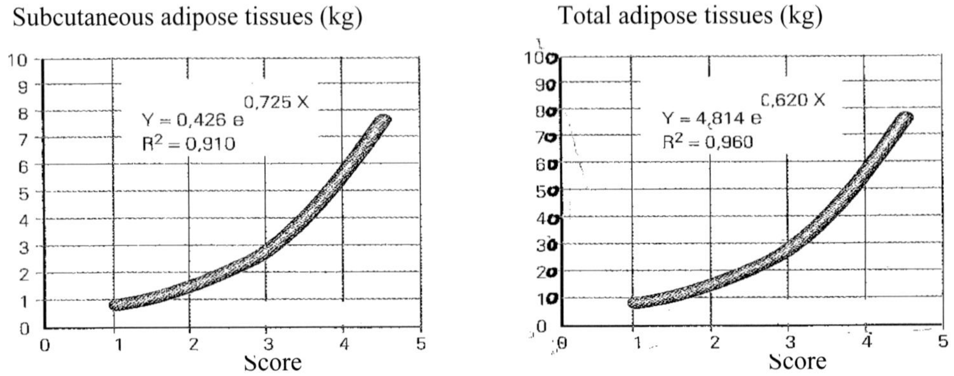

Figure 7. Relationship between body condition score (BCS) and the weight of total or subcutaneous adipose tissues (Martin-Rosset et al., method in progress) to predict BCS using (INRA-HN-IE scoring, 1997).

Variation of empty body weight, digesta content and weight of the conceptus over the annual reproductive cycle of the mare

Using the experimental data of the variation in body weight obtained at INRA, and the estimated variation in conceptus, body reserves and digesta content predicted by the INRA respective models; the variation over the annual cycle in body weight of a mare, in empty body weight, weight of conceptus, and in the wet weight of the gut content has been attempted (Figure 8). Such a model of variation in body weight is very useful to estimate the requirements and to design feeding strategies (Martin-Rosset and Doreau, 1984a).

Body weight of the mares in moderate body condition fed to meet the requirements can gain 10 to 15 percent during the last 4 month of pregnancy whereas birth weight of the foal average for 70 p. 100 of this gain (Figure 6). But gain can be very low if the mares are in high body condition without any negative effect on the foal body weight (Martin-Rosset *et al.*, 1986; Kowalski *et al.*, 1990).

A comparison of the body weight of mares in good condition fed either 100 percent (HL), or 80 percent (LL) of INRA requirements 70 days before foaling lost 82 and 118 kg respectively at foaling. This difference of 36 kg BW would be largely due to the mobilisation of body reserves as far the mare were fed the same limited amount of dry matter one week before foaling to reduce the interaction between the variation of body weight and the variation of dry matter intake.. This variation of BW would represent 5 percent of the body weight of the LL mares (Martin-Rosset and Doreau, 1980).

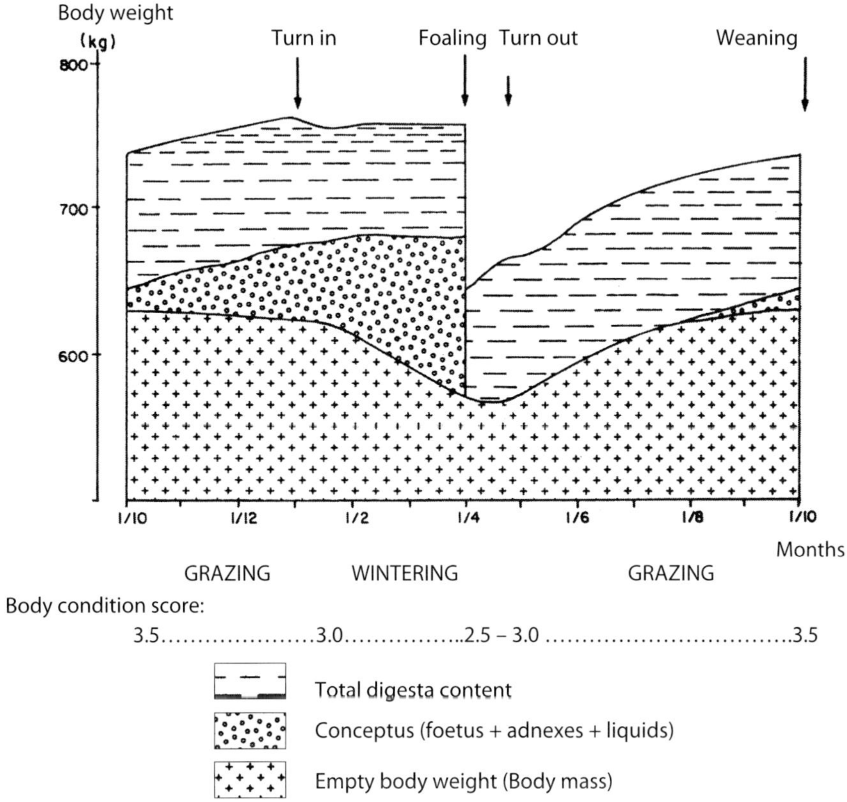

Figure 8. Variation of the weight of the different main components of body weight in the mare of the heavy breed over the annual reproductive cycle (Martin-Rosset and Doreau, 1984a).

The restriction in energy did not cause any significant effect on the length of pregnancy and foals birth weight (Table 23). A more drastic restriction in energy allowances (35 percent to INRA requirements) has no significant effect too (Table 23). This observations were confirmed by Henneke *et al.*,1984.

Table 23. Effect of energy restriction in late pregnancy in heavy mares (700 kg BW) (from Martin-Rosset and Doreau, 1980).

Energy level[1]	100[1]	80	100	65
Number of mares	30	26	5	5
Foal birth weight (kg)	63.5	67.8	68.5	67.7
Length of pregnancy	342	340	345	335

The mares in moderate (3.0 – 3.5) or good (> 3.5) condition (Scale 0 – 5: INRA – HN – IE, 1997) is capable to mobilise body reserves as highlighted by the rise of non esterified fatty acids plasma concentration of mares between two evening and morning subsequent meals (Doreau *et al.*, 1981).

Recommended allowances in relation to changes in body weight and body reserve

In most countries, except France, the requirements are proposed to cover all the needs (e.g. 100 percent) INRA propose allowances which are related to body condition score according to the goal of production (Table 24).

Table 24. Daily energy and protein allowances for pregnant mares according to INRA (1990).

	UFC		g MADC	TDMI
	HL[1]	LL[2]	NL[5]	kg DM
500 kg BW				
Dry mares and early pregnancy	3.8	4.8	295	6.0 – 8.5
Late pregnancy				
8th – 9th Months	4.1	5.0	340	6.5 – 9.0
10th Month	4.7	5.7	460	7.0 – 10.5
11th Month	4.8	5.8	485	7.5 – 11.0
700 kg BW				
Dry mares and early pregnancy	4.2	5.2	380	6.5 – 9.5
Late pregnancy				
8th – 9th Months	4.5	5.6	445	7.0 – 10.0
10th Month	5.2	6.5	610	8.0 – 12.0
11th Month	5.3	6.7	645	8.0 – 12.0

UFC: Horse Feed Unit; MADC = Horse Digestible Crude Protein
1 UFC = 9.20 MJ NE (INRA, 1990)
TDMI: Total Dry Matter Intake
[1]HL: High Level = 110 percent requirement BCS < 3.5
[2]LL: Low Level = 90 percent requirement BCS ≥ 3.5
} optimum 3.5, 2 months before foaling for light breeds (500 kg BW)
[3]HL: Normal Level = 100 percent requirement BCS < 3
[4]LL: Low Level = 90 percent requirement BCS ≥ 3
} optimum 3.0, 4 months before foaling for heavy breeds (700 kg BW)
[5]NL: Normal Level = 100 percent requirement for all breeds

Discussion and conclusion

Harmonisation of requirements in Europe

The average requirements for the 8-9-10-11th months of pregnancy in European Countries are: 1.09 – 1.13 – 1.18 and 1.23 times maintenance for energy respectively and 1.13 – 1.28 – 1.39 – 1.61 times maintenance for protein respectively. The main discrepancy between countries in the evaluation of the requirements is related to the growth curve of the foetus.

The requirements should be estimated in Europe using the same amount of nutrients fixed in the foetus and efficiency rates. The same growth curve of the foetus could be fitted to the data of (Dusek, 1966; Fowden *et al.*, 2000; Meyer and Ahlswede, 1976; Platt, 1978; Guissani *et al.*, 2005). And chemical composition of the foetus determined from Meyer and Ahlswede (1976) is the reference. It would be relevant to assume that 20 percent of additional energy and protein deposition in the adnexes, using the weight of adnexes determined by Douglas and Ginther (1975), should be added to estimate consistent accretion rate for energy and protein in the conceptus during the last four months of pregnancy. Additional energy maintenance requirement of the foetus could be considered as well – 0.28 MJ/kg/d (Fowden *et al.*, 2000). The efficiency rates for energy and protein deposition should be respectively the same as far as those proposed are so close: 20 – 25 percent for energy and 50 – 55 percent for protein.

Allowances vs requirements

Requirements should be validated using experimental data from feeding trials to check that all the models, which have been stated, are consistent. This validation has been carried out in France by INRA (and in USA by NRC to some extend). It could contribute to the harmonisation of the recommendations. But data from feeding trials conducted in other countries would be very useful to take into account the effects of breeds and environmental factors due to local conditions, then to propose allowances in the different European Countries.

Recommended allowances should refer to the variation in Body weight and in body condition score as far as they can vary with month of pregnancy, feeding level and diet composition. The true variation in body weight (empty body weight) can be estimated as far as the weight of the digesta content or/and its variation have been determined. Body reserves and its variation can be estimated using the body condition score method as amount of total body fat can be predicted from body condition score. As a result a description of the variation of the empty body weight of the mare using the data related to the variation of digesta content weight, body reserves and of the conceptus, might be attempted to estimate energy and protein allowances in late pregnancy. At present the relationship between body condition score and the content of adipose tissue was implemented by INRA to determine the optimal body condition score to be met by the mare at foaling, and to state the recommended allowances in late pregnancy.

References

Allen, W.R., S. Wilsher, C. Turnbull, F. Stewart, J. Ousey, P.D. Rossdale and A.L. Fowden, 2002. Influence of maternal size on placental, foetal and postnatal growth in the horse. I. Development in utero. Reproduction, 123, 445-453

Argenzio, R.A. and H.F. Hintz, 1971. Energy utilisation in the horse. Proc. Cornell Nut. Conf., 86-92.

Arthur, G.H., 1969. The foetal fluids of domestic animals. J. Reprod. Fert., Suppl. 9, 45-52.

Austbo, D., 2004. The Scandinavian adaptation of the French UFC System. In Proceedin 3rd European Workshop Equine Nutrition. V. Julliand and W. Martin-Rosset Eds. Nutrition of the performance Horse. EAAP publication no. 111. Wageningen Academic Publishers. The Netherlands, 69-78.

Barth, K.M., J.W Williams and D.G. Brown, 1977. Digestible energy requirements of working and non-working ponies. J. Anim. Sci., 44, 585-589.

Barone, R. and C. Monnet, 1955. Les mamelles des équidés domestiques. Bull. Soc. Sci. Vet. Lyon, 57, 73-92.

Baur, R., 1977. Morphometry of the placental exchanges area. Advances in Anatomy, Embryology and Cell Biology, 53, 3-65.

Bell, A.W., J.M. Kennaugh, F.C. Battaglia, E.L. Makowski and G. Meschia, 1986. Metabolic and circulatory studies of the foetal lamb at mid gestation. American Journal of Physiology, 250, 538-544.

CVB, 1996. Documentatierrapport Nr 15, Het definitieve VEP en VRE system, Centraal veevoederbureau.

CVB, 2005, New Dutch recommendations for horses (personal communication from M. Block)

Den Engelsen, 1966. Het gewicht van de landbouwhuisdieren. Veteelt Ziuvelber, 9, 293-310.

Doreau, M., W. Martin-Rosset and J.P. Barlet, 1981. Variations au cours de la journée des teneurs en certains constituents plasmatiques chez la jument.Reprod. Nutr. Dévelop. 21, 1-17.

Doreau, M. and S. Boulot, 1986. Evolution of voluntary intake in the mare during late pregnancy and early lactation, effect of diet. In Proceedings. 37th Animal EAAP Meeting, Budapest, Hungary, Horse Commission. Session I, p. 13.

Doreau, M., C. Moretti and W. Martin-Rosset, 1990. Effect of quality of hay given to mares around foaling on their voluntary intake and foal growth. Ann. Zootech., 39, 125-131.

Douglas, R.H. and O.J. Ginther, 1975. Development of the equine foetus and placental. Journal of Reproduction and Fertility, Suppl. 23, 503-505.

Dusek, J., 1966. Notes sur le développement prenatal des chevaux (in Czech Language). Ved. Pr. Vysk. San. Chov. Keni., Slatinany, 2, 1-25.

Forbes, J.M., 1970. The voluntary food intake of pregnant and lactating ruminants: a review. Brit. Vet. J., 126, 1-111.

Fowden, A.L., L. Mundy, J.C. Ousey, A. Mc Gladdery and G., Silver, 1991. Tissue glycogen and glucose-6-phosphate activity in the foetal and new born foal. J. Reprod. Fertility, Suppl. 44, 537-542.

Fowden, A.L. and M. Silver, 1995a. Glucose and oxygen metabolism in the foetal foal during late gestation. American Journal of Physiology, 268, 1455-1461.

Fowden, A.L. and M. Silver, 1995b. The effects of thyroid hormones on oxygen and glucose metabolism in the sheep foetus during late gestation. American Journal of Physiology, 482, 203-213.

Fowden, A.L., P.M. Taylor, K.L. White and A.J. Forhead, 2000a.Ontogenic and nutritionally induced changes in foetal metabolism in the hors. Journal of Physiology, 528, 209-219.

Fowden, A.L., A.J. Forhead, K.L. White and P.M. Taylor, 2000b. Equine uteroplacental metabolism at mid-and late gestation.Exp. Physiol, 85, 5, 539-545.

GEH, 1994. Gesellschaft fur Ernährungphysiologie. 2. Empfehlungen zur Energie und Nährstoffversorgung der Perfde. DLG Verlage Frankfurt/Main. ISBN 3.7690.0517.1.

Giussani, D.A., A.J. Forehead and A.L. Fowden, 2005. Development of cardiovascular function in the horse foetus. J. Physiol., 565, 1019-1030.

Hay, 1997. Regultion of placental metabolism by glucose supply. Reproduction, Fertility and Development, 7, 365-375.

Henneke, D.G., G.D. Potter and J.L. Kredier, 1984. Body condition during pregnancy and lactation and reproductive efficiency in mares. Theriogenology, 21, 897-909.

Hines, K.K., S.L. Hodge, J.L. Kreider, G.D. Potter and P.G. Harms, 1987. Relationship between body condition and levels of serum luteinizing hormone in postpartum mares. Theriogenology, 28, 815-825.

Hoffman, L., W. Klippel and R. Schiemann, 1967. untersuchungen über den Energieumsatz beim Pferd unter besonderer Berücksichtigung der Horizontal bewegung. Archiv. Tierern., 17, 441-449.

INRA, 1984. Le Cheval. E. Jarrige and W. Martin-Rosset (Ed.) INRA Publications, Route de St Cyr, 78000 Versailles. pp 687.

INRA, 1990. Alimentation des Chevaux. W. Martin-Rosset (Ed) INRA Publications, Route de St Cyr, 78000 Versailles. pp. 232.

INRA – HN – IE, 1997. Notation de l'état corporel des chevaux de selle et de sport. Guide pratique. Institut de l'Elevage Ed., 149, rue de Bercy, 75595 Paris Cedex 12, pp. 40.

Ker, 2001. Advances in Equine Nutrition II. J D Pagan and RJ Geor Eds. Nottingahm University Press, Nottingahm, UK.

Knox, K.L., D.C. Crownover and G.R. Wooden, 1970. Maintenance energy requirements of mature idle horses. In: Proceedings 5th Symposium Energy Metabolism of Farm Animals. Witznau (Suisse) Shurch, A., Wenk, C. Editors, 181-184. Juris-Druck Verlag Zurich.

Kowalski, J., J. Williams and H. Hintz, 1990. Weight gains of mares during the last trimester of gestation. Equine Prac., 12(7), 6-10.

Lawrence, L., J. Di Pietro, K. Ewert, D. Parrett, L. Moser and D. Powell, 1992. Changes in body weight and condition in gestating mares. J. Equine Vet., Sci., 12, 355.

Martin-Rosset, W. and M. Doreau, 1980. Effect of variations in level of feeding of heavy mares during late pregnancy. Proc. 31st Animal Meeting EAAP. Munich. Horse Commission, Session 6, p. 4.

Martin-Rosset, W., R. Boccard, M. Jussiaux, J. Robelin and C. Trillaud-Geyl, 1983. Croissance relative des différents tissues, organs et regions corporelles entre 12 et 30 mois chez le cheval de boucherie de différentes races Lourdes. Ann. Zootech., 32, 153-174.

Martin-Rosset, W. and M. Doreau, 1984a. Besoins et alimentation de la jument. In R. Jarrige et W. Martin-Rosset. Ed. Le Cheval – Reproduction- Sélection – Alimentation – Exploitation". INRA Publications, route de St Cy, 78000 Versailles, 355-370.

Martin-Rosset, W. and M. Doreau, 1984b. Consommation d'aliments et d'eau par le cheval. In R. Jarrige et W. Martin-Rosset. Ed. Le Cheval – Reproduction- Sélection – Alimentation – Exploitation". INRA Publications, route de St Cy, 78000 Versailles, 333-354.

Martin-Rosset, W., M. Doreau and C. Espinasse, 1986a. Alimentation de la jument lourde allaitante. Evolution du poids vif des juments et croissance des poulains. Ann. Zootech., 35, 21-36.

Martin-Rosset, W., M. Doreau and C. Espinasse, 1986b. Relations entre la variations de poids vif et les quantités ingérées chez la jument.. Ann. Zootech.,

Martin-Rosset, W., M. Doreau, S. Boulot and N. Miraglia, 1990. influence of level of feeding and physiological state on diet digestibility in light and heavy breed horses. Livest. Prod. Sci., 25, 257-264.

Martin-Rosset, W., M. Vermorel, M. Doreau, J.L. Tisserand and J. Andrieu, 1994. The French horse feed evaluation systems and recommended allowances for energy and protein. Livest. Prod. Sci., 40, 37-56.

Meyer, H. and L. Ahlswede, 1976. Uber das intrauterine wachstum und die Körperzusammensetzung won Fohlen sowie den Hährstoffbedarf tragender stuten ubers; Tierernähr., 4, 263-292.

Meyer, H., S. Vom Stein and M. Schmidt, 1985. Investigations to determine endogenous faecal and renal N Losses in horses. p. 68. In: Proc. 9th Eq. Nutr. Physiol. Soc. Symp. East Lansing Mich.. University of Michigan.

Meyer, H. and B. Stadermann, 1991. Energie-und Nährstoffbedarf hochtragender Stuten. Pferdeheilkunde 7, 11-20.

Miraglia, N., C. Poncet and W. Martin-Rosset, 1992. Effect of feeding level, physiological state and breed on the rate of passage of particulate matter through the gastrointestinal tract of the horse. Ann., Zootech., 41, 69.

Molina, R.D., G. Meschia, F.C. Battaglia and W.W. Hay, 1991. Gestional maturation of placental glucose transfer capacity in sheep. American Journal of physiology, 261, 697-704.

MTT, 2004. Rehutaulukot ja Ruokintasinar-tukset. WWW.artturi.fi/rehutaulukot.

Nett, T.M., D.W. Holtan and V.L. Estergreen, 1973. Plasma estrogens in pregnant and postpartum mares. J. Anim. Sci., 37, 962-970.

NRC, 1978. Nutrient requirements of horse, 4th rev. ed. Washington, DC: National Academy Press.

NRC, 1989. Nutrient requirements of horses. 5th Revised Edition. Subcommittee on Horse Nutrition Board on Agriculture national Academy Press. Washington D.C..

Olsson, N.A. and A. Ruudvere, 1955. The nutrition of the horse. Nutr. Abstr. Reviews, 25, 1-18.

Platt, H., 1978. Growth and maturity in the equine foetus. Journal of the Royal Society of Medicine, 71, 658-661.

Platt, H., 1984. Growth of the equine foetus. Equine Veterinary Journal, 16, 247-252.

Quinn, C.R., 1975. Isobutyldene diurea as a protein substitute for horses. PhD. Dissertation, Colorado State University.

Robelin, J., R. Boccard, W. Martin Rosset, M. Jussiaux and C. Trillaud-Geyl, 1984. Caracteristiques des carcasses et qualités de la viande de cheval. In: Le cheval. R. Jarrige and W. Martin-Rosset (Eds.) INRA Editions, Route de St Cyr, 78026 Versailles, p. 602-610.

Slade, L.M., D.W. Robinson and K.E. Casey, 1970. Nitrogen metabolism in non-ruminant herbivores. I – The influence of non-protein and protein quality on the nitrogen retention of a diet in mares. J. Anim. Sci., 30, 753-760.

SLU, 2004. Utfordring rekimmendationer för häst. Sversiges lantbruks Universitet Publikation. Stjänst, Uppsala, Sweden, pp. 43.

Stammers, J.P., D. Hill, M. Silver and A.L. Fowden, 1995. Foetal and maternal plasma lipids in chronically catheterized mares in late gestation: effects of different nutritional states. Reproduction, Fertility and Development, 7, 1275-1284.

Teeter, S.M., M.C. Stillions and W.E. Nelson, 1967. Recent observations on the nutrition of mature horses. In Proc.: Am. Assoc. Eq. Pract., December, New-Orleans, LA, USA.

Wooden, G.R., K.L. Know and C.L. Wild, 1970. Energy metabolism of light horses. J. Anim. Sci., 30, 544-548.

Apparent digestibility of two diets in the Amiata breed of donkey in late pregnancy

L. Casini[1]*, M. Sgorbini*[2]*, L. Magni*[1]*, M. Corazza*[2] *and D. Gatta*[1]
[1]*Department of Animal Productions, University of Pisa, Viale delle Piagge 2, 56124 Pisa, Italy*
[2]*Department of Veterinary Clinic, University of Pisa, 56121 S. Piero a Grado, Pisa, Italy*

Abstract

Four pregnant donkeys at approximately 10-11 month of pregnancy were used. The aim of the trial was to compare the apparent digestibility of two different rations: a low quality meadow hay based diet versus a diet with hay and a cereal commercial concentrate feed (CM). Diet 1 consisted of 9 kg of meadow hay whereas in Diet 2 hay was partially replaced by the CM (70:30 hay:CM ratio). The animals were randomly divided into two groups and the trial was conducted according to a change-over design for two periods of 20d. Measurements of apparent digestibility were made on the last 6d of each period. Size of fibre particles in faeces was evaluated too. Donkeys fed with Diet 1 consumed significantly more of DM per metabolic weight unit than animals fed with Diet 2. Higher apparent digestibility of dietary DM, energy and fibre fractions were observed in donkeys fed with Diet 2. Intakes of both diets exceeded the estimated energy requirement, whereas protein needs were not satisfied by Diet 1. The percentages of different size fibre particles recovered in faeces showed no significant differences in both diets.

Keywords: nutrition, digestibility, pregnancy, donkey

Introduction

Donkeys are nutritionally adapted to life in semiarid areas as they are for example, efficient users of low quality, high fibre food, and are able to tolerate up to 30 per cent body dehydration (Yousef, 1991). These adaptations contribute to the donkey's reputation for being able to eat anything and survive on very little.

Many donkeys are fundamentally fed by being turned out onto common land to search for their own food. Most research on animal nutrition has focused on horses and ruminants. Donkeys differ from both these groups. Although there has been some work exploring differences between horses and donkeys (Pearson and Merritt, 1991; Suhartanto *et al.*, 1992; Ouedraogo and Tisserand, 1996; Pearson *et al.*, 2001) there is a need of improving scientific knowledge on autochthonous donkey breeds at risk of extinction.

The Amiata Donkey Breed is probably the only Italian breed derived from the African ones and introduced into Italy by Etruscan or Phoenician merchants. There are no studies looking at digestibility in Amiata donkeys in particular during pregnancy where digestive efficiency may be influenced by the presence of foetus. The aim of the trial was to evaluate the apparent digestibility of two traditional different rations used by the Amiata donkey breeders in the last part of pregnancy: a diet with hay versus a diet with hay and commercial cereal-mix.

Material and methods

Four adult pregnant Amiata Breed donkeys (aged 4-8) at approximately 10-11 month of pregnancy were used for the trial (body weight -BW- 294 ± 39 kg and body condition score -BCS- 4.5 evaluated according Pearson and Ouassat, 2000). The animals were at rest and fed according to a change-over design so that all animals received both the experimental diets. Experimental periods composed of a period of two weeks, to adapt the animals to the new diet, were followed by a 6 day sampling period. During the experimental periods donkeys were stabled in individual stalls and each animal was weighed at the start and at the end of each experimental period. The two diets consisted of 9 kg of a low quality meadow hay (Diet 1) or 5 kg of the same forage plus 2 kg of a flaked cereal based commercial feed (CM) composed of corn, oat, barley, soybean meal and carobs (Molitoria Val di Serchio, Lucca, Italy) (Diet 2). The donkeys didn't receive any mineral-vitamin supplement in addition to the diets. Feed and diet composition are showed in Table 1.

Due to the lack of information specifically available on the energy and protein requirements of donkeys, energy and protein requirements were estimated using the horse National Research Council (1989) recommendations as the guideline for the trial. The estimated requirements used are shown in Table 2.

The diets were offered twice a day in equal quantities at 8 am and 4 pm. Clean drinking water was available *ad libitum*. Before the trial a dental evaluation was performed on each animal and no abnormality were found.

During sampling periods faeces were collected from the rectum twice a day at the same time. Ash insoluble acid (AIA) was used as an indigestible marker to calculate the apparent digestibility. Both feed and faeces were analysed for dry matter (DM), organic matter (OM), crude protein (CP), crude fibre (CF), ash, neutral-detergent fibre (NDF), acid-detergent fibre (ADF), AIA and gross energy (GE) according to the methods reported by Martillotti *et al.* (1987).

The faecal particles size deriving from undigested fibre was determined by passing the dried faeces (65 °C for 48 hours) through a set of wire sieves with grids of different diameters (10, 4, 2, 1 and <1 mm) (Retch, Haan, Germany). Data were expressed as mean ± std (standard deviation). Results were subjected to ANOVA with a level of significance of $P < 0.05$ using a SAS Institute software package (2002).

Table 1. Chemical feed and diets composition (% on DM basis).

	Diet 1 (100% hay)		Diet 2 (70% hay-30% mix)
	Hay	CM	
DM	92.13	91.57	91.90
OM	91.58	98.19	93.36
CP	6.20	14.77	8.75
CF	36.95	6.66	33.24
NDF	73.36	25.56	54.10
ADF	46.64	11.26	36.01
GE (MJ/kg)	16.97	18.02	17.20
DE (MJ/kg)	8.94		12.25

Table 2. Requirements, on DM basis, estimated for 300 kg BW pregnant mares (9-11 months).

DE (Mcal)	11.9 – 13.1
DE (MJ)	49.81 – 54.84
CP (g)	507 – 550

Results and discussion

The voluntary DM intake (Table 3) was significantly different between the diets ($P < 0.05$), with the higher intake for Diet 1 (7.28 ± 0.83 kg *vs* 6.18 ± 0.30 kg). Hay intake was 88% and 94% of that provided in Diet 1 and Diet 2 respectively, whereas the CM was entirely consumed.

The daily intake of dry matter per metabolic weight (kg/$BW^{0.75}$) was 103.3 ± 10.1 and 86.6 ± 5.2 for Diet 1 and 2 respectively.

A lot of reports pointed out on DM intakes in donkeys but no information on pregnant donkeys was available. Pearson *et al.* (2001) reported similar results in working donkeys consuming alfalfa hay *ad libitum* (100 g/kg DM/BW0.75), while Ouedraogo and Tisserand (1996) reported values of DM intakes of 81.9 g/kg DM/BW0.75 in maintenance donkeys consuming prairie hay. Other works reported values ranging from 67 to 88 g/kg DM/BW0.75 in donkeys consuming grass and grass-legume-hay mixtures (Person and Merritt, 1991; Tisserand *et al.*, 1991; Mueller *et al.*, 1994).

DM intakes was higher in pregnant mares than non-breeding animals as reported by Miraglia *et al.* (2003) (116 and 104 g/kg DM/BW0.75 respectively). Gatta *et al.* (1995) reported an higher intakes of DM in pregnant mares (119.9 and 93.4 g/kg DM/$LW^{0.75}$) fed with hay and hay and oats respectively. Our results seem to suggest that pregnant donkeys had a lower DM intakes in comparison with pregnant horses.

Energy requirement was basically satisfied by both of the diets. Intakes exceeded the estimated energy needs by 24% and 45% in Diet 1 and 2 respectively.

Feeding level (FL = ratio between the actual energy intake and energy maintenance requirement) was significantly ($P < 0.05$) higher in Diet 2 compared with Diet 1 (1.5 *vs* 1.7). The FL of Diet 1 was similar (1.5) as reported in pregnant mares fed with a meadow hay based diet by Gatta *et al.* (1995).

Body weight and BCS were slightly lower in donkeys fed with hay based diet but no significant differences between diets were observed as shown in Table 4.

The donkeys fed with Diet 1 had a lower intake of hay than expected, consequently the actual crude protein intake was significantly lower in Diet 1 compared with Diet 2 (451.25 ± 51.16 g *vs* 540.25 ± 18.55 g; $P < 0.05$). Therefore the estimate protein requirements were no satisfied with Diet 1 and

Table 3. Feeding level, DM, CP and DE intake (mean± std).

	Diet 1		Diet 2		Sign
	Mean	Std	Mean	Std	
Feeding Level	1.5	0.1	1.7	0.1	<0.05
Daily intake of:					
DM (kg)	7.28	0.83	6.18	0.30	<0.05
CP (g)	451	51	540	18	<0.05
DE (MJ)	65.0	7.4	75.7	3.6	<0.05
DM (g/kg $BW^{0.75}$)	103.3	10.1	86.6	5.2	<0.05
CP (g/kg $BW^{0.75}$)	6.4	0.7	7.6	0.5	<0.05

Table 4. Body weight and BCS during experimental period (mean± std).

	Diet 1				Diet 2				
	Start		End		Start		End		Sign
	Mean	Std	Mean	Std	Mean	Std	Mean	Std	
Body weight (kg)	294	39	292	38	294	42	296	37	n.s.
BCS	4.5	0.18	4.0	0.25	4.5	0.21	4.5	0.26	n.s.

only just met with Diet 2. Possibly the lower CP content of hay, lower OM digestibility, higher NDF content and greater faecal bulk (Pearson *et al.*, 2001; Cuddeford, 2005), together with the effect of presence of foetus, were contributing factors to the low intake of the hay based diet.

Coefficients of apparent digestibility are shown in Table 5. The donkeys had significantly (P <0.01) higher apparent digestibility for the main dietary component in Diet 2 compared with Diet 1. The increase in digestibility ranged from 24% (NDF) to 34% (GE). The hay replacement with CM seems to be associated with the improvement in OM, CF, ADF, NDF and GE digestibility according to the experimental trial of Suhartanto *et al.* (1992) where straw was partially replaced with urea and corn grain, but in contrast to the same authors where straw was partially replaced with corn grain and soy bean meal.

The apparent digestibility of crude protein showed not significant differences between the two diets. It is possible that the lack of an expected increase in BW with increasing gestational period could perhaps be attributed to the low actual protein intake if we consider the moderate digestibility coefficient for protein in both diets (53.8 ± 9.8 and 54.1 ± 8.9 respectively for Diet 1 and 2).

The digestibility of fibre fractions was higher compared with the digestibility values reported by Suhartanto *et al.* (1992) and Ouedraogo and Tisserand (1996) in resting donkeys when straw based diet was fed. The fibre fractions apparent digestibility coefficients of Diet 1 were higher compared with those reported in pregnant mares (Gatta *et al.*, 1995) fed with similar meadow hay (CF 57.0 *vs* 52.9; ADF 49.9 *vs* 48.4; NDF 56.5 *vs* 48.6). Donkeys seem to retain food residues in the gastrointestinal tract longer than do other equids and could consequently digest fibre more efficiently than other equids (Cuddeford *et al.* 1995; Tisserand and Pearson, 2003).

Table 5. Coefficient of apparent digestibility as percentage (mean± std).

	Diet 1		Diet 2		Sign
	Mean	Std	Mean	Std	
DM	51.0	2.1	68.1	3.2	<0.01
OM	56.3	4.7	70.9	2.7	<0.01
CP	53.8	9.8	54.1	8.9	n.s.
CF	57.0	4.7	71.4	2.9	<0.01
NDF	56.4	4.4	70.2	2.7	<0.01
ADF	49.9	5.3	62.9	4.2	<0.01
GE	52.7	4.2	71.2	2.6	<0.01

The percentages of fibre particles recovered in faeces (Table 6) showed no significant differences between the two diets, with a prevalence of ≤ 2 mm particles (about 80%) in both diets, whereas Gatta *et al.* (1995) observed in pregnant mares a prevalence (about 60%) of > 4 mm particles. In our study the great percentage of smaller fibre particles (from 2 mm to <1 mm) compared with the longest ones could be attributed to a good mastication efficiency of donkeys. The mastication efficiency could be a contributing factor to the good apparent digestibility of fibre fractions.

Table 6. Percentage of different size fibre particles in faeces (mean± std).

	Diet 1		Diet 2		Sign
mm	Mean	Std	Mean	Std	
>10	0	0	0	0	n.s.
10 > 4	19.68	2.55	20.67	2.70	n.s.
2	29.48	4.99	36.23	8.67	n.s.
1	26.21	3.87	16.08	8.15	n.s.
<1	24.63	6.42	27.02	4.14	n.s.

Conclusions

The Amiata Breed seems to be have apparent digestibility of nutrients similar to that reported for other donkey breeds.

The present study shows that intake of the low quality hay alone was unlikely able to provide sufficient protein to meet the pregnancy requirements of donkeys. The concentrate supplementation improved protein intake and apparent digestibility of all nutrients with the exception of protein.

The lack of information on pregnant donkey did not allowed a complete comparison for all investigated parameters, therefore more scientific information is needed to evaluate the effects of different kind of concentrate supplementation on donkeys' intake and digestibility, especially in pregnant and lactating donkeys.

Acknowledgements

The study was carried out with financial support from National Grant (PRIN 2004). The authors thank dr. Riccardo Impeduglia, Istituto Incremento Ippico of Pisa, for providing the donkeys for the trial.

References

Cuddeford, D., 2005. Voluntary food intake by equids. Equine nutrition conference, Pferdeheilkunde, 21, p 7-8

Cuddeford, D., R.A. Pearson, R.F. Archibald and R.H. Muirhead, 1995. Digestibility and gastro-intestinal transit time of diets containing different proportions of alfalfa and oat given to Thoroughbreds, Shetland ponies Highland ponies and donkeys. Animal Science 61, 407-417.

Gatta, D., L. Krusic, L. Casini and B. Colombani, 1995. Influence of corrected teeth on digestibility of two types of diets in pregnant mares. In: Proceedings 14th Equine Nutrition and Physiology Symposium, 326-331

Martillotti, F., M. Antongiovanni, L. Rizzi, E. Santi and G. Bittante, 1987. Metodi di analisi per la valutazione degli alimenti di interesse zootecnico. CNR-IPRA, Roma, Italy.

Miraglia, N., C. Poncet and W. Martin-Rosset, 2003. Effect of feeding level, physiological status and breed on the digesta passage of forage based diet in the horse. In: Proceeding 18th Equine Nutrition and Physiology Symposium, 275-280
Mueller, P.J., H.F. Hintz, R.A. Pearson, P.R. Lawrence and P.J. Van Soest, 1994. Voluntary intake of roughage diets by donkeys. In Working Equine, 137-148.
National Research Council, 1989. Nutrient requirement of horses. Washington, DC: National Academic Press, pp 101.
Ouedraogo, T. and J.L. Tisserand, 1996. Etude comparative de la valorisation des fourrages pauvres chez l'ane et le mouton. Ingestibilité et digestibilité. Ann. Zootech., 45, 445-453.
Pearson, R.A. and J.B. Merritt, 1991. Intake, digestion and gastrointestinal transit time in resting donkeys and ponies and exercised donkeys given ad libitum hay and straw diets. Equine Vet. J., 23, 339-343
Pearson, R.A. and M. Ouassat, 2000. A guide to live weight extimation of body condition scoring of donkey. Centre for tropical veterinary medicine, University of Edimburgh, pp21
Pearson, R.A., R.F. Archibald and R.H. Muirhead, 2001. The effect of forage quality and level of feeding on digestibility and gastrointestinal transit time of oat straw and alfalfa given to ponies and donkeys. Br. J. Nutr., 85, 599-606.
SAS, 2002. JMP ® User's Guide, Version 5, SAS Institute Inc., Cary, NC, USA, pp 292.
Suhartanto, B., V. Julliand, F. Faurie and J.L. Tisserand, 1992. Comparison in digestion of donkey and ponies. In Proceed. First European Conference on Eq. Nutrition. Pferdeheikunde, 158-161
Tisserand, J.L. and R.A. Pearson, 2003. Nutritional requirements, feed intake and digestion in working donkeys: a comparison with other work animals. In: Working animals in agriculture and transport. Edited by R.A. Pearson, pp210.
Tisserand, J.L., F. Faurie and M. Toure, 1991. A comparative study of donkey and pony digestive physiology. In Donkeys, Mules and horses in tropical agricultural development, pp 67-72.
Yousef, M.K., 1991. Physiological responses of the donkey to heat stress (abstract). In Fielding D. and Pearson R.A. (eds). Donkeys, Mules and Horses in Tropical Agricultural Development, 96.

Part B – Lactation

Physiology of lactation in the mare

G.R. Starbuck
Department of Animal and Equine Science, Nottingham Trent University, Brackenhurst, Southwell, Nottinghamshire, NG25 0QF, United Kingdom

Abstract

As a predated eutherian herd mammal producing precocious offspring, lactation in the horse serves the purpose of keeping the foal in close proximity to its mother until nutritionally independant, so facilitating protection, development, skill transfer and social organization. The more obvious benefits of lactation come in the provision of the antibody rich colostrum and milk to the foal during its nutritionally dependant early life, the aquired immunity conferred by the former being of particular importance in the horse. The composition of milk is species specific, and alters throughout lactation to support the development and nutritional needs of the offspring. The mare synthesizes milk in the lobuloalveolar tissue of two pairs of mammary glands in the inguinal region, each pair of glands exiting through one teat. Lobuloalveolar growth occurs during pregnancy under the influence of progestagens and oestrogens, progestagens inhibiting milk synthesis until the periparturient period. Placental lactogen has not been detected in the mare and is not believed to play a part in equine mammary development. In addition to the decline in progestagens, the rise in prolactin during the last few days of pregnancy, peaking at parturition, drives lactogenesis. However, prolactin is not believed to have a role to play in the maintenance of established lactation, despite positive correlations between suckling and circulating maternal prolactin concentrations in some mares. Milk ejection is stimulated by oxytocin secreted from the posterior pituitary gland in response to mechanical stimulation of the teat, although milk secretion can occur in the absence of oxytocin, the capacious duct system of the glands making milk ejection less important. Lactational anoestrous is not a feature of the mares reproductive physiology. Under natural conditions, weaning occurs when the foal is around 8-10 months of age. The glands begin a gradual process of involution as demand for milk declines, an autolytic process that replaces parenchyma with connective and adipose tissue.

Keywords: mare, lactation

Introduction

A mammal is defined by the female of the species possessing mammary glands with which they nourish their offspring. The strategy of adults feeding their offspring a secretory product is not the exclusive domain of mammals; other vertebrates, most notably the pigeon, produce such secretions, interestingly also under the influence of the hormone prolactin, with which to nourish their young. This therefore leaves the specialist secretory organ of the mammary gland as the defining feature.

Lactation is now speculated to have played a crucial role in the evolutionary success of mammals. Most importantly, it enabled mammals to adapt to the major climatic and vegetation changes that occurred during the transition from the Cretaceous to the Tertiary period which led to the mass extinction of the dinosaurs. The major benefit to this ends is the need for the environment to only provide food for the adult, freeing the young from the necessity to seek food that is appropriate for their own needs. Instead, milk from the female provides the young with a reliable, consistent and readily available food source, enabling them to concentrate their energy on growth and development (Pond, 1977). The ability of mammalian herbivores to convert a cellulose rich diet into nutritionally rich milk has been capitalized on by humans for thousands of years, resulting in the domestication and management of cows, goats, sheep, camels, reindeer and horses for dairy purposes.

In addition to nutrition, benefit to the young also comes in the acquired immunoprotection conferred by the immunoglobulin rich colostrum and sustained immunoglobulin component of milk. In comparison with other domestic species, the foal is probably most reliant on this protection, without which its chance of survival would be significantly compromised (McClure, 1992).

Eutherian mammals typically produce either altricial young, born after short gestation in a helpless state and often confined to a nest, or precocious young that are born in an advanced state of development and, especially in the case of foals, are able to stand and run soon after birth (Martin, 1984). For altricial offspring, lactation supports them through the nest phase, a phase which is almost an extension of gestation. Lactation keeps precocious offspring in close proximity to their mothers at least until they are nutritionally independent, providing additional benefits that relate to protection, development, skill transfer and social organization, a benefit that is particularly important for a predated herd animal such as the horse.

Milk

For most species, milk is largely composed of water. Within this are hundreds of different compounds, the major components of which being fats, proteins and carbohydrates. Many of these compounds, such as milk fats, milk caseins and lactose, are unique to milk, requiring synthesis in the mammary gland from substrates derived from the blood. This seems obvious now, but historically, mammary glands were thought to have only a passive role in milk production, acting as filters to remove preformed substrates from the blood (Mepham, 1986). Our current understanding is that the synthetic and secretory activity of the alveolar epithelium makes functioning mammary tissue one of the most metabolically active tissues of the body.

Whilst the constituents of milk are largely common between species, the relative concentrations of these constituents is species variable (Table 1). Evolution has clearly had a role to play in this variation, ensuring the composition of milks that best suit the offspring of particular species within the constraints of the environment (Dugdale, 1986). Whilst this variation is complex, some trends have been identified; a positive correlation appears to exist between the gross energy output in milk and maternal mass (Oftedal, 1984) and for most species, there is a positive correlation between milk protein and fat concentration (Martin, 1984). There is also a trend by which precocious offspring, born at in advanced state of development (ungulates), receive milk which is comparatively lower in protein concentration than that received by their more altricial counterparts (rodents). With this in

Table 1. Average concentrations of some constituents in the milk of a number of species (source: Davies et al., 1983).

Species	Fat ($g.l^{-1}$)	Casein ($g.l^{-1}$)	Milk serum protein ($g.l^{-1}$)	Lactose (mM)	Calcium (mM)
Cow	37	28	6	133	30
Goat	45	25	4	114	22
Sheep	74	46	9	133	58
Pig	68	28	20	153	104
Horse	19	13	12	172	17
Human	38	4	6	192	7
Rat	103	64	20	90	80
Guinea-pig	39	66	15	83	41
Rabbit	183	104	32	60	214

mind, it must be said that most data on milk composition relates to milk at peak lactation, and that milk composition can vary appreciably throughout the lactation period.

Structure of the mammary gland

The equine mammary glands are located in the inguinal region. The mare has four distinct glands (Turner, 1939), two pairs on either side of the midline, each pair being served by two teats. Each teat is served by two teat canals and two teat cisterns; each of these being consistent with a gland cistern that has its own ductal and alveolar system.

In common with all exocrine glands, the parenchyma of mammary glands comprises two types of tissue, secretory and ductal. The secretory cells form a simple epithelium arranged into numerous pear-shaped alveoli, into the lumen of which the milk is secreted. Surrounding each alveolus is a network of myoepithelial cells which, upon contraction, force milk from the alveolar lumen into the ductal system. Racemose groups of alveoli empty milk into common ducts of progressively larger diameter. Groups of alveoli form lobules and groups of lobules form the lobes that are characteristic of mammary tissue (lobuloalveolar). The larger ducts converge into storage spaces or cisterns beneath the teat, from which milk is removed by the suckling offspring. The relative size of these cisterns is species variable, some of the largest being found in dairy animals where up to 50% of the available milk can be stored, as such, it is thought that the active ejection of milk may be less important in these species.

Mammary growth and function

Following each successive mating, the mammary gland enters a cycle of growth and differentiation. Of this cycle, three phases are apparent: growth of the mammary gland during pregnancy, secretion of milk during lactation (which may still contain some component of mammary growth), and involution following weaning. Changes in the mammary gland are under hormonal control, a control that is plagued with inter-species differences, possibly due to the late arrival of the mammary gland on the evolutionary scene.

Mammary development

Embryonic development

Mammary glands first appear in the embryo, arising from two parallel lines of raised ectoderm running down the ventral surface, one either side of the midline. From these, mammary buds develop, as a result of morphogenic movements of cells, in numbers and positions that correspond to those seen in the mature animal. Isometric growth of mammary tissue then ensues resulting in the formation of rudimentary nipples, a limited ductal system, some stromal tissue development and formation of a mammary fat pad. Development at this stage does not appear to be hormonally influenced, with the exception of the transitory function of androgens in the suppression of mammary development in the male, it being largely stimulated by mesenchymal factors.

Juvenile development

Prior to puberty, mammary growth continues to be isometric and is largely confined to a limited extension of the ductal system into the fat pad. From puberty onwards, allometric growth begins. This is primarily ductal rather than lobuloalveolar growth and is apparent in the follicular phase of the oestrous cycle under the influence of oestrogen. It is followed by regression in most species during the luteal phase of the cycle, so the net gain in mammary gland size is minimal. The post-pubertal mammary development of which we humans are accustomed is largely due to fat deposition and does not occur in other species.

Development in pregnancy

In most species, lobuloalveolar growth only occurs during pregnancy, with cell division in the gland increasing dramatically as lobules grow into the stromal tissue, displacing adipose tissue. This increase in tissue growth is controlled by progesterone and oestrogen; high progesterone and oestrogen concentrations during pregnancy initiating lobuloalveolar development, but the elevated progesterone concentration inhibiting milk production.

This steroidal control differs slightly in the mare as circulating progesterone concentration is typically low during the third trimester of pregnancy. Progesterone is released by the foetoplacental unit but is metabolized to 5α-pregnanes in the maternal circulation (Hamon *et al.*, 1991; Holtan *et al.*, 1991), 5α-pregnane-3,20-dione being presumed to be the most bioactive due to its high concentration and affinity for the progestagen receptor (Chavatte *et al.*, 1997). Of the oestrogens, the biologically inactive equilin and equilenin are most in evidence in late pregnancy (Pashen, R.L., 1984) with the bioactive oestradiol 17-α increasing in concentration prior to parturition (Barnes *et al.*, 1975). Placental lactogen has not been detected in the pregnant mare and is not believed to play a part in equine mammary development (Forsyth *et al.*, 1975).

The decline in progestagens at the end of gestation and the rise in prolactin leading up to parturition are probably the basis of the trigger for lactation to begin. The progestagen block on lactation is not absolute, highlighted by the fact that horses commonly show premature onset of lactation and leakage of milk prepartum, when circulating progestagen concentrations are still high. Also, if it were, simultaneous pregnancy and lactation would not be possible. Lactational anoestrus is not a feature of the mares reproductive physiology and follicular growth and ovulation resumes soon after parturition.

Prolactin appears to play a major role in lactogenesis and the initiation of lactation in the mare. Plasma concentrations of prolactin increase suddenly during the last few days of pregnancy and peak around the time of parturition (see Figure 1; Lothrop *et al.*, 1987; Worthy *et al.*, 1987) remaining elevated until some three months after parturition (Worthy *et al.*, 1986). This increase is probably instigated by the cessation of release of an inhibitory factor in the hypothalamus (Forsythe *et al.*, 1975). Inhibition of endogenous prolactin release in late pregnant mares by the administration of the dopamine agonist bromocriptine results in agalactica (Ireland *et al.,* 1991).

Development during lactation

It was originally believed that mammary development was essentially complete at the time of parturition, especially in dairy ruminant species. However, this belief is now not upheld and the extent of lactational mammary growth shows wide species variation, from 10% in ruminants to as much as 50% in rodents (Forsyth, 1986), supporting the significant increase in milk production seen in the first weeks of lactation. The control of this growth is not fully understood.

Galactopoiesis

Despite having a role to play in the initiation of lactation in the mare, prolactin does not appear to be required for the maintenance of established lactation. Administration of bromocriptine during established lactation, whilst reducing circulating prolactin concentrations, had no effect on milk yield or mammary size (Neuschaefer *et al.,* 1991) despite a positive relationship between suckling

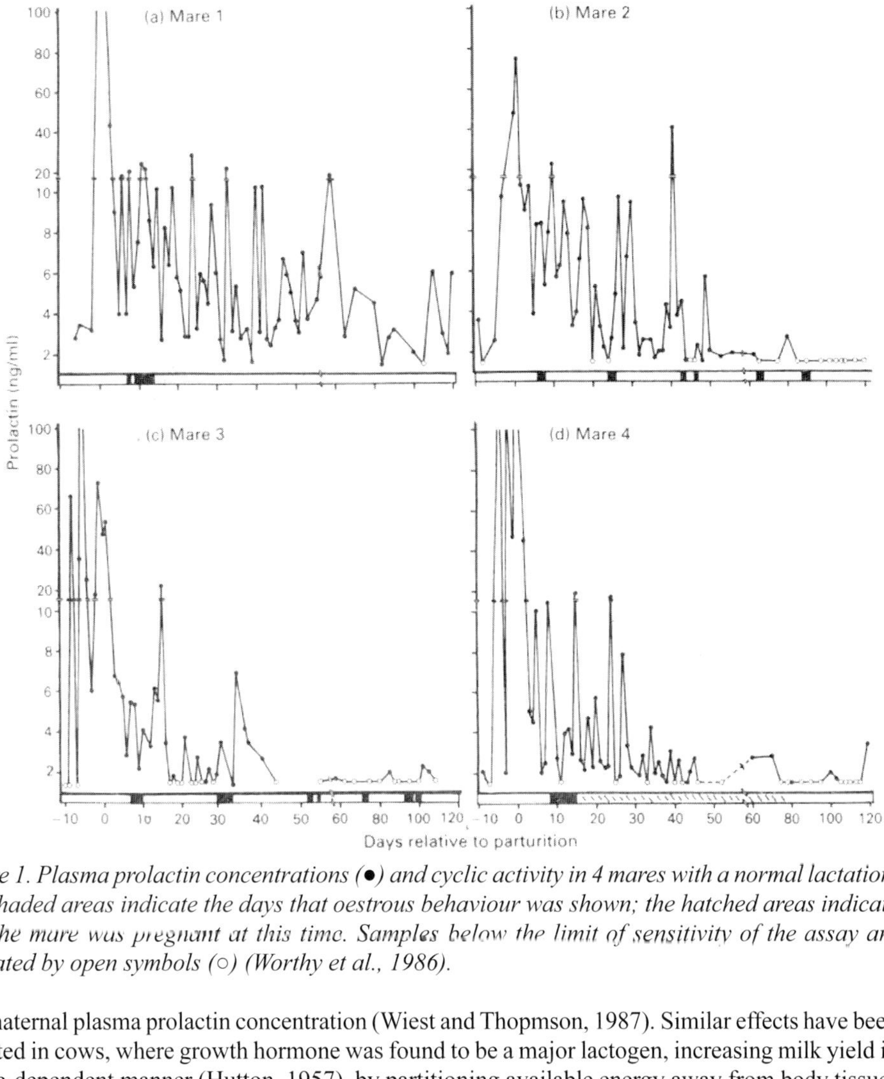

Figure 1. Plasma prolactin concentrations (●) and cyclic activity in 4 mares with a normal lactation. The shaded areas indicate the days that oestrous behaviour was shown; the hatched areas indicate that the mare was pregnant at this time. Samples below the limit of sensitivity of the assay are indicated by open symbols (○) (Worthy et al., 1986).

and maternal plasma prolactin concentration (Wiest and Thopmson, 1987). Similar effects have been reported in cows, where growth hormone was found to be a major lactogen, increasing milk yield in a dose-dependent manner (Hutton, 1957), by partitioning available energy away from body tissues and towards milk production (Forsyth, 1986), a finding that has led to commercial exploitation in this species.

Milk yield is determined by the number of secretory epithelial cells in the mammary gland and secretory activity per cell. Post-partum regulation of milk yield adjusts production to the demands of the young and has been related to litter size or milking frequency in a number of species (Archer, 1983; Henderson *et al.*, 1985), indicating that the secretory capacity of cells can be increased. The controlling factors are not fully understood, but are likely to act locally and may involve inhibitors present in milk such as those suggested in ruminants (Wilde and Peaker, 1990).

Milk ejection

As with most mammals, milk ejection in the horse is stimulated by oxytocin secreted from the posterior pituitary gland in response to mechanical stimulation of the teat during suckling (Sharma,

1974). Oxytocin causes contraction of the myoepithelial cells and ejection of milk into the duct system and teat sinus, increasing intramammary pressure and the proportion of mammary milk for removal by the suckling young. However, milk secretion can occur in the absence of any detectable oxytocin in the circulation (Ellendorf and Schams, 1988), a fact that has also been noted in dairy ruminants. It has been postulated that this is due to the capacious duct system making milk ejection less important in these species, although alternative mechanisms have been postulated (Mepham, 1987).

Mammary involution

Under natural conditions, weaning occurs when the foal is around 8-10 months of age, when the foal is gaining most of its nutrition from sources other than milk and milk production by the mare is quite low. As the foals demand for milk declines, the mammary glands begin a gradual process of involution. Most domesticated systems enforce weaning at between five to six months when milk production is comparatively higher, this abrupt termination of suckling exaggerating the involutionary effects. The increase in alveolar and intramammary pressure caused by the accumulation of milk, in addition to the effects of postulated inhibitors contained in milk, suppresses milk secretion. The initial distension of the glands usually subsides within a few days and the glands visibly shrink. Involution is essentially an autolytic process facilitated by lysosomes and phagocytic cells, progressively replacing parenchyma with connective and adipose tissue. Management of the mare at weaning is important due to the risk of intramammary inflammatory damage and mastitis resulting from gland distension.

Conclusion

The mammary gland has an important role to play in equine reproduction. There is no doubt that the early immunoprotection conferred by the immunoglobulin rich colostrum dramatically increases the chances of survival of the foal. Furthermore, milk provides a dynamic food source that adapts to the needs and demands of the foal, providing ideal nutrition in early life. Despite the importance of mammary function in the survival of the foal, research is limited on the control of lactation in the mare when compared to humans, guinea pigs and dairy ruminants. What work has been done has brought to light some features; such as the absence of placental lactogen, the non-requirement of prolactin for the maintenance of established lactation, the absence of lactational anoestrous and the ability for milk to be made available to the foal in the absence of detectable oxytocin, that combined lead to a unique control of mammary function. The mare is occasionally prone to lactational disorders such as agalactica, particularly of the maiden mare, and premature lactation which, without an adequate understanding of lactational physiology, will remain frustrating to treat and will continue to compromise the foal.

References

Archer, P., 1983. Milking three times a day. Milk Marketing Board Report 34.

Barnes, R.J., P.W. Nathanielsz, P.D. Rossdale, R.S. Comline and M. Silver, 1975. Plasma progestagens and oestrogens in fetus and mother in late pregnancy. Journal of Reproduction and Fertility Supplement 23: 617-623.

Chavatte, P., D. Holtan, J.C. Ousey and P.D. Rossdale, 1997. Biosynthesis and possible biological roles of progestagens during equine pregnancy and in the newborn foal. Equine Veterinary Journal Supplement 24: 89-95.

Davies, D.T., C. Holt and W.W. Christie, 1983. The composition of milk. In: Biochemistry of Lactation, T.B. Mepham (editor), Elsevier, Amsterdam.

Dugdale, A.E., 1986. Evolution and infant feeding. Lancet i: 670-673.

Ellendorf, F. and D. Schams, 1988. Characteristics of milk ejection, associated intramammary pressure changes and oxytocin release in the mare. Journal of Endocrinology 119: 219-227.

Forsyth, I.A., 1986. Variation among species in the endocrine control of mammary growth and function: the roles of prolactin, growth hormone and placental lactogen. Journal of Dairy Science 69: 886-903.
Forsythe, I.A., P.D. Rossdale and C.R. Thomas, 1975. Studies on milk composition and lactogenic hormones in the mare. Journal of Reproduction and Fertility Supplement 23: 631-635.
Hamon, M., S.W. Clarke, E. Houghton, A.L. Fowden, M. Silver, P.D. Rossdale, J.C. Ousey and R.B. Heap, 1991. Production of 5α-dihydroxyprogesterone during late pregnancy in the mare. Journal of Reproduction and Fertility Supplement 44: 529-535.
Henderson, A.J., D.R. Blatchford and Peaker, M., 1985. The effects of thrice-daily milking on milk secretion in the goat. Quarterly Journal of Experimental Physiology 68: 645-652.
Holtan, D.W., E. Houghton, M. Silver, A.L. Fowden, J. Ousey and P.D. Rossdale, 1991. Plasma progestagens in the mare, foetus, and newborn foal. Journal of Reproduction and Fertility Supplement 44: 517-528.
Hutton, J.B., 1957. The effect of growth hormone on the yield and composition of cows' milk. Journal of Endocrinology 16:115-125.
Ireland, F.A., W.F. Loch, K. Worthy and R.V. Anthony, 1991. Effects of bromocriptine and perphenazine on prolactin and progesterone concentrations in pregnant pony mares during late gestation. Journal of Reproduction and Fertility 92, 179-186.
Lothrop, C.D., J.E. Henton, B.B. Cole and H.L. Nolan, 1987. Prolactin response to thyrotrophin-releasing hormone in normal and agalactic mares. Journal of Reproduction and Fertility Supplement 35: 277-280.
McClure, J.J., 1992. The immune system. In: Equine Reproduction, A.O. McKinnon and J.L. Voss (editors). Lea and Febiger, Philidelphia, 1003-1016.
Martin, R.D., 1984. Scaling effects and adaptive strategies in mammalian lactation. Symposia of the Zoological Society of London 51: 87-117.
Mepham, T.B., 1986. The development of ideas on milk protein secretion. Vlaams Diergeneeskundig Tijdschrift 55: 228-238.
Mepham, T.B., 1987. Physiology of Lactation. Open University Press, Milton Keynes.
Neuschaefer, A., V. Bracher and W.E. Allen, 1991. Prolactin secretion in lactating mares before and after treatment with bromocriptine. Journal of Reproduction and Fertility Supplement 44: 551-559.
Oftedal, O.T., 1984. Milk composition, milk yield and energy output at peak lactation: a comparative review. Symposia of the Zoological Society of London 51: 33-85.
Pashen, R.L., 1984. Maternal and foetal endocrinology during late pregnancy in the mare. Equine Veterinary Journal 16, 233-238.
Pond, C.M., 1977. The significance of lactation in the evolution of mammals. Evolution 31: 177-199.
Sharma, O.P., 1974. Release of oxytocin elicited by suckling stimulus in mares. Journal of Reproduction and Fertility Supplement 37: 421-423.
Turner, C.W., 1939. The Comparative Anatomy of the Mammary Glands. Missouri University Cooperative Store, Columbia.
Wiest, J.J. and D.L. Thompson, 1987. Plasma prolactin, LH and FSH concentrations after suckling in post-partum mares. Journal of Reproduction and Fertility Supplement 35: 731-732.
Wilde, C.J. and M. Peaker, 1990. Autocrine control in milk secretion. Journal of Agricultural Research 114: 235-238.
Worthy, K., R. Escreet and J.P. Renton, 1986. Plasma prolactin concentrations and cyclic activity in pony mares during parturition and early lactation. Journal of Reproduction and Fertility Supplement 77: 569-574.
Worthy, K., K. Colquhoun, R. Escreet, M. Dunlop, J.P. Renton and T.A. Douglas, 1987. Plasma prolactin concentrations in non-pregnant mares at different times of the year and in relation to events in the cycle. Journal of Reproduction and Fertility Supplement 35: 269-276.

Milk yield of nursing and dairy mares

M. Doreau[1] *and F. Martuzzi*[2]
[1]*INRA-Department of Animal Science, Research Center of Clermont-Ferrand/Theix, 63122 Saint Genès Champanelle, France*
[2]*Dept. PABVQSA, Parma University, Via del Taglio 8, 43100 Parma, Italy*

Abstract

This paper reviews main characteristics of milk yield in nursing and dairy mares, and the main factors of variation. Milk yield is generally reached between 2 and 3.5 kg per 100 kg liveweight in nursing mares. Peak of lactation is generally comprised between 1 and 3 months of lactation, and lactation persistency is high. Generally, milk yield of dairy mares is lower, with an earlier peak and a lower persistency of lactation than nursing mares. However, experimental data are sometimes questionable, because a reliable measurement of milk yield is difficult, due to the high frequency of sucklings by foal. In dairy mares, milk yield depends on frequency and conditions of milking, because of the small capacity of the udder. Differences in milk yield of nursing mares depends to a large extent on their liveweight. For dairy mares, between-breed differences are important for a same liveweight. Influence of diet on liveweight is limited. A moderate effect of energy level is observed. Few data are available on the effect of diet composition, which appears moderate too. Thin mares at foaling may produce less milk than mares in good condition. Further research is necessary to improve the knowledge of factors of variation of milk yield.

Keywords: mare, milk, milking, lactation, suckling

Introduction

Maternal milk is the main source of energy for foals in the first months of their life, and milk intake determines foal growth. Besides this, mare milk is a more or less usual beverage for approximately 30 million people throughout the world, especially in the former USSR and in Mongolia, and is now consumed in Western Europe for its nutritional quality. This results in a large geographical distribution of dairy and non dairy mares (Doreau and Martin-Rosset, 2002), and in a wide number of genotypes, adapted, or not, to milking. Mares from most breeds weigh on average between 500 and 750 kg, but Mongolian mares may weigh less than 400 kg, and some European breeds weigh more than 850 kg. In nursing mares, milk yield is leaded by suckling behaviour of foal, whereas in dairy mares it depends on the efficiency of milking. All these differences result in a broad variation in milk yield. The objective of this review is to point the main characteristics of milk production from mares, whether they are milked or nursing, and to determine the main factors of variation. A limited amount of new and original publications has been published since the review by Doreau and Boulot (1989a). This paper summarizes available information for a better understanding of mechanisms that control milk yield both in nursing and dairy mares.

Suckling and milking

The suckling behaviour of foal is characterized by a very large number of bouts in early nursing period. According to different authors, among others Bouwman and Van der Schee (1978), Martin-Rosset *et al.* (1978) and Trottier *et al.* (2006), foals suck about 70 times per day at birth, 30 times per day at 1 month of age and 25 times per day at 4 months. The mean duration of each suckling is 80-90 seconds (Ellendorff and Schams, 1988). This may be due in part to the low volume of the udder, estimated from the amount of milk obtained in one milking, which is generally lower than 2 L (reviews by Le

Du, 1986, and Doreau and Boulot, 1989b), in part to a low capacity of foal to extract milk from the udder in early lactation. Although no direct relationship exists between sucking behaviour and milk intake by foals (Cameron *et al.*, 1999), it is clear that the maximal milk intake in one bout or one milking is limited. This explains why dairy mares have to be milked with a high frequency, in order to maximise the amount of milk obtained. A milking every 2 or 3 h is often performed.

Methods of measurement of milk yield

Determination of mare milk yield can be biased by methodological problems in nursing mares. In dairy mares, actual milk yield is the sum of milk obtained by milking and of milk consumed by the foal. Conditions of milking may influence the achievement of milk secretion potential. Methods of measurement have been analysed in detail by Doreau and Boulot (1989b). Briefly, it is concluded that for nursing mares the estimation of milk yield by milking, with or without oxytocin injection, may lead to important biases, because the amount of milk harvested does not correspond to the milk intake by the foal. If mares are milked without oxytocin injection to the mare, only a part of milk present in the udder is harvested (Doreau *et al.*, 1986), owing to the duration of manual milking (Caroprese *et al.*, 2006) in relation with the fleeting action of naturally released oxytocin. Milking with oxytocin probably overestimates actual milk intake by foal in early lactation: it can be expected that the very young foal does not completely empty the udder when suckling. The measurement by weighing before and after foal suck, performed several times per day, is more reliable. However the quality of the method is very variable. Measurement can be made throughout day and night or only during the day, and the number of hours between two weigh-suck-weigh measurements can be close to natural conditions of suckling, or higher, reaching sometimes 3 hours. In order to mimic natural behaviour, this interval may be shorter in early lactation than later. Nevertheless, it is likely not necessary to reduce too much the interval between sucks. Indeed, milk secretion rate in the udder is constant until maximal udder capacity is near to be reached. This method suffers from some drawbacks. It disturbs the normal behaviour of foals. When the method is performed only during the day, it hypothesises that milk intake by foal is the same during the night as during the day, whereas foals suck a longer time during the day than at night (Duncan *et al.*, 1984, Trottier *et al.*, 2006).

The most accurate method for early lactation is probably the use of deuteriated or tritiated water as a tracer (Doreau and Dussap, 1980). Isotopic water is injected to foal and dilutes immediately in total body water. Decrease in isotopic water concentration in blood is proportional to water intake by foal, arising from milk. This method is not biased because it measures the milk yield without disturbing the natural sucking frequency of the foal, but it can be used only when milk can be considered as the only source of water for the foal, i.e. the first 2 months of lactation. Milk yield can be measured later by a double isotope technique, as it has been done by Martin *et al.* (1992).

Data on milk yield of dairy mares are often questionable or difficult to interpret, especially the very numerous data published in the former USSR, but also more recent data. First, it is sometimes difficult to be sure that published figures include the amount of milk fed by the foal when mares are not milked. Secondly, the number of daily milkings and the interval between milkings is generally not mentioned in publications. At least, conditions of milking are not specified, and the amount of milk harvested in one milking depends on pulsation and vacuum level of the milking machine, which can be variable (Le Du, 1986), and on the adaptation of mare to milking.

Milk yield throughout lactation

Nursing mares generally produce between 2 and 3.5 kg milk daily per 100 kg liveweight during the first months of lactation. Despite the low capacity of the udder, this yield is high because foal sucks are very frequent. Such a production allows a high liveweight gain of the foal, which can reach 2 kg

/ day for mares weighing 700 kg (*e.g.* Martin-Rosset *et al.*, 1978). The peak of lactation is probably reached between the 2nd and the 3rd month. All measurements performed by the isotope dilution method (Oftedal *et al.*, 1983, Doreau *et al.*, 1990, 1992, 1993, Martin *et al.*, 1992) have shown an increase until 2 months, but unfortunately, these measurements were not carried out later. Milk yield measurements occurring during the whole lactation, with the suck–weigh–suck method (Gibbs *et al.*, 1982, Santos *et al.*, 2005) show either flat curves of lactation, with a moderate increase between the 1st and the 3rd month (Neseni *et al.*, 1958, Bouwman and Van der Schee, 1978) or a slight decrease as soon as lactation goes forward (Gibbs *et al.*, 1982, Santos *et al.*, 2005) (Figure 1). By modelling milk yield of 7 mares, Santos and Silvestre (2006) determined that lactation reached the peak between 19 and 48 days for 5 mares, whereas two mares had atypical curves. This discrepancy between experiments probably arises from the method of measurement, due to the above mentioned limitation of the milking technique. We made an attempt of modelling from literature data, accounting for experiment effect (Figure 1), with the model of Wood (1967) which is used for dairy ruminants. This modelling results in a peak of lactation at 50 days, and a high persistency. However the reliability of the model is limited because i) it may be inappropriate for lactating mares; ii) there is a high interaction between experiment effect and lactation stage.

The lactation curve of milked mares is rather different with an early peak (28 days according to Wood's model) and a lower persistency of lactation, but few data are available (Alaguzhin, 1974, Fedotov and Akimbekov, 1983, Pinto *et al.*, 2001) (Figure 1). It is to be noted that the conditions of milking and estimation of milk yield are not specified in these publications, and thus that the reliability of the typical lactation curve obtained by modelling (Figure 2) could be questioned. In particular, the extent of persistency could differ from that of the curve: Medvedev and Yavorskii (1984) have shown large differences in persistency from one breed to another for a same average yield.

A comparison between nursing and dairy mares on one hand, nursing and dairy cows of the same weight on the other hand, shows that nursing mares produce more milk than dairy mares, whereas nursing cows produce much less milk than dairy cows (Figure 2). This can be explained by a lesser genetic selection in mares than in cows. It is likely that, in mares, selection has been made on easiness of milking. This characteristic is difficult to reach: a number of dairy mares require the presence of the foal for a maximal milk ejection (Cherepanova and Belokobylenko, 1974). Indeed in mares 70 to 85% of milk is alveolar (Le Du, 1986) due to a very limited size of the cisterns, whereas in cows most milk is cisternal. Moreover, selection in the former USSR has often been made on morphological

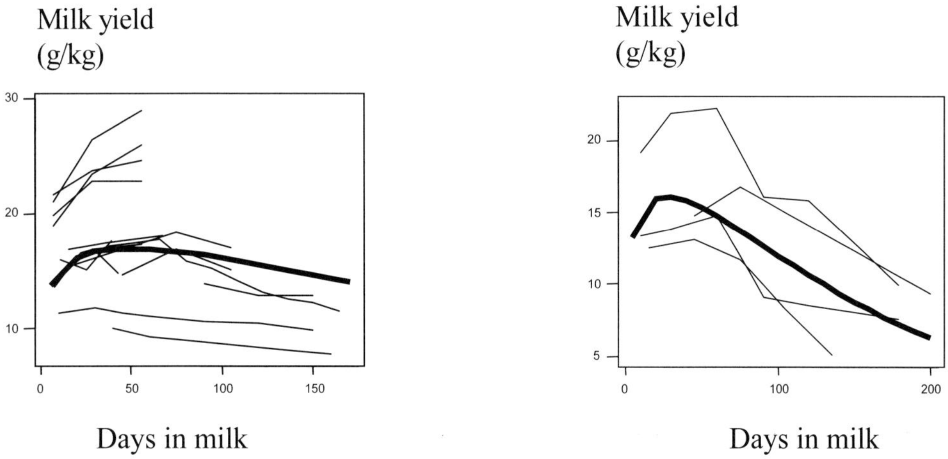

Figure 1. Milk yield of nursing and milked mares. Effect of lactation stage.

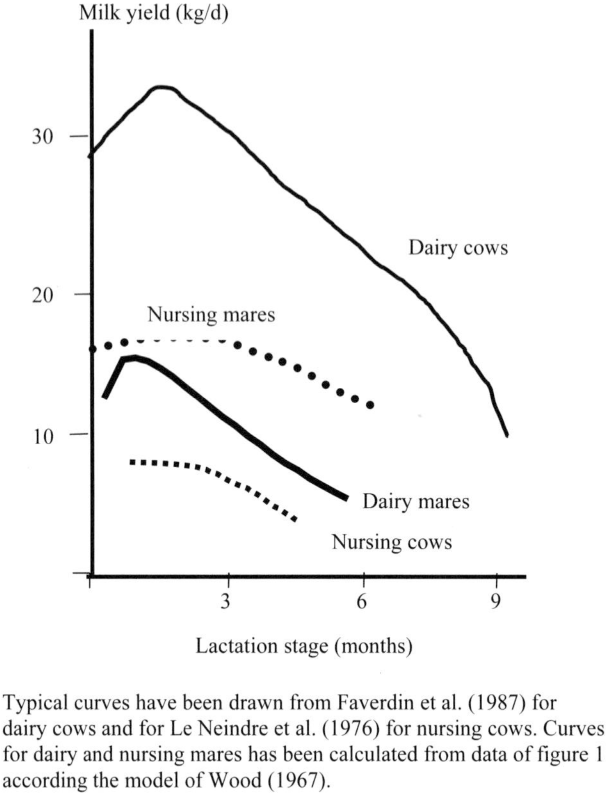

Figure 2. Typical curves of lactation of nursing and dairy mares and cows weighing on average 600 kg.

characteristics to the udder (Tarasevich, 1979). This may explain that for a same mare liveweight, milk yield is higher in nursing mares than in dairy mares. Milk yield is also higher in nursing mares than in nursing cows of the same weight. It is likely that milk yield of nursing cows is limited by the moderate growth potential of calf compared to foal, and thus by the moderate milk intake by calf, which generally sucks twice a day (Le Neindre *et al.*, 1976).

Effect of genotype, age and parity on milk yield

Among nursing mares, differences in milk yield are explained first by mare liveweight. Figure 3 shows the milk yield of mares either of heavy breeds (Breton and Comtois) or of saddle breeds (Anglo-Arabian and Selle Français), receiving a diet based on 85 to 95% hay, in good body condition. The mean milk yield per kg liveweight is of the same extent for saddle and heavy mares. Within a category, individual variation is high, but no difference was observed between Comtois and Breton on one hand, Anglo-Arabian and Selle Français on the other hand. More recently, Pinto *et al.* (2001) compared Murgese breed of 480 kg and Tiro Pesante Rapido (TPR) breed of 880 kg fed comparable diets, and obtained differences in milk yield, measured by milking, throughout 6 months of lactation, but milk yield per 100 kg liveweight was higher for the small size than for the large size mares (3.0 and 2.5 kg, respectively). In nursing mares, it can be supposed that for a given diet, milk secretion is controlled by growth potential of the offspring, as it has been demonstrated in nursing cows (Le Neindre *et al.*, 1976); moreover nursing mares have not been selected for milk yield or maternal

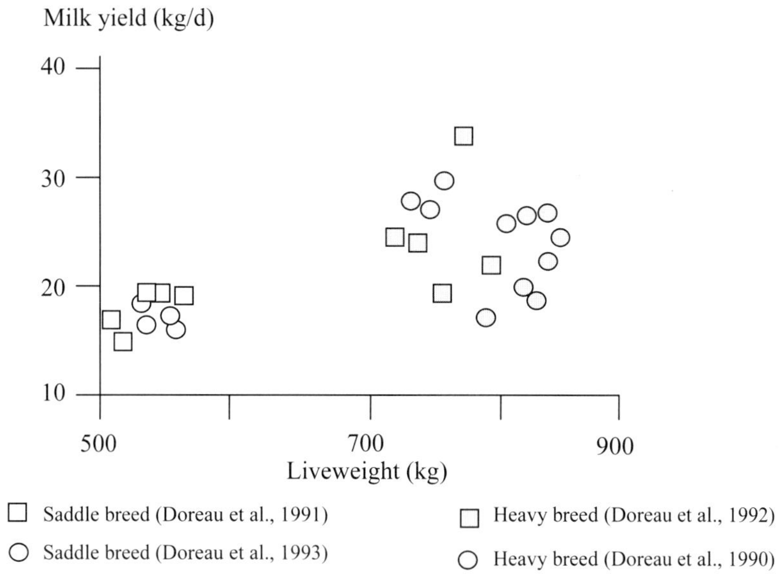

Each symbol represents one mare. Only mares fed a hay diet, multiparous and in good body condition have been kept

Figure 3. Relationship between milk yield and mare liveweight at 2 months of lactation.

ability. Unfortunately, there is no reliable information on milk yield in pony mares, so that it is not possible to expand his relationship between weight and milk secretion: indeed the two references on Shetland pony mares mention daily milk yields of 5 and 10 kg, respectively.

Publications in the former USSR (quoted by Doreau and Boulot, 1989a) showed that differences between dairy breeds or within breed individual variations were high for a same liveweight. Contrary to nursing mares, it cannot be assumed that foal milk intake is a major factor explaining differences due to liveweight, and the efficiency of selection for milk production could have been different among breeds. Very few information is available concerning the level of milk production of non-dairy breeds when they are milked. Haflinger breed is sometimes considered as adapted to milking, but no experimental data allows to confirm this thought.

Milk production did not significantly vary between 1st and 2nd lactation in experiments by Gibbs *et al.* (1982) and Doreau *et al.* (1991) but the number of mares was low. Several authors quoted by Doreau and Boulot (1989a) observed an increase in production of dairy mares until a very late maximum, between 11 and 15 years, whereas the maximum could be around 7 years in nursing mares (Duncan and Gleize, 1985).

Dietary effects on milk yield

When comparing two extreme diets (95% hay and 5% concentrates vs 50% hay and 50% concentrates, given ad libitum, Doreau *et al.* (1992) showed a positive effect of energy and/or concentrates supply on milk yield. Nevertheless, with the forage-based diet, milk yield reached 3 kg per 100 kg liveweight, evidencing that a high yield could be reached with a diet short in glucose precursors, which are theoretically necessary to lactose synthesis and thus to milk secretion. With less different diets than in this experiment, Pinto *et al.* (2001) observed that an increase in concentrates, which increased both energy and protein supply, resulted in a non significant increase in milk yield (Table 1). The

Table 1. Effect of energy and/or protein supply on milk yield of mares at 2 months of lactation.

Reference	Mare breed and weight	Diet composition and intake	Milk yield (kg/d)
Doreau *et al.*, 1992	Breton, Comtois, 726 kg	95% hay, 5% soybean meal, ad lib. (CP1 12.9% DM1). Intake: 24 kg DM	26.0
		50% hay, 50% concentrates, ad lib. (CP 14.1% diet). Intake: 22 kg DM	29.0
Pinto *et al.*, 2001	Tiro Pesante Rapido, 880 kg	18 kg hay, 3,5 kg oats, 0.3 kg bran (CP: 9.8% DM)	17.6
		20 kg hay, 8 kg concentrates (CP 11.5% DM)	18.7

1CP: crude protein; DM: dry matter

Data for nursing mares from heavy and saddle breeds: Nordstrom (1970), Bouwman and Van der Schee (1978), Gibbs *et al.* (1982), Oftedal *et al.* (1983), Doreau *et al.* (1982, 1990, 1992, 1993), Sigler *et al.* (1989), Santos *et al.* (2005).

Data for milked mares: Alaguzhin (1974), Fedotov and Akimbekov (1983) and Pinto *et al.* (2001)

effect of energy level is generally of low extent. Sutton *et al.* (1977) with a diet given at two levels of intake and Pagan *et al.* (1984) with diets increasing in energy content, did not show any variation in foal growth. It can be supposed that when energy intake is lower than requirements, body reserves mobilization provides supplementary energy for milk production.

The effect of protein content of the diet has not been directly determined on milk yield, but only on foal growth. From several data summarized by Doreau (1994) it appears that protein level of the diet increases milk yield until ca. 14% of crude protein. However, ad libitum feeding allows to meet protein requirements, as it has been shown by Doreau *et al.* (1992) with mares fed a hay diet containing less than 9% crude protein.

Very few data deal with the effect of the composition of concentrate. A non significant trend to an increase in foal growth when fat was added to the diet was mentioned by Davison *et al.* (1987), but further research should be carried out to confirm this data.

Level of feeding in late pregnancy determines the body condition at foaling. A positive effect of the extent of mare body reserves at foaling on foal growth (and thus mare milk production) in the first months of lactation has been shown first by Martin-Rosset and Doreau (1980) and Henneke *et al.* (1981) comparing fat and thin mares, but not by Kubiak *et al.* (1989) comparing fat and medium body condition mares. In these experiments, food intake was given in restricted amounts so that thin mares probably did not achieve their milk potential due to an insufficient energy supply, whereas fat mares could, due to lipid mobilization. In an experiment in which mares were fed ad libitum, no difference in milk production was observed between fat and thin mares, these latter eating more (Doreau *et al.*, 1993), and the high intake even allowed thin mares to restore their body reserves in early lactation. This specificity of mares demonstrates the interest of ad libitum feeding in early lactation.

Conclusion

In horses, data on milk yield are much less numerous than data on milk composition, due to the difficulty for a reliable measurement in nursing mares, and to the small number of well-designed experiments in dairy mares. However, it has been possible to evidence the high milk yield of nursing mares, compared to nursing cows or dairy mares. Dietary factors seem to have a moderate effect on milk yield, and it can be thought for available data that at libitum feeding allows to meet milk secretion potential, even with diets low in energy. Facing the increase in the use of mares from non-dairy breeds for milk production in many European countries, further research is needed to evaluate their milk potential.

References

Alaguzhin, A., 1974. Variation of milk production of mares of the Lokai breed throughout lactation (in Russian). Trudy Tadz. Sel'skokzyaistevennyi Inst., 19:216-226.

Bouwman, H. and W. Van der Schee, 1978. Composition and production of milk from Dutch warmblooded saddle horse mares. Z. Tierphysiol. Tierernähr. Futtermittelk., 40:39-53.

Cameron, E.Z., K.J. Stafford, W.L. Linklater and C.J. Veltman, 1999. Suckling behaviour does not measure milk intake in horses, Equus caballus. Anim. Behav., 57:673-678.

Caroprese, M., M. Albenzio, A. Santillo, R. Marino, S. Pelosi and F. D'Emilio, 2006. Behaviour and milk yield of Murgese mares subjected to machine or hand milking. This book.

Cherepanova, V.P. and V.T. Belokobylenko, 1974. Milk ejection characteristics in machine milking of mares. Proc 3rd all-union Symp. Physiol. Principles of machine milking, in Dairy Sci. Abstr., 37, 691.

Doreau, M., 1994. La lait de jument et sa production: particularités et facteurs de variation. Lait, 74:401-418.

Doreau, M. and G. Dussap, 1980. Estimation de la production laitière de la jument allaitante par marquage de l'eau corporelle du poulain. Reprod. Nutr. Dev., 20:1883-1892.

Doreau, M. and S. Boulot, 1989a. Recent knowledge on mare milk production: a review. Livest. Prod. Sci., 22: 213-235.

Doreau, M. and S. Boulot, 1989b. Methods of measurement of mare milk yield and composition in nursing mares: a review. Lait, 69: 159-171.

Doreau, M. and W. Martin-Rosset, 2002. Dairy Animals I. Horse. In: Encyclopedia of Dairy Sciences. Roginski H., Fuquay J.W. Fox P.F. Eds. Academic Press, London (GBR), 1, 630-637.

Doreau, M., S. Boulot, J.P. Barlet and P. Patureau-Mirand, 1990. Yield and composition of milk from lactating mares: effect of lactation stage and individual differences. J. Dairy Res., 57: 449-454.

Doreau, M., S. Boulot, D. Bauchart, J.P. Barlet and W. Martin-Rosset, 1992. Voluntary intake, milk production and plasma metabolites in nursing mares fed two different diets. J. Nutr., 122: 992-999.

Doreau, M., S. Boulot and Y. Chilliard, 1993. Yield and composition of milk from lactating mares: effect of body condition at foaling. J. Dairy Res., 60: 457-466.

Doreau, M., S. Boulot and W. Martin-Rosset, 1991. Effect of parity and physiological stage on intake, milk production and blood parameters in lactating mares differing in body size. Anim. Prod., 53:111-118.

Doreau, M., S. Boulot, W. Martin-Rosset and H. Dubroeucq, 1986. Milking lactating mares using oxytocin: milk volume and composition. Reprod. Nutr. Dev., 26: 1-11.

Doreau, M., W. Martin-Rosset and H. Dubroeucq, 1982. Production laitière de la jument. Liaison avec la croissance du poulain. Proc. 8th Journée d'Etude CEREOPA, Paris, France, 88-100.

Duncan, P. and J.C. Gleize, 1985. Nutrition and growth of horses in a mediterranean wetland, the Camargue. Proc. 36th Ann. Meet. EAAP, Thessaloniki, Greece, 11 pp.

Duncan, P., P.H. Harvey and S.M. Wells, 1984. On lactation and associated behaviour in a natural herd of horses. Anim. Behav., 32:255-263.

Ellendorff, F. and D. Schams, 1988. Characteristics of milk ejection, associated intramammary pressure changes and oxytocin release in the mare. J. Endocr., 119: 219-227

Faverdin, P., A. Hoden and J.B. Coulon, 1987. Recommandations alimentaires pour les vaches laitières. Bull. Tech. CRZV Theix, INRA, 70:133-152.

Fedotov, P.A. and B.R. Akimbekov, 1983. Increasing milk production of kushum mares (in Russian). Konevodstvo Konnyi Sport, 11, 6-7.

Gibbs, P.D., G.D. Potter, R.W. Blake and W.C. McMullan, 1982. Milk production of Quarter Horse mares during 150 days of lactation. J. Anim. Sci., 54:496-499.
Henneke, D.R., G.D. Potter and J.L. Kreider, 1981. Rebreeding efficiency of mares fed different levels of energy during late gestation; Proc. 7th Eq. Nutr. Phsiol. Symp., Virginia State Univ., USA, 101-104.
Kubiak, J.R., J.W. Evans, G.D. Potter and P.G. Harris, 1989. Milk production and composition in the multiparous mare fed to obesity. Proc. 11th Eq. Nutr. Physiol. Symp., Stillwater, Oklahoma, USA, 295-296.
Le Du, J., 1986. Mechanical milking of mares. Proc. 37th Ann. Meet. Europ. Assoc. Anim. Prod., Budapst, Hungary, 12 pp.
Le Neindre, P., M. Petit, R. Tomassone and C. Roux, 1976. Production laitière des vaches allaitantes et croissance de leurs veaux. Ann. Zootech., 25:533-542.
Martin, R.G., N.P. McMeniman and K.F. Dowsett, 1992. Milk and water intakes of foals sucking grazing mares. Equine Vet. J., 24:295-299.
Martin-Rosset, W. and M. Doreau, 1980. Effect of variations in the level of feeding of heavy mares during late pregnancy. Proc. 31st Ann. Meet. Europ. Assoc. Anim. Prod., München, Germany, 6 pp.
Martin-Rosset, W., M. Doreau and J. Cloix, 1978. Etude des activités d'un troupeau de poulinières de trait et de leurs poulains au pâturage. Ann. Zootech., 27:33-45.
Nordstrom, A., 1970. On the growth of young horses and on factors affecting the growth (in Finnish). MsSci Thesis, Univ. Helsinki.
Medvedev, V. and V. Yavorskii, 1984. Milk yield of draft-type mares. Konevodstvo Konnyi Sport, 11:11.
Neseni, R., E. Flade, G. Heidler and H. Steger, 1958. Milchleistung und Milchzusammensetzung von Stuten im Verlaufe der Laktation. Arch. Tierzucht., 1, 91-129.
Oftedal, O.T., H.F. Hintz and H.F. Schryver, 1983. Lactation in the horse: milk composition and intake by foals. J. Nutr., 113:2196-2206.
Pagan, J.D., H.F. Hintz and T.R. Rounsaville, 1984. The digestible energy requirements of lactating pony mares. J. Anim. Sci., 58:1382-1387.
Pinto, F., M. Faccia, A. Di Summa and G. Mastrangelo, 2001a. Mare's milk: early result concerning quality and quantity from Murgese and TPR mares. Riv. Ippiatria Ippologia, 7: 7-19.
Santos, A.S. and A.M. Silvestre, 2006. The lactation curve in Lusitano mares – a preliminary study. This book.
Santos, E.M., F.Q. de Almeida, A.A. Vieira, L.F.B. Pinto, A. Corassa, R.R. Moreira Pimentel, V. Pimentel Silva and L. Galzerano, 2005. Lactaçao em eguas da raça Mangalarga Marchador: produçao e composiçao do laite e ganho de peso dos potros lactentes. R. Bras. Zootec., 34: 627-634.
Sigler, D.H., D.E. Ericson, P.G. Gibbs, G.H. Kiracofe and J.S. Stevenson, 1989. Reproductive traits, lactation and foal growth in mares fed altrenogest. J. Anim. Sci., 67: 1154-1159.
Sutton, E.I., J.P. Bowland and W.D. Ratcliff, 1977. Influence of level of energy and nutrient intake by mares on reproductive performances and blood serum composition of the mares and foals. Can. J. Anim. Sci., 57:551-558.
Tarasevich, L.F., 1979. The relationship of milk production of White-Russian coach mares with udder shape and measurements; Sbornik Trudov. Belorusskii Nauchno-Issledovatel'skii Inst. Zhivotnovodtsva, 20:110-114, in Anim. Breed. Abstr., 1980, 48:512.
Trottier N., Stamper T., Moore J., Liesman J. and Nielsen B.D., 2006. A weigh-suckle-weigh approach for estimating milk yield in the Arabian mare. Proccedings 3rd EWEN Congress, Campobasso, June 20th – 22nd, EAAP Publication 120, Wageningen Academic Publishers, the Netherlands.
Wood, P.D.P., 1967. Algebraic models of the lactation curves for milk, fat and protein production, with estimates of seasonal variation. Anim. Prod., 22:35-40.

Mare milk composition: recent findings about protein fractions and mineral content

F. Martuzzi[1] *and M. Doreau*[2]
[1]*Dept. PABVQSA, Parma University, Via del Taglio 8, 43100 Parma, Italy*
[2]*INRA, Department of Animal Science, Research Center of Clermont-Ferrand/Theix, 63122 Saint Genès Champanelle, France*

Abstract

This review deals with the most recent studies about mare milk composition regarding protein and mineral content and some of their causes of variations. Mare milk is studied for two main purposes: human consumption and nutrition for foals. In particular the studies about milk proteins characterization are summarized. Other studies considered: differences and similarities between human and mare milk regarding main protein fractions, differences in colostrum and milk composition or in milk components trends during lactation in several horse breeds, effects of protein and mineral supplementation of the lactating mare on milk composition. The results of recent trials regarding the effects of mare milk use in the treatment of some health problems in adults are presented. A wide variability appears in milk protein quality, especially where whey protein concentrations are concerned. The considered studies regarding mineral elements in milk confirmed what observed in previous research: supplementing a lactating mare's diet with minerals will have scarce effect on the macro- and microelements levels in her milk.

Keywords: mare milk, protein, casein, whey proteins, minerals

Introduction

Aim of this review is to show the most recent advancements in mare milk composition research, regarding protein and mineral content and some of their causes of variation, considering mainly the studies conducted in the last five years.

The most recent studies regarding mare milk composition with respect to protein and mineral content deal with the following issues:

- Human nutrition:
  - as a substitute of cow milk for children with intolerance or allergy: identification and characterization of caseins and whey proteins;
  - as fermented milk (koumiss or airag): studies regarding production technologies and lactic acid bacteria involved in the fermentation process;
  - as "functional food" for several health problems.
- Foal nutrition:
  - feeding and the administration of mineral supplements of the lactating mare;
  - variations in the composition of precolostrum, colostrum and milk.

Protein fractions

Main components

In comparison to ruminant milk, equine milk has been less studied, and until few years ago the knowledge of the protein system of mare milk was limited: while whey proteins were well known, the study concerning casein regarded mainly the concentration variations, the main properties of the whole protein and its amino acid composition, rather than the characterization of the individual fractions, probably due to the major difficulties in the separation and identification of the casein components by means of conventional separative methods (Malacarne *et al.*, 2000).

Recently, several studies investigated the protein profile of mare milk to provide information on fractions of casein and whey proteins, because it could be interesting from the nutritional point of view and in particular to assess differences and similarities with human milk, to find a substitute for cow milk for children with cow milk intolerance or allergy. Studies on the allergenicity of mare milk in children suffering of an IgE-mediated cow milk allergy have shown that mare milk is much better tolerated (Businco *et al.*, 2000; Curadi *et al.*, 2001; Docena *et al.*, 2002; Katz, 2004; Muraro *et al.*, 2002). Docena *et al.* compared milk samples from mare, sheep and goat with immunoenzymatic methods and noticed after several *in vitro* tests that mare milk proved to be the least antigenic and allergenic substitute for people allergic to cow milk. However some remarks about the validity of the transposition of the *in vitro* test into the *in vivo* situation were made by Vandenplas and Hauser (2002).

Main nitrogen fractions in mare's milk could be so described: casein 50%, true whey protein 39%, non protein nitrogen 11% (Table 1).

Table 1. Main nitrogen fractions of mare milk (modified from Malacarne et al., 2002).

		Mare		Human		Cow	
Crude protein	g/kg	21.4	(15-28)	14.2	(9-17)	32.5	(31-38)
True wheyprotein	g/kg	8.3	(7.4-9.1)	7.6	(6.8-8.3)	5.7	(5.5-7.0)
Casein	g/kg	10.7	(9.4-12.0)	3.7	(3.2-4.2)	25.1	(24.6-28.0)
NPN x 6.38	g/kg	2.4	(1.7-3.5)	2.9	(2.6-3.2)	1.7	(1.0-1.9)
True wheyprotein	%	38.8		53.5		17.6	
Casein	%	50.0		26.1		77.2	
NPN x 6.38	%	11.2		20.4		5.2	

Mean value and, between brackets, minimum-maximum values reported in literature
References only for mare milk: Csapò-Kiss *et al.*, 1995; Doreau, 1994; Malacarne *et al.*, 2002; Mariani *et al.*, 1993; Martuzzi *et al.*, 2000; Pagliarini *et al.*, 1993.
References for human and cow milk: Doreau, 1994; Alais, 2000

Caseins

In mare's milk, casein represents about 50-65% of true protein. In the past, the proportion of casein in mare milk may have been underestimated, because most determinations have been made by precipitation at pH 4.6 as in cow's milk, whereas for mare's milk the maximum of casein precipitation is obtained at pH 4.2 (Egito *et al.*, 2002). The fractionation and characterization of the individual equine caseins appears to be more difficult than fractionation and characterization of casein from ruminants. The electrophoretic profiles of horse caseins show a great heterogeneity suggesting a high level of post translational modifications (Miranda *et al.*, 2004).

Evidence of the presence of α_{s1}-, α_{s2}-, and β- casein-like in mare's milk were provided between the years 1982 and 1999, while κ-casein was identified in 2001. Recently, physical mapping of equine α_{s1}-, β -and κ-casein genes was performed by fluorescent *in situ* hybridization (FISH) (Lenasi *et al.*, 2005).

α_{s1} – and α_{s2} caseins

From the evolutionary point of view, calcium sensitive caseins (α_{s1} -, α_{s2} -, and β - casein) originate from the same ancestral gene, consisting of four exons. The degree of evolutionary conservation of α_{s1} - and α_{s2} caseins is lower compared to that of β - and κ- casein. In mare's milk, α_{s1}casein is the least conserved when compared to α_{s1}casein from other species. The only highly conserved parts of this casein are signal peptide and sites which ensure sufficient supply of Ca and P to the newborn. Comparing the amino acid sequence of α_{s1} casein from mare's milk with the same casein from other species, the sequence identity is 54% between human and equine protein, the highest among the considered species (Table 2) (Lenasi *et al.*, 2003). The difference among species is probably due to different patterns of splicing from one species to another (Milenkovic *et al.*, 2002). A high polymorphism in equine αs casein was demonstrated since the nineteen-eighties (Doreau *et al.*, 2002). Fractionation and purification by anion-exchange chromatography and by reverse-phase HPLC showed evidence in the αs1casein of at least 7 electrophoretic bands (Egito *et al.*, 2002) which probably differ in their degrees of phosphorilation. The presence of α_{s2} casein was evidenced by urea PAGE but not sufficiently characterized, this probably due to its very low amount in equine milk (Egito *et al.*, 2002). In human milk this casein has not yet been identified.

Table 2. Pair-wise amino acid sequence alignment of α_{s1} -, β - and κ-casein. For each casein, equine amino acid sequence (left hand column) and human amino acid sequence (right hand column) are pair-wise compared with corresponding sequences in other species. Sequence identities are shown in percents (from Lenasi et al., 2003).

	α_{s1} – casein		β - casein		κ-casein	
	horse	human	horse	human	horse	human
horse	100	54	100	59	100	65
camel	46	43	53	60	67	58
pig	44	38	59	60	62	56
human	54	100	59	100	65	100
cow	42	34	55	54	57	52
sheep	40	31	55	56	60	51
goat	42	34	54	55	57	51

β - casein

The β- and κ- casein are responsible for micelle formation and strongly influence micelle size and curd firmness. This function requires conserved structure of the whole protein and represents, due to the importance of curd formation in the gut of suckling animals, permanent selection pressure conserving the structure of these caseins (Lenasi *et al.*, 2003). In mare's milk β- casein is the major casein component, similarly to human milk, and was the first casein fraction to be isolated in mare's milk (Visser *et al.*, 1982). Polymorphism of this casein was demonstrated in two studies, where the presence of 5 and 6 β- like-caseins was found (Visser *et al.*, 1982; Ochirkhuyag, *et al.*, 2000). These caseins differ one from the other not only in the number of phosphate groups but also in their content of some amino acid residues. Human milk also contains 6 β- like-caseins, which differ in their phosphorus content.

In equine milk there is a large quantity of γ- like caseins, probably due to a high plasmin activity on β- casein, whose amount decreases after the milk is stored. The plasmin activity seams to be about 5 times higher than that measured in bovine milk (Humbert *et al.*, 2005). This would explain the large quantity of γ-like caseins in equine milk; γ2- and γ3-casein-like, not phosphorylated, where detected by Visser *et al.* (1982) and Egito *et al.* (2002).

κ-casein and micelles size

κ-casein was the last to be identified: it was isolated by Miranda *et al.* in 2000 (Miranda *et al.*, 2004) by reverse phase HPLC and the terminal sequence was determined, then its primary structure was entirely determined by Iametti *et al.* in 2001. κ-casein is present in very small amounts in mare's milk, less than half of the κ-casein found in cow milk. It seems more glycolsylated than cow's κ-casein, while non-glycolsylated κ-casein was not detected in mare's milk. Thus, equine κ-casein has similarities to human κ-casein. This casein is mainly located at the surface of the casein micelle, which stabilises by electrostatic repulsion. From the evolutionary point of view, equine κ-casein proved to be the most conserved casein, closely followed by β-casein, in agreement with the physiologically important function of these caseins in micelle formation and with the role of κ-casein in milk coagulation (Lenasi *et al.*, 2003). The different amounts of κ-casein cause considerable differences in micelle size distribution: equine micelles have an average diameter of 255 nm, 1.5 times larger than cow milk micelles (182 nm), while human milk the micelles size are much smaller: the average size is 64 nm (Buchheim *et al,* 1989; Egito *et al.*, 2001) (Table 3).

Table 3. Caseins distribution of mare's milk in comparison to human and cow's milk (modified from Malacarne et al., 2002).

	Mare		Human		Cow	
Casein (g/kg)	10.7		3.7		25.1	
αs_1-casein (%)	46.65	(40.2-59.0)	11.75	(11.1-12.5)	38.46	(48.3-48.5)
αs_2-casein (%)					10.00	
β-casein (%)	45.64	(40.1-51.4)	64.75	(62.5-66.7)	35.77	(35.8-37.9)
k-casein (%)	7.71		23.50	(22.2-25.0)	12.69*	(12.7-13.9)
Micelles diameter (nm)	255		64		182	

* 100% reached with γ-casein fraction (3.08%).
Mean value and, between brackets, minimum–maximum values reported in literature.
Reference for micelles size: Buchheim *et al.*, 1989.
References for mare, human and cow: Ochirkhuyag *et al.*, 2000, Malacarne *et al.*, 2002.

Whey proteins

In mare's milk whey protein and casein contents are similar. Whey proteins include α–lactalbumin, β–lactoglobulin, serum albumin, immunoglobulins and also proteose-peptones, lysozyme, transferrin, lactoferrin and other lesser proteins. α-lactalbumin and β-lactoglobulin are the two main whey proteins, both of mammary origin, while serum albumin and immunoglobulins are of hematic origin. Available data regarding the amounts are very variable for the main whey proteins and also for the components of hematic origin, *e.g.* for serum albumin. Said variability may be due to the different methods utilised for the quantifications of fractions (Doreau and Boulot, 1989; Martuzzi *et al.*, 2000). The percentage distribution of whey proteins in mare's milk is reported in Table 4. β-lactoglobulin exists predominantly as a monomer in equine milk, whereas this protein is dimeric in milk of ruminants (Selo *et al.*, 1999; Fessas *et al.*, 2001). Two molecular forms of β-lactoglobulin have been distinguished in horse milk, and they have been named type I and II. The complete amino acid sequences of both proteins are known (Herrouin *et al.*, 2000). Three different kinds of α-lactalbumin,

Table 4. Whey proteins distribution of mare milk.

		Mare		Human		Cow	
True wheyprotein	g/kg	8.3		7.6		5.7	
β-Lactoglobulin	%	32.4	(25.3- 63.5)	Absent		53.6	(50-62)
α-Lactalbumin	%	28.6	(25.2-48.6)	42.4	(30.3-45.4)	20.1	(19-22)
Immunoglobulins	%	19.8	(4.3-21.0)	18.1	(15.1-19.7)	11.7	(11-12)
Serum albumin	%	4.4	(2.0-18.7)	7.5	(4.5-9.1)	6.2	(5-7)
Lactoferrin	%	8.2	(6.6-9.9)	30.3		8.4	
Lysozyme	%	6.6	(5.4-10.8)	1.7		Trace	

Proteose-peptone fraction was not reported in the considered references.
Mean value, and between brackets, minimum–maximum values reported in literature.
References common to human and cow: Malacarne *et al.*, 2002 and Solaroli *et al.*, 1993.
References only for mare: 13 references quoted in Summer *et al.*, 2003; Malacarne *et al.*, 2002, Martuzzi *et al.*, 2000; Summer *et al.*, 2005; Pagliarini *et al.*, 1993.

named A, B and C have been isolated in mare's milk. Comparison of the sequence of B and C with that of A indicates 3 and 4 amino acids exchanges, respectively. The primary structures of equine α-lactalbumin B and C have been determined (Godovac-Zimmermann, *et al.*, 1987).

Comparing the SDS-PAGE patterns obtained for equine and human milks, the main features of mare's milk are the presence of two β-lactoglobulins (type I and II) and of lysozyme at a sufficiently high level to be visualized, as it is in human milk, while β-lactoglobulin is apparently lacking in human milk, where, in contrast, lactoferrin is present in high levels (Miranda *et al.*, 2004). The primary structure of equine lysozyme has been determined and has been reported as occurring in at least two forms by electrophoresis, but these do not appear to be genetic variants (Bell *et al.*, 1980-81 cited by Herrouin *et al.*, 2000). The elevated content of lysozyme and lactoferrin compared to cow milk could be involved in the beneficial aspects observed in mare milk consumption. As in human milk, antimicrobial defence in mare milk is mainly due to lysozyme, and its activity is highly thermo-stable (Di Cagno *et al.*, 2004).

Since in human milk β-lactoglobulin is absent, this protein is one of the major allergens in children who are allergic to cow's milk (while in adults the predominant allergen is considered to be casein) (Carroccio *et al.*, 1999). Some cases have been reported of IgE-mediated allergy caused by low molecular weight heat-labile proteins, most likely α-lactalbumin and β-lactoglobulin, when mare's milk was used for human nutrition in adults (Gall *et al.*, 1996; Fanta and Ebner, 1998).

Mare's milk for human nutrition and health

For centuries, mare's milk has been one of the most important food for the nomadic populations of central Asia and former Soviet Union, where it is used mainly for the manufacture of a lactic-alcoholic beverage, named koumiss, chigee or airag in Mongolia. Fermentation takes place with the contribution of a mixed indigenous microbial population mainly consisting of various species of *Lactobacillus* and *Saccharomyces* (Di Cagno *et al.*, 2004). About the particular healing properties attributed since centuries to koumiss, probably some merits are to be ascribed to the lactic acid bacteria involved in its fermentation. This bacteria can play a role in improving intestinal microflora and preserving the homeostasis of human health and are therefore considered probiotics in human nutrition. Some recent studies deal with the classification of lactic acid bacteria isolated from fermented mare's milk collected in Mongolia (An *et al.*, 2004).

At present, koumiss is manufactured also at an industrial level in the countries where its use is traditional. There has been an increasing interest in the consumption of mare's milk in the western countries as well, in particular in Germany, where mare's milk production and commerce for human use is now regulated by law (Schüppel and Kny, 2001). Quality control of milk from species other than the cow is not yet a reality in many countries, but some parameters are starting to be considered for mare's milk, like antimicrobial residues (Barbosa *et al.*, 2004). In Germany, the high cost of mare's milk seems a limiting major factor for its use. Some recent studies deal with milk conservation (Liu *et al.*, 2005) or with production technique of fermented mare's milk in western countries (Kücükcetin *et al.*, 2003; Di Cagno *et al.*, 2004).

The benefits of mare's milk for human health, documented not always rigorously in the abundant literature from the former URSS, have been summarized by Lozovich (1995), while the characteristics of mare's milk that may play a role in these supposed healing properties were described by Doreau *et al.* (2002). At present the use of mare's milk regards mainly the treatment of gastrointestinal ulcers and chronic hepatitis, while in the past also tuberculosis was treated. Mare's milk possible healing properties are the object of some recent trials in the western world as well, regarding the treatment of skin diseases or inflammatory processes: at the University of Jena (Germany) it was documented in a controlled study that consumption of mare's milk can improve the skin condition of patients with neurodermatitis. In one-third of the patients drinking mare's milk, the severity of the condition improved by 30%, while the control group, which drank "other milk", not specified, showed no improvement. The effectiveness of the treatment was comparable to that of medication (Kaatz, cited by Anonymus, 2005). In another study on 18 healthy volunteers, the results suggest that drinking deep frozen mare's milk modulates inflammation processes by decreasing chemotaxis and respiratory burst, which might be favourable for giving relief to diseases with recurrent inflammation, while immunostimulating effects accredited to mare's milk consumption could not be observed in healthy volunteers, at least concerning phagocytosis (Ellinger *et al.*, 2002).

Causes of variations in milk composition regarding protein and minerals

Effect of lactation stage

The main variations in milk protein are due to the stage of lactation and have been extensively studied (Doreau and Boulot, 1989; Doreau, 1994; Summer *et al.*, 2000; Martuzzi *et al.*, 2004) and are quite well known, even if not many studies took into account six months of lactation. Considering the whole lactation period has scarce significance for foal nutrition, but could be of some interest if an industrial exploitation of mare's milk is expected. Protein content decreases rapidly in the first 2 months of lactation, then the decrease is less accentuated: in a study regarding Haflinger mares, protein in milk was 3.3 g/100g of milk at day 4, then 1.8g at day 40 and 1.6 at day 180. Crude protein content was about 50% lower at the 6th lactation month (Mariani *et al.*, 2001). Casein decreases of about 48% at the 5th month. In studies regarding Haflinger mares' milk, from day 4 to day 180 of lactation, casein nitrogen decreased by 54% and true whey protein nitrogen by 40%. These values are in agreement with most Authors (Summer *et al.*, 2003). Casein number (casein nitrogen x 100/total nitrogen) represents an index of the protein profile of the milk. According to most Authors (cited by Formaggioni *et al.*, 2003), excluding colostrum and the short transition phase, lactation stage shouldn't have a significant effect on casein number trend, its values ranging around 67%. In a study on milk of Haflinger and Italian Saddle mares regarding a lactation period of 5 months, a decrease of 5 percent was observed for casein number at the end of lactation (Formaggioni *et al.*, 2003).

With regard to mineral content in milk, the highest ash concentration is observed during the 1st week of lactation (Grace *et al.*, 1999; Schryver *et al.*, 1986; Summer *et al.*, 2004) afterwards, the total ash regularly decreases, due to a decrease of all minerals: the ash content in the later stages of lactation is about 39% lower than that of the earlier stages: 0.5 g/100g of milk in the 1st lactation month *versus* 0.3 in the 8th month in Haflinger and Italian Saddle mares milk (Martuzzi *et al.*, 2002; 2004). Similar variations were observed by Summer *et al.* (2004) in an extensive study regarding the trends of mineral during 6 lactation months in Haflinger mares milk. Models are proposed to describe the trends of macro-mineral levels: in global lactation the trends are curvilinear, well defined by cubic equations, while in early lactation are linear for calcium, and curvilinear for ash and phosphorus (quadratic equations) and for magnesium, potassium, sodium and chloride (cubic equations).

Another study was designed to model the variations of nine mineral element concentrations in the mammary secretions of Arabian mares *pre*-and *post partum*, using a non-linear spline regression to model time-varying fluctuations (Lloyd *et al.*, 2000).

Effect of mare's diet on milk protein

Recently, very few experiments have been carried out in this area. The main effects have been summarized by Doreau and Boulot (1989) and Doreau (1994): according to studies presented in the reviews, protein content in milk decreases when the energy supply of the diet increases above requirements. By increasing the level of energy fed, it appears that the amount of milk produced by a mare can be increased, but apparently there is a dilution effect on nitrogen components, as demonstrated in women, and contrary to results in cows (Doreau *et al.*, 1992). An increase in energy supply and/or proportion of concentrate in the diet can decrease protein content by 4g/L. A protein supplementation in the diet has inconsistent effects: it may result in no change in milk protein content, but in an experiment a supplement of protein in the concentrate in a hay-based diet increased milk protein content from 17 to 22 g/kg. This inconsistency between trials could be due to a low protein content of the control diet, which inhibited an optimal protein secretion in milk (Doreau *et al.*, 1988). In a study conducted by Martin *et al.* (1993) administering 2 kg of high protein pellets (24% crude protein) everyday to grazing mares had no effect on their milk composition.

Protein concentration in milk from mares fed hays with different crude protein levels was studied in an experiment. Two groups of Quarter horse mares were fed Matua bromegrass hay (*Bromus willdenowii* Kunth) with 11.5% crude protein, and alfalfa hay (*Medicago sativa* L.) with 15.4% crude protein, both as the roughage portion of the diet with a grain supplement, starting one month before parturition up to the 70th lactation day. On day one of lactation, colostrum from mares fed alfalfa contained significantly less crude protein than colostrum from mares fed Matua hay, but until the 70th day of lactation, no significant differences in milk protein content and rate of decline during lactation between treatments were observed anymore (Guay *et al.*, 2002).

Australian Authors, studying Thoroughbred mares, reported that the quality of protein in the diet can affect the protein content in the mare's milk. An increase in milk protein occurs when higher quality soybean protein constitutes 50% of the protein intake, with a corresponding increase in the growth rate of suckling foals. It has been shown that mares grazing mature grass based pasture may receive adequate energy, but may be marginally protein deficient, in particular with reference to the amino acid threonine, to satisfy the needs of heavy lactation (McMeniman, 1996; Kohnke, 2000).

Effect of mineral supplementation on mare milk

Some recent researches studied the effects on milk of mineral supplements given to lactating mares. Thoroughbred and Quarter Horse late gestating and lactating mares were supplemented with trace minerals at levels higher than those indicated by NRC (1989) (Kavazis *et al.*, 2002). The results are in agreement with previously published results, which indicated that the concentration of Cu, Zn and Fe in mare milk could not be elevated by providing higher dietary levels of trace minerals during late gestation and lactation (Csapó-Kiss *et al.*, 1995). Grace *et al.* studied the concentrations of macro-and micro-elements in the milk of pasture-fed Thoroughbred mares. The study confirmed in particular that mare milk is low in Fe, and research has indicated that the level couldn't be increased by feeding higher concentrations of Fe to the lactating mares (Grace *et al.*, 1999).

Lang *et al.* studied the effects of silicon supplement on Arabian mares. The mares received 44.29 g/d of Si in supplemental diet. Results indicated that supplemental Si increases the concentration of this element in milk (Lang *et al.*, 2001). Currently, Si recommendations for horses are not included in the 1989 NRC guidelines, but neither it has been demonstrated that Si is of nutritional value.

Differences between breeds

Some differences between breeds concerning mare's milk composition have been reported in studies made mainly in eastern Europe, where dairy mares breeding is a tradition (see review of Doreau and Boulot, 1989). However, knowledge regarding this aspect is quite limited. Generally, it is difficult to differentiate the effect of a certain feeding regimen or herd conditions from that of the breed. Moreover, a large individual variability complicates the assessment of a breed effect. Therefore, differences in milk composition due to the breed appear only incidentally in some studies. In the following experiments, unless otherwise specified, the compared mares received the same diet, in some cases with slight differences in quantity to suit different body weights.

Protein in general

In a study conducted on Murgese and Italian Heavy Draft (T.P.R.) breeds considering the variations during a whole lactation, the average percentage values of all nitrogen fractions were higher in the milk of Murgese mares compared to T.P.R. mares: *e.g.* crude protein at 30d was 2.30 in Murgese milk versus 1.90 in the T.P.R. mares, casein nitrogen was 0.17 in Murgese and 0.12 in T.P.R. (Pinto *et al.*, 2001). These findings appear in contrast with the results of Neseni *et al.* (1958) who found higher protein values in heavy mares' colostrum and lesser protein values in lighter mares, but other factors than breed could have interfered.

Curadi *et al.* (2000) studied protein concentration in colostrum by means of different separative procedures based on electrophoretic and immunochemical principles in milk of Haflinger, Thoroughbred and Anglo-Arab mares. Differences among breeds were found both in the protein content and its trend: the highest protein concentration at foaling was recorded in the colostrum of Haflinger mares (154 g/L) while the lowest was in Thoroughbred colostrum (134.6 g/L). The variation of protein level within the first 12 h after parturition was similar for Thoroughbred and Anglo-Arab mares, whereas in the colostrum of Haflinger mares the drop in protein content was very marked already 6 h after foaling. However, no indication was given regarding the diets of the different breeds, except that the requirements were satisfied.

Casein

In a study comparing Haflinger and Italian Saddle mares, during a lactation period of 5 months, significant differences were found regarding total nitrogen (mg/100g of milk), casein nitrogen (mg/100g of milk), and casein number (CNx100/TN): all values were higher in the milk from Italian Saddle mares, from the 15th to the 90th day in milk: *e.g.* for casein N: 140 mg/100g in Haflinger milk versus 188 mg/100g in Italian Saddle milk (Formaggioni *et al.*, 2003).

Whey proteins

Regarding the identification of whey proteins: in a study α-lactalbumin was isolated from the colostrum of a mare of Arab-Persano breed and during the determination of the amino-acid sequence it appeared that it consisted of two components and that both differed in sequence from that isolated from samples of milk from Thoroughbred horses in Australia. The two α-lactalbumins from the Italian mare were designated as α-lactalbumin B/C and that from the Australian milk as α-lactalbumin A (Godovac-Zimmermann *et al.*, 1987).

In a study regarding pony mare's milk using proteomic tools, the protein identified as pony α-lactalbumin produced the same score as donkey and horse α-lactalbumins. On the other hand, β-lactoglobulin II was identified through the tryptic peptide fingerprint as matching with the donkey protein rather than with its horse counterpart. This result suggests that pony β-lactoglobulin II is structurally more closely related to the donkey protein than to that of the horse (Miranda *et al.*, 2004).

As for quantitative analysis of whey fractions, obtained comparing capillary electrophoresis and Kjeldahl methods, in a study conducted by Civardi *et al.* milks from Haflinger, Norico, Arabian, and Trotter mares were compared. Differences were found between the milks: Norico milk showed significant quantitative differences compared to the other milks, in particular lower α-lactalbumin, higher lysozyme and β-lactoglobulin content (Civardi *et al.*, 2002). No indication regarding diet was given in this study.

The average lysozyme content during a whole lactation, in another study conducted on Murgese and T.P.R. breeds, resulted higher in the Murgese breed: 0.52 g/L *versus* 0.50 g/L in T.P.R. milk. (Faccia *et al.*, 2001).

Ash content and minerals

In a study regarding Italian Saddle and Haflinger mares during the first 6 months of lactation, ash content was always significantly higher in the milk of Italian Saddle mares: in the first lactation month 0.55 g/100g of milk in Italian Saddle *versus* 0.45 g/100g in Haflinger mares (Martuzzi *et al.*, 2004).

Conclusions

Many of the most recent studies about mare's milk are aimed to the characterization of its protein fractions. This issue could seem more interesting for researchers involved in mare's milk use in human allergology, or in general in a comparison between human and dairy species milks, than for horse nutritionists or breeders. Studies on mare milk protein variations might provide useful information when the objective is an industrial exploitation of this milk, and might give some indication for the choice of the breed to use, or which is the best period of the lactation to obtain milk with desired characteristics. If the use of mare milk in human nutrition will spread in western Europe, there could be a new employment possibility for ancient work horse breeds, traditionally bred in disadvantaged areas. Some differences among breeds in milk composition regarding protein and minerals have been found, but clear breed effects remain to be assessed by more experiments on a larger number of animals.

Considering the aspect of foal nutrition, a wide variability appears in milk protein quality, in particular concerning whey protein concentrations. Due to the important biological and functional properties of these specific proteins, a very low concentration of these compounds could arouse a certain degree of worry. Further studies could be carried out to investigate the causes of variation of these proteins and to deepen the knowledge about their influence on metabolic processes.

Experiments carried out recently regarding the influence of diet on milk of nursing mares are really scarce: few advancements appear in the knowledge of the effect of different concentrates or hays on milk.

The considered studies regarding mineral elements in milk confirmed the concentration trends during lactation observed in previous studies. Supplementing gestating or lactating mares with minerals, with the aim to increase the concentrations of macro- and microelements in milk, appears of scarce utility.

Acknowledgement

A special thank to Massimo Malacarne for his precious suggestions.

References

Alais, C., 2000. Scienza del latte. 3rd ed. Ed. Tecniche nuove, 239 pp.

An, Y., Y. Adachi and Y. Ogawa, 2004. Classification of lactic acid bacteria isolated from chigee and mare milk collected in Inner Mongolia. Animal Sci. J., 75: 245-252.

Anonymous, 2005. Success with mare's milk against neurodermatitis. Deutsche Ärztezeitung, 7.12.2005.

Barbosa, M., G. Suhren and R. Beukers, 2004. Suitability and application of available test kits for the detection of residues of antimicrobials in milk from species other than the cow – a review. Bull. of the Intern. Dairy Federation, 390: 30-40.

Buchheim, Von W., S. Lund and J. Scholtissek, 1989. Vergleichende Untersuchungen zur Struktur und Größe von Caseinmicellen in der Milch verschiedener Species. Kieler Milchwirtschaftliche Forschungsberichte, 41: 253-265.

Businco, L., P.G. Giampietro, P. Lucenti, F. Lucaroni, C. Pini, G. Di Felice, P. Iacovacci, C. Curadi and M. Orlandi, 2000. Allergenicity of mare's milk in children with cow's milk allergy. J. Allergy Cli. Immunol., 105, 5: 1031-1034.

Carroccio, A., F. Cavataio and G. Iacono, 1999. Cross-reactivity between milk proteins of different animals. Clinical and Experimental Allergy, 29: 1014-1016.

Civardi, G., M.C. Curadi, M. Orlandi, T.M.P. Cattaneo and R. Giangiacomo, 2002. Capillary electrophoresis (CE) applied to analysis of mare's milk. Milchwissenschaft, 57, 9/10: 515-517.

Csapó-Kiss, Zs., J. Stefler, T.G. Martin, S. Makray and J. Csapó, 1995. Composition of mares' colostrum and milk. Protein content, amino acid composition and contents of macro-and micro-elements. Int. Dairy Journal, 5: 403-415.

Curadi, M.C., P.G. Giampietro, P. Lucenti and M. Orlandi, 2001. Use of mare milk in pediatric allergology. Proc. A.S.P.A. XIV Congress, 647-649.

Curadi, M.C., M. Orlandi, G.F. Greppi, P.M. Toppino, S. Barzaghi and T.M.P. Cattaneo, 2000. Identification of protein fractions in mare's colostrum and milk. Milchwissenschaft, 55, 8: 446-449.

Di Cagno, R., A. Tamborrino, G. Gallo, C. Leone, M. de Angelis, M. Faccia, P. Amirante and M. Gobbetti, 2004. Uses of mare's milk in manufacture of fermented milks. Int. Dairy J., 14: 767-775.

Docena, G., P. Rozenfeld, R. Fernández and C.A. Fossati, 2002. Evaluation of the residual antigenicity and allergenitics of cow's milk substitutes by in vitro tests. Allergy, 57: 83-91.

Doreau, M., 1994. Le lait de jument et sa production: particularités et facteurs de variation. Lait, 74: 401- 418.

Doreau, M. and S. Boulot, 1989. Recent knowledge on mare milk production: a review. Livest. Prod. Sci., 22: 213-235.

Doreau, M., S. Boulot, D. Bauchart, J.P. Barlet and W. Martin-Rosset, 1992. Voluntary intake, milk production and plasma metabolite in nursing mares fed two different diets. J. Nutr., 122: 992-999.

Doreau, M., J.P. Bruhat and W. Martin-Rosset, 1988. Effet du niveau des apports azotes chez la jument en début de lactation. Ann. Zootech., 37: 21-30.

Doreau, M., J.L. Gaillard, J.M. Chobert, J. Léonil, A.S. Egito and T. Haertlé, 2002. Composition of mare and donkey milk fatty acids and proteins and consequences on milk utilisation. Proc. 4th Meeting New findings in equine practice, 51-71.

Egito, A.S., L. Miclo, C. López, A. Adam, J.-M. Girardet and J.-L. Gaillard, 2002. Separation and characterization of mare's milk α_{s1} -, β-, κ-caseins, γ-casein-like, and proteose peptone component 5-like peptides. J. Dairy Sci., 85: 697-706.

Egito, A.S., J.-M. Girardet, L. Miclo, D. Mollè, G. Humbert and J.-L. Gaillard, 2001. Susceptibility of equine κ- and β- caseins to hydrolysis by chymosin. Int. Dairy J., 11, 11-12: 885-893.

Ellinger, S., K.P. Linscheid, S. Jahnecke, R. Goerlich and H. Enbergs, 2002. The effect of mare's milk consumption on functional elements of phagocytosis of human neutrophil granulocytes from healthy volunteers. (abstract) Food and Agricultural Immunology, 14, 3: 191-200.

Fanta, E. and C. Ebner, 1998. Allergy to mare's milk. Allergy, 53: 539-540.

Faccia, M., F. Pinto, M. Veronico and V.A. Liuzzi, 2001. Lisozyme in milk of Murgese and Italian Heavy T.P.R. mares and of Martina Franca donkey. Proc. 3° Convegno "Nuove acquisizioni in materia di alimentazione, allevamento e allenamento del cavallo", 149-154.

Fessas, D., S. Iametti, A. Schiraldi and F. Bonomi, 2001. Thermal unfolding of monomeric and dimeric β-lactoglobulins. Eur. J. Biochem., 268: 5439-5448.

Formaggioni, P., M. Malacarne, F. Martuzzi, A. Summer and P. Mariani, 2003. Casein number variability of mare milk from Haflinger and Italian Saddle Horse breeds. Proc. of the A.S.P.A. XV Congress: 601-603.

Gall, H., C.M. Kalveram, H. Sick and W. Sterry, 1996. Allergy to the heat-labile proteins α-lactalbumin and β-lactoglobulin in mare's milk. J. Allergy Clin. Immunol. 97, 6: 1304-1307.

Godovac-Zimmermann, J., D. Shaw, A. Conti and H. McKenzie, 1987. Identification and the primary structure of equine α-lactalbumin B and C. Equus caballus, Perissodactyla. Biol. Chem. Hoppe-Seyler, 368: 427-433.

Guay, K.A., H.A. Brady, V.G. Allen, K.R. Pond, D.B. Wester, L.A. Janecka and N.L. Heninger, 2002. Matua bromegrass hay for mares in gestation and lactation. J. Anim. Sci., 80: 2960-2966.

Herrouin, M., D. Mollé, J. Fauquant, F. Ballestra, J.L. Maubois and J. Léonil, 2000. New genetic variants identified in donkey's milk whey proteins. J. of Protein Chemistry, 19, 2: 105-115.

Iametti, S., G. Tedeschi, E. Oungre and F. Bonomi, 2001. Primary structure of κ-casein isolated from mare's milk. J. of Dairy Research, 68: 53-61.

Katz, Y. and G. Zadik-Mnuchin, 2004. Individuals with cow's milk allergy are sensitized to milk from deer and ibex but not to milk from pork. Is there a kosher epitope? J. Allergy Clin. Immunol., 113, 2, suppl.1: S156.

Kavazis, A.N., J. Kivipelto and E.A. Ott, 2002. Supplementation of brood mare with copper, zinc, iron, manganese, cobalt, iodine and selenium. J. of Equine Veterinary Science, 22, 10: 460-464.

Kohnke, John, 2000. Poor Feed - Poor Fertility. Review presented at the 2nd Asian Thoroughbred Breeders Conference May 27-30th 2000, Gold Coast, Queensland.

Kücükcetin, A., H. Yaygin, J. Hinrichs and U. Kulozik, 2003. Adaptation of bovine milk towards mare's milk composition by means of membrane technology for koumiss manufacture. Int. Dairy J., 13: 945-951.

Lang, K.J., B.D. Nielse, K.L. Waite, G.M. Hill and M.W. Orth, 2001. Supplemental silicon increases plasma and milk silicon concentrations in horses. J. Animal Sci., 79: 2627-2633.

Lenasi, T., N. Kokalj-Vokac, M. Narat, A. Baldi and P. Dovc, 2005. Functional study of the equine β-casein and κ-casein gene promoters. J. of Dairy Research, 72: 34-43.

Lenasi, T., I. Rogelj and P. Dovc, 2003. Characterization of equine cDNA sequences for α_{s1}-, β- and κ-casein. Journal of Dairy Research, 70: 29-36.

Lloyd, J.W., J.S. Rook, E. Braselton and M.E. Shea, 2000. Use of a non-linear spline regression to model time-varying fluctuations in mammary secretion element concentrations of periparturient mares in Michigan, USA. Preventive Veterinary Medicine, 43: 211-222.

Liu, H.Y., K. Gao and Y.H. Xue, 2005. Development on keeping mare's milk for a longer time. (English abstract) China Dairy Industry, 33, 7: 13-17.

Lozovich, S., 1995. Medical uses of whole and fermented mare milk in Russia. Cultured Dairy Products Journal, 30: 18-21.

Malacarne, M., F. Martuzzi, A. Summer and P. Mariani, 2002. Nitrogen fractions and fat composition of mare milk: some nutritional remarks with reference to woman and cow milk. Int. Dairy Journal, 12, 11: 869-877.

Malacarne, M., A. Summer, P. Formaggioni and P. Mariani, 2000. Observations on percentage distribution of the main mare milk caseins separated by reversed-phase HPLC. Annali Fac. Medicina Veterinaria Parma, XX: 143-152.

Mariani, P., F. Martuzzi and A.L. Catalano, 1993. Composizione e proprietà fisico-chimiche del latte di cavalla: variazione dei costituenti azotati e minerali nel corso della lattazione. Annali Fac. Medicina Veterinaria Parma, XIII: 43-58.

Mariani P., A. Summer, F. Martuzzi, P. Formaggioni, A. Sabbioni and A.L. Catalano, 2001. Physicochemical properties, gross composition, energy value and nitrogen fractions of Haflinger nursing mare milk throughout 6 lactation months. Animal Research, 50: 415-425.

Martuzzi, F., A. Summer, P. Formaggioni and P. Mariani, 2002. Mare milk at drying-off: chimico-physical characteristics, nitrogen composition and mineral elements in Italian Saddle and Haflinger nursing mares. Proc. 53rd Annual Meeting of EAAP, Cairo, 6 pp.

Martin, R.G., N. McMeniman and K.F. Dowsett, 1992. Milk and water intakes of foals sucking grazing mares. Equine Vet. Journal, 24, 4: 295-299.

Martuzzi, F., A. Summer, P. Formaggioni and P. Mariani, 2004. Milk of Italian Saddle and Haflinger nursing mares: physico-chemical characteristics, nitrogen composition and mineral elements at the end of lactation. Italian Journal of Animal Science, 3: 293-299.

Martuzzi, F., A. Tirelli, A. Summer, A.L. Catalano and P. Mariani, 2000. Ripartizione delle sieroproteine nel latte dei primi due mesi di lattazione in giumente Sella Italiano. Rivista di Ippiatria e Ippologia. VI, 1: 21-27.

McMeniman, N., 1996. Nutrition of grazing broodmares and growing horses. Aust. Vet. Journal 74: 64-70.

Milenkovic, D., P. Martin, G. Guérin and C. Leroux, 2002. A specific pattern of splicing for the horse α_{s1}-casein mRNA and partial genomic characterization of the relevant locus. Genet. Sel. Evol., 34: 509-519.

Miranda, G., M.F. Mahé, C. Leroux and P. Martin, 2004. Proteomic tools to characterize the protein fraction of Equidae milk. Proteomics, 4: 2496-2509.

Muraro, M.A., P.G. Giampietro and E. Galli, 2002. Soy formulas and nonbovine milk. Ann. Allergy Asthma Immunol., 89, suppl.: 97-101.

NRC, 1989. Nutrient requirements of horses. 5th ed., National Academic Press, Washington D.C.

Ochirkhuyag, B., J.M. Chobert, M. Dalgalarrondo and T. Haertlé, 2000. Characterization of mare caseins. Identification of α_{s1} and α_{s2} caseins. Lait, 80: 223-235.

Pagliarini, E., G. Solaroli and C. Peri, 1993. Chemical and physical characteristics of mare's milk. Ital. J. Food Sci., 4: 323-332.

Pinto, F., M. Faccia, A. Di Summa and G. Mastrangelo, 2001. Mare's milk: early results concerning quality and quantity from Murgese and TPR mares. Rivista di Ippiatria e Ippologia, 7, 2: 7-19.

Schryver, H.F., O. T., Oftedal, J. Williams, L.V. Soderholm and H.F. Hintz, 1986. Lactation in the horse: the mineral composition of mare milk. Journal of Nutrition, 116: 2142-2147.

Sélo, G., H. Clément, J.-M. Bernard, C. Chatel, C. Créminon and G. Peltre, 1999. Allergy to bovine β-lactoglobulin: specificity of human IgE to tryptic peptides. Clinical and Experimental Allergy, 29: 1055-1063.

Schüppel, H and G. Kny, 2001. Food legal aspects with regard to marketing of mare milk. (in German) Tierärztl Prax, 29: 108-113.

Solaroli, G., E. Pagliarini and C. Peri, 1993. Composition and nutritional quality of mare's milk. Ital. J. Food Sci., 1: 3-10.

Summer, A., A. Sabbioni, P. Formaggioni and P. Mariani, 2004. Trend in ash and mineral element content of milk from Haflinger nursing mares throughout six lactation months. Livestock Production Sci., 88: 55-62.

Summer, A., A. Tirelli, P. Formaggioni, M. Malacarne and P. Mariani, 2005. Mare milk nitrogen fractions during lactation and determination by reversed-phase HPLC of the major whey proteins. Canadian J. of Animal Science, 85: 93-99.

Summer, A., A. Tirelli, P. Formaggioni, F. Martuzzi and P. Mariani, 2003. Variation of mare milk nitrogen fractions distribution of the main whey proteins in relation to lactation stage. Proc. 54th Annual Meeting EAAP, 8 pp.

Vandenplas, Y. and B. Hauser, 2002. Has in vitro allergenicity testing any clinical relevance? Allergy, 57: 73-75.

Visser, S., R. Jenness and R. J. Mullin,1982. Isolation and characterization of β- and γ-caseins from horse milk. Biochemical Journal, 203: 131-139.

Fat content and composition of mare's milk

M. Doreau[1] *and F. Martuzzi*[2]
[1]*INRA, Department of Animal Science, Research Center of Clermont-Ferrand/Theix, 63122 Saint Genès Champanelle, France*
[2]*Dept. PABVQSA, Parma University, Via del Taglio 8, 43100 Parma, Italy*

Abstract

This review summarises knowledge on fat and fatty acid composition in mare milk. The fat content is very low in mare milk, generally comprised between 10 and 20 g/kg, but can sometimes be lower than 5 g/kg, with diets rich in concentrates. Milk fat strongly decreases during the first 2 - 3 months of lactation then remains stable or slightly decreases. Fat composition is characterised by a high content in polyunsaturated fatty acids: linoleic and α-linolenic acid. The proportion of this latter fatty acid, known for a positive effect on human health, is very variable but can reach 25% especially when mares are on pasture. No other fatty acids beneficial to human health, as conjugated linoleic acid, are found in significant amounts.

Keywords: mare, milk, fatty acids, linolenic acid, lactation

Introduction

Mare milk is known as especially poor in fat. According to Jenness (1974) who summarised data on milk fat content in a very large number of mammals, the only species of which milk is poorer in fat than horse is white rhinoceros. Besides that, it can be supposed that good conditions of sampling, i.e. complete milking, was not obtained in a bad-tempered species as rhinoceros. In mares, most data range between 10 and 20 g/kg (reviews by Doreau and Boulot, 1989b and Martuzzi *et al.*, 2001), compared to 35-40 g/kg in cow and human milk. The objective of this article is to provide the main features of mare milk fat, in comparison with cow and human milk, and to analyse the main factors of variation of mare milk fat content and milk fatty acid composition, especially stage of lactation and feeding, in the light of the mechanisms of synthesis and of general knowledge on milk fat secretion in mammals.

Milk fat synthesis

In horses as in other mammals, milk fat has a double origin: circulating fatty acids (FA), transported in lipoproteins, and FA synthesised in the udder. Circulating FA mainly come from dietary 16- and 18-carbon FA which, in horses as in other species, are absorbed in the small intestine. As in other monogastric species, they are not metabolised before absorption, contrary to ruminants, in which FA are transformed prior to absorption by isomerisation and hydrogenation, and to a low extent synthesised, in the rumen. In the large intestine, FA metabolism occurs due to bacterial activity. In ruminants it has been shown that large intestine is not a site of FA absorption (Doreau and Ferlay, 1994). In the absence of experimental data, the same hypothesis can be formulated for horses. As a consequence, in horse milk long-chain FA composition is close to dietary FA composition.

De novo mammary synthesis arises from glucose in most monogastric species. On the contrary, in ruminants it arises from two of the three main volatile fatty acids: acetate and butyrate, this latter being transformed in β-hydroxybutyrate in the rumen wall. The amount of glucose absorbed in ruminants is very low in most dietary conditions. In horses, acetate and butyrate are produced in the large intestine from forage carbohydrates, and butyrate is converted in β-hydroxybutyrate mainly in the liver. As in ruminants, FA are synthesised in mare udder from acetate and β-hydroxybutyrate (Linzell *et al.*, 1972). Glucose is absorbed in the small intestine of horse with diets rich in concentrates, but glucose does not contribute to *de novo* FA synthesis. This could be due to the inhibition by acetate of ATP-citrate lyase, an enzyme which is involved in FA synthesis from glucose.

The main difference in the mechanisms of *de novo* synthesis between ruminants and horses is that in ruminants *de novo* synthesis accounts for 4- to 14-carbon FA, and about half of 16-carbon FA, whereas in horses *de novo* synthesis results in addition in a part of 18-carbon FA (Linzell *et al.*, 1972).

Mare milk fat globule and lipid classes

In mare, milk fat is organised in globules of 2-3 μm diameter (Kharitonova, 1978, Welsch *et al.*, 1988), i.e. a lower size than in cow and humans (3-3.5 μm). The structure of mare milk fat globule membrane, composed of three layers, and its composition are close to that of human milk and differs from that of ruminants. Horse and human milk fat globule membrane have in common a filamentous glycocalyx with high molecular weight glycoproteins (Welsch *et al.*, 1988).

The main specificity of mare milk lipid classes compared to cow or human milk is the lower proportion of triglycerides (around 80%), compensated for by a high percentage of free fatty acids (9 – 10%) and of phospholipids (5 – 19%) (Kharitonova, 1978; Pastukhova and Gerbeda, 1982). According to this former author, phospholipids are made of sphingomyelin (34%), phosphatidylethanolamine (31%), phosphatidylcholine (19%) and phosphatidylserine (16%) but not phosphatidylinositol. The high proportion of free fatty acids may explain that Forsyth *et al.* (1975) have found in mare milk free glycerol (0.0056%) that has not been reported in other species.

Milk fat content and fatty acid composition: average and extreme values

Mare milk content is very variable, compared to cow, so that it is difficult to give an average value. In their well-documented reviews, Neseni *et al.* (1958) and Neuhaus (1959) reported extreme values of 0 and 79 g/kg of fat in milk. Nil or very low values are probably due to incomplete milking, because cisternal milk contains less fat than alveolar milk, and because hand milking in unaccustomed mares does not allow to obtain all alveolar milk (Doreau *et al.*, 1986, review by Doreau and Boulot, 1989a). Nevertheless, Doreau and Boulot (1989b), on 131 samples obtained with a standardised milking procedure leading to the emptying of the udder, recorded extreme values of 0.2 and 3.5% fat in milk. This low milk fat results in a low content in gross energy of horse milk (2.0 to 2.5 MJ/kg, review by Doreau *et al.*, 1988), and in a part of fat in milk gross energy close to 25%, whereas fat represents about 50% of milk gross energy in bovine and humans (review by Oftedal, 1984).

Mare milk composition is very different from ruminant milk composition, because of the above mentioned extensive hydrogenation of dietary FA in ruminants. The main difference in composition with other monogastric species is that horses consume grass, which is rich in α-linolenic acid, whereas feedstuffs consumed by non herbivorous monogastric species are most often poor in this acid. Compared to human milk, mare milk is richer in short- and medium-chain FA and in α -linolenic acid, and poorer in oleic acid (Table 1).

Concentrations in individual FA in milk fat, based on literature data, are very variable. These results are often biased by different analytical factors: 1) the loss of short-chain FA when methyl esters are used instead of butyl esters; 2) imperfect chromatographic conditions; 3) the expression of FA generally in weight percentages, but sometimes in molar percentages; when it is expressed in weight, it can be on FA basis or on ester basis, which changes the result, especially for butyl esters of very short-chain FA. In many published papers, the mode of expression is not specified.

Table 1. Milk fat from mares, cows and humans. Mean and extreme values of the literature, in % of total FA.

Fatty acid	Mare milk[1] Mean and extreme values	Cow milk[2] Mean value	Human milk[2] Mean value
C4:0 butyric acid	0.6 (0.3 – 0.9)	3.3	-
C6:0 caproic acid	0.7 (0.3 – 1.4)	1.6	traces
C8:0 caprylic acid	3.1 (0.8 – 6.1)	1.3	traces
C10:0 capric acid	7.2 (2.3 – 16.7)	3.0	1.3
C12:0 lauric acid	7.6 (3.8 – 14.6)	3.1	3.1
C14:0 myristic acid	7.5 (4.7 – 19.2)	14.2	5.1
C14:1 n-5 myristoleic acid	0.7 (0.1 – 2.6)	1.3	0.5
C15:0 pentadecanoic acid	0.4 (0.2 – 0.9)	1.3	traces to 0.4
C15:1 pentadecenoic acid	0.4 (0.3 – 0.6)	0.3	traces
C16:0 palmitic acid	20.8 (12.4 – 28.5)	42.7	20.2
C16:1 n-7 palmitoleic acid	5.6 (2.2 – 9.7)	3.7	5.7
C17:0 margaric acid	0.4 (0.0 – 1.2)	0.8	0.6
C17:1 heptadecenoic acid	0.4 (0.0 – 1.1)	0.3	0.3
C18:0 stearic acid	1.2 (0.3 – 3.0)	5.7	6.0
C18:1 n-9 oleic acid	19.8 (9.4 – 31.6)	16.7	46.4
C18:2 n-6 linoleic acid	11.3 (3.6 – 20.3)	1.6	13.0
C18:3 n-3 linolenic acid	11.9 (2.2 – 26.2)	1.8	1.4

[1]From 17 publications quoted by Doreau and Boulot, 1989b, and 8 more recent publications: Doreau *et al.* (1990), Doreau *et al.* (1992), Doreau *et al.* (1993), Csapo *et al.* (1995), Zeyner *et al.* (1996), Martuzzi *et al.*, 1998, Hoffman *et al.*, 1998, Curadi *et al.*, 2001, Doreau *et al.* (2003).
[2]From Jensen *et al.*, 1990

Mare milk is rich in short- and medium-chain FA (Table 1). Butyric and caproic acid are present in low amounts (less than 1%), caprylic acid represents about 3%, capric, lauric and myristic acids about 7.5% each. The proportion of short and medium chain FA is higher that that of cow or human milk fat (ca. 20 and 25%, respectively, see Martuzzi *et al.*, 2001). Palmitic acid represents 12 to 28% of total FA. This is less than in cow milk and human milk. A specificity of mare milk fat is the very low concentration of stearic acid, between 0.3 and 3.0% of total FA. Among mammals, only seals have such a low concentration. For mares, it can be attributed to 1) the low content of stearic acid in the diet, and 2) a possible high activity of Δ 9 desaturase, which converts stearic acid into oleic acid (C18:1 n-9, i.e.Δ9) in the udder. This latter hypothesis is enhanced by the high content in palmitoleic acid (C16:1 n-7, i.e. Δ 9), which varies between 4 and 8% in most experiments.

Mare milk is rich in polyunsaturated FA. The important proportion of linoleic acid, between 5 and 20% of total FA in most data, is due to the presence of this acid in the diet, which is the major FA in cereals and their by-products. However, a major specificity of mare milk is the high content in α-linolenic acid (ALA), on average 12%, between 2 and 26% according to the authors. A high concentration of ALA can be reached in milk from animals with are both nonruminants and herbivorous, that is when the diet contains large amounts of α-linolenic acid, as grass, and when no hydrogenation occurs before absorption. The effect of diet on concentration of ALA will be detailed below.

Non dietary effects on fat content and fatty acid composition

The effect of the availability in end-products of digestion, and thus of dietary composition, is the major determinant of FA composition for a given animal species. Non-dietary factors generally play a minor role, except for lactation stage.

Mare milk fat decreases with lactation stage, on average from 15 - 25 g/kg at the beginning of lactation to 5 - 15 g/kg at 6 months of lactation (Figure 1). As in other species, colostrum is higher in fat, and colostrum fat is higher in long-chain FA than milk (Doreau *et al.*, 1993, Csapo *et al.*, 1995, Curadi *et al.*, 2001), but after 1 week of lactation, the composition of fat is not modified to a large extent when mares are fed a constant diet (Doreau *et al.*, 1993, Hoffman *et al.*, 1998, Curadi *et al.*, 2001). Results on the whole lactation are sometimes difficult to interpret, due to the change in feeding during lactation which interferes with the effect of lactation stage. However, it can be considered that fat content decreases until 3 months of lactation then remains stable or slightly decreases until 6 months. Figure 1 shows that milk fat content is very variable from a trial to another during this period, but the general trend from pooling literature data is an inverse function of lactation stage, as proposed for cows by Freeze and Richards (1992). This model may be more adapted to mares than to cows because fat content does not increase in late lactation, contrary to cows, and thus more appropriate that the curvilinear model used for mares by Cabrera *et al.* (1990). At 6 months of lactation, milk fat can be between 8 and 10 g/kg (Intrieri and Minieri, 1969, Santos *et al.*, 2005) or lower than 5 g/kg (Tomczynski *et al.*, 1999, Mariani *et al.*, 2001). This variability is certainly caused by feeding (see below).

Genetic effects have seldom been studied. Csapo *et al.* (1995) found no difference in fat composition between Breton, Boulonnais, Haflinger and Hungarian Draught, and Pinto *et al.* (2001a) found no significant difference between fat content of Tiro Pesante Rapido and Murgese, although fat content tended to be higher and more sensitive to diet for this latter breed. Differences obtained by

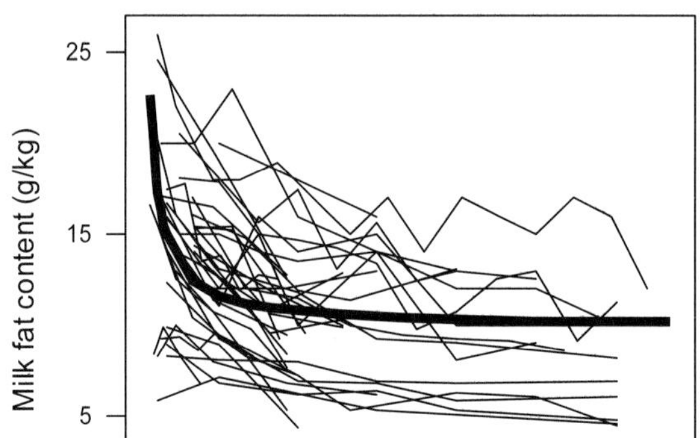

Figure 1. Effect of lactation stage on milk fat: summarising literature data[1] and determining the theoretical variation of fat content with lactation stage[2].

[1]Data come from 36 series from 22 publications: 10 references quoted in Doreau and Boulot (1989b), and Davison *et al.*, 1987, Sigler *et al.*, 1989, Cabrera *et al.*, 1990, Smolders *et al.*, 1990, Doreau *et al.*, 1990, Burns *et al.*, 1991, Doreau *et al.*, 1992, Doreau *et al.*, 1993, Mariani *et al.*, 1993, Tomczynski *et al.*, 1999, Mariani *et al.*, 2001, Pinto *et al.*, 2001a, Santos *et al.*, 2005. Data from Hoffman *et al.* (1998) have not been included, because fat content increased with lactation stage, contrary to other data.

[2]The fitting of experimental data was performed considering that fat content (F, g/kg) is an inverse function of lactation stage (D, days of lactation): $F = 51.26/D + 9.88$ ($R2 = 0.82$, $RMSE = 2.02$)

Kulisa (1977) between Arabian, Malopolski and Huculski breeds, and by Tomczynski *et al.* (1999) between Wielkopolska and Konik Polski breeds are likely due to their situation in different herds, with different feeding conditions: for example, the lower fat content for Wielkopolska breed in this latter experiment (4.9 vs 5.8 g/kg corresponds to a higher concentrate intake (6 vs 2 kg/day).

It can be wondered whether low milk fat is related to high production levels, as it occurs in cows. Such relationship was not observed by Gibbs *et al.* (1982); Doreau (1994) obtained contradictory results by analysing two different trials. In both experiments, the number of animals was probably too low to evidence a genetic relationship between fat content and milk yield.

Dietary effects on milk fat content and FA composition

Several authors failed to show an effect of energy concentration or of crude fibre content of the diet on milk fat (Zimmerman, 1985, Pagan and Hintz, 1986), probably because diets were not enough different. However, replacing a hay diet by a hay-concentrate (50:50) diet resulted in a strong decrease in fat content and in a decrease in short- and medium-chain FA (Doreau *et al.*, 1992), probably owing to a shortage in precursors of de novo synthesis with concentrate diets. This could explain that Goryaev (1970) observed a much higher proportion of short- and medium-chain FA (from 4 to 14 carbons) in December than in July: 35 vs 26%. Curiously, probiotics seem to have an effect on de novo FA synthesis, depending on the yeast strain (Yocum *et al.*, 2002).

The most obvious dietary effect on FA composition is the effect on ALA, of which proportions in milk fat can be 5 times higher with herbage than with winter diets. Fresh grass contains 1 to 3% FA, of which more than 50% is made of ALA. Almost all measurements made with fresh grass result in proportions of ALA comprised between 15 and 25%, whereas all measurements made with winter diets give values lower than 10% (e.g. Goryaev, 1970, Jamsranjav, 1982, Csapo *et al.*, 1995, Hoffman *et al.*, 1998, Orlandi *et al.*, 2004); unfortunately no direct comparison is available. Among winter diets, a hay diet has given a higher proportion of ALA than a hay-concentrate diet (Doreau *et al.*, 1992), probably due to a higher ALA content in hay than in concentrate. This higher proportion, together with a higher fat secretion, resulted in a higher daily secretion of ALA with the hay diet (15 vs 5 g/d, respectively).

Logically, a protein supplement does not modify milk fat (Peltonen *et al.*, 1980). The replacement of a concentrate rich in starch and sugar by a concentrate rich in fibre and fat from maize oil did not modify fat content but resulted in an increase in linoleic acid from 10 to 15% of total FA, and to a lower extent in a decrease in ALA and in an increase in transvaccenic acid, the other FA being unmodified (Hoffman *et al.*, 1998). The high content in linoleic acid is a consequence of maize oil addition, but other variations cannot be explained, especially because of concomitant variations in starch, sugar, fibre and fat in the diet. In some cases, fat addition in the diet may increase fat content (Davison *et al.*, 1987, with 5% unspecified fat). The addition of soybean oil in the diet also increased linoleic acid in a trial by Zeyner *et al.* (1996) but to a lower extent, due to a low amount of oil given to animals. More recently, Pinto *et al.* (2001b) showed a decrease in saturated FA from 63 to 56% of total FA, and an increase in linoleic acid from 20 to 24% when 1.2% safflower oil was supplied in the diet; Bontempo *et al.* (2000) observed an increase in different n-3 FA and a decrease in n-6 FA when cod liver oil was supplied.

Mare feeding in pregnancy may have an effect on milk composition through body condition at foaling. Compared to milk of thin mares, milk of fat mares is higher in fat, and this fat is slightly higher in long-chain FA and poorer in short- and medium-chain FA (Doreau *et al.*, 1993). This is a consequence of a lower mobilisation of the long-chain FA of body reserves in thin mares.

Minor fatty acids

The composition of milk fat is generally much more complex than that of feedstuffs from vegetal origin, suggesting transformations in animal organism. This is particularly true for cow milk, due to the high microbial metabolism in the rumen, which results not only in an extensive hydrogenation of dietary FA, but also in specific FA (Doreau and Ferlay, 1994). In particular, odd-chain FA, with 15 and 17 carbons, are characteristics of bacteria. Moreover trans monounsaturated 18-carbon FA and conjugated linoleic acids (CLA) are intermediate compounds of hydrogenation of polyunsaturated FA. On another hand, specific dietary FA, as 20- and 22-carbon FA, present in fish and algae fat, can be found in milk. Most milk FA analyses have been carried out with rather rough methods allowing to analyse main FA. For a few years, the increasing interest for minor FA leads to analyse FA with more accuracy, but until now few data are available for horse milk.

Odd-chain FA, which are characteristic of bacteria, are present in small amounts. From 12 publications in which they are determined, their concentration is generally comprised between 0.2 and 0.9% for 15:0, between 0.3 and 0.6% for 15:1, between 0 and 1.2% for 17:0, and between 0.0 and 1.1% for 17:1. The concentration seems to be reduced by dietary fat (Zeyner *et al.*, 1996). This concentration is only 2 to 3 times lower than in cow milk fat for saturated FA, and in the same range of concentration for monounsaturated FA (Jensen *et al.*, 1990), whereas absorption of FA of microbial origin occurs in ruminants and not in monogastric animals.

Transvaccenic acid has been found in mare milk, at concentrations of 0.9% (Curadi *et al.*, 2001) or 0.2% (Hoffman *et al.*, 1998). Other data (Zeyner *et al.*, 1996, Doreau *et al.*, 2003 and Table 2) suggest that the main isomer of trans monounsaturated 18-carbon FA is elaidic acid (n-9) and not transvaccenic acid (n-7) as it occurs in cow. In fact, in ruminants transvaccenic acid arises from the ruminal hydrogenation of polyunsaturated FA; there is no reason to assume the same importance of this trans isomer in horses.

In cow, the main isomer of CLA (18:2 cis 9 trans 11) is produced in the rumen but is mainly synthesised in the udder from transvaccenic acid (18:1 trans 11, i.e. n-7) of ruminal origin; its concentration is within 0.5% for normal diets to 2% with diets rich in lipids (Doreau *et al.*, 1999). It has been first observed by Park and Pariza (1998) that CLA was present in mare plasma, but concentrations were very low, strengthening the hypothesis of the absence of absorption of FA of microbial origin produced in the large intestine. In mare milk, its concentration has recently been found as 0.05% by Curadi *et al.* (2001) and as 0.09% by Jahreis *et al.* (1999). A more specific determination by separation of isomers has shown a mean concentration of 0.05%, mainly composed of the cis 9 trans 11 isomer, and of different trans trans isomers (Doreau *et al.*, 2003 and Table 2). This pattern is similar to that of absorbable CLA in ruminants (Loor *et al.*, 2004), after the action of rumen microbes but before the mammary desaturation of transvaccenic acid in the cis 9 trans 11 isomer. The very low concentration in CLA in mares compared to cows is due to the quasi absence of absorption of both CLA and transvaccenic acid in mares.

An isomer of ALA, γ-linolenic acid of the n-6 series, is generally present in very small amounts (0.02% according to Curadi *et al.*, 2001) but Csapo *et al.* (1995) observed a concentration of 0.6%. This may be due to the intake at pasture of plants rich in γ-linolenic acid. This FA was present as traces in determinations by Doreau, Chabrot and Loor (unpublished).

Very long-chain FA have also been found in mare milk. In normally fed mares, the two acids of the n-3 series, eicosapentaenoic acid (EPA, 20:5) and docosahexaenoic acid (DHA, 22:6) are present in very small amounts (less than 0.02%) but partially hydrogenated 20-carbon FA are present in higher amounts, especially 20:3, 20:2 and 20:1 (0.3 to 0.5% each) (Curadi *et al.*, 2001, Doreau *et*

Table 2. Concentration in isomers of some minor FA[1] of nutritional importance, as % of total FA methyl esters (Doreau et al., 2003 and unpublished).

	Extreme values (6 milks)
Isomers of conjugated linoleic acid	
cis 9 trans 11	0.021 – 0.043
trans 8 cis 10	0.003 – 0.006
trans 9 cis 11 + cis 10 trans 12	0.004 – 0.006
cis 9 cis 11	0.005 – 0.015
trans 11 trans 13	0.000 – 0.003
trans 8 trans 10 + trans 9 trans 11 + trans 10 trans 12	0.013 – 0.043
Isomers of trans octadecenoic acid	
trans 5	0.001 – 0.007
trans 6 + trans 7 + trans 8	0.002 – 0.059
trans 9 (elaidic acid)	0.028 – 0.180
trans 10	0.001 – 0.077
trans 11 (transvaccenic acid)	0.002 – 0.063
trans 12	0.009 – 0.067
trans 13 + trans 14	0.008 – 0.028
20- and 22-carbon FA	
20:0	0.022 – 0.037
20:1 n-3	0.124 – 0.291
20:2	0.071 – 0.204
20:3 n-3	0.155 – 0.515
20:5 n-3 (eicosapentaenoic acid, EPA)	0.009 – 0.043
22:0	0.004 – 0.010
22:1 n-9	0.013 – 0.033
22:6 n-3 (docosahexaenoic acid, DHA)	0.004 – 0.019

[1]Milks were 5 commercial milks and 1 milk of INRA research centre, from herds of different regions of France, composed of Haflinger (3 milks), Breton (1 milk), Auxois (1 milk) and Merens (1 milk). Fatty acids have been determined by gas chromatography, using a 100 m column CPSil 88, with temperatures from 70 °C to 225 °C with a step at 175 °C.

al., 2003, Table 2). On the contrary, among 22-carbon FA, only 22:0 (Intrieri and Minieri, 1970) and 22:1 have been found, in very low amounts. All these results have been obtained with classical diets. Supplying mare diets with sources of EPA and DHA, as fish oil, may increase these two FA in milk as it occurs in human (Jensen *et al.*, 1990), unless they are not incorporated in milk triglycerides. A trial by Bontempo *et al.* (2000) showed an moderate increase in n-3 FA with a cod liver supply, but authors did not specify the chain length of these FA.

Are fat components involved in mare milk nutritional quality?

The nutritional quality of mare milk for human health or as replacement of maternal milk is mainly due to nitrogen fraction of milk. The main interest of mare milk fat is related to its high content in polyunsaturated FA, especially in ALA, of which nutritional quality for human health is demonstrated (Williams *et al.*, 2000): prevention of cardiovascular diseases, synthesis of prostaglandins and long-chain FA which have different actions on the immune system, on infant growth, and anti-inflammatory properties. Some populations traditionally consume mare milk to a large extent as koumiss which is the product obtained after alcoholic fermentation of mare milk, in Russia, in some countries of Central Asia as Kazakhstan, and in Mongolia. Although no direct comparison of composition between milk and koumiss made from this milk is available, general data on milk and koumiss composition suggest the absence of modification in fat content and FA composition (Goryaev *et al.*, 1970). This contributes to the good nutritional value of koumiss, which may have a positive action on health, provided it is consumed regularly.

The high level of FA unsaturation could make mare milk oxidisable. In fact, it is much less sensitive to oxidation than expected (Sidhu *et al.*, 1976), perhaps due to natural antioxidants in milk. On the contrary, mare milk is sensitive to lipolysis and thus tends to become rancid, because of a high content in free fatty acids, and of a lipase in milk (Chilliard and Doreau, 1985). For this reason, mare milk cannot be easily consumed as fresh milk. In some countries of Western Europe, mare milk is thus sold frozen or lyophilised. One of the main arguments in advertising is the high content in polyunsaturated FA of the n-3 series. However, the high price does not allow the consumption of significant amounts of ALA from mare milk. Mare milk is sometimes sold as pills of less than 0.5 g, which obviously cannot have any effect. Moreover, 1 kg of milk from mares fed a concentrate diet does not contain more ALA (ca. 10 g/kg fat containing 5% ALA) than 1 kg of milk from cows fed on pasture (35 g/kg fat containing 1.5% ALA). In addition, the main source of FA from the n-3 series for humans is fish, and other foods as rapeseed oil contain significant amounts of ALA. It is thus likely that a regular but low consumption of mare milk is not the best way to enhance the intake of n-3 FA, and that a major issue to improve the nutritional value of mare milk fat is to enhance the content in n-3 FA. Some nutritional ways exist. Increasing EPA and DHA may be achieved by the consumption by mares of fish oil or fish meal, but it is not an acceptable way for the consumer. Algae, which contain EPA and DHA are more acceptable provided that their innocuousness is proven. Increasing ALA in winter diets may be obtained by linseeds, which are the major vegetal source of this FA, but no experimental results are available. Moreover, the sensorial quality of mare milk may be reduced, as it has been shown in milk or meat of cows fed linseeds.

Another interest of mare milk fat is the use for the care of some diseases. The lipid fraction could be involved in the treatment of ulcers (Sharmanov *et al.*, 1981), due to the high content in phospholipids which is assumed to favour healing. However, recent findings have shown that the cause of gastric ulcer is a bacteria, *Helicobacter pylori*. The treatment by antibiotics which is now recommended is probably the most efficient way to cure this disease.

Conclusion

A main feature of mare milk fat is the high variability of fat content and of fatty acid composition. In particular, the content in ALA varies in an important range, due to feeding. Until now, few experiments controlled the relationship between dietary fatty acid intake and milk fatty acids, so that it is difficult to predict milk composition. The use of mare milk as a supplier of n-3 FA needs to guarantee a minimal content of this FA. This could be achieved by nutritional means, but requires additional research.

References

Bontempo, V., B. Chiofalo, M. Polidori, D. Tedesco and E. Salimei, 2000. Somministrazione di olio di fegato di merluzzo a giumente in lattazione: studio sul profilo acidico del latte e del tessuto adipose. Atti 2nd Convegno Soc. Ital. Ippol., Campobasso, Italy, 53-55.

Burns, H.D., G.D. Potter and P.G. Gibbs, 1991. Milk energy production by lactating mares. Proc. 12th Eq. Nutr. Physiol. Symp., Calgary, Canada, 257-259.

Cabrera, L., L.C. de O. Fernandes and C.M.M. de Moraes, 1990. Composiçao de leite de éguas P.S.I. e desenvolvimento ponderal de suas crias. A Hora Veterinaria, 55, 24-29.

Chilliard, Y. and M. Doreau, 1985. Characterization of lipase in mare milk. J. Dairy Sci., 68: 37-39.

Csapo, J., J. Stefler, T.G. Martin, S. Makra and Z. Csapo-Kiss, 1995. Composition of mare's colostrum and milk. Fat content, fatty acid composition and vitamin content. Int. Dairy J., 5: 393-402.

Curadi, M.C., G. Civardi, G. Contarini and M. Orlandi, 2001. Long chain polyunsaturated fatty acids (LCPS) variation during early lactation in mares. Proc. 52nd Ann. Meet. EAAP, Budapest, Hungary (poster).

Davison, K.E., G.D. Potter, L.W. Greene, J.W. Evans and W.C. McMullan, 1987. Lactation and reproductive performance of mares fed added dietary fat during late gestation and early lactation. Proc. 10th Eq. Nutr. Physiol. Symp., Colorado State Univ., USA, 87-92.

Doreau, M., 1994. Le lait de jument et sa production: particularités et facteurs de variation. Lait, 74: 401-418.

Doreau, M. and S. Boulot, 1989a. Methods of measurement of mare milk yield and composition in nursing mares: a review. Lait, 69: 159-171.

Doreau, M. and S. Boulot, 1989b. Recent knowledge on mare milk production: a review. Livest. Prod. Sci., 22: 213-235.

Doreau, M. and A. Ferlay, 1994. Digestion and utilisation of fatty acids by ruminants. Anim. Feed Sci. Technol., 45: 379-396.

Doreau, M., S. Boulot, W. Martin-Rosset and H. Dubroeucq, 1986. Milking lactating mares using oxytocin: milk volume and composition. Reprod. Nutr. Dev., 26: 1-11.

Doreau, M., W. Martin-Rosset and S. Boulot, 1988. Energy requirements and the feeding of mares during lactation: a review. Livest. Prod. Sci., 20: 53-68.

Doreau, M., S. Boulot, J.P. Barlet and P. Patureau-Mirand, 1990. Yield and composition of milk from lactating mares: effect of lactation stage and individual differences. J. Dairy Res., 57: 449-454.

Doreau, M., S. Boulot, D. Bauchart, J.P. Barlet and W. Martin-Rosset, 1992. Voluntary intake, milk production and plasma metabolites in nursing mares fed two different diets. J. Nutr., 122: 992-999.

Doreau, M., S. Boulot and Y. Chilliard, 1993. Yield and composition of milk from lactating mares: effect of body condition at foaling. J. Dairy Res., 60: 457-466.

Doreau, M., Y. Chilliard, H. Rulquin and D. Demeyer, 1999. Manipulation of milk fat in dairy cows. In: Recent Advances in Animal Nutrition. Garnsworthy P.C., Wiseman J., Eds, Nottingham Univ. Press, 81-109.

Doreau, M., J., Chabrot and J.J. Loor, 2003. Horse milk composition in minor fatty acids, including CLA. Proceedings 25th World Cong. Intern. Soc. Fat Science, Bordeaux, France, 45-46.

Forsyth, I.A., P.D. Rossdale and C.R. Thomas, 1975. Studies in milk composition and lactogenic hormones in the mare. J. Reprod. Fert., Suppl., 23: 631-635.

Freeze, B.S. and T.J. Richards, 1992. Lactation curve estimation for use in economic optimization models in the dairy industry. J. Dairy Sci., 75:2984-2989.

Gibbs, P.G., G.D. Potter, R.W. Blake and W.C. McMullan, 1982. Milk production of quarter horse mares during 150 days of lactation. J. Dairy Sci., 54: 496-499.

Goryaev, M.I., L.K. Shafieva and L.G. Denisova, 1970. Fatty acid composition of fat in mare milk and koumiss (in Russian). Molotshnaya Promyshlennost, 31: 22-24.

Hoffman, R.M., D.S. Kronfeld, J.H. Herbein, W.S. Swecker, W.L. Cooper and P.A. Harris, 1998. Dietary carbohydrates and fat influence milk composition and fatty acid profile of mare's milk. J. Nutr., 128: 2708s-2711s.

Intrieri, F. and L. Minieri, 1969. Sulla composizione chimica del latte di cavalla: indagini su soggetti di razza avelignese. Atti Soc. Ital. Sci. Veter., 23: 558-561.

Intrieri, F. and L. Minieri, 1970. Sul contenuto in acidi grassi della quota lipidica del colostro e del latte di cavalla. Indagini su soggetti di razza avelignese. Acta Med. Vet. Napoli, 16: 89-98.

Jahreis, G., J. Fritsche, P. Möckel, F. Schöne, U. Möller and H. Steinhart, 1999. The potential anticarcinogenic conjugated linoleic acid, cis-9,trans-11 C18:2, in milk of different species: cow, goat, ewe, sow, mare, woman. Nutr. Res., 19: 1541-1549.

Jamsranjav, N., 1982. Cow and mare milk fatty acid composition. XXI Int. Dairy Congr., 2, Moskow, Russia, MIR Publishers, 195-196.

Jenness, R., 1974. The composition of milk. In: "Lactation", vol 3, B.L. Larson, V.R. Smith, Eds, Acad. Press., London, UK, 3-107.

Jensen, R.G., A. M. Ferris, C.J. Lammi-Keefe and R.A. Henderson, 1990. Lipids of bovine and human milks: a comparison. J. Dairy Sci., 73: 223-240.

Kharitonova, I., 1978. Fatty acids and phospholipids in mare's milk (in Russian). Konevodstvo Konnyi Sport, 12 (24): 24.

Kulisa, M. 1977. The content of some free amino acids and fatty acids in the milk of Arabian, Malopolski and Huculski mares. Rocz. Nauk Zoot., 4: 79-89.

Linzell, J.L., E.F. Annison, R. Bickerstaffe and L.B. Jeffcott, 1972. Mammary and whole-body metabolism of glucose, acetate and palmitate in the lactating horse. Proc. Nutr. Soc., 31: 72A-73A.

Loor, J.J., K. Ueda, A. Ferlay, Y. Chilliard and M. Doreau, 2004. Biohydrogenation, duodenal flow and intestinal digestibility of trans fatty acids and conjugated linoleic acids in response to dietary forage:concentrate ratio and linseed oil in dairy cows. Journal of Dairy Science, 87: 2472-2485.

Mariani, P., F. Martuzzi and A.L. Catalano, 1993. Composizione e proprieta fisico-chimiche del latte di cavalla: variazione dei costituenti azotati e minerali nel corso della lattazione. Ann. Fac. Med. Veter., Univ. Parma, 13: 43-58.

Mariani, P., A. Summer, F. Martuzzi, P. Formaggioni, A. Sabbioni and A.L. Catalano, 2001. Physicochemical properties, gross composition, energy value and nitrogen fractions of Haflinger nursing mare milk throughout 6 lactation months. Anim. Res., 50: 415-425.

Martuzzi, F., A. Summer, A.L. Catalano, S. Barbacini and P. Mariani, 1998. Il contenuto in acidi grassi polinsaturati del grasso del latte di cavalla prodotto nelle prime settimane di lattazione. Proc. Convegno Naz. S.I.S. Vet., 52: 537-538.

Martuzzi, F., A. Summer, M. Malacarne and P. Mariani, 2001. Main protein fractions and fatty acids composition of mare milk: some nutritional remarks with reference to woman and cow milk. Proc. 52nd Ann. Meet. Europ. Assoc. Anim. Prod., Budapest, 10pp.

Neseni, R., E. Flade, G. Heidler and H. Steger, 1958. Milchleistung und Milchzusammensetzung von Stuten im Verlaufe der Laktation. Arch. Tierzucht., 1, 91-129.

Neuhaus, U., 1959. Milch und Milchgewinnung von Pferdestuten. Z. Tierzucht., 73: 370-392.

Oftedal, O.T., 1984. Milk composition, milk yield and energy oupput at peak lactation: a comparative review. Symp; Zool. Soc. London, 51: 33-85.

Orlandi, M., J. Goracci and M.C. Curadi, 2004. Fat composition of mare's milk with reference to human nutrition. Ann. Fac. Med. Vet. Pisa, 56: 97-105.

Pagan, J.D. and H. F. Hintz, 1986. Composition of milk from pony mares fed various levels of digestible energy. Cornell Vet., 76: 139-148.

Park, Y. and M.W. Pariza, 1998. Evidence that commercial calf and horse sera can contain substantial amounts of trans-10,cis-12 conjugated linoleic acid. Lipids, 33: 817-819.

Pastukhova, Z.M. and V.V. Gerbeda, 1982. Comparative study of the lipid composition of mare's milk and koumiss mixture prepared on the basis of cow's milk (in Russian). Vopr. Pitan., 1: 34-36.

Peltonen, T., V. Kossila, V. Antila and L. Huida, 1980. Effect of protein supplement on milk composition of the mares ans growth rate of their foals. Proc. 31st Ann. Meet. EAAP, München, Germany, 5pp.

Pinto, F., M. Faccia, A. Di Summa and G. Mastrangelo, 2001a. Mare's milk: early result concerning quality and quantity from Murgese and TPR mares. Riv. Ippiatria Ippologia, 7: 7-19.

Pinto, F., M. Ragni, A. Caputi Jambrenghi, A. Vincenti, G. Marsico, L. Zezza and G. Vonghia, 2001b. Fatty acid composition of milk from mares fed on a diet containing safflower oil. Proc. Vth Intern. Safflower Conf., Williston, ND, 33-36.

Santos, E.M., F.Q. de Almeida, A.A. Vieira, L.F.B. Pinto, A. Corassa, R.R. Moreira Pimentel, V. Pimentel Silva and L. Galzerano, 2005. Lactaçao em eguas da raça Mangalarga Marchador: produçao e composiçao do laite e ganho de peso dos potros lactentes. R. Bras. Zootec., 34: 627-634.

Sidhu, G.S., M.A. Brown and A.R. Johnson, 1976. Autoxidation in milk rich in linoleic acid. II. Modification of the initiation system and control of oxidation. J. Dairy Res., 43: 239-250.

Sigler, D.H., D.E. Ericson, P.G. Gibbs, G.H. Kiracofe and J.S. Stevenson, 1989. Reproductive traits, lactation and foal growth in mares fed altrenogest. J. Anim. Sci., 67: 1154-1159.

Sharmanov, T.Sh., R.Kh. Kadyrova and B.A. Salkhanov, 1981. Effectiveness of peptic ulcer diet therapy using rations containing whole mare's and camel's milk (in Russian). Vopr. Pitan., 3: 10-14.

Smolders, E.A.A., N.G. Van der Veen and A. Van Polanen, 1990. Composition of horse milk during the suckling period. Livest. Prod. Sci., 25: 163-171.

Tomczynski, R., K. Roman and E. Szybinska, 1999. A comparative analysis of the chemical composition of milk from mares of the Wielkopolska and Konik Polski breeds. Natur. Sc., 2: 87-96.

Welsch, U., W. Buchheim, U. Schumacher, I. Schinko and S. Patton, 1988. Structural, histochemical and biochemical observations on horse milk-fat globule membranes and casein micelles. Histochemistry, 88: 357-365.

Williams, C.M., 2000. Dietary fatty acids and human health. Ann. Zootech., 49: 165-180.

Yocum, P.M., V. Fellner and B. Alston-Mills, 2002. The effect of Kluyveromyces marxianus and Saccharomyces cerevisiae on fatty acid composition of equine milk. J. Anim. Sci., 80 (suppl. 1): 57 (abstr.).

Zeyner, A., C. Geissler, I. Peschke, R. Jope and G. Kny, 1996. Beitrag zum Fettsäurenmuster in der Stutenmilch. Pferdeheilkunde, 12: 213-219.

Zimmerman, R.A., 1985. Effect of ration on composition of mare's milk. Proc. 9th Eq. Nutr. Physiol; Symp., Michigan Univ., USA, 96-102.

Energy and protein requirements and recommended allowances in lactating mares

W. Martin-Rosset[1], D. Austbo[2] and M. Coenen[3]
[1]INRA, Department of Animal Science, Research Centre of Clermont-Ferrand/Theix, 63122 St Genès Champanelle, France
[2]University of Norway, Department of Animal and Acquaculture Science, Norvegian University of Life Sciences, Box 5003, N, 1432 Aas, Norway
[3]University of Leipzig, Institute of Animal Nutrition, Nutritional Diseases and Dietetics, Leipzig, Germany

Abstract

Original feeding standards/systems were proposed in the eighties in the US (NRC, 1978-1989) and in France (INRA, 1984-1990). Several feeding standards were derived in Germany (GEH, 1994), in the Netherlands (CVB, 1996) and in Scandinavia (SCAND, 2002-2004). In all the feeding standards/systems, total energy or protein requirements are broken down in maintenance and lactation requirements. Maintenance requirements are estimated from metabolic body weight except for energy in NRC system where the requirement are related to body weight. Energy and protein requirements for lactation are estimated in all the systems using milk production, energy and protein content of milk at various months of lactation and efficiency rates of conversion of energy and protein to milk. Hence all the systems are using the factorial method. A consensus could be easily met in Europe. But recommended allowances depend on intake capacity and body reserves of the mares as well according to diet composition and goal of production: athlete horses vs leisure horses. Recommended allowances, based on experimental data, which implement these nutritional characteristics and feeding strategies should be stated. Such recommendations have been proposed by INRA and to some extend by NRC. Additional experiments should be carried out more or less for the other standard/systems to take care of the breed diversity and the local conditions in the different countries.

Keywords: mare, lactation, energy, protein, requirements, allowances

Introduction

Lactation is a critical period of the breeding cycle of the broodmare. The broodmare should nurse adequately the foal which should meet 45 p. 100 of the adult weight at weaning. And the nursing mare should be rebred during the first month following foaling to secure as much as possible an interval period of one year between two subsequent foalings and an appropriate date of foaling the next following year consistent with the aim of production - race horse – Sport horses or leisure horses – horse for meat.

Requirements are mainly related to physiological expenditure due to milk secretion. Milk production and composition have been extensively studied (see chapters by Doreau *et al.*; Martuzzi *et al.*, in this issue). Energy and protein requirements have been estimated in differents systems (NRC – INRA – GEH – CVB – SCAND). Comparison of those estimations are relevant to improve our knowledge and to suggest some harmonisation. Nutrients and feed allowances depend on intake capacity and body reserves of the mare throughout the breeding cycle, namely during lactation period. The influence of these characteristic should be determined to perform allowances which should be well adapted to the mares devoted to produce either race – sport or leisure horses – horse meat in the conditions of the different countries.

This chapter is focused on energy and protein requirements and allowances only as there are enough data to discuss the recommendations proposed in different countries. Minerals and vitamins requirements are of high concern as well, but most of the recommendations proposed are based on the same data used by NRC, 1978 – 1989; and there are not a lot of new experiments carried out at present in the world to argue new figures (see the reviews published in the Proceedings of KER, 2001).

Metabolism of nutrients

Milk synthesis in the mammary gland has a dual origin: nutrients from feeding and body reserves, or/and *de novo* synthesis. And the synthesis of milk components in the mare is very similar to that described in ruminants (Doreau and Martin-Rosset, 2002).

Lactose comes from glucose absorbed in the small intestine. Fatty acids are supplied by *de novo* synthesis and direct uptake by the udder. All fatty acids from C4 to C18 are supplied by *de novo* synthesis. The precursors of *de novo* synthesis are acetate and 3-hydroxybutyrate. The latter arises from butyrate. Acetate and butyrate are end-products of carbohydrates digestion in the large intestine. Propionate in the large intestine and glucose in the small intestine are not precursors of milk fatty acids. Acid palmitic (C16) comes from *de novo* synthesis and from fatty acids uptake in approximatively similar proportion. Unsaturated C18 fatty acid comes mainly from direct uptake (diet and body reserves) in contrast to ruminants. (Linzell *et al.*, 1972).

Adipose tissue can contribute to provide fatty acids of milk when the brood mares are fed limited energy. Fatty acids of milk come from either uptake of fatty acids circulating in the blood (Pagan and Hintz, 1986a) or/and triglycerides transported by lipoproteins via the liver to the udder. Energy (ATP) is supplied to the udder from acetate of fatty acids after fat mobilization through the Krebs cycle in the liver.

Crude protein is made of about 10% of non protein N, of which urea represent about 50 percent (Doreau and Boulot, 1989a). Among proteins, caseins represent 50 to 65 percent of true protein in the mare's milk whereas the ratio casein/protein is 80 percent in the cow (see Martuzzi and Doreau in this issue). Little is known about nitrogen metabolism in the lactating mare. Peltonen *et al.*, 1980 did not observe any relationship between the protein allowances and milk composition comparing two groups of mares fed either diets with 10.0 or 7.7% DCP kg DM. The allowances were too close to NRC, 1978 requirements used a reference: (8.4% DCP/kg DM). Meadows *et al.*, 1979 then Doreau *et al.*, 1988 observed a reduction of CP, NP-NPN content of milk respectively in 2 groups of mares fed either 6.7 and 5.5% DCP/kg DM referring to NRC, 1978 recommendations, or 8.7 and 5.4% DCP/kg DM referring to INRA, 1984 recommendations (8.8% kg DM) respectively. NP and NPN are simultaneously reduced because the content NP and NPN fractions is well linked (r = 0.80) (Doreau *et al.*, 1988). The elevation of DCP content of diet from 5.4 to 8.7% kg DM increase the urea content of milk (Doreau *et al.*, 1988) because of the amount of ammonia produced by the increase of the alimentary nitrogen degradation in the large intestine. It is well established now that ammonia is the main nitrogen end products of fermentation which is absorbed in the large intestine to contribute to the urea cycle in the horse (see review of Martin-Rosset and Tisserand, 2004). If we consider in horses as in other farm animals that urea concentration is the same in blood as in milk; the higher plasma urea concentration measured in mare fed the higher nitrogen allowances by Doreau *et al.*, 1988 supports the hypothesis made about the digestive and metabolic process.

Methods for evaluating nutrients requirements and recommended allowances

Definitions

Requirements and recommended allowances have to be clearly distinguished. The requirements stand for estimated or measured physiological expenditure of energy and protein in horses during different physiological situations. Allowances stand for the amount of nutrients, which are provided by the appropriate ration to meet the requirement of horses, and thus includes estimation of energy and protein provided by feed. Recommended allowances stand for the amount of nutrients provided by the ration optimised for meeting the goal of production and utilisation of horses – these link the breeders' goal, the physiological requirements of the horse and feed allowances. It means that the amount of nutrients required for milk of the same mare, can be lower, equal or higher than the nutritional requirements depending on husbandry or/and economical aims.

Methods for determination

Requirements are basically determined by factorial method. For maintenance, requirements are determined using balance experiments and then appropriate nutrients conversion rates for calculation. For lactation, requirements are determined using milk production, based on average daily milk yield, nutrients content of milk, and then nutrients conversion rates if these are known. Allowances are determined by global method e.g. feeding experiments carried out with a high number of animals during long period corresponding to husbandry system to include the effect of individual animal variation, environmental factors as far as animals are expected to be in good health and well managed. In these experiments energy and nitrogen intakes are related to the true milk yield and body weight, body condition score variation.

Evaluation of energy requirements

Calculation of energy requirements in different countries: data base – methodology – requirements

US

In US according to NRC, 1989 (National Research Council) daily energy requirements for maintenance and lactation are calculated by using the following equations:

DE = (Maintenance) + (Lactation)

- 200 kg of BW

DE = (1.4 + 0.3 BW) + (0.04 BW ∗ 3.311) from foaling to 3 months
+ (0.03 BW ∗ 3.311) from 3 months to weaning

- 400 – 600 kg of BW

DE = (1.4 + 0.3 BW) + (0.03 BW ∗ 3.311) from foaling to 3 months
+ (0.02 BW ∗ 3.311) from 3 months to weaning

- 600 – 900 kg of BW

DE = (1.82 + 0.0383 BW – 0.00015 BW^2)
+ 0.03 BW * 3.311) from foaling to 3 months
+ (0.02 BW * 3.311) from 3 months to weaning

Where

DE = Digestible Energy (MJ/day)
BW = Body Weight (kg)
3.311 = DE content 1 kg of milk (MJ/kg)

Milk yield of mares of light breeds are assumed to be 3 and 2 percent BW during early lactation (0 – 3 months) and late lactation (4 – 6 months) respectively from Doreau *et al.*, 1980, Gibbs *et al.*, 1982 and Oftedal *et al.*, 1983. Milk yield of pony mares was estimated to be 4 and 3 percent BW during early and late lactation respectively (Neuhaus, 1959).

Referring to NRC, 1978, GE content of one kg of milk was estimated to contain 2.056 MJ/kg (Neseni *et al.*, 1959; Ullrey *et al.*, 1966) and horses were expected to convert DE into milk energy with 60 percent efficiency. Hence 3.311MJ/kg of milk are required for each kg of milk produced whatever the stage of lactation.

Requirements of NRC, 1978 were refined using the observations of Jordan, 1979; Zimmerman, 1981; Drepper *et al.*, 1982; Pagan *et al.*, 1984; Pagan and Hintz, 1986b.
The daily energy requirements of 500 kg BW mare are stated in Table 1 using appropriate model.

Table 1. Daily energy requirement in lactating mare (500 kg BW) according to NRC, 1989 (MJ DE/day).

	Maintenance + milk yield	
Maintenance	0 – 3 Months	3 Months - Weaning
68.6	118.3	101.6

Germany

In Germany according to GEH, 1994 (Gesellschaft für Enärhungsphysiologie) daily requirements for maintenance and lactation are calculated by using the following equation

DE = (Maintenance) + (Lactation)
for mares which weight from 100 to 800 kg.

Maintenance is calculated using the equation

DE = 0.6 MJ/kg BW^{75} based on Hoffman *et al.*, 1967; Knox *et al.*, 1970; Wooden *et al.*, 1970; Argenzio and Hintz, 1971; Barth *et al.*, 1977.

Milk yield of the mares is assumed to be 0.14 – 0.17 and 0.12 BW^{75} at 1st, 3rd and 5th months of lactation respectiviely from Neseni *et al.*, 1958; Neuhaus, 1960, Bowman and Van Der Schee, 1975 and GE content is 2.44 – 2.32 and 2.12 MJ/kg milk for the corresponding stages of lactation from NRC, 1989 and Coenen, 1992. Efficiency rate of energy for milk secretion is assumed to be 66 percent (Gutte, 1972).

$$DE = (0.6\ MJ/kg\ BW^{75}) + (0.12 \text{ to } 0.17\ kg\ milk/kg\ BW^{75} * \frac{2.12 \text{ to } 2.44\ MJ/kg\ milk)}{0.66}$$

Where

DE = Digestible Energy (MJ)
BW^{75} = Metabolic body weight

The daily requirements of 500 kg BW mare are calculated using this model (Table 2).

Table 2. Daily requirements in lactating mare (500 kg BW) according to GEH, 1994 (MJ DE/day).

	Maintenance + milk yield		
Maintenance	1 Month	3 Months	5 Months
69.7	118.0	124.0	104.0

France

In France according to INRA, 1984-1990 (Institut National de la Recherche Agronomique) requirements for daily energy requirements for maintenance and lactation are calculated by using the following equations:

NE = (Maintenance) + (Lactation)

$$NE\ (MJ/d) = (0.351\ MJ * BW^{75}) + (kg\ Milk * \frac{BW}{100} * GE * \frac{km}{kl})$$

$$NE\ (UFC/d) = (0.038\ UFC * BW^{75}) + (kg\ Milk * \frac{BW}{100} * GE * \frac{km}{kl})/NEm$$

Where

NE = Net Energy expressed either in MJ or UFC
NEm = 9.2 MJ/kg: NE of 1 kg barley at maintenance (UFC system: Martin-Rosset *et al.*, 1994)
BW = Body Weight
BW^{75} = Metabolic body weight
GE = Gross Energy content/kg milk (MJ/kg)
km = Efficiency rate of energy for maintenance (UFC System) -= 0.785
kl = Efficiency rate of ME for lactation = 0.65

Milk yield of the mares is assumed to be 3.0 – 2.5 and 2.0 kg/100 kg at 1st; 2-3; and over 4 months of lactation respectively using the data drawn from the review of Doreau and Boulot, 1989a, and data from experiments of Doreau *et al.*, 1992. GE content of was estimated to be 2.404 – 2.096 and 1.986 MJ/kg of milk at the same months of lactation, and referring to the same publications. And the efficiency rate of ME to NE is assumed by INRA, 1990 (Martin-Rosset *et al.*, 1994) to be 65 percent, intermediary between the cow and the sow as previously assessed by INRA, 1984. Hence 3.698; 3.215; 3.055 MJ NE/kg of milk are required to produce 1 kg of milk at 1; 2-3 and over 4 months of lactation: or 0.316; 0.275; 0.261 UFC/kg of milk

Requirements published by INRA, 1984 were slightly reduced by INRA, 1990 as milk yield and GE content were lowered except for the 1st month. The daily requirements of a 500 kg BW mare are calculated using this model (Table 3).

Table 3. Daily requirements in lactating mare (500 kg BW) according to INRA, 1990 (MJ NE or UFC/day).

	Maintenance + milk yield			
	Maintenance	1 Month	2-3 Months	4 Months - Weaning
NE (MJ)	39.0	82.6	70.6	63.0
UFC	4.2	9.0	7.7	6.8

The Netherlands

In the Netherlands according to CVB, 1996; 2005 (Central Veevoeder Bureau) daily, requirements for maintenance and lactation are calculated by using the following equation

NE = (maintenance) + (Lactation)

$$NE = (0.348 \text{ or } 0.367 * BW^{75}) + \left(\frac{BW}{100} * \frac{\text{kg Milk}}{100 \text{ kg BW}} * GE * \frac{km}{kl}\right)$$

where

NE = Net Energy (MJ/kg BW^{75}):
0.348 MJ/kg BW^{75} for Underbred mares and 0.367 MJ/kg BW^{75} for Thoroughbred mares
BW = Body Weight (kg)
BW^{75} = Metabolic body weight
GE = Gross Energy (MJ/kg)
km = Efficiency rate at maintenance: 0.779
kl = Efficiency rate for milk: 0.62

$$\frac{km}{kl} = 1.25$$

Milk yield of light and heavy breeds was assumed to be 2.5; 3.0; 2.5 percent of BW for 1st; 2 – 3 and 4-6 months of lactation respectively. Milk yield of pony mares was estimated to be 3.0; 3.5; 3.0 percent of BW for the same stage of lactation respectively. GE per kg of milk was fixed at 2.41; 2.09; 1.99 MJ for all the breeds and the stage of lactation previously mentioned.

Kl was assumed to be 0.62 whereas km is 0.779. In CVB, 2005 system energy requirement are evaluated in NE for maintenance. Hence NE requirement calculated should be multiplied by the ratio km/kl. And NE is expressed in EWpa a Dutch unit (Energie worden paard) and 1 EWpa = 8.93 MJ Nem/kg DM).

The daily requirements of a 500 kg BW mare are calculated using this model (Table 4).

Table 4. Daily energy requirements (EWpa) for lactating mare (500 kg BW) according to CVB, 1996; 2005).

		Lactating (maintenance + milk)		
Maintenance		1 Month	2-3 Months	4-5 Months
NE MJ	36.8	74.4	76.0	67.9
Ewpa	4.1	8.3	8.5	7.6

Scandinavia

In Scandinavia according to Austbo, 2004 daily requirements for maintenance and lactation are calculated by using the following equation.

NE = (maintenance) + (Lactation)

For maintenance

NE = 0.351 MJ/kg BW^{75} referring to INRA
NE = 0.0373 UFC/BW^{75} in Denmark, Norway and Island
Me = 0.50 MJ/kg BW^{75} in Sweden (SLU, 2004)
ME = 0.0429 Fu/kg BW^{75} in Finland (MTT, 2004)

Where

NE = Net Energy (MJ)
UFC = Unité Fourragère Cheval (Horse Feed Unit) in Denmark, Norway, Island
ME = Metabolisable Energy (MJ) in Sweden (SLU, 2004)
Fu = Feed Unit (expressed in ME) in Finland (MTT, 2004) - Fu is based on the ME content of 1 kg Barley (1 Fu = 11.7 MJ ME)

The following factors should be implemented to calculate energy requirements accross the different systems

1 UFC = 13.45 MJ NE
1 UFC = 1.15 Fu
1 MJ ME = 0.0743 UFC
1 MJ ME = 0.0855 Fu
1 Fu = 11.17 MJ ME
1 Fu = 0.87 UFC

For the Nordic Countries it is suggested that the requirement for maintenance should be corrected for type of horses:

- Cold blooded ponies and draught horses: no correction
- Warm blood horse and Cold blooded trotters: + 5% correction
- Thoroughbred: + 10% correction

Milk yield is estimated to be similar to that proposed by CVB, 1996. GE content of milk is assumed to be 2.41; 2.09; 1.99 MJ/kg milk and ME or NE Content of milk expressed in the different systems is given in the Table 5

Table 5. ME or NE Content of 1 kg milk.

	Unit	1st Mont		2-3 Months		4-5 Months	
		≤ 200 kg	> 200 kg	≤ 200 kg	> 200 kg	≤ 200 kg	> 200 kg
Denmark Norway Island	UFC (NE)	0.32		0.28		0.26	
Sweden (SLU, 2004)	MJ (ME)	4.32		3.73		3.56	
Finland (MTT, 2004)	Fu (ME)	0.37		0.32		0.30	

And total daily energy requirements of a 500 kg BW mare are stated in the Table 6.

Table 6. Daily energy requirements in lactating (500 kg BW) in SCAND, 2004: Denmark; Norway; Island; Sweden (SLU, 2004); Finland (MTT, 2004).

	Unit	1st Month	2-3 Months	4-5 Months
Denmark Norway Island	UFC (NE)	8.1	8.3	7.4
Sweden (SLU, 2004)	MJ (ME)	106.9	108.9	96.9
Finland (MTT, 2004)	Fu (ME)	9.1	9.3	8.3

Comparison of the variations of energy requirements according to the month of lactation

In Table 7 the proportional increase with month of lactation in energy requirements, with requirements at maintenance set as a reference point, is shown for the different system.

Table 7. Comparison of variation of energy requirements across the different systems.

	NRC 1989	GEH 1994	INRA 1990	CVB 2005	SCAND 2004
Maintenance	100	100	100	100	100
Lactation					
1st month	173	169	212	202	200
2-3 months	173	177	182	206	204
4-6 months	149	149	162	184	182

The relative variation of total energy requirement to maintenance requirement are very similar between NRC and GEH on one hand and between CVB and SCAND on the other hand. INRA is intermediary position. The maximum variation takes place in the 1st – 3rd months of lactation for all the systems except INRA where maximum is in the 1st month of lactation.The discrepancy could be explained by the milk yield (Table 8) and the energy content per kg of milk with the 1st month of lactation sites a reference point.

Table 8. Comparison of milk yield during lactation across the different systems in a 500 kg BW mare (Milk yield/500 kg BW).

Lactation	NRC 1989	GEH 1994	INRA 1990	CVB 2005	SCAND 2004
1st month	100	100	100	100	100
	(3.0)	(3.0)	(3.0)	(2.5)	(2.5)
2-3 months	100	120	83	120	120
	(3.0)	(3.6)	(2.5)	(3.0)	(3.0)
4-6 months	67	83	67	100	100
	(2.0)	(2.5)	(2.0)	(2.5)	(2.5)

The milk yield expressed in percent kg BW during the first month is 17 percent lower in CVB and SCAND estimation than in other systems, whereas it is similar between the NRC; GEH and INRA. The maximum of milk yield, is met at the 2nd months for all the recommendations, except for NRC and INRA. The maximum is very high for GEH, and rather similar for other recommendations except INRA which is 17 p. 100 lower. Milk yield in late lactation is 20 p. 100 higher for GEH, CVB and SCAND than for NRC and INRA.

Referring to a recent synthesis of the data available, the peak of milk yield takes place at the 2nd month of lactation (Doreau and Martin-Rosset, 2002). Milk yield could be more accurately estimated for the first two months using the relationship between the milk yield determined by the reference method: delution of deuterium oxide as a marker of foal body water (Doreau and Dussap, 1980) or predicted from the average daily gain (ADG) of the foal (Doreau *et al.*, 1986b).

1st month: milk yield/kg (d) = 10.6 * ADG $r = 0.81$ $n = 19$ $P < 0.01$
2nd month: milk yield/kg (d) = 13.7 * ADG $r = 0.74$ $n = 18$ $P < 0.01$

These estimations carried out using these models are similar to those determined by Bowman and Van der Schee, 1978 and Ofledal *et al.*, 1983. Hence a consensus could be stated about milk yield.

Table 9. Comparison of energy content (GE) of 1 kg of milk during lactation across the different systems (MJ/kg milk).

Lactation	NRC 1989	GEH 1994	INRA 1990	CVB 2005	SCAND 2002
1st month	100	100	100	100	100
	(2.056)	(2.441)	(2.404)	(2.404)	(2.404)
2-3 months	100	95	87	87	88
	(2.056)	(2.320)	(2.090)	(2.090)	(2.090)
4-6 months	100	87	83	83	81
	(2.056)	(2.120)	(1.986)	(1.986)	(1.986)

Except for NRC where GE content of milk is constant throughout the lactation, the relative variation is very close for all the other recommendations at the different periods of lactation. Absolute value of GE is very close for INRA-CVB and SCAND throughout the lactation whereas GE is higher for GEH and very low for NRC.

Energy content of milk is variable between recommendations because GE was determined either with an adiabatic bomb or calculated from fat, nitrogen and lactose using general relationship (Perrin, 1958) or equations specific to mares (Doreau *et al.*, 1986). Fat and lactose content vary strongly (Doreau and Boulot, 1989b) as it depends of sampling conditions (Doreau *et al.*, 1986a), method of analysis (Doreau *et al.*, 1985). Thus the direct determination of milk gross energy content seems more reliable.

From all the studies carried out it arises that milk energy content varies inversely with milk yield (see review of Doreau *et al.*, 1988a). As a result total energy output is less variable according to the physiological stage and between diets. For example, during the first 2 months of lactation the GE output of a 500 kg BW mare ranges between 30 to 40 MJ day-1 (Bowman and Van der Schee, 1978; Oftedal *et al.*, 1983; Doreau and Boulot, 1987). In a 800 kg BW mare, the value is 50-55 MJ day-1 (Doreau *et al.*, 1986b). These measures of total output are likely the most reliable and they should be implemented in the future to state a consensus.

The efficiency rate for DE range between 60 and 66 (NRC – GEH) and 60 – 65 for NE (INRA – CVB – SCAND). The variations in each group of systems DE vs NE are very narrow and contribute to similarity of energy requirements in those two groups of recommendations.

Evaluation of protein requirements

Calculation of protein requirements in different countries: data base – methodology – requirements

US

In US according NRC, 1989, daily protein requirements for maintenance and lactation are calculated by using the following equations:

g CP = (Maintenance) + (Lactation)

Maintenance requirement is estimated to be 0.6 g DP/kg BW/day using the data of Teeter *et al.*, 1967; Slade *et al.*, 1970; Hintz and Schryver, 1972; Prior *et al.*, 1974; Quinn, 1975; Meyer *et al.*, 1985

- Foaling to 3 months
  - 200 kg of BW

$$\text{g CP} = \frac{(0.6\text{ g DCP/kg BW}) + [(0.04\text{ BW x }0.021\text{ x }1.000)/0.65]}{0.55}$$

  - 400 – 900 kg of BW

$$\text{g CP} = \frac{(0.6\text{ g DCP/kg BW}) + [(0.03\text{ BW x }0.021\text{ x }1.000)/0.65]}{0.55}$$

- 3 months to weaning:
  - 200 kg of BW

$$g\,CP = \frac{(0.6\text{ g DCP/kg BW}) + [(0.03\text{ BW x }0.018\text{ x }1.000)/0.65]}{0.55}$$

  - 400 – 900 kg of BW

$$g\,CP = \frac{(0.6\text{ g DCP/kg BW}) + [(0.02\text{ BW x }0.018\text{ x }1.000)/0.65]}{0.55}$$

Where:

CP = Crude Protein (g)/day
DCP = Digestible Crude Protein (g)/day
BW = Body Weight (kg)

Milk yield is the means of the figures mentioned in Energy section. CP Content of milk were assumed to contain 2.1 percent (0.021) and 1.8 percent (0.018) in early (foaling – 3 months) and late (3 months – weaning) lactation respectively from the data of Ullrey *et al.*, 1966; Gibbs *et al.*, 1983; Oftedal, *et al.*, 1982; Zimmermann, 1985.

Referring to NRC, 1978, digestible protein (DP) is used with an efficiency of 65 percent (0.65) for milk production and protein digestibility in lactation diets is 55 percent (0.55). The daily protein requirements of a 500 kg BW mare are calculated using the appropriate model in Table 10.

Table 10. Daily protein requirements (g CP/day) in lactating mare according to NRC, 1989 (500 gBW).

	Maintenance + milk yield	
Maintenance	0 - 3 Months	4 Months - Weaning
656	1427	1048

Germany

In Germany according to GEH, 1994, daily protein requirement for maintenance and lactation are calculated by using the following model:

gDCP = (Maintenance) + (lactation)

Maintenance is calculated using the relationship: 3 g DCP/kg BW^{75} based on Olsson and Ruudvere, 1955; Teeter *et al.*, 1967; Slade *et al.*, 1975. Milk yield is the means of the figures mentioned in Energy section. Protein content of milk is estimated to be: 27, 22, 18 g CP/kg for 1, 2, 5 months of lactation respectively. Efficiency rate of protein for milk secretion is assumed to be 50 percent (0.50).

$$g\,DCP = (3\text{ gDCP/kg BW}^{75}) + (0.12\text{ to }0.17\text{ kg milk/kg BW}^{75} * \frac{27\text{ to }22\text{ gCP/kg milk)}}{0.50}$$

Where

CP = Crude Protein (g)/day
DCP = Digestible Crude Protein (g)/day
BW^{75} = Metabolic Body weight
0.50 = Efficiency rate of protein for milk production

The daily protein requirements of a 500 kg BW mare are calculated using this model (Table 10).

Table 11. Daily protein requirements (g DCP) in lactating mares (500 kg BW) according to GEH, 1994.

	Maintenance + milk yield		
Maintenance	1 Month	3 Months	5 Months
317	799	720	457

France

In France according to INRA, 1990, daily requirements for maintenance and lactation are calculated by using the following equation

g MADC/day = (Maintenance) + (Lactation)

Maintenance is estimated to be 2.8 g MADC/kg BW^{75} according Slade *et al.*, 1970; Prior *et al.*, 1974.

Milk yield is the means of the figures mentioned in Energy Section. And the protein Content (CP) of milk is 24 g/kg for 0-3 months and then 21 g/kg.

$$\text{g MADC} = (2.8 \text{ g MADC/kg BW}^{75}) + \left(\frac{BW}{100} * \text{kg milk/100 kg BW} * \text{g CP/kg milk}\right)/0.55$$

Where

MADC = Protein value expressed in MADC system: Matières Azotées Digestibles Cheval (Horse Digestible Crude Protein) (g/day).
CP = Crude Protein Content (g/kg milk)
BW = Body Weight (kg)
BW^{75} = Metabolic Body weight (kg)
0.55 = Efficiency rate of Protein for milk production

The efficiency rate of DCP was estimated to be 55 percent (0.55). As a result the protein allowances per kg of milk stand for 44 g, 36 g for the 0 – 3 month and then for the 4th month of lactation to weaning respectively (Martin-Rosset *et al.*, 1994).

The daily protein requirements for a 500 kg BWmare are calculated using this model (Table 12).

Table 12. Daily requirements g MADC of lactating mare (500 kg BW) according to INRA, 1990.

	Maintenance + milk yield		
Maintenance	1st Month	2-3 Months	4 Months - Weaning
296	950	770	660

The Netherlands

In the Netherlands according to CVB, 1996 and 2005, daily requirements for maintenance and lactation are calculated by using the following equation

g DCP = (Maintenance) + (Lactation)

$$g\ DCP = 3.0\ g\ DCP/kg\ BW^{75} + (\frac{BW}{100} x\ kg\ milk/100\ kg\ BW\ x\ g\ DCP/kg\ milk)$$

Where:

DCP = Digestible Crude Protein (g)/day
BW = Body Weight (kg)

CP concentration of milk was assumed to vary from 25-22 to 20 g/kg milk at 1st months; 2-3 months and 4-5 months of lactation. Efficiency rate of DCP for milk production is assumed to be 50 percent (0.50) and DCP concentration of milk is 50-44-40 g/kg milk for the corresponding period.

Daily protein requirements are calculated for a 500 kg BW mare using the milk yield mentioned in energy section (Table 13).

Table 13. Daily protein requirements (gDCP) of lactating mares (500 kg BW) according to CVB, 1996, 2005 and SCAND, 2004.

	Maintenance + milk yield		
Maintenance	1st Month	2-3 Months	4-5 Months
317	942	977	817

Scandinavia

In Scandinavia according to Austbo, 2004, daily requirements for maintenance and lactation are calculated by using the following model

g DCP = (Maintenance) + (Lactation)

For maintenance 3 g DCP/kg BW^{75}/day are assumed to meet the requirements

$$g\ DCP = 3.0\ g\ DCP/kg\ BW^{75} + (\frac{BW}{100} x\ kg\ milk/100\ kg\ BW\ x\ g\ DCP/kg\ milk)$$

Where

CP = Crude Protein (g)/day
DCP = Digestible Crude Protein (g)/day
BW = Body Weight (kg)

DCP concentration of 1 kg of milk and milk yield throughout the lactation is assumed according to CVB, 1996. Hence the daily DCP requirements for a 500 kg BW mare are the same as for CVB, 1996, 2005 (Table 13).

Comparison of the variation of protein requirements with month of lactation

When maintenance is set as a reference the proportional increase with month of lactation in protein requirements has been described in Table 14.

Table 14. Comparison of variation in protein requirements across the different systems.

	NRC 1989	GEH 1994	INRA 1990	CVB 2005	SCAND 2004
Maintenance	100	100	100	100	100
Lactation					
1st month	218	252	321	298	297
2-3 months	218	227	261	308	308
4-6 months	160	144	223	258	258

Relative variation of the total protein requirements to maintenance is very close for INRA-CVB and SCAND systems whereas these variation are very low for NRC and intermediary for GEH. The maximum variation takes place in the 1st month of lactation for all the systems except NRC and where the whole early lactation is concerned.

As for energy the discrepancy in the variation of requirements is firstly explained by the milk yield stated but difference in CP content of milk is involved to some extend as well (Table 15). The relative variation of CP content are very similar in all the systems except NRC where the CP content is constant during the whole early lactation and CP content is very low. The absolute value of DCP content is very close across the lactation for all European Systems. A consensus could be stated easily in Europe as far as milk yield are close and efficiency rate of DCP very similar 50-55 percent.

Table 15. Comparison of Crude Protein Content of 1 kg of milk (gCP/kg milk) during lactation across the different systems.

Lactation	NRC 1989	GEH 1994	INRA 1990	CVB 2005	SCAND 2002
1st month	100	100	100	100	100
	(21)	(27)	(24)	(25)	(25)
2-3 months	100	81	88	88	88
	(21)	(22)	(24)	(22)	(22)
4-6 months	86	67	83	80	80
	(18)	(18)	(21)	(20)	(20)

Recommended allowances for energy and protein in different countries

A recommended allowances is the amount of nutrients which should be supplied to horses to achieve a desirable level of performance consistent with their potential: genotype, stage of lactation, ... The horses are assumed to be in good health, well managed and housed during the winter period. These should be as optimum allowances which cover the physiological expenditure of horses so called net requirements. Exceptions are mares of heavy breeds or light breeds devoted to horse meat production or leisure horse production respectively, where a moderate and controlled use of body reserves is assumed during the winter period to reduce the feed costs. In all the situations: optimum, restricted or maximum allowances according to the types of horse production: race or sport horses, leisure horses, horses for meat production, energy and protein allowances are related to the intake capacity and to the amount and ability of body reserves to be mobilised throughout the lactation period to meet a nutritional balance compatible with normal milk yield, and reproductive performances.

Intake capacity

In Europe horses are routinely fed with high proportion of forages in the diet, except race horses. The ration is formulated in three steps as follows:

- Prediction of the maximum forage dry matter intake and calculation of the quantity of nutrients that is provided.
- The calculation of the quantity of nutrients to be supplied by the concentrates from the difference between the nutrients required and those supplied by the forage.
- The choice and the relative contribution of the ingredients of the concentrates in order to balance the ration in every respect and at the lowest cost.

A question of major concern arises. Is dry matter intake a limiting factor, to allow the mare to meet their requirements when the lactating mare is fed forage based diet?

Dry matter intake depends on the characteristic of feedstuffs (chemical composition, nutritive value, ..., etc.) so called ingestibility (Martin-Rosset and Doreau, 1984b; Martin-Rosset *et al.*, 1994); and to the characteristics of animals (Body weight, requirement, ..., etc.) so called intake capacity. If we assume that ingestibility would not be limiting in our conditions as far as straw, poor silage... are not considered, intake capacity is of major concern to propose recommendations for nutrient allowances. After foaling intake capacity increase tremendously to meet a peak and plateaued between 3 and 8 weeks depending on the quality of forage and the proportion of concentrate in the diet. (Figure 1). Daily intake rises from 2.2 kg/DM/100 kg BW to 2.8 – 3.5 kg DM/100 kg BW at 1st and 6th weeks of lactation respectively where forage are fed *ad libitum*. The range of variation is high as it is related to the quality of forage whereas the proportion of concentrate in the diet is low (Figure 1).

Mares cannot meet their energy and protein requirements in early lactation whereas they are fed *ad libitum* low quality forage and limited proportion of concentrate (Table 16) even if digesta passage in the trachtus is highly reduced: 22.2 hours in lactating mares vs 36.5 hours in dry mares (Miraglia *et al.*, 1992). As a result body reserves are mobilised (Table 16).

Intake of forage is strongly reduced whereas proportion of concentrate increases in the diet. Substitution rate average 1.2 kg DM of forage for each additional kg DM of concentrate in dry forage based diet (Figure 1)

Individual variability is high: 5 to 15 percent in early lactation (Doreau *et al.*, 1990a) and variability is higher, in mares fed high proportion of concentrate than in mares fed hay based diets (Doreau *et*

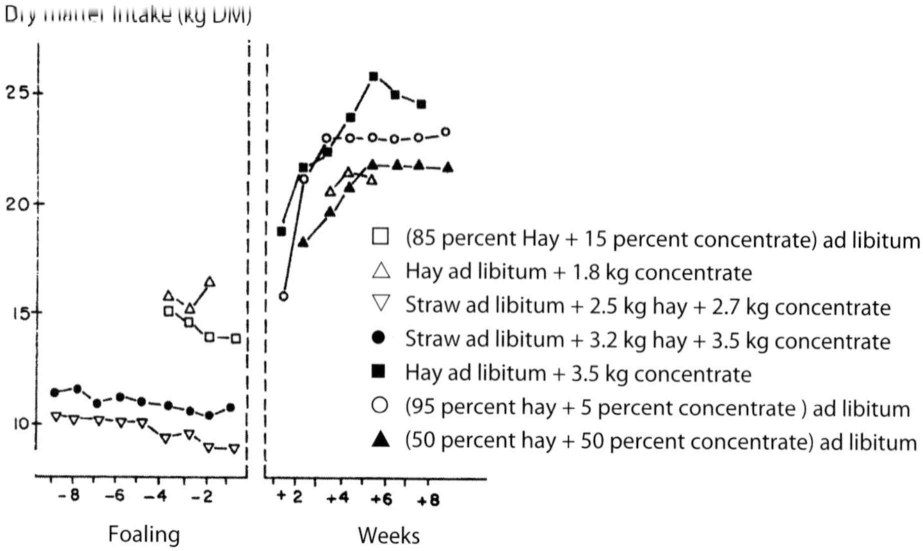

Figure 1. Dry matter intake of heavy mare in lactation (Martin-Rosset and Doreau, 1984b).

Table 16. Nutritients intake and balance in lactating mare (Anglo-Arabe and Selle Français) fed good or low quality hay based diets[1] (from Doreau et al., 1990a).

	Lactation	
	1st week	2nd – 5th weeks
Group low quality hay[1]		
Energy intake (UFC)	7.4	9.6
Protein intake (g MADC)	426	579
Energy balance[3] (percent)	76	99
Protein balance[3] (percent)	41	56
BW (kg)	575 ± 31	562 ± 35
BCS	3.20	1.93
Foal weight (kg)	-	96.9 ± 6.8
Group high quality hays[2]		
Energy intake (UFC)	11.0	14.1
Protein intake (g MADC)	1101	1431
Energy balance[3] (percent)	113	145
Protein balance[3] (percent)	106	138
BW (kg)	570 ± 34	581 ± 35
BCS	3.00	3.04
Foal weight (kg)	-	103.3 ± 7.6

[1]5.7% CP/kg DM; 38.2% ADF/kg DM
[2]11.7% CP/kg DM; 29.5% ADF/kg DM
[3]Ratio between intakes and theoretical requirements (INRA, 1990)

al., 1992). Parity would not influence significantly intake when comparing primiparous (less than 5 years at first foaling) to multiparous (Table 17).

Table 17. Effect of parity on intake and nutritient balance in mares of light breeds (Anglo Arab, Selle Français) (from Doreau et al., 1991).

	Primiparous	Multiparous
BW (kg): at foaling	510	529
Intake		
kg DM: week 1	12.8	12.5
kg DM: week 4	17.8	17.7
kg DM/100 kg BW: week 4	3.36	3.27
g DM/kg BW^{75}: week 4	161	158
Energy balance		
week 1	96	83
week 4	133	118
Protein balance		
week 1	98	90
week 4	137	127

Voluntary intake is strongly affected by body condition at foaling (Doreau, 1994). Compared to fat mares, thin mares can increase dry matter intake when they are fed ad libitum to compensate partially the deficit of energy balance during the first month of lactation (Figures 2 and 3).

Intake capacity is affected by the climatic environnement. Intake capacity of the mare conducted in the stables fed the same diet as mares managed in paddocks would increase by 20 p. 100 (Martin-Rosset, 1982). NRC, 1989 and INRA, 1990 proposed feed intake to meet the requirements in their recommendations (Table 18).

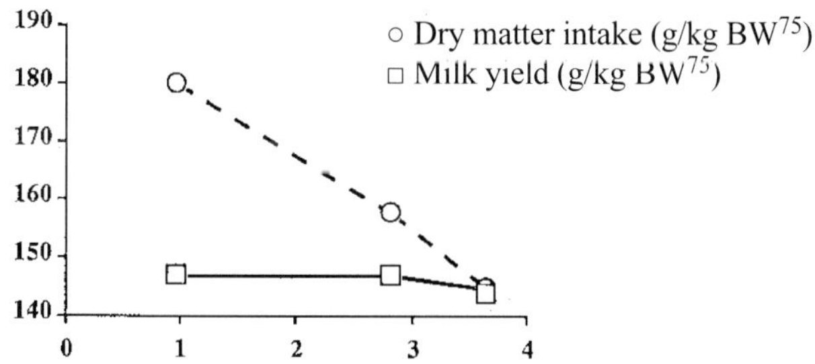

Figure 2. Influence of body condition score at foaling on voluntary feed intake and milk yield at one month of lactation (from Doreau et al., 1991a and Doreau et al., 1993).

Table 18. Feed intake (percent BW) of lactating mares to meet the requirements.

	Forage		Concentrate		F/C		Total	
	NRC	INRA	NRC	INRA	NRC	INRA	NRC	INRA
Early lactation	1.0-2.0	1.3-2.2	1.0-2.0	0.7-1.8	40/60	60/40	2.0-3.0	2.0-3.2
Late lactation	1.0-2.0	1.3-1.8	0.5-1.5	0.3-0.6	60/40	80/20	2.0-2.5	1.6-2.5

Total feed intake seems to be close. Hintz and Cymbaluk, 1994 concluded that calculations based on either systems when expressed in terms of feed intake rather than DE or UFC units yield similar values. Indeed the difference between NRC and INRA systems are much greater that mentioned whereas the composition of diet expected to meet the requirements in each system is calculated using the appropriate procedure described by Martin-Rosset and Vermorel, 2004.
The procedure is to calculate the quantities of feeds and the composition of diets necessary to meet the energy and protein requirements of the lactating mare. The characteristics of the feeds used are given in the Table 19.

Table 19. Chemical composition and nutritive value of feeds (for NRC/INRA systems).

		/kg DM							
Feeds	DM g/kg	DE (Mcal)	NE (Mcal)	CF (g)	CP (g)	DCP (g)	MADC (g)	CP/ DE	MADC/ NE
Good grass hay (n° 62)*	850	2.34	1.34	333	102	59	50	44	37
Poor grass hay (n° 70)*	850	1.69	0.92	382	76	37	31	45	34
Barley grain (n° 120)*	860	3.56	2.55	54	117	92	92	33	36
Soyabean meal extracted 48-50 (n° 130)*	883	4.20	2.40	39	545	496	496	130	207

*Tables INRA, 1990

The energy value (DE or NE per kg DM) and nitrogen value (CP or MADC, per kg DM) of each diet and the amount of feed required to meet energy and nitrogen requirements were computed in each energy and nitrogen system. In a first approach, the hay to concentrate ratio was that proposed by NRC, 1989. Then, in a second step, the hay to concentrate ratio tested was that proposed by INRA, 1990.

For the lactating mare fed a hay and concentrate diet supplemented with the same concentrate percentage proposed by NRC, TDMI of rations are 10 to 13 percent higher with INRA rations than with NRC rations at 1st month of lactation, according to quality of hay. Thereafter differences come to be erratic (0.1 to 7.2 percent). For mares fed a hay and concentrate diet supplemented with the concentrate percentage proposed by INRA, TDMI of INRA rations are 14 to 18 percent higher than the NRC ration in early lactation, according to hay quality. The differences decrease as late lactation approaches. As a result DE provided by balanced rations calculated in the INRA system supplemented with concentrate percentage proposed by INRA are 5 to 24% lower than DE requirement (NRC) in the first and fourth months of lactation; NE provided by a NRC ration calculated in the NRC system supplemented by adequate concentrate percentage in the NRC approach are 3 to 10% lower than NE requirements (INRA) (Table 20). And NE requirements can be nearly met because NRC ration is supplemented with 50 percent concentrate whereas INRA ration is supplemented with 39 percent concentrates only.

Discrepancies are very difficult to interpret further, as there are strong interactions either with the relative NRC/INRA requirements (energy and protein), and the evolution of the requirement during lactation (Table 21), or with the hay and concentrate substitution rate on DM basis and to the respective protein/energy ratios of hay, barley and soybean in each system.

Table 20. Comparison of balanced ration calculated in either NRC and INRA systems balanced for energy and protein for the lactating mare (500 kg BW).

		DM (kg)	C (%)	DE (MJ)	CP (g)	NE (MJ)
NRC	Hay (good)	5.00		48.91	510	28.01
	Barley	4.30		64.00	503	45.81
	Soyabean	0.70	50	16.47	382	7.02
Requirements NRC:		10.00		129.38	1395	80.84
118.29 MJ/DE DE						
1427 g CP			NE provided by NRC ration			= - 9.28 MJ
2.0 < TDM1 % BW < 3.0		(2.0% BW)	NE requirements (INRA)			(- 10%)

		DM (kg)	C (%)	DE (MJ)	CP (g)	NE (MJ)
INRA	Hay (good)	7.26	(%)	40.67	363	71.06
	Barley	4.27		45.47	392	63.54
	Soyabean	0.36	39	3.60	179	6.31
Requirements NRC		11.89		89.74	934	140.91
90.12 MJ NE						
950 g MADC			DE provided by INRA ration			= - 28.55 MJ
2.4 < TDM1 % BW < 3.0		(2.4% BW)	DE requirements (NRC)			(- 24%)

Table 21. Energy and protein requirements of mare (500 kg BW) related to maintenance in DE and CP system (NRC, 1989) and NE and MADC systems (INRA, 1990). Relative difference between the systems.

	Energy			Protein		
	NRC	INRA	% NRC/INRA	NRC	INRA	% NRC/INRA
Maintenance	100	100	100	100	100	100
Lactation						
1st month	173	212	82	218	321	68
2-3 months	173	182	95	218	261	84
4-6 months	148	162	92	160	223	72

Role of body reserves

Fat content of adult horses range between 8 to 14 percent of body weight that means 40 to 70 kg of body reserves in mares of 500 kg BW (Martin-Rosset *et al.*, 1983; Robelin *et al.*, 1984). In lactating mare the manipulation of dietary energy intake significantly affects body weight and body fat content (Martin-Rosset and Doreau, 1980; Doreau *et al.*, 1981; Henneke *et al.*, 1981). Hence body condition score systems were proposed by NRC, 1989 and INRA, 1990 to estimate the relative variation of body reserves in horses (NRC, 1989; INRA-HN-IE, 1997).

The optimal level of energy to be supplied to lactating mares has to be defined to recommend energy allowances. The aim of recommended allowances should be to maximize foal growth and/or to maximize the reproductive rate. Henneke *et al.*, 1981 observed that the live weight gain of the foals was higher when mares were fat at foaling, than when mares were thin, even they were overfed in lactation. In this case, the rebuilding of body reserves seemed to take priority over milk yield and subsequent foal growth. This result was also observed by Martin-Rosset and Doreau, 1980: mares either fat or thin at foaling, fed the same level of feeding during lactation, which correspond to the expected requirements increased their body weight, by 13 and 35 kg during the first month of lactation respectively, while foals of thin mares grew more slowly than foals of fat mares (Table 22).

Table 22 Effect of body reserves at foaling on weight gain of the foals (from Martin-Rosset and Doreau, 1980).

	Years of experiments		1978		1979	
Mares			HL	LL	HL	LL
Level of energy intake in pregnancy[1]			100	80	100	80
	Number of mares at foaling		10	7	12	12
Level of energy intake in lactation[1]			100	100	100	100
	Variation of Body weight (1st month) (kg)		+ 2	+ 28	+ 24	+ 41
Foals						
	Birth	Date (days)	14/4	12/4	13/4	17/4
			(± 23)	(± 18)	(± 13)	(+ 24)
		Body weight/kg	63.6	70.3	63.3	65.3
			(± 5.9)	(± 7.7)	(± 5.8)	(+ 5.5)
		0-1 month	1991	1741	1793	1656
			(± 619)	(± 411)	(± 394)	(+ 345)
	Growth (g/day)	Birth to Weaning	1511	1539	1480	1472
			(± 186)	(± 95)	(± 163)	(+ 156)

[1]Relative to nutrient requirement (NRC, 1978)
HL: High Level; LL: Low Level

Comparing 2 groups of mares fed either 65 or 100 percent of requirements in late pregnancy, and then 100 percent of requirement in early lactation, daily gain of foals of restricted mares was lower (21 percent) than the foals of mares always well fed (Martin-Rosset and Doreau, 1984a). In another experiment thin an fat mares at foaling fed ad libitum the same diet during the first two months of lactation were compared (Table 23).

Dry matter intake of thin mares was higher but milk energy output was lower than those of fat mares respectively. Body reserves were therefore rapidly but partially restored. In fat mares, a part of milk energy output came probably from body reserves (Figure 3).

In thin mares the body condition score increased when the level of plasma non estrefied fatty acids suggests fat mobilisation (Table 23). This means that, in thin mares, both lipolyses and lipogenesis could take place in early lactation. Owing to their high level of intake, mares seem to be able to gain body lipid after foaling and to maintain a high level of milk yield. The occurrence of lipid mobilisation even when there was a positive energy balance supports that part of the milk originates from adipose tissue even in thin mares.

Table 23. Effect of body condition of mares (Selle Français, Anglo-arabe) at foaling on subsequent performances in early lactation (from Doreau et al., 1993).

		Body conditions at foaling	
		Fat	Thin
Body condition score[1]		> 3.5	< 1.5
Number of mares		5	6
Intake (kg DM/d)	1st week	13.7*	15.1*
	4th week	16.1*	19.6*
	8th week	18.0*	21.2*
Milk yield (kg/d)	1st week	15.1	13.2
	8th week	17.8	16.8
Milk gross energy output (MJ/d)	1st week	33.4	29.9
	8th week	36.1	31.3
Energy balance (UFC/d)	1st week	- 0.44**	1.13**
	4th week	0.78**	3.53**
	8th week	1.78**	4.48**
Body condition score	1st week	3.65**	0.96**
	8th week	3.40**	1.38**
Body weight change (kg/d)	1st – 4th week	- 0.33	+ 0.16
	4th - 8th week	+ 0.22	+ 0.46
Non esterfied fatty acids (mMol/l)	1st week	0.486**	0.176**
	8th week	0.251**	0.090**

* P < 0.05; ** P < 0.01

[1]According to method INRA – HN – IE, 1997

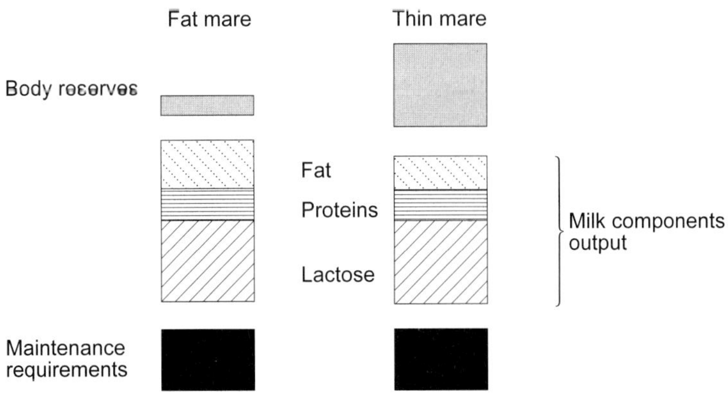

Figure 3. Utilisation of metabolisable energy intake: distribution between requirements for maintance, lactation and storage of body reserves (calculations from Doreau et al., 1993 experiments).

All these experiments point out that milk yield and energy output (and related ADG of foals) are strongly related to body condition score at foaling and feeding level in early lactation.

Effect of feeding level or/and body reserves on reproductive performance

Mares fed during the fall and winter to be maintained in moderately fat to fat body condition (6.5 < BCS < 8.0 according to NRC, 1989 scale: 0 to 10) continued to cycle throughout the winter (Gentry *et al.*, 2002). Mares which enters the breeding season with a BCS over than 5 ovulated sooner than mares with BCS lower than 5 (Kubiak *et al.*, 1987). Intervals from parturition to foal heat ovulation and from parturition to the second post partum ovulation are similars in mares in fat or moderate conditions (Carvinder *et al.*, 2005). Anovulatory period was extended in mares with moderate or fat body conditions fed restricted amount of energy (Gentry *et al.*, 2002) or in mare maintained in thin conditions (Kubiak *et al.*, 1987).

Low BCS at foaling did not affect reproductive efficiency of mares if they are well fed in early lactation (Banach and Evans, 1981; Henneke *et al.*, 1981). But fertilization rate decreased whereas embryonic mortality increased whereas the mares were underfed in late pregnancy and early lactation (Henneke *et al.*, 1981a). The number of cycle for conception is higher and the conception rate is higher as well in mares entering the breeding season in moderate body condition than in thin mares (Henneke *et al.*, 1984). Similarly the number of cycles for conception is higher in thin mares at foaling and fed only their theoretical requirements in early lactation which did not allow the restoration of body reserves (Martin-Rosset and Doreau, 1984a).

Mechanisms which are involved in the influence of energy status and reproductive performance are described in the chapter entitled: Interaction of nutrition and ovarian activity of this issue (see Guillaume *et al.*).

Recommended allowances for energy

The allowances recommended by NRC, 1989, GEH, 1994, CVB, 1996; 2005, SCAND, 2004 correspond to the requirements (tables 1, 2, 4, 6), whereas the allowances proposed by INRA, 1990 are related to body condition score of the mare at foaling and goal of production: sport horses vs leisure horses or heavy breeds (Table 24) based on energy balance performed in feeding experiments.

Recommended allowances for protein

The allowances recommended by all the systems correspond to the requirements (Tables 10, 11, 12, 13) as the effects of protein allowances on mare milk yield and foal daily gain are not very well stated.

In early lactation milk yield would be reduced in mares fed isoenergetic diet with 5.5 vs 6.7 percent of DCP (Meadows *et al.*, 1979). Daily gain of foals would be improved as far as DCP intake of the mares reaches 10 g/kg BW75 (Ott, 1970). Comparing two diets with 10 and 7.7 percent of DCP Peltonen *et al.*, 1980 observed an improvement of foals daily gain too whereas Rogers *et al.*, 1981 did not determine significant effect. Jordan, 1985 did not observe any significant effect on daily gain of foals whereas the mares were fed isoenergetic diet with 11.2 or 14.7 percent DCP. Comparing three groups of lactating mares fed during the whole lactation either 100 p. 100 (group 1) or 160 p. 100 (groups 2 – 3) of NRC, 1989, requirements Van Niekerk and Van Niekerk, 1997a, showed that the mares of group 1 lost 25 kg and the body weight of their foals at weaning were 24 p. 100 lighter, NRC, 1989 recommendation would be too low. Similarly average daily gain of foals during the 30 days following birth was lower when nursing mares weres fed only 60 percent of INRA, 1984 requirements (Table 25). No difference was observed at weaning with foals nursed by mares fed 100 percent of INRA, 1984 requirements. Body weight of the mare was not affected by the restriction of protein allowances (Table 25).

Table 24. Recommended total daily energy allowances (UFC and MADC) of lactating mares according to INRA, 1990.

	UFC		gMADC	TDMi[10]
	HL	LL	NL[9]	kg DM
500 kg BW				
Dry mares	4.6[3]	3.8[4]	295	6.0 – 8.5
Lactation				
1st month	10.7[1]	8.9[2]	950	12.0 – 15.0
2-3 months	9.2[1]	7.6[2]	770	10.0 – 15.0
4 months - weaning	7.5[3]	6.1[4]	660	8.0 – 12.5
700 kg BW				
Dry mares	5.2[7]	4.2[8]	380	6.5 – 9.5
Lactation				
1st month	13.0[5]	10.7[6]	1295	14.5 – 21.5
2-3 months	11.0[5]	9.0[6]	1045	12.0 – 18.5
4 months - weaning	8.9[7]	7.1[8]	890	9.5 – 15.0

UFC: Horse Feed Unit; MADC: Horse Digestible Crude Protein
1 UFC = 9.20 MJ NE (INRA, 1990)

[1]HL: High Level:	120 p. 100 requirements: BCS < 3	Optimum BCS: 3.0 – 3.5 at foaling for light breeds (500 kgBW)
[2]LL: Low Level:	110 p. 100 requirements: BCS ≥ 3	
[3]HL:	110 p. 100 requirements: BCS < 3	
[4]LL:	90 p. 100 requirements: BCS ≥ 3	
[5]HL:	110 p. 100 requirements: BCS < 3	Optimum BCS: 2.5 - 3.0 at foaling for heavy breeds (700 kg BW)
[6]LL:	90 p. 100 requirements: BCS ≥ 3	
[7]HL:	100 p. 100 requirements: BCS < 3	
[8]LL:	80 p. 100 requirements: BCS ≥ 3	
[9]NL:Normal Level:	100 p. 100 requirements for all breeds	

[10]TDMi: Total Dry Matter Intake

Table 25. Effect of protein allowances in nursing mares of heavy breeds fed isoenergetic diet on mare and foal performances (from Doreau et al., 1988).

	HL[1]	LL[2]
Number of mares	10	10
Body weight (kg) (at foaling)	743	743
Energy intake (UFC/d)	10.38	10.77
Protein intake (gMADC/d)	1291[1]	805[2]
Average daily gain of foals (g/d)		
0 – 30 d	1923	1706
0 – 160 d	1640	1631
Mare body weight		
0 – 30 d (kg/d)	- 0.213	- 0.203
Time interval between foaling and fertilisation	25.0	18.3
Plasma urea of the mare (mg/100 ml)	41.6	25.1

[1]HL: 100 percent protein requirements (INRA, 1984)
[2]LL: 60 percent protein requirements (INRA, 1984)

The effect of dietary protein on reproduction in the mare is much less documented than for energy. The mares fed 160 p. 100 of NRC, 1989 requirement during lactation ovulated 2 - 3 weeks earlier than mares fed 100 p. 100 of NRC, 1989, but the duration of the subsequent oestrous cycle was not affected (Van Niekerk and Van Niekerk, 1997b). 40 p. 100 restriction of protein allowances would not affect time interval between foaling and first heat or time interval between foaling and fertilisation (Doreau *et al.*, 1988).

Discussion and conclusion

Harmonisation of requirements in Europe

In Europe Energy requirements are 1.7 – 2.1; 1.8 -2.0; 1.5 – 1.9 times maintenance for 1st; 2 – 3 months; 4 – 6 months of lactation respectively. Similarly protein requirements are 2.5 – 3.0; 2.3 – 3.0; 1.4 – 2.5 times maintenance for the same periods of lactation.

A consensus could be met easily in Europe about the estimation of energy and protein requirements of brood mares as all the systems used a factorial approach. There is evidence now that milk yield peaks at the second month of lactation and variation of milk yield with other physiological stages is very similar. Energy and protein content per kg of milk are very close. Efficiency rates for energy and protein synthesis range very closely. Maintenance requirements are very similar. As a result energy and protein requirements relative to maintenance should be maximum at the second month of lactation; higher at the first month than in late lactation (3 – 6 months).

Allowances vs requirement

Requirements should be validated using experimental data from feeding trials carried out to check that all the models which have been stated are consistent. This validation was carried out for INRA systems and this could contribute to the harmonisation of the recommendations.But additional data from feeding trials should be carried out to take in to account the effects of breeds diversity and environmental factors due to local conditions to perform specific allowances in the different European Countries.

Interaction between feed allowances and reproductive efficiency should be considered to determine the optimal allowances in different situations as well, namely for Thoroughbred, Standardbred mares which are devoted to foal early in the year and to other breeds to secure a foal each year and a short interval foaling-fertilisation post partum (see Guillaume *et al.*, Ellis *et al.*, Falaschini *et al.*, in this issue).

For all these purposes allowances should be related to optimal body condition score at key points: foaling and drying. Hence allowances should be adapted to the breed and goal of production: athlete horses vs leisure horses, vs heavy breed bred for races or sport, hacking and horse meat respectively.

References

Argenzio, R.A. and H.F. Hintz, 1971. Volatile fatty acid tolerance and effect of glucose and VFA on plasma insulin levels in ponies. J. Nutr., 191, 723.

Austbo, D., 2004. The Scandinavian adaptation of the French UFC system. In European Workshop: Nutrition of the performance horse. V. Julliand and W. Martin-Rosset (eds.), EAAP publication no. 111, Wageningen Academic Publishers, The Netherslands, 69-78.

Banach, M.A. and J.W. Evans, 1981. Effects of inadequate energy during gestation and lactation on the oestrous cycle and conception rates of mares and on their foal weights. In: Proceedings 7th Nutrition Physiology Symposium, Warrenton, W.V., 97-100.

Barth, K.M., J.W. Williams and D.G. Brown, 1977. Digestible energy requirements of working and non-working ponies. J. Anim. Sci., 44, 585-589.

Bowman, H. and W. van Der Schee, 1978. Composition and production of milk from dutch warmblooded saddle horse mares. Z. Tierphysiol., Tierenärhg. Futtermittelk, 40, 39-53

Cavinder, C.A., M.M. Vogelsang, D.W. Forrest, P.G. Gibbs and T.L. Blanchard, 2005. Reproductive parameters of fat vs moderately conditioned mares following parturition. Proc. 19th Equine Science Soc., Tucson, AZ, 65-70.

Coenen M., 1992. CI-Haushalt und CI Bedarf des Pferdes. Habilschrift, Tierärztliche Hochschule Hannover.

CVB, 1996. Documentatierrrapport Nr 15, Het definitieve VEP en VRE system, Centraal veevoederbureau, pp.

CVB, 2005. Revision of CVB, 1996 (Personal communication of Blok M.).

Doreau, M. and G., Dussap, 1980. Estimation de la production laitière de la jument allaitante par marquage de l'eau corporelle du poulain. Reprod. Nutr. Dev., 20: 1883.

Doreau, M., W. Martin-Rosset and J.P. Barlet, 1981. Variations de quelques constituents plasmatiques chez la jument allaitante en fin de gestation et en début de lactation. Ann. Rech. Vét., 12, 219-225.

Doreau, M., S. Boulot, R. Jeunet and J.M. Trin, 1985. Comparaison de différentes methods de dosage des matières grasses et des matièrs azotées du lait de jument. Le Lait, 65, 149-161.

Doreau, M., S. Boulot, W. Martin-Rosset and H., Dubroeucq, 1986a. Milking lactating mares using oxytocin:milk volume and composition. Reprod. Nutr. Dev., 26, 1-11.

Doreau, M., S. Boulot, W. Martin-Rosset and J. Robelin, 1986b. Relationship between nutrient intake, growth and body composition of the nursing foal. Reprod. Nutr. Develop., 26 (2B), 683-690.

Doreau, M. and S. Boulot, 1987. Milk yield and composition in mares either fat or thin at foaling. Proc. 10th Equine Nutrtion and Physiology Symp. Colorado State University, Fort Collins, CO, 1 p.

Doreau, M., W. Martin-Rosset and S. Boulot, 1988a. Energy requirements and the feeding of mares during lactation: a review. Livest. Prod. Sci., 20: 53-68.

Doreau, M., J.P. Bruhat and W. Martin-Rosset, 1988b. Effets du niveau des apports azotés chez la jument en début de lactation. Ann. Zootech., 37(1), 21-30.

Doreau, M. and S. Boulot, 1989a. Recent knowledge on mare milk production. A review Livest. Prod. Sci., 22: 213-235.

Doreau, M. and S. Boulot, 1989b. Methodes of measurement of milk yield and composition in nursing mares: a review. Le lait, 69, 159-171.

Doreau, M., S. Boulot, J.P. Barlet, P. Patureau Mirand, 1990a. yield and composition of milk from lactating mares: effect of lactation stage and individual differences. J. of Dairy Res., 57: 449-454.

Doreau, M., C. Moretti and W. Martin-Rosset, 1990b. Effect of quality of hay given to mares around foaling on their voluntary intake and foal growth. Ann. Zootech., 39: 125-131.

Doreau, M., S. Boulot and W. Martin-Rosset, 1991. Effect of parity and physiological state on intake, milk production and blood parameters in lactating mares differing in body size. Anim. Prod., 53: 111-118.

Doreau, M., S. Boulot, D. Bauchart, J.P. Barlet and W. Martin-Rosset, 1992. Voluntary intake milk production and plasma metabolites in nursing mares fed two different diets. J. Nutr., 122: 992-999.

Doreau, M., S. Boulot and Y. Chilliard, 1993. Yield and composition of milk from lactating mares: effect of body condition at foaling. J. Dairy Sci., 60, 457-466.

Doreau, M., 1994. Le lait de jument et sa production: particularités et facteurs de variation. Lait, 74, 401-418.

Doreau, M. and W. Martin-Rosset, 2002. Dairy Animals. Horse. In: H. Roginski, J.W. Frequay, P.F. Fox (editors) Encyclopedia of Dairy Sciences Academic Press, London –GB), 1, 630-637.

Drepper, K., J.O. Gutte, H. Meyer and F.J. Schway, 1982. Empfehlungen zur Energie und Nahorstoffversong der Pferde. Frankfurt: DLG Verlag.

Gentry, L.R., D.L. Thompson, G.T. Gentry Jr., K.A. Davis, R.A. Godke and A. Cartmill, 2002. The relationship between body condition, leptin and reproductive and hormonal characteristics of mares during the seasonal anovulatory period. J. Anim. Sci., 80: 2695-2703.

GEH, 1994. Langerwirtschafts für Enährungphysiologie 2. Empfehlungen zur Energie und Nährstoffversorgung der Perfde. DLG. Verlage Frankfurt/Main. ISBN 3.7690.0517.1, pp.

Gibbs, P.G., G.D. Potter, R.W. Blake and W.C. McMullan, 1982. Milk production of Quarter Horse mares during 150 days of lactation. J. Anim. Sci., 54: 496-499.

Gutte, J.O., 1972. Energiebedarf laktierender Stuten, in: W. Lenkeit, K. Breirem, E. Crasemann: Hdb. Tierernährg., 393-398, Verlag Paul Parey, Berlin-Hamburg.

Henneke, D.R., G.D. Potter and J.L. Kreider, 1981. Rebreeding efficiency in mares fed different levels of energy during late gestation. In: Proceedings 7th Equine Nutrition Physiology Symposium, 101-104.

Henneke, D.R., G.D. Potter and J.L. Kreider, 1984. Body condition during pregnancy and lactation and reproductive efficiency in mares. Theriogenology, 21: 897-909.

Hintz, H.F. and H.F. Schryver, 1972. Nitrogen utilization in ponies. J. Anim. Sci., 34: 592.

Hintz, H.F. and N.F. Cymbaluk, 1994. Nutrition of the horse. Annu. Rev. Nutr., 14, 243-267.

Hoffman, L., W. Kippel and R. Schiemann, 1967. Untersuchungen über den Energieumsatz beim Pferd unter besonderer Berücksichtigung der Horizontal bewegung. Archiv. Tierern., 17, 441-449.

INRA, 1984. Le Cheval. R. Jarrige and W. Martin-Rosset (Eds), Editions INRA Publications, Route de St Cyr, 78000 Versailles.

INRA, 1990. Alimentation des chevaux. W. Martin-Rosset (Ed), Editions INRA Publications, Route de St Cyr, 78000 Versailles.

INRA, HN, IE, 1997. Notation de l'état corporel des chevaux de selle et de sport. Guide Pratique. Institut de l'Elevage Ed., 149, rue de Bercy, 75595 Paris cedex 12.

Jordan, R.M., 1979. Energy requirements for lactation of pony mares. In: Proc. 6th Eq. Nutr. Physiol. Soc. Symp. College Station, Tex.: Texas A&M University., 27.

Jordan, R.M., 1985. Effect of energy and crude protein intake on lactating pony mares. pp. 90-94. In Proc. 8th Equine Nutr. Phys. Soc..

Knox, K.L., D.C. Crownover and G.R. Wooden, 1970. Maintenance energy requirements of mature idle horses. In: Proceedings 5th Symposium Energy Metabolism of Farm Animals. Witznau (Suisse) Shurch. A., Wenk, C. Editors, 181-184. Juris Druck Verlag Zurich.

Kubiak, J.R., B.H. Crawford, E.L. Squires, R.H. Wrigley and G.M. Ward, 1987. The influence of energy intake and percentage of body fat on the reproductive performance of nonpregnant mares. Theriogenology, 28: 587-598.

Linzell, J.L., E.F. Annisson, R. Bickerstaffe and L.B. Jeffcott, 1972. Mammary and whole-body metabolism of glucose, acetate and palmitate in the lactating horse. Proceed.Nutr. Soc., 31, 72A.

Martin-Rosset, W. and M. Doreau, 1980. Effect of variations in level of feeding of heavy mares during late pregnancy. In: Proceedings 31st Annual Meeting EAAP, Munich (Germany). Horse Commision, Session 6, 1-4.

Martin-Rosset, W., 1982. Exploitation de troupeaux de juments lourdes en plein air. In: Actions du climat sur l'animal au pâturage, 45-48, Ed. INRA Publications, 78000 Versailles.

Martin-Rosset, W., R. Boccard, M. Jussiaux, J. Robelin and C. Trillaud-Geyl, 1983. Croissance relative des différents tissus, organes et regions corporelles entre 12 et 30 mois chez le cheval de boucherie de différentes races lourdes. Ann. Zootech., 32, 153-174.

Martin-Rosset, W. and M. Doreau, 1984a. Besoins et alimentation de la Jument. In «Le Cheval»: R. Jarrige et W. Martin-Rosset (editors) «Reproduction – Sélection – Alimentation – Exploitation». INRA Publications, route de St Cyr, 78000 Versailles, 355-370.

Martin-Rosset, W. and M. Doreau, 1984b. Consommation d'aliments et d'eau par le cheval. In «Le Cheval» R. Jarrige, W. Martin-Rosset, (editors). INRA Publications, Route de St-Cyr, 78000 Versailles, 333-354.

Martin-Rosset, W., M. Vermorel, M. Doreau, V. Tisserand and J. Andrieu, 1994. The French horse feed evaluation systems and recommended allowances for energy and protein. Livest. Prod. Sci., 40: 37-56.

Martin-Rosset, W. and M. Vermorel, 2004. Evaluation and expression of energy allowances and energy value of feeds in the UFC system for the performance horse. In: Nutrition of the Performance Horse, V. Julliand and W. Martin-Rosset (eds.). EAAP Publication, 111, Wageningen Academic Publishers, The Netherlands. 29-60.

Meadows D.G., G.D. Potter, W.B. Thomas, J.H. Hesby and J. Anderson, 1979. Foal growth from mares fed supplemental soybean meal or urea. In: Proc. 6th Eq. Nutr. Physiol. Soc., 16.

Meyer, H., S. Vom Stein and M. Schmidt, 1985. Investigations to determine endogenouse faecal and N losses in horses. In: Proc. 9th Eq. Nutr. Physiol. Soc. Symp. East Lansing. Mich., University of Michigan, 68.

Miraglia, N., C. Poncet and W. Martin-Rosset, 1992. Effect of feeding level, physiological state and breed on the rate of passage of particulate matter through the gastrointestinal tract of the horse. Ann., Zootech., 41, 69.

MTT, 2004. Rehutaulukot ja Ruokintasinar-tukset. www.artturi.fi/rehutaulukot.

Neseni, R., E. Flade, G. Heiddler and H. Steger, 1958. Milchleistung und Milchzusammensetzung von Stuten in Verlaufe der Laktation. Arch. Tierzucht, 1, 91-129.

Neuhaus, U., 1959. Milch un Milchgewinnung von Pferdestuten. Z. Tierz. Zuechtungsbiol, 73: 370.

NRC, 1978. Nutrient requirements of horse, 4th rev. ed. Washington, DC: National Academy Press.

NRC, 1989. Nutrient requirements of horse, 5th rev. ed. Subcommittee on Horse Nutrition Board on Agriculture National Academey Press - Washington, DC.

Oftedal, O.T., H.F. Hintz and H.F. Schryver, 1983. Lactation in the horse: Milk composition and intake by foals. J. Nutr. 113: 2196-2206.

Olsson, N.A. and A. Ruudvere, 1955. The nutrition of the horse. Nutr. Abstr. Reviews, 25: 1-18.

Ott, E.A., 1970. Energy and protein for reproduction in the horse. Proc. 2nd Eq. Nutr. Physiol. Soc. Symp., 6-10.

Pagan, J.D., H.F. Hintz and T.R. Rounsaville, 1984. The digestible requirements of lactating pony mares. J. Anim. Sci., 58: 1382.

Pagan, J.D. and H.F. Hintz, 1986a. Composition of milk from pony mares fed various levels of digestible energy. Cornell Veterinarian, 76, 139-148

Pagan, J.D. and H.F. Hintz, 1986b. Equine energetics. I. Relationship between body weight and energy requirements in horses. J. Anim. Sci., 63: 815.

Peltonen, T., V. Kossila, V. Antila and L. Huida, 1980. Effect of protein supplement on milk composition of the mares and growth rate of their foals. C.R. 31e Réunion F.E.Z., Munich, 6 p.

Perrin, D.R., 1958. The caloric value of milk of different species. J. Dairy Res., 25, 215-220.

Prior, R.L., H.F. Hintz, J.E. Lowe and V.H. Visek, 1974. Urea recycling and metabolism of ponies. J. Anim. Sci., 8: 565.

Quinn, C.R., 1975. Isobutylidene diurea as a protein substitute for horses. Ph. D. dissertation, Colorado State University.

Robelin, J., R. Boccard, W. Martin-Rosset, M. Jussiaux and C. Trillaud-Geyl, 1984. Caracteristiques des carcasses et qualités de la viande de cheval. In: Le cheval. R. Jarrige and W. Martin-Rosset (Eds.). INRA Editions, Route de St Cyr, 78026 Versailles, p. 602-610.

Rogers, P., W.W. Albert and G.C. Fahey, 1981. Blood amino acid profiles of gestating and lactating mares fed diets with and without lysine and methionine. In: Proc. 7th Eq. Nutr. Physiol. Soc. Symp., 73-78.

Slade, L.M., D.W. Robinson and K.E. Casey, 1970. Nitrogen metabolism in nonruminant herbivores. II. Comparative aspects of protein digestion. J. Anim. Sci., 30: 761.

Slade, L.M., L.D. Lewis, C.R. Quinn and M.L. Chandler, 1975. Nutritional adaptation of horses for endurance typeperformance. In: Proc. 4th Eq. Nutr. Physiol. Soc. Symp. Pomona, Calif., 114.

SLU, 2004. Utfordring rekimmendationer för häst. Sversiges lantbruks Universitet Publikation. Stjänst, Uppsala, Sweden, pp. 43.

Teeter, S.M., M.C. Stillions and W.E. Nelson, 1967. Recent observations on the nutrition of mature horses. In: Proc. Am. Assoc. Eq. Pract., New Orleans, La., 39.

Ullrey, D.E., R.D. Struthers, D.G. Hendricks and B.E. Brent, 1966. Composition of mare"s milk. J. Anim. Sci., 25: 217.

Van Niekerk, F.E. and C.H. Van Niekerk, 1997a. The effect of dietary protein on reproduction in the mare. II. Growth of foals, body mass of mares and serum protein concentration of mares during the anovulatroy, transitional and pregnant periods. J. S. Afr. Vet. Assoc., 68(3): 81-85.

Van Niekerk, F.E. and C.H. van Niekerk, 1997b. The effect of dietary protein on reproduction in the mare. III. Ovarian and uterine changes during the anovulatroy periods in the non-pregnant mares. J. S. Afr. Vet. Assoc., 68(3): 86-92.

Wooden, G.R., K.L. Know and C.L. Wild, 1970. Energy metabolism of light horses. J. Anim. Sci., 30, 544-548.

Zimmerman, R.A., 1981. Energy needs of lactating mares. In: Proceedings 7th Eq. Nut. Physiol. Soc. Symposium, Warrenton, West Virginie, USA, 127.

Zimmerman, R.A., 1985. Effect of ration on composition of mare's milk. In: Proc. 9th Eq. Nutr. Physiol. Soc. Symp. East Lansing. University of Michigan, USA, 96.

Asses: milk yield and composition

E. Salimei[1] *and B. Chiofalo*[2]
[1]*Dept. STAAM, University of Molise 86100 Campobasso, Italy*
[2]*Dept. MoBiFiPA, University of Messina, Polo Universitario Annunziata, 98168 Messina, Italy*

Abstract

Hypoallergenicity of ass's milk protein have been recently confirmed, allowing ass's milk to be considered a valid substitute to the available hypoallergenic infant formulas. Following the medical suggestion, this paper deals with the feasibility of ass's milk production and some of its essential traits, reviewing experimental data from studies carried out in different "dairy" conditions. Daily milk yield, obtained milking the asses twice, ranges between 1250 and 1700 $mL{\cdot}d^{-1}$ and shows a gradual decline in the first 120 – 150 days of lactation. As a hypoallergenic food for infants, the recommended high standard of hygiene is supported in raw ass's milk by the presence of antimicrobial proteins. Studies on nitrogenous and lipid fractions are then reviewed in order to clarify the hypoallergenic and functional (antimicrobial, hormonal, trophic, immunomodulant) possible role of ass's milk in human nutrition. Data on ass's milk composition substantially confirm the resemblance to human milk except for the low (<1 $g{\cdot}100\ g^{-1}$ milk) and highly variable fat content, that needs to be appropriately integrated. Studies on the effects of physiology, nutrition, milking and reproduction management of the animals, as well as of eventual physical treatments of milk could contribute to the exploitation of the innovative "dairy donkey" food chain, also preserving animal biodiversity and marginal areas of the Country.

Keywords: ass's milk, milk yield, milk composition, infant food

Introduction

The ass or donkey (*Equus asinus*, Order *Perissodactyla*, Family *Equidae*) has been domesticated before horses, probably in Numidia, since ancient times. The docile and humble species has been involved in the humankind history, as also the monoteistic Holy Texts remind (El-Razzaz, 2002). The main utilisation of donkeys as animal power, sustained in fact for thousand of years the development of Countries and still today represent a very important component of the rural domestic economy in many developing countries (El-Razzaz, 2002; Tisserand and Pearson, 2003). As a consequence of the animal work replacement by mechanisation, asinine species is showing a serious decrease in industrialised countries, where some breeds are considered extinct or strongly threatened by extinction (Gandini and Rognoni, 1997; Miraglia *et al.*, 2003).

Besides animal draught source, the role of donkey as a "milk and meat producer" species is also known from the popular knowledge (El-Razzaz, 2002; Tisserand and Pearson, 2003); as far as milk utilization is concerned, it is interesting to note that an Italian law promulgated in 1929 (Regio Decreto n. 994/29) in its art. 43 specifically provides for the case of ass's milk selling. Moreover, D'Arval (1912) reported that "according to few researches carried out in French orphanages, infants fed ass's milk grew well and showed lower mortality than babies fed cow's milk"; the author, on the other hand, pointed out the lack of more in depth studies on this issue. That lack lasted about eighty years.

More recently, in the effort to investigate on new hypoallergenic foods for infant with cow's milk protein allergy (CMPA), an increasing disease involving between 1.8 to 7.5% of the general infant population (Host, 2002), clinical studies revalued ass's milk feeding as a safe and valid treatment of the most complicated cases of allergy in infants (Iacono *et al.*, 1992; Carroccio *et al.*, 2000a; Monti, 2004).

Hypoallergenicity of ass's milk protein have been recently confirmed (Restani *et al.*, 2002), allowing ass's milk to be considered a valid substitute to the available hypoallergenic infant formulas, which have several drawbacks (Muraro *et al.*, 2002; Seppo *et al.*, 2005). Efficacy of ass's milk feeding is also related to the consistent probability for CMPA subjects to develop a multiple food allergy, i.e. to soy (Host, 2002); allergy may also persist up to the adult life, with a severe impact on patients health and well being status (Carroccio *et al.*, 2000b). On this regard, both some food components and enteric microbes are reported to affect the tight junctions of epithelial cell through a number of different factors; the so-called "leaky intestin" is also reported to be involved in diseases such as inflammatory bowel disease, type I diabetes, allergies, asthma and even autism (Liu *et al.*, 2005).

Due to the possible role of ass's milk in human nutrition, the aim of the paper is to review the recent findings on ass's milk characteristics, as related to an innovative hypoallergenic food chain for infancy.

Ass's milk yield

Feasibility of ass's milk production has been proved and experimental data summarised in Table 1 show the daily milk production, observed lower in asses than in dairy mares (Doreau and Boulot, 1989; Drogoul *et al.*, 1992; Dell'Orto *et al.*, 1993). Since management of dairy equids could influence the amount of milk extracted by the mammary gland, characterised by low capacity (Doreau, 1991), it has to be noted that throughout all the studies reviewed in Table 1 milk produced the first month of lactation has been totally devoted to the foals and milking was carried out in average 3 hours after foals were separated by their dams, as already experienced on mares (Drogoul *et al.*, 1992). Interestingly, asses always showed a quick adaptation to the "dairy management" routines, in all the quoted studies.

Variability in milk yield could be related to genetic diversities in investigated Italian donkey populations (Martina Franca, Ragusano, Romagnolo and Grigio Siciliano) even though Blasi *et al.* (2005) defined genetically similar the Romagnolo, Ragusano and Martina Franca populations; the Authors also showed reciprocal influences, confirming the hypothesis formulated by Gandini and Rognoni (1997).

Table 1. Daily ass's milk yield, observed in different "dairy" management conditions (mean values, mL milk·d^{-1}).

Author	Year	Milking technique	d[1]	milkings/24 h	Milk yield
Salimei *et al.*	2000	Mechanical	300[2]	2	1500
Simoni *et al.*	2004	Mechanical	2	1	810
Chiofalo *et al.*	2004	Manual	150	3	2150
Chiofalo *et al.*	2005b	Manual	1	1	1130
Alabiso *et al.*	2005	Mechanical	320	2	1700
Salimei *et al.*	2005b	Mechanical	84	2	1350
Salimei *et al*	2006	Mechanical	150	2	1250

[1] d= length of the study, in days. - [2] 2 lactations.

Milk ejection of asses machine milked has been observed to be incomplete, being the residual milk after oxytocin injection about 37% of total milk produced, and milk fat is the main retained milk component (Salimei *et al.*, 2004b), consistently with data on mares (Doreau *et al.*, 1986).

Lactation curve proposed for dairy asses (Figure 1) shows high individual variability, explained by the total absence of any form of genetic selection of the animals; starting at 30 d post partum, milk yield constantly decreases up to 4th – 5th month of lactation (Salimei *et al.*, 2005a). This trend is substantially confirmed by data on Ragusana population (Alabiso *et al.*, 2005), also showing seasonal variation of milk yield, as presumably due to foaling period and the related different availability of pasture at the onset of lactation.

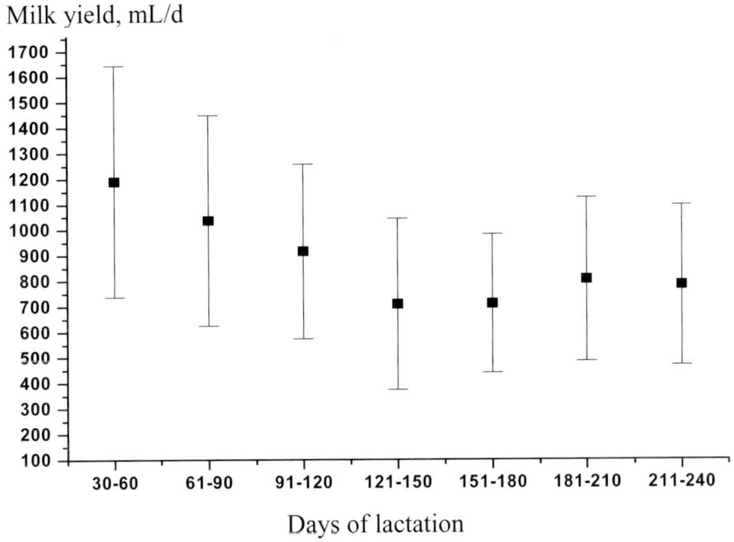

Figure 1. Average ass's milk yield (± s d) (from Salimei et al., 2005a).

Ass's milk hygiene

As already mentioned, ass's milk is considered a promising alternative hypoallergenic food for infancy (Restani *et al.*, 2002) when appropriately evaluated from the hygienic point of view: since the innovative food chain has been so far experimented only in Italy, where the already mentioned 994/1929 law (Regio decreto) only allows its direct sale, data on raw ass's milk production should be considered inseparable from its hygienic status (Albertini *et al.*, 2002).

As summarised in Table 2, raw ass's milk shows a general good hygienic standard quality, when observed values are compared with the EC Dir. 92/46 and the EC Reg. 853/2004. The overall low microbial counts seems to be related to the high content of lysozyme (Coppola *et al.*, 2002; Salimei *et al.*, 2004a; Chiavari *et al.*, 2005), a nitrogenous milk components with useful antimicrobial properties (Lonnerhdal, 2003), discussed later. Variability of total bacteria counts (Table 2) also underline the importance of cleaning and disinfection in both manual and mechanical milking procedures.

The low somatic cell count (SCC) of ass's milk (Table 2) suggest an average good mammary health status with both manual and machine milking. Even if mastitis is rare in equine (Svendsen, 1997), more in depth studies should investigate the effect of a more intensive exploitation of dairy asses.

Table 2. Milk hygiene and mammary healthy status of asses: total bacterial and somatic cell count of ass's milk (means ± s.d.).

Author	Year	Milking technique	Total Bacteria count, logCFU/mL	somatic cell count, logSCC/mL
Salimei *et al.*	2000	Mechanical	4.46 ± 0.08	3.68 ± 0.05
Coppola *et al.*	2002	Mechanical	4.60 ± 0.02	n.a.
Conte *et al.*	2003	Manual	3.66 ± 0.15	4.55 ± 0.10
Simoni *et al.*	2004	Mechanical	3.74 ± 0.50	3.83 ± 0.5
Salimei *et al.*	2004b	Mechanical	5.51 ± 0.06	3.52 ± 0.08
Alabiso *et al.*	2005	Mechanical	n.a.	3.90 ± 0.40
Sorrentino *et al.*	2005	Mechanical	3.95 ± 0.09	n.a.
Salimei *et al.*	2005b	Mechanical	4.00 ± 0.06	3.85 ± 0.05
Conte *et al.*	2004	Manual	4.21 ± 0.06	4.36 ± 0.41
		Mechanical (n=1)	5.87	4.48
Salimei *et al.*	2006	Mechanical	3.89 ± 0.39	3.92 ± 0.61

n.a. – not available

The recent EC legislation on raw milk (EC Reg. 853/2004), exceeding discrimination among dairy species, supports the innovative production but asses' reproductive management could interfere with a constant supplying of milk throughout the year (Chiofalo *et al.*, 2004; Alabiso *et al.*, 2005): studies of new technologies for extending the shelf-life of the products seem therefore to be of a considerable practical interest when applied to ass's milk, whose microbiologic characteristics have been investigated up to 14 days storage at 4 °C (Sorrentino *et al.*, 2005). Besides a lower microbial total count than reference levels reported by the cited EC Reg. 853/2004 (Table 3), the authors observed in raw ass's milk the rare presence of undesirable groups like enterobacteria, faecal and total coliforms; Clostridium spp. were absent in ass's milk. Moreover, data reported in Table 3 seem to confirm ass's milk as an optimal growth medium for lactic acid bacteria, as already observed with some *Lactobacillus rhamnosus* strains (Coppola *et al.*, 2002). On this purpose it has to be noted that antimicrobial activity of some proteins has been proved also in human milk, notwithstanding the suggested "bifidogenic" role of several milk oligosaccharides (Lonnerdal, 2003).

Ass's milk could therefore be also valorised as a very good base ingredient for "health promoting" foods based on its probiotic and other functional activities (Coppola *et al.*, 2002; Chiavari *et al.*, 2005).

Table 3. Microbiological characteristics of raw ass's milk machine milked at t=0 and during storage at 4 °C (log CFU/mL milk) (from Sorrentino et al., 2005).

Storage, d	TBC[1]	Psychrotropic microflora	Lactic acid bacteria	Total coliforms	Faecal coliforms	Enterobacteria
0	3.48	3.00	3.00	1.48	1.48	1.48
3	5.84	5.30	3.48	1.70	1.78	1.70
7	6.00	5.70	4.00	1.84	1.48	1.90
14	6.00	5.48	4.48	1.30	1.30	1.30

[1]TBC: total bacteria count.

Ass's milk composition

Experimental data (Table 4) substantially confirm the compositional resemblance of ass's milk to human milk, even though more in depth studies should consider the high variability of milk fat content, ranging from 1.82 to 0.28 g·100g^{-1} milk.

As a comment to the wide variability of the ass's milk fat content (Table 4), it has to be noted that the highest values are observed both in those trials carried out up to 1998, where milking techniques are not described, and after oxjtocin injection (Salimei *et al.*, 2004a); if we exclude those trials, ass's milk fat content shows average values (< 0.7 g·100g-1 milk) significantly lower than those observed in mare's (Doreau *et al.*, 2002; Malacarne *et al.*, 2002) and human milk (Malacarne *et al.*, 2002). According to studies on equine (Doreau and Boulot, 1989; Doreau, 1991), a decline of milk fat content has been observed during lactation in Ragusana donkeys fed a hay-based diet (Chiofalo *et al.*, 2004; Alabiso *et al.*, 2005).

The alternative infant feeding with ass's milk, as a hypoallergenic food, requires therefore appropriate modifications in composition (Restani *et al.*, 2002): because the interesting profile of ass's milk components and their nutraceutical role, as also reviewed by Chiofalo and Salimei (present *EWEN*), more specific researches are needed to determine the relevance of breed, milking (and sampling) techniques, besides of nutrition, on the milk fat fraction.

Average total solids and lactose content of donkey's milk (Table 4) are consistent with values reviewed in equine and human milk (Solaroli *et al.*, 1993); similarly, total protein and salt content of milk are comparable to mare's and human milk, while cow's milk is characterised by a higher content of both milk components (Malacarne *et al.*, 2002).

Table 4. Average composition of ass's milk (mean values, g·100g^{-1} milk).

Author	Year	Milking technique	Total solids	Fat	Protein	Lactose	Ash
Nigro	1982	n.a.	n.a.	1.00	1.60	6.00	0.50
Schryver *et al.*	1986	Manual	10.1	n.a.	n.a.	n.a.	n.a.
Oftedal and Jenness	1988	Manual	10.8	1.82	1.74	5.87	0.44
Polidori	1994	n.a.	9.61	1.10	1.74	6.23	0.43
Pinto *et al.*	1998	Manual	11.07	1.68	1.76	7.25	0.37
Salimei *et al.*	2000	Mechanical	8.84	0.38	1.72	6.88	0.39
Coppola *et al.*	2002	Mechanical	8.86	0.52	1.66	7.03	0.41
Conte *et al.*	2003	Manual	9.31	0.45	1.70	6.3	n.a.
Chiofalo *et al.*	2004	Manual	n.a.	0.50	1.67	6.90	n.a.
Salimei *et al.*	2004b	Mechanical	n.a.	1.00	1.63	7.02	0.38
Simoni *et al.*	2004	Mechanical	n.a.	0.51	1.60	7.20	n.a.
Alabiso *et al.*	2005	Mechanical	n.a.	0.44	1.90	6.40	n.a.
Chiofalo *et al.*	2005b	Manual	8.1	0.57	1.50	5.10	n.a.
Salimei et al	2005b	Mechanical	8.9	0.30	1.52	6.63	0.36
Chiavari *et al.*	2005	Mechanical	8.9	0.28	1.59	6.73	0.32
Sorrentino *et al.*	2005	Mechanical	9.2	0.66	1.36	7.25	n.a.
Salimei et al	2006	Mechanical	9.2	0.52	1.57	6.53	0.43

n.a. - not available

In particular ass's milk protein content, ranging between 1.36 and 1.90 $g \cdot 100g^{-1}$ milk (Table 4), is slightly closer to human than mare's milk (Malacarne *et al.*, 2002). The protein milk percentage has been observed to decline during lactation (Salimei *et al.*, 2004a; Alabiso *et al.*, 2005; Salimei *et al.*, 2005b; Salimei *et al.*, 2006), as already described for milk yield and its fat percentage.

With regard to the ash content of donkey's milk, it has to be highlighted that the mineral composition was observed closer to human milk than other milks except for calcium and phosphorus absolute levels; on the other hand, the Ca:P ratio resulted intermediate between the values of human milk and cow's milk (Salimei *et al.*, 2004a).
According to the knowledge on the relationship between cow's milk salts content and stability and properties of the milk protein system (Fox, 2001), more in depth studies should be carried out on factors affecting the mineral profile in donkey's milk.

The pH values range from 7.00 and 7.30 (Salimei *et al.*, 2000; Conte *et al.*, 2003; Chiofalo *et al.*, 2004; Sorrentino *et al.*, 2005; Chiavari *et al.*, 2005), as also reported for mares' milk (Solaroli *et al.*, 1993); moreover, density (Salimei *et al.*, 2000; Chiavari *et al.*, 2005) and freezing point (Conte, 2005) were consistent with values of mare and cow's milk (Solaroli *et al.*, 1993).

Deepening the knowledge on functional properties of foods seems very interesting when related to the possible role of ass's milk as a hypoallergenic food for infancy; on this purpose a special regard has been addressed to nitrogenous and lipid fractions.

Nitrogenous fraction

Regarding the nitrogenous component, the main dietary antigens source in food allergy reactions (Muraro *et al.*, 2002), the average casein and whey protein contents of ass's milk were found similar to the respective levels in equine and human milk (Solaroli *et al.*, 1993, Roncada and Greppi, 2001; Lonnerdal, 2003; Salimei *et al.*, 2004a).

A large variability has been observed in ass's milk non-protein nitrogen (NPN) and casein content, ranging respectively from 0.18 to 0.41 g/100g milk and from 0.18 to 1.18 g/100g milk (Salimei *et al.*, 2004a; Sorrentino *et al.*, 2005; Alabiso *et al.*, 2005; Chiavari *et al.*, 2005; Fantuz *et al.*, 2006). The presence of NPN compounds in mares' colostrum and milk already raised questions about their functional significance to the foal, as a possible further functional dimension of milk (Salimei *et al.*, 2002). Besides the high content of NPN, Fantuz et al (2006) report for ass's milk a lower casein index (averaging 43%) compared to mare's milk; a negative trend in donkey's milk casein content has been evidenced during lactation (Alabiso *et al.*, 2005).

SDS-PAGE of donkey milk showed one major band in the area of casein and three proteins in the area of whey proteins (Restani *et al.*, 2002) while lactoferrin (4.48% total whey protein), serum albumin (6.18% total whey protein), β-lactoglobulin (29.85% total whey protein), lysozyme (21.03% total whey protein) and α- lactalbumin (22.56% total whey protein) have been determined (Salimei *et al.*, 2004a).

Genetic variants for lysozyme and β-lactoglobulin I and II have been identified in donkey milk (Godovac-Zimmerman *et al.*, 1990; Herrouin *et al.*, 2000) and an additional protein with a molecular weight of approximately 23.5 kDa has been shown (Fantuz *et al.*, 2001).

The observed presence of β-lactoglobulin in donkey's milk, at level comparable to mare's milk (Fantuz *et al.*, 2001; Civardi *et al.*, 2002; Malacarne *et al.*, 2002) but at higher level than that reported for human milk (Malacarne *et al.*, 2002), could explain the weak allergenic cross-reactivity observed by immunoblotting of donkey's milk sample, obtained after incubation with an anti β-lactoglobulin monoclonal antibody, while among ruminants even goat's milk has been associate to the high risk of cross reactivity (Muraro *et al.*, 2002; Restani *et al.*, 2002). These findings seem to confirm β-lactoglobulin as an important milk allergen in infants and small children unlike casein is the predominant allergen in adults, as reported by Carroccio *et al.* (1999). On the other hand, studies on genetic polymorphism of milk proteins could clarify some controversial results, as reported in literature for goat's milk (Bevilacqua *et al.*, 2001).

With regard to the consumption of donkey's milk by adults, it is important to consider that a connection between inhalant sensitization to animal products and food allergens derived from the same animals is described in literature in a case of allergy to mare's milk in a allergic woman (Fanta and Ebner, 1998): for this reason, ass's milk consumption should be specifically tested (Prick tests, RAST, CAST, ALCATEST, etc.) before offering to adults with allergies (DeBlasis MT, authorised personal communication).

The presence of α_S-, β-, κ- and γ- like caseins have been reported in donkey's milk samples differently among the quoted studies (Fantuz *et al.*, 2001; Iametti et al, 1998; Vincenzetti *et al.*, 2005; Restani *et al.*, 2002) probably because of different methodological approaches. However, ass's milk casein cold precipitated fraction separated, in anion exchange chromatography followed by reversed phase, into 2 subfractions while the thermally precipited casein fraction separated in 3 subfractions, identified as αS- like caseins, β-like caseins and γ- like caseins (Fantuz *et al.*, 2001); the presence of both αS1- caseins (MW 30.9 and 33.0 kDa), having the N-terminal sequence RPKLPHRXPE, and β-caseins (MW 34.0 and 35.4 kDa), having N-terminal sequence REKEELNVS have been detected in donkey's milk (Vincenzetti *et al.*, 2005). At this time, studies are needed for a better understanding of ass's milk casein components, especially those involved in the hypoallergenic potentiality of equid's milk.

Besides its hypoallergenic characteristics, the healthy properties traditionally recognised to ass's milk could be related to the presence of enzymes with antibacterial activities also recovered in human milk (Lonnerdal, 2003); among the whey proteins observed in ass's milk, lysozyme, also called muramidase, inhibits the growth of many bacteria, particularly Gram-positives, and may release hydrolytic products to support the growth of bifidobacteria (Modler, 1994). The lysozyme content of ass's milk, approximatively 1.5 g/L as measured by semi-quantitative analysis on SDS-PAGE (Fantuz *et al.*, 2001), is equal or higher than in mare milk (Civardi *et al.*, 2002; Doreau *et al.*, 2002; Malacarne *et al.*, 2002) and much higher than in bovine milk (Solaroli *et al.*, 1993). The assay of lysozyme used in cheese making technology, evaluating the lytic activity on *Micrococcus lysodeikticus* compared to a purified standard extracted from egg (Lodi *et al.*, 1984), when tested on ass's milk showed much higher levels of lysozyme-like activity (>3 g/L) (Coppola *et al.*, 2002; Chiavari *et al.*, 2005). As a possible explanation of the difference between analytical methods, the glycoprotein lactoferrin, almost absent in cow's milk (Solaroli *et al.*, 1993), is reported to act mainly as an antimicrobial factor in human milk (Lonnerdal, 2003); on the other hand, lactoferrin has also shown its role in gut growth regulation, according to *in vitro* cell lines studies (Playford *et al.*, 2000; Kanyshkova *et al.*, 2003).

Milk is considered a functional food: besides its nutritive value, mammary secretions also provide a number of biologically active substances (Table 5), most of them characterised by interspecific activity, that may be inactivated by the technological processing used in manufacture and storage of infant formulas, leading to either a greater susceptibility to infection and/or the development of allergies (Donnet-Hughes *et al.*, 2000).

Table 5. Biologically active substances in mammary secretions (adapted from R.J. Xu, 1996 and A. Donnet-Hughes et al., 2000).

Adrenal steroids	
Ovarian steroids	Plasminogen activator inhibitor
Prostaglandins	GRP (gastrin releasing peptide)
Insulin	GRP-like factor
Cortisol	Vasoactive intestinal peptide
Triiodothyronine, thyroxine	Granulocyte-macrofage colony stimulating factor
Thyroid-stimulating hormone	Hepatocyte growth factor
Thyrotropin-releasing hormone	EGF (epidermal growth factor)
Calcitonin	TGF (tranforming growth factor)
Growth hormone-binding protein	NGF (nerve growth factor)
Somatostatin	IGF (insulin like growth factor) I and II
Leptin	IGF-binding proteins
Prolactin	FGF (fibroblast growth factor)
Oxytocin	VEGF (vascular endotelial growth factor)
Erythropoietin	Nucleotides
Betacasomorphin and opioid peptides	Polyamines
Bombesin	Lactoferrin
Neurotensin	

As Table 5 shows, the milk protein fraction also provides peptides with trophic or protective activity and growth factors, such as insulin like growth factors, epidermal growth factor, TGF-β2, etc., playing an important role in growth, differentiation and permeability of intestinal epithelium, according to studies on adults patients with either celiac or Crohn's disease (Donnet-Hughes *et al.*, 2000; Liu *et al.*, 2005).

Among the hormones listed in Table 5 as natural bioactive substances found in mammary secretion, leptin, a 16 kDa protein recently discovered in human milk is reported to be involved in mammary cell proliferation, differentiation and apoptosis but it might also act on neonate physiology before and after absorption (Bonnet *et al.*, 2002). The fascinating issue involving leptin in milk needs to be more studied: as a contribute to knowledge on this regard, leptin levels were measured for the first time in ass's skimmed milk (Salimei *et al.*, 2005a) and observed values (3.16 – 3.46 ng immunoreactive human equivalent/mL milk) were comparable to data reported in literature for many mammalians (Bonnet *et al.*, 2002; Salimei *et al.*, 2002).

Lipid fraction

As already discussed, the main limits of ass's milk are represented by the low fat content, observed variable in relation to various genetic and environmental factors, and the consequent low energetic value of this food (Salimei *et al.*, 2004a). However, when considering the lipid fraction of donkey's milk, it has to be noted that in immunonutrition, besides the antioxidant properties of certain nutrients, *e.g.* vitamins, increasing available evidences suggest that dietary lipids, especially long-chain polyunsaturated fatty acids, regulate the immune function (Cocchi e Turchetto, 1999) and therefore they may be involved in the development and severity of symptoms of allergic disease (Hoppu *et al.*, 2002). Food is in fact considered not only a source of dietary antigens causing sensitization but it may contain protective factors, that may both counteract with the oxidative stress and diminish the inflammatory response in allergic disease by regulating the immune function (Laiho *et al.*, 2002).

Sorrentino *et al.* (2005) determined lower levels of both trans retinol and α-tocopherol in donkey's raw milk than in cow's and mare's milk (Marconi and Panfili, 1998); the Authors also showed that the low content of vitamin A was unaffected by heat treatments (Table 6), which on the other hand reduced the α-tocopherol content of milk.

As already suggested with respect of the native nitrogenous fraction of milk, eventual physical treatments on ass's milk should therefore consider with care the related effects also on the lipid bioactive substances in milk. With regard to milk fatty acids composition, saturated fatty acids are the most represented class in ass's milk compared to monounsaturated and polyunsaturated fatty acid levels, even though an ample variability is observed among the experimental data (Table 7), most likely related to dietary and/or body condition differences, as already observed in non ruminant herbivores (Doreau and Boulot, 1989; Salimei *et al.*, 1996; Jahreis *et al.*, 1999; Doreau *et al.*, 2002; Chiofalo *et al.*, 2005c).

More in details, the equine large intestin (cecum, ventral colon, distal colon and small colon) mucosa exhibits significant differences in relative rate of transport of volatile fatty acids compared with rumen mucosa (Van Soest, 1994). Moreover, from equine studies (Linzell *et al.*, 1972 in Doreau *et al.*, 2002) it is known that *ex novo* synthesis of part of C18 fatty acids occurs, besides that of 4- to 14 carbon FA and part of 16-carbon FA, from the products of the large bowel fermentations, as described for other non ruminant herbivorous species (Van Soest, 1994).

In Ragusana ass's milk both total saturated and monounsaturated fatty acids did not vary during lactation, even though significant variations has been observed for caprylic ($C_{8:0}$) and capric ($C_{10:0}$)

Table 6. Ass's milk Trans retinol and α Tocopherol content (mean values ± s.d.) (Sorrentino et al., 2005).

Milk treatment	Trans retinol µg/100g of milk	α Tocopherol µg/100g of milk
Raw milk	1.67 ± 0.15	5.14 ± 0.35
63 °C*30min	1.64 ± 0.01	4.73 + 0.24
66 °C*10min	1.39 ± 0.10	4.35 ± 0.00
70 °C*1min	1.42 ± 0.08	4.67 ± 0.00
90 °C*1min	1.41 ± 0.00	3.03 ± 0.02

Table 7. Donkey's milk fatty acid composition (mean values reported by quoted Authors).

		Fatty acids (g· 100 g^{-1} total FA)			
Authors	Year	Saturated	Monounsaturated	Polyunsaturated	UFA:SFA ratio
Pinto *et al.*	1998	49.31 - 49.66	28.2 - 27.7	21.9 - 22.6	1.03 - 1.01
Chiofalo and Salimei	2001	67.7	15.3	16.0	0.48
Chiofalo *et al.*	2005a	46.7	35.0	18.3	1.18
Chiofalo *et al.*	2005b	64.2	20.7	15.2	0.56
Chiofalo *et al.*	2005c	55.3 - 49.3	23.1 - 20.2	21.6 - 30.5	0.81 - 1.07
Chiofalo *et al.*	2006a	52.8 - 56.2	24.43 - 22.8	22.8 - 21.0	0.89 - 0.78

UFA:SFA ratio – unsaturated fatty acids: saturated fatty acids ratio.

as well as for eicosanoic ($C_{20:1}$) acid (Chiofalo *et al.*, 2005a), among "major" components (≥ 1 g/100g total fatty acids).

Notwithstanding the highly variable UFA:SFA ratios of ass's milk, it is interesting to note the high values reported for the polyunsaturated fraction of milk fat, whose n3:n6 ratio ranges between 0.31 and 1.50 (Table 7). A high content (<6 g·100g^{-1} fatty acids) of linoleic ($C_{18:2\ n6}$) and linolenic ($C_{18:3\ n3}$) acids has been observed in ass's milk (Pinto *et al.*, 1998; Chiofalo and Salimei, 2001; Chiofalo *et al.*, 2005a) while conjugated linoleic acid group has not been detected, according to data on mares' milk (Jahreis *et al.*, 1999; Doreau *et al.*, 2002; Malacarne *et al.*, 2002). Among "minor" PUFA (<0.5 g·100g-1 fatty acids), ass's milk contains the eicosadienoic (C20:2 n6), arachidonic (C20:4 n6), eicosapentaenoic (C20:5 n3) and docosaesaenoic (C22:6 n3) acids (Chiofalo and Salimei, 2001; Chiofalo *et al.*, 2005a), which are considered essential in the development of the neonatal brain and retina (Al *et al.*, 1995) but also involved in the inflammatory response (Laiho *et al.*, 2002; Liu *et al.*, 2005).

Acccording to the role attributed to dietary long chain fatty acids (Cocchi and Turchetto, 1999), the potential immune-modulator properties of ass's milk could be emphasised by animal nutrition, since the PUFA content is likely related to the type of consumed forages and feeds, as data in Table 8 indicate.

With regard to nutrients digestibility and its close relationship with triglyceride distribution (Morera Pons *et al.*, 1998; Dugo *et al.*, 2005), further studies should be carried out on this lipid fraction of ass's milk in order to clarify both the typology and the stereospecific distribution of the fatty acids, some quali-quantitative differences with values observed in human and cow's milk, as reviewed by Chiofalo *et al.* (present *EWEN*), and their variation during lactation (Chiofalo *et al.*, 2006b).

Table 8. Total polyunsaturated fatty acids in ass's milk: series n3 and n6 (mean values reported by quoted Authors).

Authors	Year	PUFA n3	PUFA n6	n3/n6 ratio	AI	TI
		g· 100 g^{-1} total FA				
Chiofalo and Salimei	2001	7.4	8.7	0.85	1.42	0.52
Chiofalo *et al.*	2005a	8.0	10.3	0.77	0.89	0.72
Chiofalo *et al.*	2005b	3.6	11.6	0.31	1.48	0.99
Chiofalo *et al.*	2005c	9.3 - 18.3	12.2 - 12.2	0.76 - 1.50	1.11 - 0.83	0.68 - 0.32
Chiofalo *et al.*	2006a	9.6 - 9.4	13.1 - 11.6	0.73 - 0.81	0.93 - 1.12	0.54 - 0.59

PUFAn3, n6 - Polyunsaturated fatty acids series n3, n6; AI – Atherogenic index; TI – Thrombogenic Index.

Conclusions

Reviewed data suggest the feasibility of the innovative food chain "ass's or donkey's milk", whose hypoallergenic and compositional characteristics confirm the resemblance with human milk. A good hygiene level has been evidenced in raw ass's milk, produced in different "dairy donkey" systems. Genetic diversities among donkey populations could have also contributed to the observed variability of reviewed data on milk yield.

Besides its hypoallergenic properties for infancy, mainly related to the low presence of β-lactoglobulin, some nutraceutical components have been determined in the nitrogenous fraction of ass's milk: it is the case of lysozyme and lactoferrin, whose antimicrobial activity in human milk is recognised, or leptin, a hormon-like peptides probably involved in the neonate physiology.

The main limits of ass's milk as an infant food are represented by the low fat content, which appears to vary in relation to environmental and genetic factors, and the related low energetic value: notwithstanding ass's milk has to be integrated, from a nutritional point of view it has to be noted the interesting profile of both fatty acids, that includes long chain polyenes, such as arachidonic acid, docosaesaenoic acid and eicosapentaenoic acid, and tryglicerides.

The potential bio-dietetic value of ass's milk requires more in depth studies, also considering the influence of animal physiology, nutrition, reproduction and management in the innovative food chain, as well as the effects of physical treatments of milk for extending its shelf-life, as they may affect the natural properties of the raw product. As a final consideration, the negative trend generally occurring in donkey population of industrialised Countries could be counteracted by the proposed donkey's production system, also contributing to the preservation of marginal areas of our Country, where the total number of residents, besides raised animals, is declining.

The Authors have no conflict of interest.

Acknowledgements

Research funded by PRIN 2003.

References

Al, M.D.M., A.C. Van Houwelingen, A.D.M. Kester, T.H.M. Hasaart, A.E.P. De Jong and G. Hornstra, 1995. Maternal essential fatty acids pattern during normal pregnancy and their relationship to the neonate essential fatty acid status. Br. J. Nutr., 71, 55-68.

Alabiso, M., G. Russo, C. Giosuè, M.L. Alicata and C. Torrisi, 2005. La produzione di latte nell'arco di una intera lattazione in asine allevate in Sicilia. In: Proc. 7th Congress New Findings In Equine Practices, Lodi (LO, Italy) 22-23 july: 153-160.

Albertini, A., G. Menguzzato and E. Salimei, 2002. La riscoperta del latte di asina – Aspetti igienico-sanitari per la produzione e la vendita di un alimento alternatico. Igiene alimenti – Disinfestazione e Igiene Ambientale: sett/ott, 5-10.

Bevilacqua, C., P. Martin, C. Candalh, J. Fauquant, M. Piot, AM. Roucayrol, F. Pilla and M. Heyman, 2001. Goats' milk of defective α (s1)-casein genotype decreases intestinal and systemic sensitization to β-lactoglobulin in guinea pigs. J Dairy Res, 68: 217–227

Blasi, M., G. Perrotta, A. Lanza, D. Iamartino and F. Pilla, 2005. Genetic diversity in three Italian donkey populations assessed by microsatellite markers. Ital. J. Anim. Sci. 4 (suppl.2): 127.

Bonnet, M., C. Delavaud, K. Laud, I. Gourdou, C. Leroux, J. Diane and Y. Chilliard, 2002. Mammary leptin synthesis, milk leptin and their putative physiological roles. Reprod. Nutr. Dev., 42: 399-413.

Carroccio, A., F. Cavataio and G. Iacono, 1999. Cross-reactivity between milk proteins of differents animals. Clin. Exp. Allergy, 29: 1014:1016.

Carroccio, A., F. Cavataio, G., Montaldo, D. D'Amico, L. Alabrese and G. Iacono, 2000a. Intolerance to hydrolised cow's milk proteins in infants: clinical characteristics and dietary treatments. Clin. Exp. Allergy, 30: 1597-1603.

Carroccio, A., G. Montalto, N. Custro, A. Notarbartolo, L. Alabrese and G. Iacono, 2000b. Evidence of very delayed clinical reactions to cow's milk in cow's milk-intolerant patients. Allergy 55, 574-579.

Chiavari, C., Coloretti F., M. Nanni, E. Sorrentino and L. Grazia, 2005. Use of donkey's milk for a fermented beverage with lactobacilli. Lait 85: 481-490.

Chiofalo, B. and E. Salimei, 2001. Ass's milk: exploitation of an alimentary resource. Folium per l'ambiente e la sicurezza sul lavoro 3: 235-241;

Chiofalo, B., V. Azzarra, L.Liotta and L. Chiofalo, 2004. The chemical and physical parameters of the Ragusana ass's milk during lactation. In: Proc. 6th Congress New Findings In Equine Practices, Campobasso (I), july 2004: 77-84.

Chiofalo, B., V. Azzara, D. Piccolo, L. Liotta and L. Chiofalo, 2005a. Il latte d'asina al traguardo della ricerca. Gli acidi grassi nel corso della lattazione. Large Animal Rewiew, 1, 39-44.

Chiofalo, B., D. Piccolo, V. Azzara, G. Cascone, L. Liotta and L. Chiofalo, 2005b. L'asino "Grigio Siciliano": risultati preliminari sulle caratteristiche composizionali del latte. In: Proceedings In Proc. 7th Congress New Findings In Equine Practices, Lodi (LO, Italy) 22-23 july (pp. 168-172).

Chiofalo, B., M. Polidori, R. Costa and E. Salimei, 2005c. Fresh forage in dairy ass's ration: effect on milk fatty acid and composition and flavours. Ital.J.Anim.Sci., 4(suppl.2): 433-435.

Chiofalo, B., D. Piccolo, E.B., Riolo, C. Maglieri and E. Salimei, 2006a. Different fiber sources in dairy ass's diet: I. Effects on milk fatty acid composition. In Proc. 3rd European Workshop on Equine Nutrition, Campobasso (Italy), june 20th – 22nd, 2006: in press.

Chiofalo, B., E. Salimei, P. Dugo, T. Kumm, D. Piccolo and L. Mondello, 2006b. Evaluation of triglycerides in donkey milk during lactation. In Proc. 3rd European Equine Health and Nutrition Congress, Ghent (Belgium), 17-18 march, 102-104.

Civardi, G., M.C. Curadi, M. Orlandi, T.M.P. Cattaneo and R. Giangiacomo, 2002. Capillary electrophoresis (CE) applied to analysis of mare's milk. Milchwiss 57: 515-517.

Cocchi, M. and E. Turchetto, 1999. Polyunsaturated fatty acids (LCPs) and perinatal development. Progress in nutrition, 1: 3-27.

Conte, F., A. Calabrò and G. Monsù, 2003. Il latte di asina: alimento per il futuro. Il progresso veterinario, 2/2003: 63-68.

Conte, F., ML Scatassa, G. Monsù, V. Loverde, A. Finocchiaro, M. DeFino, 2004. Monitoring of safety and quality of donkey's milk. In Int. Conf. on Veterinary Public health and Food safety toward a risk based chain control, Roma, Italy, 22nd – 23rd October: 58-59.

Conte, F., 2005. Osservazioni sul punto crioscopico del latte di asina. Il latte, dic. 2005: 42-45.

Coppola, R., E. Salimei, M. Succi, E. Sorrentino, M. Nanni, P. Ranieri, R. Belli Blanes and L.Grazia, 2002. Behaviour of Lactobacillus rhamnosus strains in ass's milk. Annals of Microbiology, 52: 55-60.

D'Arval, C., 1912. Il latte nella produzione e nell'igiene dell'alimentazione. Antonio Vallardi Ed., Milano (Italy), pp. 115.

Dell'Orto, V., E. Salimei, V. Bontempo, F. Fantuz, P.M. Toppino and G. Contarini, 1993. Produzione e composizione di latte equino: osservazioni sperimentali. In: Proc. XLVII Congress Società Italiana delle Scienze Veterinarie, 47: 2073-2077

Doreau, M., 1991. Le lait de jument. INRA Prod. Anim. 4: 297-302.

Doreau, M. and S. Boulot, 1989. Recent knowledge on mare milk production. Liv. Prod. Sci., 22: 213-235.

Doreau, M., S. Boulot, W. Martin-Rosset and H. Dubroeucq, 1986. Milking lactating mares using oxjtocin: milk volume and composition. Rep. Nutr. Dev., 26: 1-11.

Doreau, M., J.L. Gaillard, J.M. Chobert, J. Léonil, A.S. Egito and T. Haertlé, 2002. Composition of mare and donkey milk fatty acids and proteins and consequences on milk utilisation. In proceedings of 4th Congress "New findings in equine practice", Campobasso (Italy) 7th -9th July: 51-71.

Donnet-Hughes, A., N. Duc, P. Serrant, K. Vidal and E.J. Schiffrin, 2000. Bioactive molecules in milk and their role in health and disease: the role of transforming growth factor-β. Immunol. and Cell Biol. 78, 74-79.

Drogoul, C., H. Prevost and J.L. Maubois, 1992. Le lait de juments un produit, une filière a développer? In Proceedings 18ème Journée d'Etude, CEREOPA (editor), Paris, France. 37-51.

Dugo, P., T. Kumm, M. Lo Presti, B. Chiofalo, E. Salimei, A. Cotroneo and L. Mondello, 2005. Determination of triacylglycerols in donkey milk by using high performances liquid chromatography coupled with atmospheric pressure chemical ionization mass spectrometry. J. Separation Science, 28: 1023-1030.

El Razzaz, M., 2002. Donkeys in Egypt. In Proc. Congress EAAP, 1-3 September 2002, Cairo, Egypt, pp. 29.

Fanta, C. and C. Ebner, 1998. Allergy to mare's milk. Allergy, 53: 539-540.

Fantuz F., S. Vincenzetti, P. Polidori, A. Vita, F. Polidori and E. Salimei, 2001. Study on the protein fractions of donkey milk. In: Proc. XIV Congress of Associazione Scientifica di Produzione Animale, Firenze (Italy) 12-15 June, 635-637.

Fantuz, F., P. Polidori, C. Maglieri, G. Varisco, S. Vincenzetti and E. Salimei, 2006. Ass's milk nitrogen distribution: effects of different dietary fibre source, In: Proc. 3rd European Workshop on Equine Nutrition, Campobasso (Italy) 20th – 22nd june: in press.

Fox, P.F., 2001. Milk proteins as food ingredients. Int. J. Dairy Technol., 54: 41-55

Gandini, G. and G. Rognoni, 1997. An ethnographic atlas of Italian horse and ass populations. Città degli Studi Edizioni, Milano (Italy), pp. 142.

Godovac-Zimmermann, J., A. Conti, M. Sheil and L. Napolitano, 1990. Covalent structure of the minor monomeric beta-lactoglobulin II component from donkey milk. Biological Chemistry Hoppe-Seyler, 371: 871-879.

Herrouin, M., D. Molle, J. Fauquant, F. Ballestra, JL Maubois and J. Leonil, 2000. New genetic variants identified in donkey's milk whey proteins. J. of Protein Chemistry, 19: 105-115.

Hoppu, U., M. Kalliomaki and E. Isolauri, 2002. Cow's milk allergy – a matter of fat. Allergy 57, 61-62.

Høst, A., 2002. Frequency of cow's milk allergy in childhood. Ann. Allergy Asthma Immunol., 89 (Suppl.): pp. 33-37.

Iacono, G., A. Carroccio, F. Cavataio, G. Montalto, M. Soresi and V. Balsamo, 1992. Use of ass's milk in multiple food allergy. J. Pediatric Gastroent. Nutr., 14: 177-181.

Iametti, S., F. Sessa, F. Bonomi, G.F.Greppi, M. Feligni and G. Enne, 1998. Biochemical methods for the characterisation of mare and donkey casein. IDF Bulletin, issue Milk protein polymorphism, 1998: 268–274.

Jahreis, G., J. Fritsche, P. Mockel, F. Schone and U. Moller, 1999. The potential anticarcinogenic conjugated linoleic acid, cis-9, trans-11 C18:2, in milk of different species: cow, goat, ewe, sow, mare, woman. Nutr. Res., 19: 1541 – 1549.

Kanyshkova, T.G., S.E. Babina, D.V. Semenov, N. Isaeva, A.V. Vlassov, K.N. Neustroev, A.A. Kul'minskaya, V.N. Buneva and G.A. Nevinsky, 2003. Multiple enzymic activities of human milk lactoferrin. Eur. J. Biochem., 270: 3353-3361.

Laiho, K., A. Ouwehand, S. Salminen and I. Isolauri, 2002. Inventing probiotic functional foods for patients with allergic disease. Ann. Allergy Asthma Immunol., 89 (Suppl.): 75-82.

Liu, Z., N. Li and J. Neu, 2005. Tight junctions, leaky intestines, and pediatric diseases., Acta Paediatrica, 94: 386-393.

Lodi, R., R. Todesco and S.Carini, 1984. Indagine preliminare sull'impiego del lisozima nella tecnologia del formaggio Provolone. Ind. Latte, 20: 37–50.

Lonnerdal, B., 2003. Nutritional and physiologic significance of human milk proteins. Am. J. Clin. Nutr. 77(suppl): 1537S–43S.

Malacarne, M., F. Martuzzi, A. Summer and P. Mariani, 2002. Protein and fat composition of mare's milk: some nutritional remarks with reference to human and cow's milk. Int Dairy J. 12: 869-877.

Marconi, E.and G. Panfili, 1998. Chemical composition and nutritional properties of commercial product of mare's milk powder. J. of Food Comp. and Analysis, 11: 178-181.

Miraglia, N., M. Polidori and E. Salimei, 2002. A review of feeding strategies, feeds and management of equines in Central-Southern Italy, In In: Ed. R.A. Pearson, P.Lhoste, M. Saastamoinen, W. Martin-Rosset, Working animal in agriculture and transport, EAAP Technical Series n°6, Wageningen Academic Publishers, The Netherlands, 103-112

Modler, H.W., 1994. Bifidogenic factors – sources, metabolism and applications, Int Dairy J., 4, 389-407.

Monti, G., 2004. Contro l'allergia il latte d'asina. Notiziario Azienda Ospedaliera O.I.R.M., S. Anna, Torino, marzo: 29-31.

Morera, Pons S., A.I. Castellote Bargallò and M.C. Lòpez Sabater, 1998. Evaluation by high-performance liquid chromatography of the hydrolysis of human milk triacylglycerides during storage at low temperatures. J. of Chromatography A, 823: 467-474.

Muraro, A.A., P.G. Giampietro and E. Galli, 2002. Soy formulas and nonbovine milk. Ann. Allergy Asthma Immunol., 89 (Suppl.): 97-101.

Nigro, N., 1982. Puericulture. Minerva Italica ed., Torino (Italy).

Oftedal, O.T. and R. Jenness, 1988. Interspecies variation in milk composition among horses, zebras and asses (Periossidactyla: Equidae). J Dairy Res., 55: 57-66.

Pinto, F., A. Lestingi, A. Caputi Jambrenghi, G.Marsico and G. Vonghia, 1998. Conservazione e valorizzazıone dell'asino di Martina Franca: influenza dell'integrazione alimentare su alcuni aspetti quanti-qualitativi del latte. I. Indagine preliminare. In: Proc. 4th National Congresss on Biodiversity, Alghero (SS, Italy), 1173-1176.

Playford, R.J., C.E. Macdonald and W.S. Johnson, 2000. Colostrum and milk derived peptide growth factors for the treatment of gastrointestinal disorders. Am.J.Clin. Nutr. 72: 5-14.

Polidori, F. 1994. Il latte dietetico. In: Symposium "Aspetti dietetici della produzione del latte, un alimento antico proiettato verso il futuro", Torino 4th November: 16 pp.

Restani, P., B. Beretta, A. Fiocchi, C. Ballabio and C.L. Galli, 2002. Cross-reactivity between mammalian proteins. Ann Allergy Asthma Immunol. Suppl. 89:11-15.

Roncada, P. and G.F. Greppi, 2001. Il progetto proteoma: confronto fra latte d'asina e latte per neonati. In: Proc. LV Congr. Ital. Soc. Vet. Sci. (S.I.S.V.E.T.), Rimini, Italy, pp. 29-30.

Salimei, E., M. Cattaneo, B. Chiofalo and V. Dell'Orto, 1996. Exploitation of mare's milk by poliunsaturated fatty acids enrichment. In: Food & health: role of animal products, G. Enne and GF Greppi editors: 223-227.

Salimei, E., R. Belli Blanes, A. Marano, E. Ferretti, G. Varisco and D. Casamassima, 2000. Produzione quanti-qualitativa di latte di asina: risultati di due lattazioni. In Proc. 35th Int. Symp. of Società Italiana per il Progresso della Zootecnia, Ragusa Ibla (RG), may 25th, 2000: 315-322.

Salimei, E., G. Varisco and F. Rosi, 2002. Major constituents, leptin, and non-protein nitrogen compounds in mares' colostrum and milk. Reprod. Nutr. Dev. 42:65-72.

Salimei, E., Fantuz F., Coppola R., Chiofalo B., Polidori P. and Varisco G., 2004a. Composition and characteristics of ass's milk. Anim. Res., 53: 67-78.

Salimei, E., F. Fantuz, A. Simoni, G. Varisco and C. Chiari, 2004b. Ass's milking machine: first results on residual milk. In Proc 6th New Findings In Equine Practices Congress, Campobasso, Italy, 7-9 july: 93-98.

Salimei, E., Rosi F., Maglieri C., Polidori M., Fantuz F. and Varisco G., 2005a. Effetti di differenti fonti fibrose nella dieta di asine sul contenuto di leptina e dei principali costituenti del latte. In Proc. 7th Congress New Findings In Equine Practices, Lodi (LO, Italy) 22-23 july: 160-165.

Salimei, E., F. Fantuz, G. Varisco, C. Maglieri and M. Polidori, 2005b. Different fiber sources in dairy ass's diet: effects on milk yield and composition. Ital. J. Anim. Sci. 4 (suppl. 2): 430-432.

Salimei, E., C. Maglieri, M. Polidori, R. Socci, B. Chiofalo, M. Gambacorta and G. Varisco, 2006. Machine milking of dairy asses as related to milk production and body condition. In: Proc. 3rd European Workshop on Equine Nutrition, Campobasso (Italy) 20th – 22nd june: in press.

Schryver, H.F., O.T. Oftedal, J. Williams, N.F. Cymbaluk, D. Antczak and H.F. Hintz, 1986. A comparison of the mineral composition of milk of domestic and captive wild equids (Equus przewalski, E. zebra, E. burchelli, E. caballus, E. asinus). Comp. Biochem. Physiol. 85A:233-235.

Seppo, L., R. Korpela, B. Lonnerdal, L. Metsaniitty, K. Juntunen-Backman, T. Klemola, A. Paganus and T. Vanto, 2005. A follow-up study of nutrient intake, nutritional status, and growth in infants with cow milk allergy fed either a soy formula or an extensively hydrolysed whey formula. Am. J. Clin. Nutr., 82: 140-145.

Simoni, A., E. Salimei, G. Varisco, 2004. Struttura e routine di mungitura e caratteristiche della produzione di latte di asina, alimento ipoallergenico per l'infanzia. In Proc. 6th New Findings In Equine Practices Congress, Campobasso, Italy, 7-9 july: 85-91

Solaroli, G., E. Pagliarini and C. Peri, 1993. Composition and nutritional quality of mare's milk. Ital. J. Food Sci. 1: 3-10.

Sorrentino, E., E. Salimei, M. Succi, D. Gammariello, T. Di Criscio, G. Panfili and R. Coppola, 2005. Heat treatment of ass's milk, a hypoallergenic food for infancy. In: Proc. Congress on Technological innovation and enhancement of marginal products, Foggia (Italy) 6th -8th april, 6 pp

Svendsen, E.D., 1997. The professional handbook of the donkey, 3rd Ed. For the donkey sanctuary, Whittet Books Limited, London, 400 pp.

Tisserand, L.-L. and R.A. Pearson, 2003. Nutritional requirements, feed intake and digestion in working donkeys: a comparison with other work animals. In R.A. Pearson, P. Lhoste, M. Saastamoinen and W. Martin-Rosset (editors) Working animals in agriculture and transport, EAAP Technical Series n.6, 63-73

Van Soest, P.J., 1994. Nutritional ecology of the ruminant – 2nd ed. Comstock Publishing Associates, Cornell University Press, Ithaca & London, 476 pp.

Vincenzetti, S., P. Polidori, E. Salimei, P.L. Mariani, S. Allegri, N. Cammertoni and A.Vita, 2005. Purification and identification of alfa s1- and beta caseins from asses milk. Vet. Res. Comm., 29 (suppl. 2): 211-213.

Xu, R.J., 1996. Development of the newborn GI tract and its relation to colostrum/milk intake: a review. Reprod. Fertil. Dev., 8: 35-48.

Other utilisation of mare's and ass's milk

B. Chiofalo[1], C. Drogoul[2] and E. Salimei[3]
[1]Dept. Morphology, Biochemistry, Physiology and Animal Production, University of Messina, Polo Universitario Annunziata, 98168 Messina, Italy
[2]Experimental farm LEGTA Semur Chatillon, 21400 Chatillon sur Seine, France
[3]Dept. S.T.A.A.M., University of Molise, Via De Sanctis, 86100 Campobasso, Italy

Abstract

This review summaries the recent knowledge on the mechanisms of some bioactive substances, observed in the mare and donkey milk, in favour of the human health. The first studies on equine's milk composition have focussed the attention on the protein fraction showing a casein and whey protein content very similar to human milk and a higher presence of functional substances, hormones, immunoglobulin, nitrogenous compounds characterized by antibacterial action, *e.g.* lysozyme or lactoferrin. For the probiotic and prebiotic activities on the intestinal microflora, mare's and ass's milk, are traditionally known as an alternative food for infants affected by allergic reactions on immunological basis to cow's milk proteins. More recently, some bioactive substances are also identified in the category of lipids. Among these, the essential fatty acids, found in higher quantity, are capable to interact in the development of the neonatal nervous system as well as to condition indirectly or directly the intestinal environment and the immune-inflammatory system, being involved, through the synthesis of eicosanoids (prostaglandins, thromboxanes and leukotrienes), in the prevention and cures of some pathologies not only of infants but also of adults (osteogenesis process, arteriosclerosis, premature senescence, coronary disease). Moreover, thanks to the qualitative composition of triglycerides, the equine milk has a similar digestibility to human milk and higher than that of cow milk.

Keywords: mare, ass, milk, lipid, human health

Introduction

Although equid (mare's and ass's) milk is mainly devoted to foal feeding, the use of this milk for human consumption is increasing thanks to its nutritional and dietetic properties (Doreau and Martuzzi, 2006; Salimei and Chiofalo, 2006).

In the former USSR and Mongolia, there is a tradition of the utilisation of this milk, e.g. as koumiss (alcoholic fermented milk), based on its therapeutic qualities, suggested by empirical knowledge, but which has never been scientifically assessed (Doreau *et al.*, 2002).

In Western Europe, equid milk utilisation is developing, on hand for drinking, on the other hand for cosmetic. With regard to equid's milk feeding, fermented, not fermented and milk derivatives, the positive experimental results of paediatric studies on the treatment of the allergies (Carroccio *et al.*, 2000; Curadi *et al.*, 2001; Iacono and D'Amico, 2001), and the recent issue on genetically modified production of soy, one of the most important ingredient of hypoallergenic food for early infancy, have stimulated new researches in this direction for different reasons: i) for a better knowledge of equid's milk composition; ii) for analysing the origin of the positive effects for human and iii) for evaluating the effects of nutrition on productive (qualitative and quantitative) and nutritional response of the animals (Doreau *et al.*, 2002; Salimei *et al.*, 2005a).

Considering the bio-dietetic value of equid milk thanks to some complex bio-nutritional and extra-nutritional compounds, this review will describe some of the mechanisms of bioactive substances in favour of human health. In this context, its utilisation in dermatology, well known since ancient Rome, probably related to its lysozyme content, efficacious in soothing skin and scalp inflammations, seems to be less interesting.

Incidence of cow's milk allergy in childhood

In Western Countries it is well-known that the cow's milk proteins allergy (CMPA), a reaction on immunological basis, represents the most frequent case of alimentary allergy in the infants with an incidence that varies between 0,3 and 7% (Iacono and D'Amico, 2001); in these subjects it is possible to distinguish approximately: a 50-70% of cutaneous symptoms, a 50-60% of gastrointestinal problems and a 20-30% of respiratory symptoms (Høst, 2002). Although most children will recover by the age of 3 years, it is reported that up to 30% of children are still symptomatic after 4 years of age (Muraro *et al.*, 2002). In these patients the CMPA condition becomes a serious problem of alimentary emergency from the first infancy to the schooling years and it could develop towards a multiple alimentary intolerance in the 10% of the cases (Iacono and D'Amico, 2001; Host, 2002).

The rational treatment of the alimentary allergies in infants requires the substitution in the diet of the injurious food with other hypoallergenic formulas. The most diffuse substitutes are soy and hydrolyzed protein formulas, unfortunately often characterized by low palatability ("cooked taste") because of high temperatures during the technologic treatments, by risks of cross-reactivity in highly sensitive patients, by high costs and by nutritional deficiencies (A.A.P., 1998). In these cases the therapeutic treatment represents a problem of difficult solution, object of recent studies of the paediatric medicine, which is searching a valid alternative. In clinical practice, a widespread alternative to these hypoallergenic formulas, are the animal proteins (goat's milk, mare's-ass's milk, lamb/chicken meat based formulas) (Muraro *et al.*, 2002; Restani *et al.*, 2002). However, babies affected by CMPA have also manifested allergic reactions to the goat's milk proteins (approximately 25-30%) and to the meat proteins of herbivorous species (Greco, 2001).

A developing therapeutic approach of alimentary allergies is based on the use of immunotherapy that modulates the hypersensitivity reactions and promotes the function of barrier of the intestine. In fact, the microflora represents a crucial component of the gut environment, which is altered by the inflammatory processes. Therefore, a normal microflora contributes to the development of the oral tolerance suggesting, therefore, that a probiotic therapy could have positive effects in the hypersensitivity (Troncone and Borrelli, 2001).

Alternative treatment of multiple food allergy: Mare' s and Ass's milk

Amongst the new food, as a replacement for human breast milk for infants affected by food allergies and intolerances, particular interest is addressed to equid milk, already used since Erodoto times (5th century B.C.) for its composition much more similar to human milk than can be said of cow's milk. In 1881, the French Welfare Services set up in Paris a herd of asses to nurse syphilitic children, asses being impervious to syphilis contamination (Delahaye, 1990).

As regard mare's milk utilisation, Businco *et al.* (2000) have demonstrated the low allergenic potential of mare's milk in a population of 25 selected children with severe IgE-mediated cow's milk allergy. All the children had strong positive skin test responses to cow's milk; two children had positive test reactions to mare's milk, too. All children were positive to double-blind, placebo-controlled food challenge (DBPCFC) for cow's milk, but only one was positive for mare's milk.

The primary structures of equine α-lactalbumin have been determined and the phylogenetic difference between equine α-lactalbumin and bovine α-lactalbumin has been shown to be related to 39- and 40- amino acid substitution, respectively (Godovac-Zimmermann *et al.*, 1987). These differences in the amino acid sequences of bovine and mare proteins could account for different levels of inhibition obtained by immunoblotting techniques with the two types of milk tested: the critical amino acid sequence relevant for IgE binding to cow's milk could be in fact different in mare's milk (Businco *et al.*, 2000).

Several studies report that the addition of γ-linolenic acid in the human diet improves the degree of eczematous involvement of the skin in some atopic dermatitis patients (Horrobin, 1993; Berth-Jones *et al.*, 1995; Horrobin, 2000). Doreau and Boulot (1989) evaluated the variability of the fatty acid composition and of the nutritional content of mare's milk from a variety of breeds with a view to its potential use as a good linoleic and linolenic source; the HUFA content was also found quite high in mare's milk (Bontempo *et al.*, 2000), when compared to cow's milk, These data suggest that mare's milk can also be considered a potential nutritional source in the future for children suffering from atopic dermatitis. Moreover, the high level of linoleic and linolenic acids in mare's milk underline the role of this product in the premature senescence and the hypocholesterolemic diets (Dell'Orto *et al.*, 1993).

Because the donkey has the same phylogenetic origin as the mare, but different from that of the cow, some trials have been conducted in patients with diagnosis of CMPA, based on the use of ass's milk (Iacono and D'Amico, 1992). The results of these studies showed, in the treated patients, a growth trend similar to those obtained with other formulas, total disappearance of the symptoms and its persistency in the follow-up (15-20 months), no allergic type reactions when cow's milk was reintroduced in the infant's diet (Muraro *et al.*, 2002), indicating ass's milk as a promising alternative protein source in the severe IgE-mediated cow's milk allergy.

The "virtues" attributed to the ass's and mare's milk, could be also referable to the presence of functional factors, hormones, immunoglobulin, as well as to nitrogenous compounds characterized by antibacterial and immune-modulator activity, e.g. lysozyme and lactoferrin (Coppola *et al.*, 2002; Di Cagno *et al.*, 2004; Salimei *et al.*, 2004) and by some other bioactive components. Among the bioactive protein of milk, leptin is a hormone probably involved in the neonates growth besides its influence on dam's adiposity and feed intake, as reviewed by Bonnet and coll. (2002); the leptin content of both mare's and ass's milk were close to those observed in human milk (Salimei *et al.*, 2002; Salimei *et al.*, 2005b).

Moreover, among the protein components involved in the CMPA, Salimei *et al.* (2004) showed the lower content of casein in ass's milk (0.64% - 1.03 g/100g milk) than in mare's milk at the beginning of lactation (Martuzzi *et al.*, 2000) but it was intermediate between human and ruminant milk values (Travia, 1986); the whey proteins content of ass's milk (0.49 – 0.80 g/100g milk), was very similar to that observed in mare's milk (Doreau *et al.*, 2002; Malacarne *et al.*, 2002), and α-lactalbumin and β-lactoglobulin levels of ass's milk were 22.56% and 29.85% of the total whey protein, respectively,(Salimei *et al.*, 2004; 2006). It has to be noted that β-lactoglobulin is considered the probable major milk allergen in infants and small children, whereas the casein is considered the predominant allergen in adults (Carroccio *et al.*, 1999).

Together with the allergenic properties, also the organoleptic characteristics have contributed to the spread of this product as the good palatability, because of the high lactose content (Oftedal and Jennes, 1988; Chiofalo *et al.*, 2004) and its flavour constituents, carbonylic compounds, alcohols, terpenes, even if variable in relation to the feed, mainly fibrous, of the animal diet (Chiofalo *et al.*, 2005a).

Because of its hypoallergenic role, the properties of the ass's milk protein fraction are investigated widely while few attention is paid to the lipid composition which, instead, appears to be a particularly importance considering the pivotal role of fat-derived anti-inflammatory substances (Chiofalo, 2001; Doreau *et al.*, 2002). According to the proved efficacy of the lipid fraction on the regulation of the immune-inflammatory system, on the neonatal development (Caramia *et al.*, 2000) as well as on the digestibility of a product intended for human (Morera Pons *et al.*, 1998), this study aims to deepen the knowledge on some lipid components of ass' milk.

Bioactive substances in ass's and mare's milk: the lipids

Recently, ass's milk has been proposed as a functional food thanks to some bioactive compounds interesting not only in the diet of the infants but also for that of the "elders"; these substances are lipids characterized by particular functional properties because of their indirect or direct effects on both the intestinal environment and the immunity, involved in the prevention and cures of some pathologies (Chiofalo, 2001; Chiofalo *et al.*, 2003).

Few references concerning the fat composition show the main specificities of equine milk fat compared to cow or human milk, that can be synthesised as: i) the higher content of PUFA n-3 fatty acids, in particular the level of linolenic acid; ii) the lower proportion of tryglicerides (TAGs), compensated for by high percentage of both free fatty acids and phospholipids (Doreau *et al.*, 2002). On the other hand, new data concerning the fatty acid and the triacylglycerol components of ass's milk may allow a better understanding of the positive effect of this product on human health.

I. Milk fatty acid composition

Recent studies (Laiho *et al.*, the 2002) on the immunomodulatory properties of fatty acids and antioxidant, including alfa-tocopherol, of certain nutrients, have shown that food not only is a source of dietary antigens causing sensitization but also may contain protective factors, that through the regulation of the immune function, may counteract with the oxidative stress and may diminish the inflammatory response in allergic disease. In fact, frequently, the problems of bronchial reactivity, allergic asthma and inflammation, are reported in patients with imbalanced intake between of n-3 and n-6 polyunsaturated fatty acids in favour of the latter, with consequent greater production of prostaglandin E2 (PGE2), and with low concentrations of plasma antioxidants (Laiho *et al.*, 2002). Whereas, it has been demonstrated that high intake of vitamin E and of n-3 series fatty acid levels, of which are well known the anti-inflammatory, antiaggregant and non immunosuppressant properties, cause a decrease of the haematic IgE synthesis (Laiho *et al.*, 2002). This underlines the necessity to assure the intake of both fatty acids (n-6 and n-3) series for a re-balance between pro-inflammatory and anti-inflammatory factors, together with adequate vitamin E levels in order to neutralize the possible peroxide production, balancing oxidants and anti-oxidants, as well as in order to maintain the immunity (Caramia *et al.*, 2000).

As regard to ass's milk, the fatty acids more represented are on average: capric ($C_{10:0}$= 11.19 g/100 g fatty acids), lauric ($C_{12:}0$= 10.29 g/100 g), palmitic ($C_{16:0}$ = 16.55 g/100 g), oleic ($C_{18:1n9}$ = 14.55 g/100 g), linoleic ($C_{18:2n6}$ = 11.14 g/100 g) and linolenic ($C_{18:3n3}$ = 8.62 g/100 g) acids (Chiofalo *et al.*, 2006a). The levels of these acids are indicative, being this lipid fraction significantly influenced by the experimental methodologies such as breed, stage of lactation (Chiofalo *et al.*, 2005b), milking system and management, etc..

Compared to the mean values of monounsaturated (23.62 g/100 g) and polyunsaturated (21.90 g/100 g) classes (Figure 1), saturated milk fatty acids are the most represented (54.52 g/100 g) (Chiofalo *et al.*, 2006a); the SFA and MUFA levels are comparable to those observed in mare milk (Salimei *et al.*,

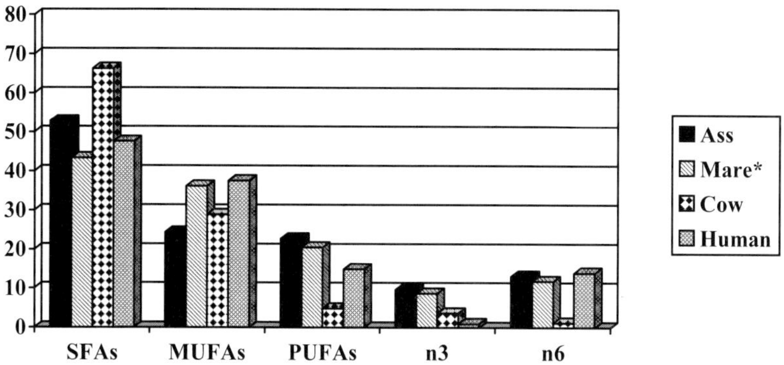

*Figure 1. Acidic class percentages in the milk of different animal species and human (Chiofalo et al., 2006a; *Salimei et al., 1996).*

1996; Goracci *et al.*, 2004), and lower than those observed in ruminant milk. According to Others' observations on mare's milk, the relatively high content of fatty acids with 16 and less carbons could be due to a synthesis of these fatty acids from acetate and 3-hydroxybutirate, as in ruminants, and not from glucose, as monogastrics (Doreau and Boulot, 1989).

The level of polyunsaturated fatty acids in ass's milk resulted higher than that observed in ruminant milk: these data, consistent with values observed in mare's milk, confirms that in monogastric herbivora, the amount of unsaturated long chain fatty acids in milk is related to the amount consumed with the diet Doreau and Boulot (1989). The absence of hydrogenation of fatty acids in the digestive tract before absorption, otherwise occurring in ruminants, may then explain the high content in linoleic and linolenic acids in milk samples (Figure 2).

High and equilibrate essential fatty acid content, together with the low atherogenic (0,80) and thrombogenic (0,32) indices (Table 1) observed by Chiofalo and coll. (2005a), underline the immune-modulator properties of this product. In fact, compared with ruminants' milk, the considerable presence of unsaturated fatty acids found in ass's milk make it very interesting in the prevention of the cardiovascular, auto-immune and inflammatory diseases (Kinsella *et al.*, 1990). The n-3 polyunsaturated fatty acids content, characteristic constituents of the fish oils, can counteract the above-mentioned pathologies through the synthesis of antiinflammatory, antiaggregant and non immunosuppressant substances, like lipid mediators (eicosanoids), prostaglandins (PGE_3) and

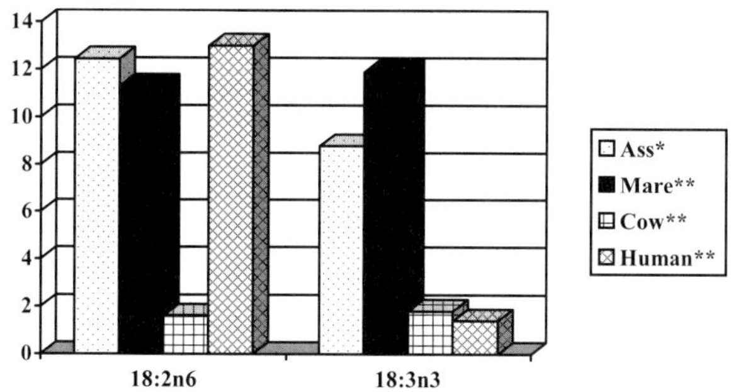

*Figure 2. Essential fatty acid percentages in the milk of different animal species and human (*Chiofalo et al., 2006a; **Doreau et al., 2002).*

Table 1. Quality indices of some products for human consumption.

Feed	Atherogenic index*	Thrombogenic index*
Ass's milk**	0.80	0.32
Olive oil***	0.14	0.31
Butter***	2.07	2.42
Lard***	0.47	1.20
Pork***	0.83	0.68
White meat***	0.51	1.06
Trout fillet***	0.50	0.35

*Calculated using equations proposed by Ulbricht and Southgate (1991);
** From Chiofalo *et al.*, 2005a;
*** From Amerio and Elli, 1996

Questionnaire. Evaluation of the acceptability of two types of fermented mare milk (Koumis and yogurt) according to the knowledge of the consumer.

Fermented milk tasted	Koumiss			Yogurt		
	No	Yes	Out of which Very much	No	Yes	Out of which Very much
Question 1: After having tasted the product: would you say you like this product?						
Group 1 *	44.9%	55.1%	10.1%	23.0%	77.0%	23.0%
Group 2**	33.3%	66.7%	15.4%	9.2%	90.8%	33.6%
Question 2: After having heard about the mare milk qualities: How often would you drink it ?***						
Group 1	45.4%	44.4%	10.2%	22.3%	50.6%	33.6%
Group 2	36.5%	53.1%	10.4%	14.5%	58.6%	26.9%

*Group 1: consumer did not know the origin of the milk before tasting it
**Group 2: consumer knew he (or she) was tasting mare's fermented milk
*** For this question, group 1 was informed that they just had tasted mare's milk.
From Drogoul and Bigand, 1996

leukotrienes (LTB_5), and protein mediators (cytokines), interleukins (IL_4, IL_{10}, IL_{13}, IL_{1ra}), tumor necrosis factor, etc (Williams, 2000).

In this direction some Authors pointed out the role of ass's milk both in the osteogenesis process (Wolter, 1996) and in the atherosclerosis dietotherapy, in the rehabilitation of the patients with coronary hearth disease (Chiofalo, 2001).

However, the results obtained in the last years also have evidenced some limits of the ass's milk that, if supplemented by appropriate nutrients, could optimize the role of "functional food" of this product, making it a valid and alternative protein source. The major limit is represented by its low fat content, as described elsewhere (Salimei and Chiofalo, 2006): ass's milk is also characterised by the low presence of some long chain polyunsaturated fatty acids as conjugated linoleic acids (CLA) (Doreau *et al.*, 2002), responsible for the wide variety of beneficial effects (e.g. anticarcenogenic effect, antiatherosclerotic effects, antidiabetic effects), as well as arachidonic (C20:4n6) and docosaesaenoic (C22:6n3) acids, particularly represented in the membranes of the nervous cells, in the external segments of the retinal photoreceptor and in the acrosome of the spermatozoa, therefore essential during the neonatal development (Cocchi, 2000).

II. Milk triacylglycerols

The knowledge of the composition of milk lipids, in terms of molecular species of triacylglycerols (TAGs), is fundamental in order to explain the physical properties, nutritive (action of lipolytic enzymes)/organoleptic (palatability) characteristics and the biosynthetic pathways of milk fat (Morera Pons *et al.*, 1998). The large number of fatty acids present in the lipid fraction of milk makes it one of the most complex naturally occurring fats with an overwhelming variety of different TAG species (Morera Pons *et al.*, 2003). The analysis of the TAG composition of milk fat appears to be a particularly challenging and important task, also considering the pivotal role of fat-derived inflammatory substances.

Moreover, considering the close correlation between triglyceride distribution and digestibility of a food (Morera Pons *et al.*, 1998), and considering the main destination of the ass's milk, more information are necessary relatively to this lipid component. In fact, the little literature at disposal on this subject (Dugo *et al.*, 2005) underline some quali-quantitative differences in the fatty acid typology that form the ass's milk triglycerides in comparison with those of human' and cow' milk.

In the past, several chromatographic methods (Parody, 1982; Morera Pons *et al.*, 1998) were used for the determination of triacylglycerols in the milk of large and small animals, of monogastric and ruminant species and of human but no data have been found about ass's milk.

Recently (Dugo *et al.*, 2005), the analysis of the ass's milk by using reversed-phase and silver ion performance liquid chromatography coupled with atmospheric pressure chemical ionization mass spectrometry (RP-HPLC-Ag+-HPLC/APCI-MS) has permitted the separation of more than 50 triacylglycerols in less than 80 min., as Figure 3 shows. The totally and partially separated TAGs content of Ragusana ass's milk fat with corresponding retention time (tR), partition number (PN = CN – 2DB), total carbon number (CN) and number of double bonds in the TAG molecule (DB) are reported in Table 2 and 3 respectively (Dugo *et al.*, 2005).

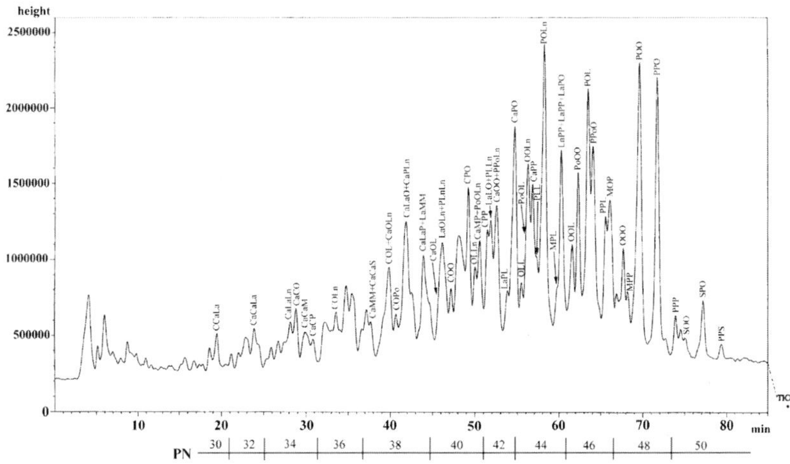

Figure 3. RP-HPLC-APCI-MS chromatogram of donkey milk TAGs (Dugo et al., 2005).

Table 2. Totally separated triacylglycerols with corresponding retention time (t_R), partition number (PN) total carbon number (CN), double bond number (DB) and quantitative results of donkey milk TAGs.

TAG*	t_R (min)	PN	CN	DB	% of total **
CCaLa	19.32	30	30	0	0.71
CaCaLa	23.66	32	32	0	0.81
CaLaLn	27.95	34	40	3	1.08
CaCo	28.62	34	36	1	0.96
CaCaM	29.65	34	34	0	1.18
CaCP	30.55	34	34	0	0.58
COLn	33.25	36	44	4	1.32
COPo	40.44	38	42	2	0.84
COO	47.01	40	44	2	1.21
CPO	49.05	40	42	1	2.70
OLLn	49.87	42	54	6	1.38
CPP	51.28	40	40	0	1.82
LaPL	53.69	42	46	2	1.21
CaPO	54.52	42	44	1	4.63
OLL	55.31	44	54	5	1.14
POLn	58.10	44	52	4	6.69
OOL	61.49	46	54	4	2.40
PoOO	62.21	46	52	3	2.80
POL	63.30	46	52	3	4.48
PPoO	64.25	46	50	2	4.18
PPL	65.49	46	50	2	1.85
MOP	65.97	46	48	1	2.99
POO	69.52	48	52	2	6.22
PPO	71.94	48	50	1	5.25
PPP	73.71	48	48	0	0.87
SOO	74.97	50	54	2	0.68
SPO	77.22	50	52	1	1.46
PPS	79.44	50	50	0	0.51

* The nomenclature used to describe the TAGs is not stereospecific: the order of the three abbreviations does not define the position of the fatty acyl residues linked to the glycerol backbone.
** The quantitative results are calculated according to the corresponding peak area values of every TAG, considering only identified TAGs that make up to 86% of total TAG area in the RP-HPLC chromatogram.
From Dugo *et al.*, 2005

The peculiar triglyceride distribution of donkey's milk as well as horse's milk (Breckenidge and Kuksis, 1967) is largely due to the unusually high presence of Capric acid (Ca) that is recovered in 18 triacylglycerols out of 55 TAGs identified (Table 2, 3). Moreover, the milk fat of donkey showed a TAG pattern with 30-54 acyl carbon atoms (Table 2, 3) as well as horse milk (Breckenidge and Kuksis, 1967) in relation to the high content of medium- and long-chain fatty acids. The main components of the TAG fraction of donkey milk are (Table 2): Palmitic-Oleic-Linolenic (6.69%), Palmitic-Oleic-Oleic (6.22%), Palmitic-Palmitic-Oleic (5.25%), Capric-Palmitic-Oleic (4.63%), Palmitic-Oleic-Linoleic (4.48%) and Palmitic-Palmitoleic-Oleic (4.18%).

Table 3. Partially separated triacylglycerols with corresponding retention time (t_R), partition number (PN) total carbon number (CN), double bond number (DB) and quantitative results of donkey milk TAGs.

TAG*	t_R (min)	PN	CN	DB	% of total **
CaMM	36.97	38	38	0	1.77
CaCaS		38	38	0	
CaOL	39.64	38	44	3	3.07
CaOLn		38	46	4	
CaLaO	41.66	38	40	1	3.90
CaPLn		38	44	3	
CaLaP	43.83	38	38	0	3.90
LaMM		40	40	0	
CaOL	45.99		46	3	3.96
LaOLn		40	48	4	
PLnLn			52	6	
CaMP	50.41	40	40	0	2.28
PoOLn		42	52	5	
LaLO	51.72	42	48	3	1.85
PLLn			52	5	
CaOO	52.41	42	46	2	3.32
PPoLn			50	4	
PoOL	56.13	44	52	4	3.01
OOLn			54	5	
CaPP	56.81	42	42	0	
PLL	57.29	44	52	4	3.41
MPL	59.72	44	48	2	
LnPP	60.07		50	3	4.72
LaPP		44	44	0	
LaPO			46	1	
OOO	67.71	48	54	3	
MPP	68.19	46	46	0	2.89

* The nomenclature used to describe the TAGs is not stereospecific: the order of the three abbreviations does not define the position of the fatty acyl residues linked to the glycerol backbone.
** The quantitative results are calculated according to the corresponding peak area values of every TAG, considering only identified TAGs that make up to 86% of total TAG area in the RP-HPLC chromatogram.
From Dugo *et al.*, 2005

Literature data on the composition of the TAG fraction of mature human milk showed that the main components were Palmitic-Oleic-Oleic (about 24%) and Palmitic-Oleic-Linoleic (about 19%), followed by Palmitic-Palmitic-Oleic, Oleic-Oleic-Oleic, Palmitic-Palmitoleic-Oleic and Linoleic-Oleic-Oleic present in amounts ranging from 3 to 8% (Morera Pons *et al.*, 2000).

These results show a certain degree of qualitative similarity in the TAG fraction of these two products, both very dissimilar from the composition of cow milk, where the main components were reported to be Butyric-Palmitic-Oleic, Butyric-Palmitic-Palmitic and Butyric-Myristic-Palmitic, and where TAGs containing polyunsaturated fatty acids (Linoleic and Linolenic acids) were not found (Gresti *et al.*, 1993).

This observation could be explained by the absence in the small intestine of donkey of isomerization and hydrogenation processes of the fatty acids prior to absorption and esterification in blood; it also could confirm the nutritional value of donkey milk fat composition in relation to human health.

Moreover, according to Morera Pons *et al.* (2003) observations, the trend of the TAG in ass's milk during the lactation (Chiofalo *et al.*, 2006b) show a certain degree of similarity with that of TAGs profile in human milk; in fact, during the lactation some TAG species (Caprylic-Oleic-Linolenic, Caprylic-Palmitic-Oleic, Oleic-Linoleic-Linolenic and Capric-Palmitic-Oleic), also recovered in human milk, show relatively constant levels and could thus be considered as markers of the ass milk TAG profile. It has also to be noted that concentrations of other TAG species, e.g. Capric-Caprylic-Palmitic, Capric-Palmitic-Palmitic and Palmitic-Palmitoleic-Oleic, varied considerable (Chiofalo *et al.*, 2006b) and consequently these may be understood to be especially affected by external factors such as dietary intake, nutritional status, etc (Morera Pons *et al.*, 2003) which could have changed the availability of some fatty acids involved in the TAG synthesis in the mammary gland.

Figure 4 shows the numerical relationships between saturated and unsaturated TAGs on the basis of double bond (DB) numbers in ass's milk. As it can be seen, most of the identified TAGs presented no or only a few double bonds. This is obviously due to the higher frequency (expressed in percent) of saturated fatty acids present in the TAG molecules: six fatty acids out of ten identified in the glycerol molecule are saturated (Caprylic, Capric, Lauric, Myristic, Palmitic and Stearic), two are monounsaturated (Palmitoleic and Oleic), one is diunsaturated (Linoleic) while the remaining fatty acid is characterized by 3 double bonds (Linolenic).

Neverthless, in literature there is no information in relation to their stereospecific distribution, on the basis of the position of the fatty acyl residues linked to the glycerol backbone, which is an interesting characteristic in order to evidence possible analogies with the human's milk. As regard human's milk, it is well-known the esterification of the palmitic acid in position 2 on the glycerol molecule, whereas for the cow's milk the position 2 of the glycerol is esterified by the oleic acid. Consequently, for the specificity of the pancreatic lipase towards the primary ethereal bonds, the digestion of the human's milk permit a greater absorption of the palmitic acid like monoacylglycerides, while, during the digestion of the cow's milk, the palmitic acid, set free from the glycerol, bind itself to the calcium present in the intestinal lumen, precipitate as calcium soap, and therefore is excreted through the faeces with consequent a twofold nutritional damage: the loss of palmitic acid and of calcium (Fidanza and Liguori, 1988) from the body.

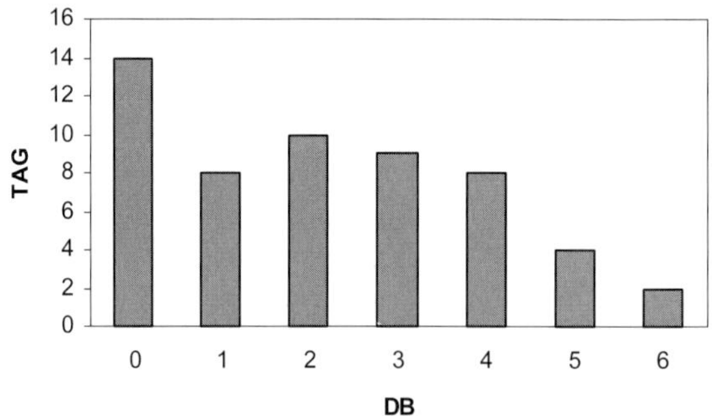

Figure 4. Distribution of TAGs on the basis of double bond (DB) numbers in donkey milk (Dugo et al., 2005).

Equid milk as fermented drink

Thanks to its chemical and microbiological characteristics, equids milk could be placed amongst the new generation drinks based on fermented milks of increasing interest in human nutrition (Drogoul *et al.*, 1992; Montanari *et al.*, 1996; Malacarne *et al.*, 2002; Di Cagno *et al.*, 2004). In particular, Koumiss, a lactic-alcoholic beverage derived from mare's milk represents an effective combination of the advantageous properties of the raw ingredient with mixed indigenous microbial population (Di Cagno *et al.*, 2004).

The incubation of ass's milk with some culture of *Lactobacillus rhamnosus*, a species which recently includes strains studied and recommended for use in probiotic foods (Jacobsen *et al.*, 1999; Shu *et al.*, 1999), appears as well very interesting: Coppola *et al.* (2002) have observed that culture of *Lactobacillus rhamnosus* inoculated in pasteurised samples of ass's milk increased slightly during the incubation phase and remained: i) substantially stable during storage and ii) highly viable after 15 days of storage at 4 °C and at low pH (3.7-3.8), thus demonstrating to be a good candidate for probiotic foods. The high lysozyme content of ass's milk has only partially influenced the growth of the strains tested; moreover its presence in the pasteurised milk can also ensure optimal features from a therapeutic and nutritional point of view.

These results testify that equids milk can be valorised as a very good base ingredient for probiotic and therapeutic foods but the production of fermented milks by the means of a standardised protocol of manufacture should be considered crucial for increasing the market and the consumption (Di Cagno *et al.*, 2004).

Sensory properties of fermented equid milk, on the other hand, may represent a limit to the diffusion of the products, so that fortification with Na-caseinate, pectin and threonine or the addition of flavors can enhance the rheological and sensory quality (Di Cagno *et al.*, 2004; Chiavari *et al.*, 2005).

On this regard, a field survey, held in 1995, by the milking mare experimental farm in France, showed that the natural lipolysis and hydrolysis of fatty acids that happens during milk collection and treatment is the main curb on is acceptance by consumers. Adaptations of the milking machine and milk treatment among the conservation chain were realized with success to limit these phenomenons (Drogoul and Bigand, 1996).

Transformation of milk through fermentation processes reduces considerably the appearance of soapy and rancid taste in the product: sensory assessment of Koumiss and yogurt produced with mare's milk were conducted on a large number (> 500 persons) of volunteers during the gastronomic fare in Dijon. Fifty percentage of the volunteers were not aware of the origin of the fermented product (group 2) before they were asked to taste it and give their opinion (Question 1). Both groups were then informed on the milk nutritional properties and asked if they would consume it (Question 2). The main results of this survey are given in the Questionnaire (see below). Whatever the group, yogurt had more favorable assessments than did koumiss, especially with youths and women. Assessments of yogurt were even better (>90% like it) for group 2 (77%) compare to group 1, because information could be given on the surprisingly unusual liquid texture of the fermented milks.

It has to be noted that, among the volunteers informed that they were tasting mare's milk, one person out of 4 flatly refused both to taste the products and to take part to the survey. Therefore, milk origin can be an obstacle for its consumption and knowledge of nutritional information is essential to commercial success of equidae milk production (Drogoul and Bigand, 1996).

Conclusions

This review puts in evidence the bio-dietetic value of the equids milk and underline the necessity of more deepened and analytic knowledge, considering the complex bio-nutritional and extra-nutritional aspects, more and more emerging, than some components of this product show in favour of the human. In this context, considering: i) the Regulation (EC) No 853/2004 of the European Parliament and of the Council, laying down specific hygiene rules for food of animal origin, includes ass's raw milk and ii) the recent significant events that have influenced negatively the European agricultural and alimentary sectors, the production "equids milk" could represent, like it is happening in some southern and island regions, an economic justification for breeding endangered domestic *Equidae* breeds and an incentive of large significance for the valorization of the autochthonous breeds with positive effects on animal biodiversity, helping to protect certain breeds from extinction in industrialised countries, and for the exploitation of the marginal areas.

Acknowledgements

Research funded by PRIN 2003.

References

A.A.P. - American Academy of Pedriatics, Committee on Nutrition, 1998. Pediatrics, 101: 148-153.

Amerio M. and M. Elli, 1996. Parliamo di acquacoltura e pesca. Ed. Edagricole, Bologna.

Breckenridge, W.C. and A. Kuksis, 1967. Molecular weight distribution of milk fat triglycerides from seven species. J. of Lipid Res. 8: 473-478.

Berth-Jones J., J. Thompson and R.A. Graham-Brown, 1995. Evening primrose oil and atopic eczema. Lancet, 345: 520.

Bonnet M., C. Delavaud, K. Laud, I. Gourdou, C. Leroux, J. Diane and Y. Chilliard, 2002. Mammary leptin synthesis, milk leptin and their putative physiological roles. Reproduction Nutrition Development, 42: 399-413.

Bontempo V., B. Chiofalo, M. Polidori, Tedesco D. and E. Salimei, 2000. Cod liver oil administration to lactating mares: effects on fat and adipose tiessue fatty acid composition. In proceedings of 2nd "New findings in equine practice", 53-55.

Businco L., P.G. Giampietro and L. Lucenti, 2000. Allergenicity of mare's milk in children with cow's milk allergy. J. Allergy Clin. Immunol., 105: 1031-1034.

Caramia G., M. Cocchi and N. Frega, 2000. Recenti progressi in nutrizione. Progress in Nutrition: 2, 25-41.

Carroccio A., F. Cavataio and G. Iacono, 1999. Cross-reactivity between milk proteins of differents animals. Clin. Exp. Allergy, 29: 1014:1016.

Carroccio A., F. Cavataio, G., Montaldo, D. D'Amico, L. Alabrese and G. Iacono, 2000. Intolerance to hydrolised cow's milk proteins in infants: clinical characteristics and dietary treatments. Clin. Exp. Allergy, 30: 1597-1603.

Chiavari C., Coloretti F., M. Nanni, E. Sorrentino and L. Grazia, 2005. Use of donkey's milk for a fermented beverage with lactobacilli. Lait 85: 481-490.

Chiofalo B., 2001. Gli acidi grassi nel latte di asina: Molecole bioattive di grande interesse. In proceedings of "L'asino: Attualità e prospettive dell'impiego in campo medico, zootecnico ed alimentare", Palermo 25 maggio, pp. 69-79.

Chiofalo B., E. Salimei E. and L. Chiofalo, 2003. Acidi grassi del latte di asina: Proprietà bio-nutrizionali ed extranutrizionali. Large Animals Review, 9, n. 6: 21-26.

Chiofalo B., V. Azzara, L. Liotta and L. Chiofalo, 2004. Influenza delle condizioni di allevamento sui parametri chimico-fisici del latte di asina Ragusana nel corso della lattazione. In proceedings of "New findings in equine practice", 77-84.

Chiofalo B., M. Polidori, R. Costa and E. Salimei, 2005a. Fresh forage in dairy ass's ration: effect on milk fatty acid composition and flavours. It. J. Anim. Sci., 4: 433-435.

Chiofalo B., V. Azzara, D. Piccolo, L. Liotta and L. Chiofalo, 2005b. Il latte d'asina al traguardo della ricerca. Gli acidi grassi nel corso della lattazione. Large Animal Rewiew, 1, 39-44.

Chiofalo B., D. Piccolo, E.B., Riolo, C. Maglieri and E. Salimei, 2006a. Different fiber sources in dairy ass's diet: I. Effects on milk fatty acid composition. In Proc. 3rd European Workshop on Equine Nutrition. Accepted, In press.

Chiofalo B., E. Salimei, P. Dugo, T. Kumm, D. Piccolo and L. Mondello, 2006b. Evaluation of triglycerides in donkey milk during lactation. In proceedings of 3rd European Equine Health & Nutrition Congress, Ghent (Belgium), 17-18 March. Accepted, In press.

Cocchi M., 2000. Acido docosaesaenoico (DHA) e funzione visiva. Progress in Nutrition, 2: 43-51.

Coppola R., E. Salimei, M. Succi, E. Sorrentino, M. Nanni, P. Ranieri, R. Belli Blanes and L. Grazia, 2002. Behaviour of Lactobacillus rhamnosus strains in ass's milk. Ann. Microbiol., 52: 55-60.

Curadi M.C., P.G. Giampietro, P. Lucenti and M. Orlandi, 2001. Use of mare milk in pediatric allergology. In proceedings of XIV A.S.P.A., 647-648.

Delahaye, M-C. 1990. Tétons et tétines: histoire de l'allaitement. Trame Way editor. Barcelone, Spain.

Dell'Orto V., E. Salimei, V. Bontempo, F. Fantuz and P.M. Toppini, 1993. Produzione e composizione di latte equino: osservazioni sperimentali. In proceedings of XLVII S.I.S.Vet., 3: 2073-2077.

Di Cagno R., A. Tamborrino, G. Gallo, C. Leone, M. De Angelis, M. Faccia, P. Amirante and M. Gobbetti, 2004. Uses of mares' milk in manufacture of fermented milks. International Dairy Journal 14: 767-775

Doreau M. and S. Boulot, 1989. Recent knowledge on mare milk production. Liv. Prod. Sci., 22: 213-235.

Doreau M., J.L. Gaillard, J.M. Chobert, J. Léonil, A.S. Egito and T. Haertlé, 2002. Composition of mare and donkey milk fatty acids and proteins and consequences on milk utilisation. In proceedings of 4th Congress "New findings in equine practice", 51-71.

Doreau M. and F. Martuzzi, 2006. Fat content and composition of mare milk. In proceedings of 3rd European Workshop on Equine Nutrition, in press.

Drogoul C., H. Prevost and J.L. Maubois, 1992. Le lait de juments un produit, une filière a développer? In Proceedings 18ème Journée d'Etude, CEREOPA (editor), Paris, France. 37-51.

Drogoul. C. and G. Brigand. 1996. Bilan technico-économique de la jumenterie expérimentale du GIS «lait de jument». In Proceedings 22ème journée de la recherche équine. Institut du cheval (editor), Paris, France. 128-133.

Dugo P., T. Kumm, M. Lo Presti, B. Chiofalo, E. Salimei, A. Cotroneo and L. Mondello, 2005. Determination of triacylglycerols in donkey milk by using high performances liquid chromatography coupled with atmospheric pressure chemical ionization mass spectrometry. J. Separation Science, 28: 1023-1030.

Fidanza F. and G. Liguori, 1988. Nutrizione Umana. Ed. Idelson (Napoli).

Godovac-Zimmermann J., D. Shaw, A. Conti and H. MacKenzie, 1987. Identification and the primary structure of equine α-lactalbumin B and C (Equus caballus, Perissodactyla). Biol. Chem. Hoppe-Seyler, 368: 427-433.

Goracci J., M.C. Curadi and M. Orlandi, 2004. Mare milk FFA composition and effects in human nutrition. In proceedings of 55th Annual Meeting of European Association for Animal Production, Wageningen Academic Publisher, The Netherlands, p. 322.

Greco L., 2001. Gestione pratica del bambino con diagnosi certa di I.P.L.V. In proceedings of "L'asino: Attualità e prospettive dell'impiego in campo medico, zootecnico ed alimentare", Palermo 25 maggio, pp. 29-42.

Gresti J., M. Bugaut, C. Maniongui and J. Bezard, 1993. Composition of molecular species of Triacylglycerols in bovine milk fat. J. Dairy Sci., 76: 18501869.

Horrobin D.F., 1993. Fatty acid metabolism in health and disease: the role of δ-6 desaturase. Am. J. Clin. Nutr., 57 (Suppl): 732S-736S.

Horrobin D.F., 2000. Essential fatty acid metabolism and its modification in atopic eczema. Am. J. Clin. Nutr., 71 (Suppl): 367S-372S:

Høst A., 2002. Frequency of cow's milk allergy in childhood. Ann. Allergy Asthma Immunol., 89 (Suppl.): pp. 33-37.

Iacono G., A. Carroccio, F. Cavataio, G. Montalto, M. Soresi and V. Balsamo, 1992. Use of ass's milk in multiple food allergy. J. Pediatric Gastroent. Nutr., 14: 177-181.

Iacono G. and D'Amico D., 2001. Utilizzo del latte di asina nel trattamento delle poliallergie alimentari: Esperienze personali. In proceedings of "L'asino: Attualità e prospettive dell'impiego in campo medico, zootecnico ed alimentare", Palermo 25 maggio, pp. 43-48.

Jacobsen C.N., V.R. Nielsen, A.E., Hayford, P.L. Moller, K.F. Michaelsen, A. Paerregaard, B. Sandstrom, M. Tvede and M. Jakobsen, 1999. Screeing of probiotic activities of forty-seven strains of Lactobacillus spp. by in vitro techniques and evaluation of the colonization ability of five selected strains in human. Applied & Environmental Microbiology, 65 (11): 4949:4956.

Kinsella J., K. Shane Broughton and J. Whelan, 1990. Dietary unsaturated fatty acids: intercationa and possible needs in relation to eicosanoid synthesis. J. Nutr. Biochem., 1: 123-141.

Laiho K., A. Ouwehand, S. Salminen and I. Isolauri, 2002. Inventing probiotic functional foods for patients with allergic disease. Ann. Allergy Asthma Immunol., 89 (Suppl.): 75-82.

Malacarne M., F. Martuzzi, A. Summer and P. Mariani, 2002. Protein and fat composition of mare's milk: some nutritional remarks with reference to human and cow's milk. Int. Dairy J., 12: 869-877.

Martuzzi F., A. Tirelli, A. Summer, A.L. Catalano and P. Mariani, 2000. Ripartizione delle sieroproteine nel latte dei primi due mesi di lattazione in giumente Sella Italiano. Soc. Ital. Ippol. 6: 21-27.

Montanari G., C. Zambonelli, L. Grazia, G.K. Kamesheva and M.K.H. Shigaeva, 1996. Saccharomyces unisporum as the principal alcoholic fermentation microrganism of traditional koumiss. Journal of Dairy Research 63: 327-331.

Morera Pons S., A.I. Castellote Bargallò and M.C. Lòpez Sabater, 1998. Evaluation by high-performance liquid chromatography of the hydrolysis of human milk triacylglycerides during storage at low temperatures. J. of Chromatography A, 823: 467-474.

Morera Pons, S.M., A.C. Bargallo, C.C. Folgoso and M.C. Lopez Sabater, 2000. Triacylglycerol composition in colostrum, transitional and mature human milk. Eur. J. Clin. Nutr. 54 (12): 878-882.

Morera Pons, S., A.I. Castellote, O. Jauregui, I. Casals and M.C. Lopez Sabater, 2003. Triacylglycerol markers of mature human milk. Eur. J. Clin. Nutr.57 (12): 1621-1626.

Muraro A.A., P.G. Giampietro and E. Galli, 2002. Soy formulas and nonbovine milk. Ann. Allergy Asthma Immunol., 89 (Suppl.): 97-101.

Oftedal O.T. and R. Jennes, 1988. Interspecies variation in milk composition among horses, zebras and asses (Periossidactyla: Equidae). J Dairy Res., 55: 57-66.

Parodi, P.W., 1982. Positional distribution of fatty acids in triglycerides from milk of several species of mammals. Lipids 17 (6): 437-442.

Restani P., B. Beretta, A. Fiocchi, C. Ballabio and C.L. Galli, 2002. Cross-reactivity between mammalian proteins. Ann. Allergy Asthma Immunol., 89 (Suppl.): 11-15.

Salimei E., M. Cattaneo, B. Chiofalo and V. Dell'Orto, 1996. Exploitation of mare's milk by polyunsaturated fatty acids enrichment. In "Food and Health: Role of Animals Products", 223-227.

Salimei E., G. Varisco and F. Rosi, 2002. Major constituents, leptin and non protein nitrogen compounds in mares' colostrum and milk. Reproduction Nutrition Development 42 (1): 65-72.

Salimei E., F. Fantuz, R. Coppola, B. Chiofalo, P. Polidori and G. Varisco, 2004. Composition and characteristics of ass's milk. Animal Research, 53: 67-78.

Salimei, E., F. Fantuz, G. Varisco, C. Maglieri and M. Polidori, 2005a. Different fibre sources in dairy ass's diet: effects on milk yield and composition. Italian Journal of Animal Science, 4 (Suppl. 2): 430-432.

Salimei, E., F. Rosi, C. Maglieri, M. Polidori, F. Fantuz and G. Varisco, 2005b. Effect of different fiber sources in dairy ass's' diet on major constituents of milk and leptin content. In proceedings of 7th Congress "New findings in equine practice", 160-165.

Salimei E., F. Fantuz, P. Polidori, R. Coppola, B. Chiofalo and G. Varisco, 2006. Ass's milk: nutritional and functional characteristics. In 6th ILFSS Proceedings Book – EAAP publication, Editors: R. Rubino, L. Sepe, A. Dimitriadou and A. Gibon. No. 118, 93-98.

Salimei E. and B. Chiofalo, 2006. Ass's milk: yield and composition. In proceedings of 3rd European Workshop on Equine Nutrition, in press.

Shu Q, J.S. Zhou, K.J. Rutherfurd, M.J. Birtles, J. Prasad, P.K. Gopal and H.S. Gill, 1999. Probiotic lactic acid bacteria (*Lactobacillus acidophilus* HN017, *Lactobacillus rhamnosus* HN 001 and *Bifidobacterium lactis* HN019) have no adverse effects on the health of mice. Intern. Dairy J., 9 (11): 831-836.

Travia L., 1986. Significato biologico e nutrizionale del latte nell'alimentazione dell'uomo. Il Latte, 9: 358-371.

Troncone R. and M. Borrelli 2001. Etiopatogenesi delle malattie allergiche del tratto gastrointestinale. In proceedings of "L'asino: Attualità e prospettive dell'impiego in campo medico, zootecnico ed alimentare". Palermo 25 maggio, 7-10.

Ulbricht, T.L.V. and D.A.T. Southgate, 1991. Coronary heart disease: seven dietary factors. The Lancet 338: 985-992.

Williams C.M., 2000. Dietary fatty acids and human health. Ann. Zootech, 49: 165-180.

Wolter R., 1996. Osteocondrosi e alimentazione del cavallo. SIDI, 2: 27-32.

The lactation curve in Lusitano mares - a preliminary study

A.S. Santos and A.M. Silvestre
CECAV, Department of Animal Science, UTAD, Apartado, 5001-909, Vila Real, Portugal

Abstract

Data concerning milk yield from seven nursing Lusitano mares (450 – 580 kg live weight and 2 – 9 parities) were used in this study (5 measurements per mare). Wood's lactation model was used to describe the individual lactation curves. From the seven lactation curves estimated, two were considered atypical in shape and were, therefore, not considered. For the five remaining curves, peak was reached at day 34.6±10.5 of lactation, with a milk yield of 14.0±2.1 kg (2.9±0.3% BW). The estimate of total milk yield in 180 lactation days was of 1975.6± 251.1kg.

Keywords: mares, lactation curve, milk yield, wood's model

Introduction

The Lusitano horse is used all over the world and it plays an important role in equine production in Portugal. With a production system based on roughage availability, the young foals depend almost exclusively, and for a long period of time, on their mother's milk, revealing the importance of available accurate information on this matter.

A better understanding of the nutrient requirements for both mare and foal requires the knowledge of mare's milk yield and composition. Information on milk composition for the Lusitano breed is presented by Santos *et al.* (2005), the same study also indicates daily milk yields. Although information on mare's milk composition is somewhat extensive (Doreau and Boulot 1989a), the information regarding milk yield is scarce, probably due to methodology limitations (Doreau and Boulot, 1989b).

The lactation curve is the graphical representation of the dairy milk yield and can be described by mathematical models (Silvestre *et al.*, 1998). It is characterized by its scale (initial and maximum yields) and shape (time of maximum yield and persistency; Gipson and Grossman, 1990). Various mathematical models have been used to describe the lactation curve. Linear regressions for representing milk yield in mares have been used (Gibbs *et al.*, 1982). The use of non linear models such as Wood's model (Wood, 1967) in dairy cows is common (Varona *et al.*, 1998; Macciota *et al.*, 2005). However, its application to the mare lactation curve has not, to the extend of our knowledge, been used until now.

The purpose of this work was to investigate the application of Wood's model to dairy data of Lusitano mares.

Material and methods

Data for this study was collected from seven multiparous nursing Lusitano mares aged from 7 to 12 years, with an average live weight after foaling of 472.1±36 kg. Milk collection was as made after a mare/foal separation and using oxytocin, with 5 observations. Milk yield was evaluated on days 15, 45, 60, 90 and 120 *post-partum.* The procedures followed were as described by Santos *et al.* (2005):

- Separation of mare and foal for 1 hour. Mare and foal where able to see, touch and smell each other, but the foal was not able to suck.
- Administration of 1.0 ml of an oxitocin solution (20 IU/ml) to the mare followed by hand-milking of the two teats as deep as possible, this was made in the presence of the foal. The foal was left to suckle, and since the efforts of the foal were unsuccessful, the udder was assumed to be empty. The milk collected was then given to the foal.
- Second mare-foal separation, that was identical to the first.
- Oxitocin administration and milking identical to the procedure b). The amount of milk collected was measured and a 200 ml sample was withdrawn. The remaining milk was offered to the foal.

Individual daily milk yield was then analysed using Wood's model (Wood, 1967) that is represented in Equation (1).

$$Y(t)=a\,t^{b}\,e^{-ct} \qquad (1)$$

Y – average daily milk yield in time unit t;
e – Neper number;
a, b and c – positive parameters that determine the curve's shape.

Wood's model represents the peak in day $t=b/c$, witch means that b and c are parameters that define the pre peak and post peak of the curve respectively. Peak yield is independent of a, that represents a scale factor (Wood, 1976). Persistency (s) definition in Wood's model (2) is a dimensionless quantity, however, it can be used for comparison of lactations (Cobby and Le Du, 1978; Silvestre *et al.*, 1996)

$$s= - (b+1)\ \ln c \qquad (2)$$

For the adjustment of the model (1), to each individual dairy data, the nonlin module of Systat program (Wilkinson *et al.*, 1992) was used, this module applies the Quasi-Newton method, with convergence criteria with a precision of 5x10-5. Total milk yield were estimated with a numeric integration process, according to Silvestre *et al.* (1996).

Results and discussion

Lactation curves obtained after application of Wood's model are represented in Figure 1. From the seven lactation curves obtained, two were considered atypical (28.6%) once b value obtained was negative and were, therefore, not considered.

This percentage of atypical lactation curves obtained by the application of this mathematical model is also referred in dairy cows and can vary considerably between 2% (Shanks *et al.*, 1981) and 45% (Schneeberger, 1981). This wide range of variation is due to differences in data set properties, namely number of test days made and different intervals of birth – 1st test day (Shanks et al.,1981; Silvestre et al., 1998).

Parameters estimated for the five mares with typical curves are represented in Table 1. Table 1 also shows values obtained for each curve concerning peak day, peak yield, total yield at 180 lactation days and persistency. We considered lactation length of 180 days since weaning in the Lusitano breed occurs around 6 months (180 days) and therefore we considered that Lusitano mare's lactation is of that duration.

Table 1. Wood's model parameters (a, b, c), adjusted coefficient of determination (R^2), peak (day and yield), total yield at 180 days and persistency (Pers) for the 5 curves (values presented for kg/100kgLW and kg/day).

	Mare	R^2	a	b	c	Peak		Total yield	Pers
						day	yield		
kg/100kgLW	A	0.94	0.85	0.461	0.00961	47.92	3.20	459.3	6.78
	D	0.75	1.00	0.401	0.01096	36.57	2.83	375.6	6.32
	E	0.88	0.94	0.453	0.01256	36.10	3.04	386.5	6.36
	F	0.89	1.38	0.289	0.00863	33.53	2.85	394.7	6.13
	G	0.60	2.27	0.028	0.00148	18.62	2.40	402.4	6.69
	$\overline{X}$	0.81	1.29	0.326	0.00865	34.55	2.86	403.7	6.46
	sd	0.14	0.58	0.181	0.00427	10.48	0.30	32.6	0.27
kg/day	A	0.94	4.44	0.461	0.00961	47.92	16.65	2388.2	6.78
	D	0.75	4.56	0.401	0.01096	36.57	12.91	1712.8	6.32
	E	0.88	4.70	0.453	0.01256	36.10	15.18	1932.6	6.36
	F	0.89	6.88	0.289	0.00863	33.53	14.24	1973.3	6.13
	G	0.60	10.57	0.028	0.00148	18.62	11.14	1871.0	6.69
	$\overline{X}$	0.81	6.23	0.326	0.00865	34.55	14.02	1975.6	6.46
	sd	0.14	2.63	0.181	0.00427	10.48	2.11	251.1	0.27

Persistency values average was 6.46±0.27. This value reflects the decrease of milk yield after the peak is reached, the higher persistency value is, the less the decrease on milk yield observed in that lactation. However, the value (6.46) *per se*, does not indicate a percentage of milk yield decrease or any other unit. Persistency of lactation after maximal yield is high for nursing mares: grater than 95% month-1 (Gibbs *et al.*, 1982).

By applying Wood's model, peak was reached at day 34.6±10.5 of lactation with a great dispersion of values, peak yield between day 18 and day 47. Gibbs *et al.* (1982) observed a maximum yield during the first month. Santos *et al.* (2005), using the same data but a different analytical methodology, observed the higher yield at day 45, while other authors refer an increase in milk yield until the 2nd month of lactation (Oftedal *et al.*, 1983; Doreau and Boulot 1989a).

The milk yield at peak was of 14.0±2.1 kg (2.86±0.30% BW). Santos *et al.* (2005) observed milk yields of 14.2 kg at day 45 (3% body weight), these values are in accordance with data reported by NRC (1989) and with results obtained for other light breeds such as Thoroughbred, French saddle and Anglo-arab (Oftedal *et al.*, 1983; Doreau *et al.*, 1993), and for Quarter horse mares (Gibbs *et al.*, 1982). In spite of higher values being mentioned for heavy mares, such as Percheron and Breton, the milk yield values here presented are comparable to majority of data available in the literature (Doreau and Boulot, 1989a).

In order to better estimate the shape of the lactation curve of Lusitano mares using this model, it would be desirable to have more data, namely milk yields before 15 d, and up to 180 d of lactation. Nevertheless, longitudinal modulation of the lactation curve allows extrapolation in order to estimate the beginning and the ending of the lactation curve, as well as the total milk yield during the 180 d of lactation. The results of this extrapolation are shown in Figure 1, and also in Table 1.

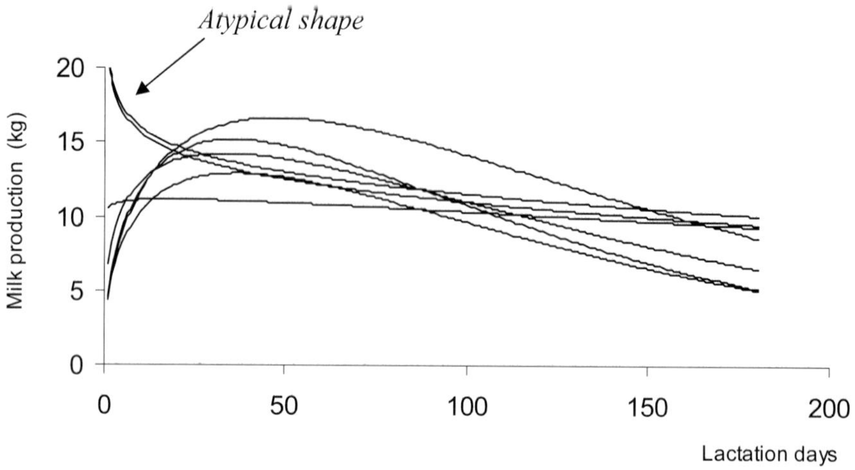

Figure 1. Lactation curves obtained from the seven mares.

The atypical curves are also shown in Figure 1. These two curves were obtained due to data set limitations and do not have biological meaning.

The estimate of total milk yield at 180 d was of 1975.6±251.1 kg. Yields of 1890 to 2225 kg in 180 days for dairy mares, and 1400 to 2200 kg in 150 days for saddle breeds are presented by Doreau and Boulot (1989a). The same authors present higher yield values for dairy mares recorded by mechanical milking (from 2060 kg to 2100 kg in 180 days). Nevertheless, values found in this study with the application of Wood's model seem suitable when compared with that of dairy mares.

Residue analysis for the 5 typical curves is represented in Figure 2. Although residues average was zero for all the curves, they show some oscillation during lactation. In day 15, residues are very close to zero for all measurements made, but their dispersion increases on the following measurements.

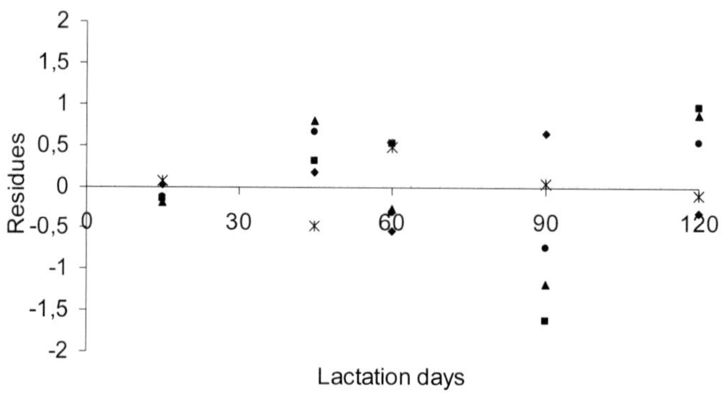

Figure 2. Residues distribution for the five typical curves.

Conclusions

To the extent of our knowledge, the application of Wood's model to study the lactation curve of the mare, results for Lusitano breed were never published. Comparing with values of other breeds, namely peak location and yield, the application of this mathematical model seems to show good results. Nevertheless, for this application to be widely used, there's a need for more data collection, namely milk yields prior to 15 d and up to 180 d, to better adjust the model to the lactation curve of the mare. Also further investigation including other mathematical functions is necessary.

References

Doreau, M. and S. Boulot, 1989a. Recent knowledge on mare milk production.: a review. Livest. Prod. Sci., 22:213-235.

Doreau, M. and S. Boulot, 1989b. Methods of measurements of milk yield and composition in nursing mares: a review. Lait 69:159- 171.

Doreau, M., S. Boulot and Y. Chilliard, 1993. Yield and composition of milk from lactating mares: effect of body condition at foaling. J. Dairy Res., 60: 457-466.

Cobby, J.M. and Y.L.P. Le Du, 1978. On fitting curves to lactation data. Anim. Prod. 26: 127-133.

Gibbs, P., G.D. Potter, R.W. Blake and W.C. McMullan, 1982. Milk production of quarter horse mares during 150 days of lactation. J.Anim.Sci., 54: 496-499.

Gipson, T.A. and M. Grossman, 1990. Lactation curves in dairy goats: a review. Small Rumin. Res., volume 3:383-396.

Macciotta, N.P.P., D. Vicario and A. Cappio-Borlino, 2005. Detection of different shapes of lactation curve for milk yield in dairy cattle by empirical mathematical models. J. Dairy Sci. 88:1178–1191.

National Research Council (NRC), 1989. Nutrient Requirements of Domestic Animals. nº 6 Nutrient Requirements of Horses, 5th revised edition. National Academy of Sciences, Washington D.C.

Oftedal, O.T., H.F. Hintz and H.F. Schryver, 1983. Lactation in the horse: milk composition and intake by foals. J. Nutr., 113:2196-2206.

Santos, A.S., B.C. Sousa, L. Chambel and V.C. Alves, 2005. Yield and composition of milk from Lusitano lactating mares. Pferdeilkunde, 21: 115-116, Suppl. S.

Schneeberger, M., 1981. Inheritance of lactation curve in Swiss Brown Cattle. J. Dairy Sci., 64: 475-483.

Silvestre, A.M.D., J. Colaço and M.F.S. Petim-Batista, 1996. Lactation curves modelling: Possibility of applying date on test day records. Revista Portuguesa de Zootecnia, Ano III (2), 45-58.

Silvestre, A.M.D., M.F.S. Petim-Batista and J. Colaço, 1998. Lactation curve sasonality. Revista Portuguesa de Zootecnia., Ano V (2), 17-27.

Shanks, R.D., P.J. Berger, A.E. Freeman and F.N. Dickinson, 1981. Genetic aspects of lactation curves. J. Dairy Sci., 64: 1852-1860.

Varona, L., C. Moreno, L.A. García Cortés and J. Altarriba, 1998. Bayesian analysis of Wood's lactation curve for Spanish dairy cows. J. Dairy Sci., 81: 1469-1478.

Wilkinson, L., M. Hill, J. P. Welna and G.K. Birkenbeuel, 1992. Systat for Windows, Version 5. Systat, Inc., Evanston, Illinois.

Wood, P.D.P., 1967. Algebraic models of lactation curve in cattle. Nature, London, 216: 164-165 (cit. by Wood, 1976).

Wood, P.D.P., 1976. Algebraic models of the lactation curves for milk, fat and protein production, with estimates of seasonal variation. Animal Production, 22: 35-40.

A novel restrictive grazing approach to enhance leptin sensitivity in obese pony mares*

P.R. Buff[1], D.H. Keisler[2], P.J. Johnson[3], N.T. Messer IV[3] and V.K. Ganjam[1]
[1]Department of Biomedical Sciences, University of Missouri-Columbia, Missouri 65211, USA
[2]The Department of Animal Sciences, University of Missouri-Columbia, Missouri 65211, USA
[3]Department of Veterinary Medicine and Surgery, University of Missouri-Columbia, Missouri 65211, USA
**Portions of this research were presented at the 19th Meeting of the Equine Science Society 2005, Tucson, AZ, USA.*

Abstract

Obesity is a pandemic within the human population with striking parallels in the equine industry. Obesity may increase the risk for certain disorders, such as insulin resistance, infertility, laminitis and equine metabolic syndrome. Horses known as "easy keepers" are metabolically efficient and will increase adiposity more readily than normal horses. Thus, the management of these individuals can be more challenging in a herd or grazing environment. Leptin plays a major role in feed intake, growth, metabolism, and reproduction. Leptin resistance (reduced receptor sensitivity to leptin) may play a role in promoting obesity and dysregulation of energy balance. It has been well documented that the circulating plasma leptin concentration decreases following feed restriction, resulting in increased appetite. We hypothesized that restricting obese pony mares to grazing pasture for 12 h during daytime (diurnal; 0700 to 1900) or 12 h during nighttime (nocturnal; 1900 to 0700) would reduce BW and alter plasma concentrations of leptin and insulin when compared to mares grazing continually (24 h). Crossbred obese pony mares (n = 15) were divided into 3 groups (diurnal, nocturnal, 24 h) and subjected to treatments for 12 weeks. No differences were observed in BW as an effect of treatment. Concentrations of leptin decreased in both diurnal and nocturnal groups compared to the 24 h group during the first six weeks of the study ($P < 0.001$), with the greater difference observed in the nocturnal group. Mean concentrations of insulin were greater following grazing compared to restriction in all mares ($P < 0.001$). These results indicate that restricting obese pony mares to grazing 12 h during the day or 12 h during the night will suppress concentrations of leptin without any change in BW. A decrease in leptin without a subsequent decrease in BW may be attributable to an increased sensitivity to leptin.

Keywords: equine, obesity, leptin resistance, insulin, feed restriction

Introduction

Some domestic horses are metabolically efficient, commonly known as "easy keepers", and often develop obesity when managed on a feeding program that would meet the maintenance requirements for "normal" horses (National Research Council, 1989). Horses that are allowed to develop and maintain an obese body condition are predisposed to developing insulin insensitivity (Jeffcott *et al.*, 1986, Hoffman *et al.*, 2003). Recent literature has discussed the potential for obesity to play a role in laminitis (Johnson *et al.*, 2004), equine metabolic syndrome (Johnson, 2002) and affect reproduction in the mare (Sessions *et al.*, 2004).

Leptin is a 16 kDa protein hormone, primarily produced and secreted by white adipose tissue to contribute to the regulation of energy homeostasis (Ahima and Flier, 2000). This hormone has been identified in horses and circulating plasma concentrations increase as adiposity increases (Buff *et al.*, 2002). Leptin works in concert with insulin to influence the neuroendocrine mediators of appetite control as signals of adiposity (Schwartz *et al.*, 2000). Circadian patterns of leptin secretion have been observed in horses (Piccione *et al.*, 2004, Buff *et al.*, 2005b), indicating that secretion of leptin may be influenced by photoperiodic, or circadian rhythms in addition to nutritional status.

The theory of leptin resistance was first suggested in humans with the discovery of elevated concentrations of leptin in obese subjects (Considine *et al.*, 1996). Briefly, leptin resistance is defined as a reduced sensitivity to concentrations of leptin within the blood brain barrier, which serves to abrogate leptin's inhibitory effect on appetite. Based on our previous findings of circadian secretion patterns of leptin in horses and elevated concentrations of leptin in obese horses, we formulated the following hypothesis. Obese pony mares managed under restrictive periods of nocturnal or diurnal grazing versus obese pony mares grazing ad libitum will undergo weight loss with altered hormonal secretion, as reflected by peripheral concentrations of leptin and insulin.

Materials and Methods

Animals

This experiment utilized 15 crossbred obese non lactating non pregnant pony mares (Quarter Horse X Shetland or Welsh type) with a mean age and SEM of 9.2 ± 1.09 yr and ranging from 5 to 15 yr of age. All mares maintained a body condition score > 7 (1 = thin to 9 = obese; Henneke *et al.*, 1983) prior to and during experimentation with a mean BCS and SEM of 8 ± 0.16 and ranged from 7 to 9. Mean initial BW and SEM of the experimental group was 259 ± 41.85 kg and ranged from 151 to 434 kg. All procedures with live animals were approved by the University of Missouri Animal Care and Use Committee.

Procedures

Experimentation was conducted in Columbia, Missouri, USA (38.9° N 92.2° W) from 19 August 2003 until 14 November 2003. To ensure that mares were evenly distributed, they were ranked by BW and then distributed by individual weight equally into each group to create a statistical block. Each group was randomly assigned to one of three treatments. The group that served as the control (24 h) was allowed to graze ad libitum for 24 h/d during the experiment. The second group was allowed to graze from 07:00 until 19:00 (diurnal) and the third group was allowed to graze from 19:00 until 07:00 (nocturnal). All horses were managed in the same pasture for at least 6 mo prior to and during experimentation. The pasture was 16.2 ha in size and consisted primarily of tall fescue grass (*Festuca arundinaceae*), which was maintained at 12 to 20 cm in lush condition throughout the experiment. When not allowed to graze, mares were maintained in a corral with no access to feed and with unlimited access to water and shelter. Mares were weighed weekly and blood samples were collected on the same day of the week at 07:00 and 19:00 to account for possible circadian secretion and effects of feeding and restriction. Three blood samples were collected beginning at 07:00 from each mare, 15 min apart and 3 more blood samples were collected at 19:00 from each mare 15 min apart to account for variation of hormone secretion, via jugular venipuncture using Vacutainer® (Becton Dickinson, Franklin Lakes, NJ) tubes containing EDTA. Blood samples were kept on ice and centrifuged at 3,000 g for 25 min at 4°C within 12 h from collection to obtain plasma, which was then stored at -20°C until assayed.

Hormonal analysis

All plasma samples collected were analyzed as individual samples in duplicate. Plasma samples were analyzed for leptin using double-antibody radioimmunoassay (RIA) procedures previously validated for equine plasma (Buff *et al.*, 2002). Serial dilutions of equine plasma were parallel to the standard curve. Minimum detectable concentration was 0.1 ng/tube and the intra- and inter-assay coefficients of variation were < 10%. Plasma concentrations of insulin were measured using a RIA kit (Diagnostic Products Corporation, Los Angeles, CA), validated for use with equine plasma (Freestone *et al.*, 1991). Serial dilutions of equine plasma were parallel to the human insulin standard curve. All samples were analyzed in a single assay. Minimum detectable mass was 4 μIU/ml and the inter-assay coefficients of variation was 5%.

Statistical analysis

An initial ANOVA was performed to determine if differences existed between samples collected at 07:00 and 19:00 for concentrations of leptin with the aid SAS V8 (SAS Inst. Inc., Cary, NC). We determined that no statistical differences in concentrations of leptin existed within individuals by sample times. Leptin values of all samples collected within a given week for individual animals were then combined for analyses, providing 6 concentrations per week per animal. To determine if concentrations of insulin were different following the periods of grazing or feed restriction an ANOVA was performed using the general linear model procedures of SAS V8. Effects used in this model were sample time (07:00 and 19:00), nutritional state (fed and restricted) and individual animal was used as a covariate. To determine effects of grazing restriction on BW, leptin and insulin over time, we performed an ANOVA using the mixed procedures of SAS V8 (Littell *et al.*, 1998). Analyses on concentrations of insulin were performed to compare animals in the fed state only. Comparisons were made between nocturnal versus 24 h on samples that were collected at 07:00 and diurnal versus 24 h on samples that were collected at 19:00. Effects used in the model were treatment (diurnal, nocturnal and 24 h), week (time), block (by BW) on plasma concentrations of hormone and BW. The variable of week was used in the repeated statement and the error term used was animal within treatment.

Results

Visible light decreased from 14.5 h to 11.4 h over the duration of the experiment. No changes were observed in BW throughout the study or due to treatment ($P = 0.69$). Changes were observed in plasma concentrations of leptin in all mares over the duration of the experiment ($P < 0.001$; Figure 1). During the first six weeks, concentrations of leptin were lower in both diurnal and nocturnal groups compared to 24 h group ($P < 0.001$; Figure 2) with few differences in the final six weeks. Mean concentrations of insulin were greater in all animals following the period of grazing (195.7 ± 9.0 μIU/mL) when compared to a period of feed restriction (96.8 ± 12.8 μIU/mL; $P < 0.001$).

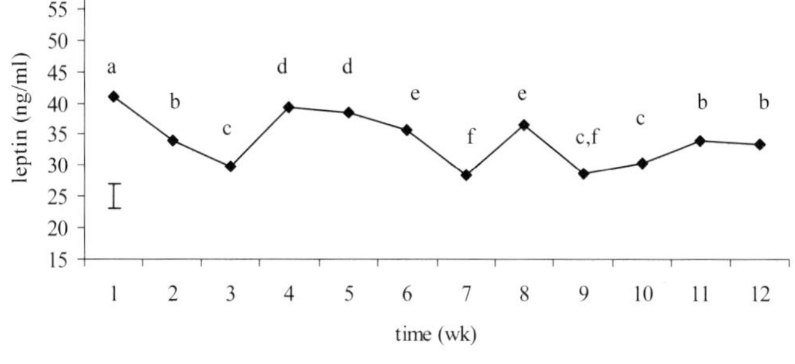

Figure 1. Concentrations of leptin in all obese pony mares over the duration of experimentation. Leptin changed in all mares over the duration of the study (P < 0.001). Data presented as LS Means and vertical bar represents ± SEM. Differences of preplanned comparisons are indicated by different letter (P < 0.05).

No differences were observed with the interaction of time of sample and nutritional state with concentrations of insulin (P = 0.46). Upon analysis of concentrations of insulin over time we found a significant model effect of treatment by time for both 24 h versus diurnal (P < 0.05) and 24 h versus nocturnal (P < 0.01). Post hoc comparisons of LS means indicated that few statistical differences existed between 24 h and diurnal or 24 h and nocturnal (Figure 3).

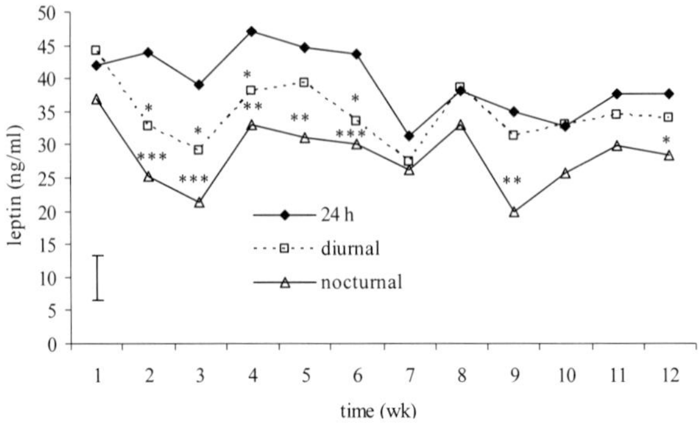

Figure 2. Concentrations of leptin in obese pony mares restricted to grazing for 12 h from 07:00 until 19:00 (diurnal) or 19:00 until 07:00 (nocturnal) versus an unrestricted grazing (24 h). Leptin decreased in both diurnal and nocturnal groups during the first six weeks of the study (P < 0.001). Data presented as LS Means and vertical bar represents ± SEM. Differences of preplanned comparisons made between 24 h and diurnal or nocturnal groups are denoted as follows: P < 0.05, P < 0.01**, P < 0.001***.*

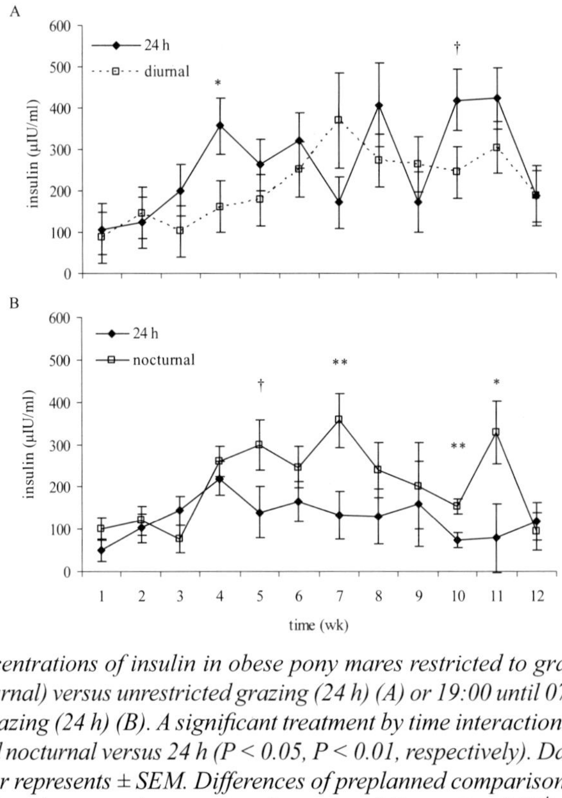

Figure 3. Concentrations of insulin in obese pony mares restricted to grazing for 12 h from 07:00 until 19:00 (diurnal) versus unrestricted grazing (24 h) (A) or 19:00 until 07:00 (nocturnal) versus an unrestricted grazing (24 h) (B). A significant treatment by time interaction was observed for diurnal versus 24 h and nocturnal versus 24 h (P < 0.05, P < 0.01, respectively). Data presented as LS Means and vertical bar represents ± SEM. Differences of preplanned comparisons made between 24 h and diurnal or 24 h and nocturnal groups are denoted as follows: P < 0.08†, P < 0.05, P < 0.01**.*

Discussion

In the present study we have shown for the first time, suppression of leptin in hyperleptinemic obese pony mares subjected to restrictive grazing. We attribute the decrease in peripheral concentrations of leptin to a decrease in leptin resistance, rather than a decrease in adiposity. By measuring BW we were able to monitor gross changes within this group of animals that reflect changes in adiposity in mature non-growing/non-exercising horses. The lack of weight loss indicates that the mares in this study did not increase or decrease in adiposity. Thus, energy homeostasis was maintained by all animals regardless of treatment.

Neel (1962) proposed a theory of a thrifty genotype in humans to explain why some humans develop obesity and subsequent related diseases more easily than others. This theory may also explain why some horses are metabolically efficient. Horses referred to as metabolically efficient or "easy keepers" may have retained these "thrifty" genes and thus have lower nutrient requirements than "normal" horses (National Research Council, 1989).

Leptin resistance has been documented, in experimental rodent models, such as db/db mice (Campfield *et al.*, 1995), fa/fa rats (Chua *et al.*, 1996) and humans (Swartz *et al.*, 1996). Previously, no reports of leptin resistance in horses or ponies have been made. However, concentrations of leptin have been reported to increase as horses increase adiposity (Buff *et al.* 2002, Gentry *et al.*, 2002) and are markedly elevated in obese mares (Buff *et al.*, 2005b). Concentrations of leptin decrease when obese mares are subjected to an acute feed deprivation (Buff *et al.*, 2005b) or during a chronic negative energy balance (Buff *et al.*, 2006). Leptin has been reported to be secreted in a circadian rhythm with a nocturnal increase in obese pony mares (Buff *et al.*, 2005b) and non-obese horses (Piccione *et al.*, 2004). Horses exhibit seasonal variations of leptin which has been reported to decrease as they transition from summer into autumn and winter without subsequent weight loss (Gentry *et al.*, 2002, Buff *et al.*, 2005b) and increase from winter to summer (Buff *et al.*, 2005a). This variation in leptin could be a mechanism to control appetite seasonally and could be induced by environmental changes. Seasonal sensitivity to leptin has been reported in Siberian Hamsters (Rousseau *et al.*, 2002) and a seasonal change in BW of up to 40% has been reported in Djungarian hamsters (Steinlechner *et al.*, 1983). Many domesticated horses are maintained under modern management practices and thus adiposity does not decrease as a result of seasonal reproduction and environmental demands. Maintaining excess energy stores throughout the year may further decrease the sensitivity to leptin and cause an even greater accumulation of adipose tissue over time.

The objective of the current study was to further investigate the effect of the circadian patterns of leptin in obese mares by restricting feeding to nocturnal or diurnal periods to coincide with the rise and fall of leptin. Both treatments induced a decrease in the plasma concentrations of leptin after the first week of the experiment, which continued through the first six weeks of the study. Concentrations of leptin were significantly lower in the group restricted to nocturnal grazing. These results indicate that leptin concentrations can be altered by restricting obese mares to grazing during diurnal or nocturnal periods and the greater reduction occurs in those subjected to nocturnal grazing activity. The nocturnal group was grazing during the period when diurnal secretion of leptin is naturally higher, which may have caused an enhanced negative feedback inhibition via neuroendocrine control of feed intake due to combined mechanisms. Grazing obese horses diurnally or nocturnally may also initiate mechanisms to down regulate leptin secretion by exposing the system to a refractory period between feeding bouts. This would allow factors regulated from the act of feeding to be controlled by an oscillation pattern of feeding behavior. From these findings we conclude that the sensitivity to circulating leptin may be increased as concentrations of leptin decreased without a subsequent decrease in adiposity. Our results agree with a report in humans where an increase in fasting period increased leptin response to a meal and thus leptin sensitivity (Elimam and Marcus, 2002). However, leptin sensitivity can not be irrefutably determined without measuring leptin receptors.

This experiment was conducted during the transient seasonal decrease in concentrations of leptin from summer to autumn where day length decreased form 14.5 to 11.4 h. Decreasing concentrations of leptin over time were observed in all mares. Within these decreasing concentrations of leptin we observed a pattern of rising and falling. We believe that this is a reset mechanism to reach homeostasis when the system is perturbed. We have previously observed this resetting in obese mares in a chronic negative energy balance (Buff *et al.*, 2006).

Concentrations of insulin were significantly greater following 12 h of grazing when compared with 12 h of restriction in all mares. A pattern of greater concentrations of insulin in the nocturnal group was observed. These results may be explained by horse's natural tendency to graze during daylight and less during night. Thus, differences would not exist between 24 h and diurnal as they would be grazing during the same time of day. The differences between 24 h and nocturnal may be due to the unnatural nocturnal grazing cycle.

The present findings elucidate the response of leptin in obese mares subjected to restrictive diurnal or nocturnal grazing periods. We suggest the suppression of leptin may be a result of decreased leptin resistance as no apparent changes in adiposity were observed. The understanding of restrictive grazing effects in obese horses may lead to further discoveries of energy homeostasis and the mechanisms involved in leptin resistance.

Acknowledgements

The authors thank Kimberly Hendrix, Jameson Scoggin and Rex Smiley for technical assistance.

References

Ahima, R.S. and J.S. Flier, 2000. Adipose tissue as an endocrine organ. Trends Endocrinol. Metab. 11:327-332.

Buff, P.R., A.C. Dodds, C.D. Morrison, N.C. Whitley, E.L. McFadin, J.A. Daniel, J. Djiane and D.H. Keisler, 2002. Leptin in horses: Tissue localization and relationship between peripheral concentrations of leptin and body condition. J. Anim.Sci. 80:2942-2948.

Buff, P.R., N.T. Messer, A.M. Cogswell, P.J. Johnson, V.K. Ganjam and D.H. Keisler, 2005a. Pulsatile and seasonal characteristics of thyrotropin and leptin in undernourished mares. In; Proceedings of the 19th Equine Science Society, 142.

Buff, P.R., C.D. Morrison, V.K. Ganjam and D.H. Keisler, 2005b. Effects of short-term feed deprivation and melatonin implants on circadian patterns of leptin in the horse. J. Anim. Sci. 83:1023-1032.

Buff, P.R., P.J. Johnson, C.E. Wiedmeyer, V.K. Ganjam, N.T. Messer, IV and D.H. Keisler, 2006. Modulation of leptin, insulin and growth hormone in obese pony mares under chronic nutritional restriction and supplementation with ractopamine hydrochloride. Vet. Ther.7:64-72.

Campfield, L,A., F.J. Smith, Y. Guisez, R. Devos and P. Burn, 1995. Recombinant mouse OB protein: evidence for a peripheral signal linking adiposity and central neural networks. Science, 269:546-549.

Considine, R.V., M.K. Sinha, M.L. Heiman, A. Kriauciunas, T.W. Stephens, M.R. Nyce, J.P. Ohannesian, C.C. Marco, L.J. McKee, T.L. Bauer and J.F. Caro, 1996. Serum immunoreactive-leptin concentrations in normal-weight and obese humans. N. Engl. J. Med. 334:292-295.

Chua, S.C. Jr, W.K. Chung, X.S. Wu-Peng, Y. Zhang, S.M. Liu, L. Tartaglia and R.L. Leibel, 1996. Phenotypes of mouse diabetes and rat fatty due to mutations in the OB (leptin) receptor. Science 271:994-996.

Elimam, A. and C. Marcus, 2002. Meal timing, fasting and glucocorticoids interplay in serum leptin concentrations and diurnal profile. Eur. J. Endocrinol. 147:181-188.

Freestone, J.F., K.J. Wolfsheimer, S.G. Kamerling, G. Church, J. Hamra and C. Bagwell, 1991. Exercise induced hormonal and metabolic changes in Thoroughbred horses: effects of conditioning and acepromazine. Equine Vet. J. 23:219-223.

Gentry, L.R., D.L. Thompson Jr, G.T. Gentry Jr, K.A. Davis, R.A. Godke and J.A. Cartmill, 2002. The relationship between body condition, leptin, and reproductive and hormonal characteristics of mares during the seasonal anovulatory period. J. Anim. Sci. 80:2695-2703.

Henneke, D.R., G.D. Potter, J.L. Kreider and B.F. Yeates, 1983. Relationship between condition score, physical measurements and body fat percentage in mares. Equine Vet. J. 15:371-372.

Hoffman, R.M., R.C. Boston, D. Stefanovski, D.S. Kronfeld and P.A. Harris, 2004. Obesity and diet affect glucose dynamics and insulin sensitivity in Thoroughbred geldings. J. Anim. Sci. 81:2333-2342.

Jeffcott, L.B., J.R. Field, J.G. McLean and K. O'Dea, 1986. Glucose tolerance and insulin sensitivity in ponies and Standardbred horses. Equine Vet. J.18:97-101.

Johnson, P.J., 2002. The equine metabolic syndrome: peripheral Cushing's Syndrome. In: The Veterinary Clinics of North America-Equine Practice, J. Vassallo (editor),. WB Saunders Co. Philadelphia, 18:271-293.

Johnson, P.J., V.K. Ganjam, S.H. Slight, J.M. Kreeger and N.T. Messer, 2004. Tissue-specific dysregulation of cortisol metabolism in equine laminitis. Equine Vet. J. 36:41-45.

Littell, R.C., P.R. Henry and C.B. Ammerman, 1989. Statistical analysis of repeated measures data using SAS procedures. J. Anim. Sci. 76:1216-1231.

National Research Council, 1989. Nutrient Requirements of Horses 5th revised edition National Academy Press Washington, D.C.

Piccione, G., C. Bertoluccci, A. Foà and G. Caola, 2004. Influence of fasting and exercise on the daily rhythm of serum leptin in the horse. Chronobiol. Int. 21:405-417.

Rousseau, K., Z. Atcha, F.R. Cagampang, P. Le Rouzic, J.A. Stirland, T.R. Ivanov, F.J. Ebling, M. Klingenspor and A.S. Loudon, 2002. Photoperiodic regulation of leptin resistance in the seasonally breeding Siberian hamster (Phodopus sungorus). Endocrinology, 143:3083-3095.

Schwartz, M.W., S.C. Woods, D. Porte, R.L. Seeley and D.G. Baskin, 2000. Central nervous system control of food intake. Nature, 404:661-671.

Sessions, D.R., S.E. Reedy, M.M. Vick and B.P. Fitzgerald, 2004. Development of a model for inducing transient insulin resistance in the mare: Preliminary implications regarding the estrus cycle. J. Anim. Sci. 82:2321–2328.

Steinlechner, S., G. Heldmaier and H. Becker, 1983. The seasonal cycle of BW in the Djungarian hamster: photoperiodic control and the influence of starvation and melatonin. Oecologia. 60:401-405.

A weigh-suckle-weigh approach for estimating milk yield in the Arabian mare

N.L. Trottier[1], T. Stamper[2], J. Moore, J. Liesman[1] and B.D. Nielsen[1]
[1]Michigan State University, East Lansing, MI 48824, USA
[2]Grand-Valley State University, Allendale, MI 49401, USA

Abstract

Six Arabian mares were used to determine milk yield using a weigh-suckle-weigh approach. Milk intake by foals was measured every 60 minutes for a total of seven hours to estimate milk yield on days 10, 20 and 30 of lactation. Behavioral nursing data were obtained on days 9, 19 and 29 of lactation over a 24-hour period. Frequency of nursing bouts (bouts/hour), duration of nursing bouts (minutes/bout), and nursing duration per hour (bouts/hour x minutes/bout) were recorded. Suckling frequency declined ($P < 0.05$) with day of lactation while duration of a single suckling bout was similar across time of day, day of lactation, and parity of mare. Total suckling duration per hour decreased (linear, $P \leq 0.1$ to $P < 0.05$) with increasing day of lactation during both WSW and Natural Nursing (NN). Suckling duration per hour during NN was higher during daytime ($P < 0.0001$) and lower during nighttime ($P < 0.01$) compared to that of WSW, but not different when averaged over the 24-hour period. Hence, WSW performed hourly and extrapolated to 24-hour may provide an estimate of milk yield close to that of NN. On a 24-hour basis, milk yield varied between 12.85 and 14.62 ± 1.43 kg across parities and day of lactation, corresponding to between 3.07 and 3.59 ± 0.40% of the mare's body weight.

Keywords: mare, lactation

Introduction

Milk yield and composition serve as important indicators of nutrients needed by both mares and foals (Oftedal *et al.*, 1983; Doreau and Boulot, 1989). Much of the information available in regards to milk production can be attributed to data obtained from large breed mares and ponies (Bouwman and Van der Schee, 1978; Doreau *et al.*, 1990) while information for modern, light-weight breeds such as the Arabian remains limited. In addition, estimation of milk production in horses is limited to costly methodology such as deuterium oxide (D2O) tracer of foal body water (Oftedal, 1983; Doreau *et al.*, 1990). Other approaches such as weigh-suckle-weigh are less costly, but have been reported so far in few studies (Gibbs *et al.*, 1982) with limited consideration for the foal's natural nursing behavior. The objectives of this study were to adapt a weigh-suckle-weigh approach to the foal's natural nursing behavior and to determine if milk yield in Arabian mares falls within ranges reported in other breeds.

Material and methods

Six mature Arabian mares, three primiparous and three multiparous, were used. Milk intake by foals was used to estimate milk yield on days 10, 20 and 30 of lactation. Foals were first observed for completion of one nursing bout beginning at 0830. Immediately thereafter, foals were muzzled to prevent suckling, but remained with dams at all times. Sixty minutes post-muzzling, the muzzle was removed, foals were weighed (Arlyn Series 320-LLA, Arlyn Scales, East Rockaway, NY) and immediately allowed to nurse until satiated. Upon completion of a nursing bout, foals were immediately reweighed, remuzzled and returned to their dams. This procedure was repeated every

60 minutes for a total of seven hours until approximately 1600 and milk intake extrapolated to a 24-hour period.

Behavioral nursing data were obtained on d 9, 19 and 29 of lactation through a time lapse videotape recorder (Panasonic® AG-TL950, Panasonic Corp. of North America, Secaucus, NJ) over a 24-hour period. Frequency of suckling bouts (bouts/hour), duration of suckling bouts (minutes/bout), and suckling duration per hour (bouts/hour x minutes/bout) were recorded. A suckling bout was defined as any uninterrupted nursing interval lasting 27 seconds or longer as described by Carson and Wood-Gush (1983).

Results and discussion

Total suckling duration per hour decreased (linear, $P \leq 0.1$ to $P < 0.05$) with increasing day of lactation during WSW and Natural Nursing (NN). Suckling duration during NN was higher during daytime ($P < 0.0001$) and lower during nighttime ($P < 0.01$) compared to that of WSW, but not different when averaged over the 24-hour period. Milk yield/suckling bout did not change with day of lactation nor differ between primiparous and multiparous mares. On a 24-hour basis, milk yield varied between 12.85 and 14.62 ± 1.43 kg across parities and day of lactation, corresponding to between 3.07 and 3.59 ± 0.40% of the mare's body weight. This is considerably higher than the 2.1% estimate reported by Gibbs *et al.* (1982) using a WSW approach in Quarter Horse mares, but close to an estimate of 3.1% reported by Oftedal *et al.* (1983) using a D2O approach in Thoroughbred and Standardbred mares. In the study by Gibbs *et al.* (1982), foals were allowed to suckle every three hours only, which may have lead to underestimation of milk yield. In this study, during NN, suckling frequency over a 24-hour period varied between 2 and 2.5 suckling bouts/hour (data not shown) and declined ($P < 0.05$) with day of lactation, while duration of a single suckling bout (data not shown) was similar

Table 1. Suckling duration (SD) per hour during weigh-suckle-weigh and natural nursing, and milk yield across days of lactation in Arabian mares.

Item	Day of lactation			SEM	P-value	
	9-10	19-20	29-30		Linear	Quadratic
Weigh-suckle-weigh						
SD, minutes/bout[1]						
Primiparous	3.191	2.476	2.048	0.355	0.045	0.741
Multiparous	2.318	1.897	2.191	0.355	0.799	0.418
Overall (primi + multi)	2.754[a]	2.187[a]	2.119[a]	0.251	0.100	0.422
Milk yield, kg/bout						
Primiparous	0.599	0.536	0.536	0.068	0.331	0.567
Multiparous	0.564	0.609	0.607	0.068	0.498	0.667
Overall (primi + multi)	0.581	0.572	0.571	0.048	0.824	0.918
Natural nursing SD[2]						
Daytime (0830 to 1600)	6.106[b]	4.698[b]	4.399[b]		0.013	0.208
Nighttime (1600 to 0830)	1.639[b]	1.455[b]	1.120[b]		0.086	0.596
24-hour	3.163[a]	2.614[a]	2.219[a]		0.027	0.881

[1]During weigh-suckle-weigh, one nursing bout is equivalent to one hour.
[2]Data for natural nursing suckling duration (SD) are for pooled parities, i.e., overall. Minutes/hour was calculated from minutes/suckling bout x number suckling bouts/hour. Data are back transformed from log.
[a,b]Comparisons are made against WSW overall SD per bout (or hour) at $P < 0.01$.

across time of day, day of lactation, and parity of mare. Thus, nursing frequency rather than duration of nursing per single suckling bout appears to be a determinant of nutrient intake by foals. Results indicate that WSW approach in mares should be conducted with a nursing frequency closer to that of natural suckling. Hence, WSW performed hourly and extrapolated to 24-hour may provide an estimate of milk yield close to that of NN.

References

Bouwman, H. and W. Van der Schee. 1978. Composition and production of milk from Dutch warmblooded saddle horse mares. Z. Tierphysiolo. Tierernaehr. Futtermitteld., 40:39-53.

Doreau, M. and S. Boulot. 1989. Recent knowledge on mare milk production: a review. Livest. Prod. Sci. 22: 213-235.

Doreau, M., S. Boulot, J. Barlet and P. Patureau-Mirand. 1990. Yield and composition of milk from lactating mares: effect of lactation stage and individual differences. J. Dairy Res. 57: 449-454.

Gibbs, P.D., G.D. Potter, J.L. Kreider, G.T. Schelling and W.L. Jenkins. 1982. Milk production of Quarter Horse mares during 150 days of lactation. J. Anim. Sci. 54: 496-499.

Oftedal, O.T., H.F. Hintz and H.F. Schryver. 1983. Lactation in the horse: milk composition and intake by foals. J. Nut. 113: 2196-2206.

Different fibre sources in dairy ass's diet: effects on body condition and plasma leptin level

C. Maglieri[1], F. Rosi[2], D. Magistrelli[2], M. Polidori[1], F. Fantuz[3] and E. Salimei[1]
[1]Dept. STAAM, Molise University, Via De Sanctis, 86100 Campobasso, Italy
[2]Milano University, Via Celoria 10, Milano, Italy
[3]Camerino University, Via Circonvallazione 93, 62024 Matelica (MC), Italy

Abstract

Ass's body condition and plasma leptin level were investigated in sixteen not pregnant pluriparous asses, divided into two groups fed two isoenergetic and isonitrogenous mixed feed including either wheat bran (group A) or dehydrated beet pulp (group B). Throughout the experiment, lasted 84 days, asses showed a good body condition unaffected by the dietary treatment. Although the investigated fibre sources did not affect plasma leptin level, measured for the first time in lactating asses, significant higher levels were observed at the end of lactation and were related to body condition score values ($R^2 = 0.42$; $P<0.01$).

Keywords: donkey, plasma leptin, body condition score, milk yield

Introduction

Leptin, the product of *ob* gene, is a metabolism modifier that plays a crucial role in coordinating food intake, energy expenditure and nutrient utilization besides regulating other physiological aspects such as reproduction, immunity, cell differentiation, proliferation, etc. (Houseknecht *et al.*, 1998). Plasma leptin concentration has been investigated in mares in relation with reproduction (McManus and Fitzgerald, 2000), however no data are available on leptinemia in lactating donkeys. Aiming to contribute to deepen the knowledge on nutritional strategies for lactating asses in an innovative food chain (Salimei *et al.*, 2005), the effects of different fibre sources in concentrate for dairy asses were investigated on asses's body condition and plasma leptin level.

Materials and methods

Sixteen not pregnant pluriparous asses (125 ± 48 days of lactation), bred in an organic farm and machine milked, were divided into two groups fed two isoenergetic and isonitrogenous mixed feed including either wheat bran (20% - group A) or dehydrated beet pulp (20% - group B). During the experimental period, lasted 84 days, asses were daily fed 8 kg coarse hay and 2.5 kg mixed feed (A or B). Asses' body condition score was monitored according to Martin Rosset (1990) every 21 days and at the same time blood samples were collected for plasma leptin determination, assayed with a multi-species leptin RIA kit (Linco Research Inc, St. Charles, MO). Intra-assay and inter-assay coefficients of variation were respectively 3.8% and 7.8%. Data were analyzed by analysis of variance, also considering the covariate effect of days of lactation (SAS Inc. Cary, NC, USA). The relations between investigated parameters were assessed by analysis of regression (SAS Inc. Cary, NC, USA).

Results and conclusion

Ass's body condition score did not differ between the two groups (A: 3.10 ± 0.05; B: 3.00 ± 0.05; $P>0.05$) and always ranged within a 3.0 – 3.25 score; moreover, body condition score increased significantly during lactation ($R^2=0.54$; $P<0.05$).

Plasma leptin levels, measured for the first time in lactating asses, ranged between 2.95 ng/mL and 14.7 ng/mL; they were also found to be higher than values reported for not pregnant mares (McManus and Fitzgerald, 2000), assayed with the same commercial multi-species leptin RIA kit. Although the investigated fibre sources did not affect plasma leptin level (A: 7.77 ± 0.44 ng/mL; B: 6.76 ± 0.45 ng/mL), statistical analysis pointed out that leptinemia was significantly related to days of lactation (R^2 = 0,8389; P<0.01) (Figure 1a), as also noted by Bonnet *et al.* (2005) in lactating not pregnant goats. Variability of the plasma leptin levels was also explained by asses's body condition, as Figure 1b shows. These results seem to confirm that body fatness strongly regulates leptinemia and its responses to other factors, along with the interesting hypothesis that physiological status could modulate plasma leptin expression (Chilliard *et al.*, 2005).
In late lactation, ass's plasma leptin concentration could in fact play a key role by increasing metabolic efficiency in both mammary secretion and body reserves reconstitution.

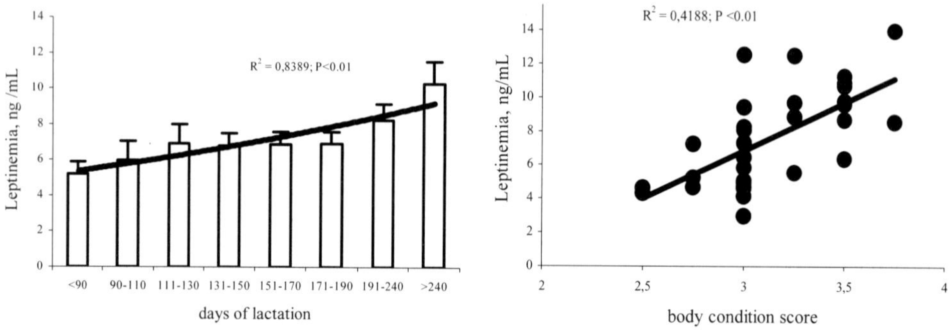

Figure 1. Relationship between plasma leptin levels and (a) days of lactation, (b) BCS in lactating, not pregnant asses (mean ± SEM).

References

Bonnet M., C. Delavaud, J. Rouel and Y. Chilliard, 2005. Pregnancy increases plasma leptin in nulliparous but not primiparous goats while lactation depresses it. Domest. Anim. Endocrinol. 28: 216-223.

Chilliard Y., C. Delavaud and M. Bonnet, 2005. Leptin expression in ruminants: Nutritional and physiological regulations in relation with energy metabolism. Domest. Anim. Endocrinol. 29 (suppl.1): 3-22.

Houseknecht K.L., C.A. Baile, R.L. Matteri and M.E. Spurlock, 1998. The biology of leptin: a review. J. Anim. Sci. 76: 1405-1420.

Mac Manus C.J. and B.P. Fitzgerald, 2000. Effects of a single day of feed restriction on changes in serum leptin, gonadotropins, prolactin, and metabolites in aged and young mares. Domest. Anim. Endocrinol. 19: 1-13.

Martin-Rosset W., 1990. Bases du rationnement. In: Martin-Rosset W., L'alimentation des chevaux, Ed. INRA, Paris.

Salimei E., F. Fantuz, G. Varisco, C. Maglieri and M. Polidori, 2005. Different fiber sources in dairy ass's diet: effects on milk yield and composition. In proceedings of the 16h ASPA Congress, Torino, June 28-30, pp. 430-432.

Nutritional status of lactating asses fed two different dietary fibre sources

C. Maglieri[1], M. Palazzo[2], D. Casamassima[2], P. Polidori[3] and E. Salimei[1]
[1]Dept. STAAM, Molise University, Via De Sanctis, 86100 Campobasso, Italy
[2]Dept. SAVA, Molise University, Via De Sanctis, 86100 Campobasso, Italy
[3]Camerino University, Via Circonvallazione 93, 62024 Matelica (MC), Italy

Abstract

The effects of different fibre sources in concentrate for dairy asses on metabolic responses of subjects were studied in an organic farming system. During experimental period (84 days), sixteen pluriparous asses divided into two groups were daily fed 8 kg coarse hay and 2.5 kg of concentrate feed including either wheat bran (20% - group A) or dehydrated beet pulp (20% - group B). Blood samples from asses were collected every 21 days for plasma metabolites determination. Although observed values were always within the normal range for *Equidae*, plasma levels of phospolipids, total protein and creatinine were significantly affected by the investigated dietary fibre sources.

Keywords: donkey, milk, dietary fibre, plasma metabolites

Introduction

Efficacy of ass's milk as a hypoallergenic food for infants have been proved (Carroccio *et al.*, 2000) and studies on this innovative food chain are becoming more frequent (Salimei *et al.*, 2006). Aiming to expand the list of fibrous feeds to be utilised in dairy asses' nutrition, dehydrated beet pulp is a by-product interesting for its soluble fibre content, a healthy component of the diet. In order to deepen the knowledge on donkeys' metabolic responses, the present study, as a part of a broader research project, is focused on the evaluation of the effects of different dietary fibre sources in concentrate for dairy asses on nutritional status of the subjects.

Materials and methods

Sixteen pluriparous asses (125 ± 48 days of lactation), bred in an organic farm, were divided into two groups fed two isoenergetic and isonitrogenous concentrates, including either wheat bran (20% - group A) or dehydrated beet pulp (20% - group B). During the experimental trial (84 days), dry matter consumption (about 3.2% of body weight) was on average characterised by 10% (d.m.) crude protein and 8.5 MJ DE/kg d.m. Jugular blood samples from asses were collected every 21 days for plasma metabolites determination; biochemical analysis were performed using commercial kits: glucose, urea, total and HDL cholesterol, triglycerides, albumin, total bilirubin, total protein, creatinine (Biotecnica Instruments, Roma, Italy), NEFA and phospholipids (Randox Laboratories Ltd, Crumlin, UK). Data were analyzed by analysis of variance, also considering the covariate effect of days of lactation (SAS Inc., Cary, NC USA).

Results and conclusion

The nutritional effects of isoenergetic and isonitrogenus replacement of wheat bran by beet pulp in mixed feed formula for lactating asses on plasma biochemical constituents are reported in Table 1; the observed values confirm the clinically healthy status of experimental subjects. As regard to the serum indices of asses' energetic metabolism, the dietary treatment did not significantly influence glucose, total and HDL cholesterol and NEFA concentrations. Instead, plasma phospholipids concentration significantly increased ($P<0.05$) in group B. The healthy benefits of high soluble dietary fibre intake in human nutrition are thought to be related to its contribution contribute in reducing plasma lipoproteins concentration (Jenkins *et al.*, 2000); on the other hand, according to Hallebeek and Beyen (2003) findings, the different effect observed in a herbivorous species could be linked to different digestion mechanisms and/or diet characteristics.

As far as the asses' nitrogenous metabolism is concerned (Table 1), plasma protein concentration was significantly increased by the dietary treatment with dehydrated beet pulp. In addition, the serum creatinine concentration seems to be affected by the dietary treatment, showing higher values ($P<0.05$) in group B. According to Van Soest (1994), this observation could be related to modifications in gut environment driven by a higher intake of fermentable fibre, i.e. pectin in dehydrated beet pulp. The different protein quality of the experimental mixed feed could have also influenced the nitrogenous plasma profile of the asses, although observed values were within the normal range of variations in both groups.

Table 1. Nutritional profile of dairy asses fed the experimental fibre sources.

Analyte	Group A	Group B	P
Glucose, mmol/L	3.44 ± 0.04	3.49 ± 0.04	ns
Triglycerides, mmol/L	0.70 ± 0.03	0.73 ± 0.03	ns
Cholesterol, mmol/L	1.81 ± 0.05	1.91 ± 0.05	ns
HDL Cholesterol, mmol/L	0.661 ± 0.018	0.694 ± 0.019	ns
NEFA, mmol/L	0.13 ± 0.004	0.14 ± 0.004	ns
Phospholipids, mmol/L	1.35 ± 0.03	1.46 ± 0.02	<0.05
Total protein, g/L	64.47 ± 0.85	67.80 ± 0.86	< 0.01
Albumin, g/L	25.53 ± 0.19	25.64 ± 0.20	ns
Urea, mmol/L	5.06 ± 0.10	5.00 ± 0.10	ns
Total bilirubin, µmol/L	8.92 ± 0.09	8.82 ± 0.09	ns
Creatinine, µmol/L	99.69 ± 1.25	104.14 ± 1.27	<0.05

References

Carroccio, A., F. Cavataio, G. Montaldo, D. D'amico, L. Alabrese and G. Iacono, 2000. Intolerance to hydrolysed cow's milk proteins in infants: clinical characteristics and dietary treatments. Clin. Exp. Allergy, 30: 1597-1603.

Hallebeek, J.M. and A.C. Beynen, 2003. Influence of dietary beet pulp on the plasma levels of triacilglycerols in horses. J. Anim. Physiol. a. Anim. Nutr. 87, 181-187

Jenkins, D.J.A., C.W.C. Kendall, M. Axelsen, L.S.A. Augustin and V. Viksan, 2000. Viscous and non viscous fibre, non absorbable and low glycaemic index carbohydrates, blood lipids and coronary heart disease. Current Opinion in Lipidology, 11, 49-56.

Salimei, E., F. Fantuz, R. Coppola, B. Chiofalo, P. Polidori and G. Varisco 2006. Ass's milk: nutritional and functional characteristics. EAAP No. 118, 2006, Wageningen Academic Publishers, 93-98.

Van Soest, P.J., 1994. Nutritional ecology of the ruminants. 2nd ed., Cornell University Press, Ithaca and London.

Values on serum metabolites in lactating jennies of Martina Franca breed

A.G. D'Alessandro[1], G. Martemucci[1], M. Palazzo[2], N. Simone[1], G.E. Colella[2], R. Pizzo[2] and D. Casamassima[2]
[1]Dept. PRO.GE.S.A., University of Bari, Via G. Amendola, 165/A, 70126 Bari, Italy
[2]Dept. S.A.V.A., University of Molise, Via De Sanctis, 86100 Campobasso, Italy

Abstract

The aim of the research was to study some parameters of the energetic (glucose, cholesterol, tryglicerides) and proteic (total proteins, urea, albumine, creatinine) metabolisms, serum hepatic profile (LDH, GOT, GGT, alkaline phosphatase, AP; total bilirubin, GPT) and ions (Ca, Mg, K, Na) in relation to physiological status of lactation in jennies of Martina Franca breed. Two experiments were performed in Southern Italy on a total of 26 jennies aged from 5 to 18 years, reared in semi-extensive conditions. Serum cholesterol, total proteins and urea proved to be higher ($0.05>P<0.01$) in lactating jennies. AP and GPT serum levels were lower ($P<0.01$) in lactating jennies (Experiment I). In the Experiment II, proteic metabolism as well as hepatic profile and mineral levels varied ($0.05>P<0.01$) with the lactation stage. Correlations were positive between milk yield and albumin ($P<0.01$), serum protein ($P<0.05$), GGT ($P<0.05$) and sodium ($P<0.01$), and negative with creatinine ($P<0.01$) and GOT ($P<0.05$).

Keywords: serum metabolities, donkey, lactation

Introduction

Knowledge of reference values of serum biochemical parameters in animals may serve as a guide to improve husbandry systems and animal welfare. It has been reported that biochemical components of blood are affected by several factors such as breed, sex, age and physiological status of the animal (Zinkl *et al.*, 1990; Cubeddu *et al.*, 1991; Jordana *et al.*, 1998; Mori *et al.*, 2003). To our knowledge, no references are available regarding biochemical serum of the Martina Franca donkey breed.

The aim of this research was to study some parameters of the energetic, proteic, hepatic and mineral profiles in relation to the physiological status of lactation in jennies of the Martina Franca breed.

Materials and methods

Two experiments were carried out in Southern Italy on a total of 26 jennies aged from 5 to 18 years, reared in semi-extensive conditions. The aim of Experiment I was to study profile of serum metabolities values in relation to lactation status. We considered a total of ten jennies subdivided into two groups (N. 5): A) non-lactating (control), and B) lactating jennies. In Group B) blood samples were collected from one animal in correspondence of each month of lactation. In Experiment II sixteen animals were used to study serum biochemical parameters during the six months of lactation (June to December). Milk yield in lactating jennies was measured once daily by machine milking, with blood samples collected monthly. Sera samples were analyzed for metabolities of the energetic (glucose - Glu, cholesterol - Cho, tryglicerides – Try) and proteic (total proteins - TP, urea - Ur, albumine Al, and creatinine - Cr) profiles, hepatic parameters (lactate dehydrogenase – LDH, glutamil-ossalacetic transaminase, GOT; γ-glutamil transferase, GGT; alkaline phosphatase, AP; total bilirubin, TB; glutamil-piruvate transaminase, GPT) and ions (Ca, Mg) in a semi-automatic biochemical analyzer (mod. ARCO), using commercially available tests. Na and K contents were estimated using a flame photometer. Statistical analysis was performed by ANOVA using the SPSS package (2003), with means compared by Scheffè's test. Correlations are also established between the biochemical parameters and milk production (SPSS, 2003).

Results and discussion

Experiment I – Lactating asses showed higher mean values of cholesterol (P<0.01), total proteins (P<0.01) and urea (P<0.05) (Table 1). Serum glucose values in this study corresponded to reference ranges in American donkeys (Zinkl *et al.*, 1990) while cholesterol and urea serum were similar to those determined in Brazilian breed donkey (Mori *et al.*, 2003). According to this study, lactation in equids causes hyperlipidemia and variations in serum protein (Mori *et al.*, 2003).

Metabolic status of lactation did not influence mineral metabolism as well as profiles of GOT, GGT and TB. Lactating jennies showed a lower mean values of AP (430.33 vs 505.25 IU/L; P<0.01) and GPT (11.50 vs 22.22 IU/L; P<0.01) (Table 2).

The serum concentrations of GGT, Ca, Na and K of this study corresponded to that stated for Italian Albino donkey (Cubeddu *et al.*, 1991) and Brazilian donkey (Mori *et al.*, 2003).

Table 1. Effect of lactation on energetic and proteic profiles.

	Group A – Control		Group B - Lactating jennies	
	x ± SD	Range	x ± SD	Range
Glu (mg/dL)	80.47 ± 6.98	74.00 - 87.10	79.67 ± 6.08	71.10 - 87.00
Cho (mg/dL)	71.37 ± 14.76^{A}	50.10 - 83.90	97.80 ± 7.51^{B}	86.90 - 110.00
Try (mg/dL)	52.47 ± 11.60	41.80 - 68.10	43.86 ± 10.01	24.30 - 52.50
TP (g/dL)	5.97 ± 0.26^{A}	5.70 - 6.20	6.73 ± 0.37^{B}	6.40 - 7.30
Ur (mg/dL)	26.90 ± 2.55^{a}	25.00 - 30.40	32.37 ± 3.21^{b}	27.80 - 37.30
Al (g/dL)	2.90 ± 0.27	2.50 - 3.10	2.98 ± 0.21	2.60 - 3.20
Cr (mg/dL)	1.30 ± 0.08	1.20 - 1.40	1.42 ± 0.26	1.10 - 1.90

A, B: P<0.01; a, b: P<0.05

Table 2. Effect of lactation on hepatic and ions profiles.

	Group A – Control		Group B - Lactating jennies	
	x ± SD	Range	x ± SD	Range
LDH (IU/L)	358.00 ± 59.09	291.00 - 413.00	396.50 ± 66.78	331.00 - 518.00
GGT (IU/L)	42.30 ± 1.31	40.80 - 43.40	39.83 ± 5.27	30.70 - 46.40
AP (IU/L)	605.25 ± 70.69^{A}	514.00 - 675.00	430.33 ± 53.20^{B}	363.00 - 521.00
TB (mg/dL)	0.46 ± 0.008	0.45 - 0.47	0.46 ± 0.04	0.42 - 0.52
GOT (IU/L)	162.50 ± 39.24	128.00 - 204.00	78.67 ± 33.68	135.00 - 213.00
GPT (IU/L)	22.22 ± 11,19^{a}	14.70 - 38.60	11.50 ± 2.32^{b}	8.90 - 14.90
Ca (mg/dL)	11.47 ± 1.08	10.00 - 12.60	11.57 ± 0.57	10.50 - 12.20
Mg (mg/dL)	2.40 ± 0.18	2.20 - 2.60	2.92 ± 0.55	2.30 - 3.70
K (mEq/L)	4.30 ± 0.22	4.10 - 4.60	4.63 ± 0.32	4.10 - 5.00
Na (mEq/L)	143.25 ± 3.86	141.00 - 149.00	145.67 ± 4.23	141.00 - 152.00

A, B: P<0.01; a, b: P<0.05

Experiment II – Energetic metabolism did not vary with lactation stage with the exception of serum glucose, which dropped (P<0.05) from the 5th to 6th month of lactation (Table 3).

Proteic metabolism (Table 3) varied with the lactation stage (0.05>P<0.01). Total protein values were higher during the 2nd to 4th month (6.74 – 7.80 g/dL; P<0.05) after foaling; albumin was at its lowest value in the 6th month of lactation (2.47 ± 0.09 g/dL; P<0.01); creatinine level was higher at the end of the lactation period (4th and 5th month, 1.44-1.56 mg/dL; 0.05>P<0.01); urea ranged from 26.25 ± 4.27 mg/dL to 34.67 ± 2.37 mg/dL (P<0.01). Correlation analysis of data showed significant positive relationships between milk production (data not shown) and albumin (r = 0.44; P<0.01) and serum protein (r = 0.33; P<0.05), and negative correlation with creatinine (r = -0.48; P<0.01).

During the lactation period significant differences (0.05>P<0.01) were found for hepatic parameters as well as ions. Results are reported in Table 4. GOT values were highest at the 6th month (241.70 ± 38.76 IU/L; P<0.01); AP values reached their peak at the 4th month (551.00 ± 80.99 IU/L; P>0.05); GGT values were lowest at 5th – 6th month of lactation (28.60 – 28.94 IU/L) (0.05>P<0.01); bilirubin proved to be quite constant (P>0.05) throughout the period (0.34 – 0.49 mg/dL) as did GPT (10.23 – 13.60 IU/L).

Mean concentrations of sera ions were not significant (P>0.05) for Ca and Na while Mg was significantly higher at the 6th month (3.19 ± 0.26 mg/dL) and K at 1st-2nd month was 4.85 – 4.87 mEq/L (P<0.05) (Table 4).

Table 3. Energetic and proteic metabolism in jennies during the lactation period (x ± SD).

	1st Month	2nd Month	3rd Month	4th Month	5th Month	6th Month
Glu (mg/dL)	74.53±2.33	77.18±5.15	80.86±9.39	81.48±3.46	84.49±10.22^a	72.79±4.32^b
Cho (mg/dL)	88.23 ±12.58	84.66±9.92	87.05±7.24	83.22±6.93	96.83±25.80	101.32±7.62
Try (mg/dL)	45.63±5.96	56.50±24.85	7.71±18.68	31.90±13.90	39.13±12.83	35.40±17.23
TP (g/dL)	6.37±0.15	6.74±0.45^a	6.67±0.36	6.80±0.49	6.18 ±0.29^b	6.12±0.41
Ur (mg/dL)	31.27±5.20	26.25±4.27^{Aa}	34.67±2.37^B	33.71±4.61^b	30.47±3.90	28.29±1.96^A
Al (g/dL)	2.93±0.06^A	2.99±0.12^{Aa}	2.99±0.13^{Aa}	3.04±0.13^{Aa}	2.77±0.21^{Ab}	2.47±0.09^B
Cr (mg/dL)	1.10± 0.00^{Aa}	1.25±0.16^A	1.25±0.13^A	1.36±0.05	1.44±0.08^b	1.56±0.20^B

A, B: P<0.01; a, b: P<0.05

Table 4. Hepatic profile and serum ions concentrations during the lactation period (x ± SD).

	1st Month	2nd Month	3rd Month	4th Month	5th Month	6th Month
LDH (IU/L)	388.33±32.39	379.18±29.24	388.55±26.5	401.80±15.90	381.00±41.04	414.00±94.98
GGT IU/L)	46.57±8.42^A	47.39±8.23^A	45.47±7.52^A	43.40±4.07^A	38.60±4.45^a	28.94±1.71^{Bb}
AP (IU/L)	383.67±23.25	413.27±109.75	439.27±71.93	551.00±80.99	490.10±93.86	420.20±69.50
TB (mg/dL)	0.43±0.02	0.49±0.04	0.49±0.03	0.48±0.02	0.47±0.03	0.46±0.03
GOT (IU/L)	168.7±32.6^A	156.73±16.1^A	161.4 ±17.5^A	177.8±21.6^A	170.5±32.0^A	241.7±38.7^B
GPT (IU/L)	11.93±0.40	13.60±3.78	11.88±1.51	12.42±3.52	11.19±1.19	10.23±1.19
Ca (mg/dL)	12.17±0.06	11.92±0.32	11.80±0.32	11.56±0.38	11.72±0.12	10.21±0.12
Mg (mg/dL)	2.33±0.06^a	2.40±0.30^A	2.95±0.56	2.54±0.18	2.87±0.39	3.19±0.26^{Bb}
K (mEq/L)	4.87±0.06	4.85±0.47^a	4.40±0.47	4.08±0.48^b	4.78±0.30	4.19±0.24^b
Na (mEq/L)	146.00±1.73	152.64±4.86	148.82±1.78	146.40±6.11	146.30±5.17	142.30±1.34

A, B: P<0.01; a, b: P<0.05

Correlation analysis between biochemical metabolities and milk yield (data not shown) proved positive for GGT ($r = 0.33$; $P<0.05$) and sodium ($r = 0.374$; $P<0.01$), and negative for GOT ($r = -0.31$; $P<0.05$).

In conclusion, the results reported in this study could serve as initial reference ranges for serum biochemical concentrations in lactating jennies of the Martina Franca breed.

Aknowledgements

This work was funded by PRIN COFIN (2004) of MIUR and University of Bari. The authors also wish to thank the Puglia Regional Government, Istituto Incremento Ippico (Foggia) and A.R.A.M.F. (Martina Franca).

References

Cubeddu G.M., P.P. Bini, B. Floris, V. Carangiu, G. Bomboi and G. Pintori, 1991. Costanti ematiche dell'asinello bianco dell'Asinara. Boll. Soc. It. Biol. Sper., 67: 577-584.

Jordana J., P. Folch and R. Cuenca, 1998. Clinical biochemical parameters of the endagered Catalonian donkey breed: normal values and the influence of sex, age, and management practises effect. Res. Vet. Sci., 64: 7-10.

Mori E., W.R. Fernandes, R.M.S. Mirandola, G. Kubo, R.R. Ferriera, J.V. Oliveira and F. Gacek, 2003. Reference values on serum biochemical parameters of Brazilian donkey (Equus asinus) breed. J. Equine Vet. Sci., 23 (8): 358-364.

SPSS, 2003. SPSS for Window, vers. 10.0.7. SPSS Inc., Chicago, IL (USA).

Zinkl J.G., D. Mae, P.G. Merida, T.B. Farver and J.A. Humble, 1990. Reference ranges and the influence of age and sex on haematological and serum biochemical values in donkeys (Equus asinus). Am. J. Vet. Res., 51: 408-413.

Different fibre sources in dairy ass's diet. I. Effects on milk fatty acid composition

B. Chiofalo[1], D. Piccolo[1], E.B. Riolo[1], C. Maglieri[2] and E. Salimei[2]
[1]Dept. MOBIFIPA, University of Messina, Polo Universitario Annunziata, 98168 Messina, Italy
[2]Dept. S.T.A.A.M., University of Molise, Via De Sanctis, 86100 Campobasso, Italy

Abstract

The effects of different fibre sources in concentrate for dairy asses on milk fatty acid composition were studied on 16 Martina Franca asses, divided into two groups fed concentrates containing either wheat bran (group A) or dehydrated beet pulp (group B). The trial lasted 84 days. On both feeds and individual milk samples, fatty acids were analysed and the quality indices calculated. The dietary treatment significantly influenced the milk content of SFAs (A:52.81% vs. B:56.23%, P=0.026). No significant differences were observed for milk MUFAs (A: 24.43% vs. B: 22.80%; P=0.065) and total PUFAs (A: 22.77% vs. B: 21.02%, P=0.075). As regard to the milk quality indices, group B showed a higher atherogenic index (A: 0.93 vs. B: 1.12, P=0.001) while no difference was observed for the thrombogenic index (A: 0.54 vs B: 0.59, P=0.179).

Keywords: dietary fibre, ass's milk, fatty acids

Introduction

Ass's milk is traditionally known as an alternative food for infants; nevertheless, scientific references on its composition have been rare for a long time. In this regard there is little information on donkey nutrition, which is a major source of variation in equid milk production (Doreau *et al.*, 2002). The recent clinical studies, confirming ass's milk feeding as a safe and valid treatment of cases of multiple food intolerance (Carroccio *et al.*, 2000), have stimulated research on the effects of feeding on productive and nutritional response of dairy asses. In this study the effects of different fiber sources (wheat bran vs. dehydrated beet pulp) in concentrate for dairy asses on both milk fatty acid composition and acidic quality indices were evaluated.

Material and methods

The research was carried out on 16 pluriparous Martina Franca dairy asses bred in an organic farm, divided into two groups (A and B; n=8) homogeneous for body weight (B.W.: 260 ± 40 kg) and day of lactation (125 ± 48 days). The asses were daily fed two isoenergetic and isonitrogenous mixed feed (2.5 kg), including either wheat bran (20% - group A) or dehydrated beet pulp (20% - group B), and meadow hay (8 kg), divided in two meals. Dry matter consumption, about 3.2% of B.W., was on average characterised by 10% of crude protein and 8.5 MJ DE/kg (Salimei *et al.*, 2005). During the trial, [which] lasted 84 days, the asses were machine milked twice within 24 hours; experimental observations were carried out every 21 days. The fatty acid composition of the feed and individual milk samples were determined by GC-FID (Chiofalo and Salimei, 2001) and the atherogenic and thrombogenic indices were calculated (Ulbricht and Southgate, 1991). The results, expressed as percentages of total fatty acid methyl esters identified, were analysed by analysis of variance for repeated measures, also considering the covariate days of lactation (proc. GLM; SAS, 2001).

Results

In spite of the similar levels of the dietary SFAs (Table 1) in the two experimental concentrates, the higher percentages of this class observed in group B milk samples (Table 2) could be related to the higher content of the soluble dietary fiber (Salimei *et al.*, 2005) in feed B than feed A (B: 17.8±0.5 vs. A: 14.9±0.3 SDF %TDF). As a possible explanation, the increase of acetate production, major precursor of the milk SFAs, could be in fact related (Vermorel *et al.*, 1993) to the observed higher levels of milk lauric (A: 9.43%± 0.42 vs. B: 11.15% ± 0.42, P=0.007) and myristic (A: 6.44% ± 0.27 vs. B: 7.71% ± 0.27, P=0.001) acids in group B. Milk MUFAs were not influenced by the dietary treatment (Table 2). Milk n6-PUFA level was higher in group A than in group B while milk n-3 PUFA content was not influenced by the dietary fibre sources (Table 2) as well as the milk linolenic acid content (A: 8.78% ± 0.50 vs. B: 8.45% ± 0.50, P=0.602), precursor of the anti-inflammatory eicosanoids. With regard to the milk quality indices (Table 2), group B showed a higher AI while no difference was observed for the TI.

Table 1. Fatty Acid class composition of feedstuffs (g/100 g fatty acids, Mean ± SD).

	Meadow Hay	Concentrate A	Concentrate B	P [1]
Saturated fatty acids (SFAs)	39.88±3.79	51.69±0.16	49.54±0.96	0.119
Monounsaturated fatty acids (MUFAs)	16.25±2.51	36.27±0.11	34.90±2.78	0.045
Polyunsaturated fatty acids (PUFAs)	43.87±4.07	12.04±0.04	15.56±1.83	0.023
n3-PUFAs	13.73±2.68	0.52±0.03	0.79±0.05	0.035
n6-PUFAs	30.13±4.41	11.53±0.01	14.77±1.80	0.011

[1] P values were calculated comparing the concentrates (A vs. B)

Table 2. Fatty acid percentages and Quality Indices of the milk in relation to the diet (LSM ± s.e.m.).

	Group A	Group B	SE	P
Saturated fatty acids (SFAs)	52.81	56.23	1.04	0.026
Monounsaturated fatty acids (MUFAs)	24.43	22.80	0.62	0.065
Polyunsaturated fatty acids (PUFAs)	22.77	21.02	0.68	0.075
n3-PUFAs	9.64	9.45	0.49	0.745
n6-PUFAs	13.09	11.57	0.39	0.008
Atherogenic Index (AI)	0.93	1.12	0.04	0.001
Thrombogenic Index (TI)	0.54	0.59	0.03	0.179

References

Carroccio, A., F. Cavataio, G., Montaldo, D. D'Amico, L. Alabrese and G. Iacono, 2000. Intolerance to hydrolised cow's milk proteins in infants: clinical characteristics and dietary treatments. Clin. Exp. Allergy, 30: 1597-1603.

Chiofalo, B. and E. Salimei, 2001. Ass's milk: exploitation of an alimentary resource. Folium I: 235-241.

Doreau M., J.L. Gaillard, J.M. Chobert, J. Léonil, A.S. Egito and T. Haertlé, 2002. Composition of mare and donkey milk fatty acids and proteins and consequences on milk utilisation. In proceedings of 4th Congress "New findings in equine practice", 51-71.

Salimei, E., F. Rosi, C. Maglieri, M. Polidori, F. Fantuz and G. Varisco, 2005. Effect of different fiber sources in dairy ass's' diet on major constituents of milk and leptin content. In proceedings of 7th Congress "New findings in equine practice", 160-165.

Ulbricht, T.L.V. and D.A.T. Southgate, 1991. Coronary heart disease: seven dietary factors. The Lancet 338: 985-992.

Vermorel, M., R. Jarrige and W. Martin-Rosset, 1993. Metabolismo e fabbisogni energetici del cavallo. Il sistema delle UFC. In: Il cavallo, R. Jarrige and W. Martin-Rosset, Masson S.p.A., Milano, Italy, 224-264.

Different fibre sources in dairy ass's diet. II. Effects on plasma fatty acid profile

B. Chiofalo[1], D. Piccolo[1], E.B. Riolo[1], C. Maglieri[2] and E. Salimei[2]
[1]Dept. MOBIFIPA, University of Messina, Polo Universitario Annunziata, 98168 Messina, Italy
[2]Dept. S.T.A.A.M., University of Molise, Via De Sanctis, 86100 Campobasso, Italy

Abstract

The effect of two different fibre sources in mixed feeds (A=wheat bran or B=dehydrated beet pulp) were investigated on the plasma fatty acid composition of 16 pluriparous Martina Franca dairy asses. Every 21 days feeds were sampled and individual blood samples were withdrawn; the trial lasted 84 days. On both feeds and individual plasma samples, fatty acid composition was analysed and the quality indices calculated. The investigated dietary fibre sources did not significantly influence the plasma levels of SFAs (A=39.30%; B=39.48%; P=0.762), MUFAs (A=18.75%; B=18.79%; P=0.968) and PUFAs (A=41.95%; B=41.73%; P=0.770). The plasma fatty acids UFA/SFA (A=1.55; B=1.54; P=0.703) ratio was unaffected by the dietary treatment as well as no differences were observed in both Atherogenic (A=0.36; B=0.37; P=0.682) and Thrombogenic (A=0.89; B=0.91; P=0.642) indices.

Keywords: dietary fibre, donkey, plasma fatty acids

Introduction

A general understanding of the influence of diet on milk production cannot be deduced from knowledge of other species. Horses as well as donkeys, being monogastric herbivorous animals, have specific mechanisms for regulating milk secretion, since nutrients absorption in equids precedes the ceco-colic fermentation (Doreau *et al.*, 1992). However, specifically to asses, the literature reports few data to establish a relationship between end-products of digestion and milk secretion. As ass's milk is increasingly considered as an effective hypoallergenic food for infants (Muraro *et al.*, 2002), studies on ass's feeding and milk composition are becoming more frequent. As a part of a larger study on the effects of the administration of different fibre sources (wheat bran vs. dehydrated beet pulp) in concentrates on productive and nutritional response of dairy asses, this study focus the attention on the plasmatic fatty acid composition of the asses.

Material and methods

The research was carried out on 16 pluriparous Martina Franca dairy asses bred in an organic farm, divided into two groups (A and B; n=8) homogeneous for day of lactation (125 ± 48 days). The asses were daily fed two isoenergetic and isonitrogenous concentrate (2.5 kg), including either wheat bran (20% - group A) or dehydrated beet pulp (20% - group B), and meadow hay (8 kg) divided in two meals. Dry matter consumption, about 3.2% of B.W., was on average characterised by 10% of crude protein and 8.5 MJ DE/kg (Salimei *et al.*, 2005). Every 21 days, feeds were sampled and individual blood samples were withdrawn in Vacutainer® containing Na-EDTA; the trial lasted 84 days. The fatty acid composition of the feed and individual plasma samples was determined by GC-FID (Chiofalo *et al.*, 2002) and the atherogenic and thrombogenic indices were calculated by Ulbricht and Southgate (1991) equations. The results, expressed as percentages of total fatty acid methyl esters identified, were analysed by analysis of variance for repeated measures, also considering the covariate days of lactation (proc. GLM; SAS, 2001).

Results

With regard to the acidic composition of the two concentrates (Table 1), the SFA class did not statistically vary and some differences were observed for the percentages of MUFAs and PUFAs. The investigated dietary fibre sources did not significantly influence the plasma levels of SFAs, MUFAs and PUFAs (Table 2). The plasmatic UFA/SFA ratio was unaffected by the dietary treatment as well as no difference was observed in both Atherogenic and Thrombogenic indices (Table 2). Results on plasma fatty acid profile are consistent with findings by Doreau *et al.* (1992) in nursing mares and could suggest sugar by-products as a safe and valid alternative fibre source in ass's diet. According to previous results observed in the milk composition (Salimei *et al.*, 2005), this by-product could in fact represent an interesting nutritional strategy for the production of donkey milk intended for infants.

Table 1. Fatty acid class percentages of feedstuffs (Mean ± SD).

	Meadow Hay	Concentrate A	Concentrate B	P [1]
Saturated fatty acids (SFAs)	39.88±3.79	51.69±0.16	49.54±0.96	0.119
Monounsaturated fatty acids (MUFAs)	16.25±2.51	36.27±0.11	34.90±2.78	0.045
Polyunsaturated fatty acids (PUFAs)	43.87±4.07	12.04±0.04	15.56±1.83	0.023
n3-PUFAs	13.73±2.68	0.52±0.03	0.79±0.05	0.035
n6-PUFAs	30.13±4.41	11.53±0.01	14.77±1.80	0.011

[1] P values were calculated comparing the concentrates

Table 2. Plasmatic fatty acid percentages, UFA/SFA ratio and Quality Indices in relation to the diet (LSM ± SE).

	Group A	Group B	SE	P
Saturated fatty acids (SFAs)	39.30	39.48	0.39	0.762
Monounsaturated fatty acids (MUFAs)	18.75	18.79	0.44	0.968
Polyunsaturated fatty acids (PUFAs)	41.95	41.73	0.55	0.770
n3-PUFAs	4.35	4.24	0.18	0.667
n6-PUFAs	37.61	37.50	0.58	0.884
Unsaturated/Saturated (UFAs/SFAs)	1.55	1.54	0.02	0.703
Atherogenic Index (AI)	0.36	0.37	0.01	0.682
Thrombogenic Index (TI)	0.89	0.91	0.02	0.642

References

Chiofalo, B., A. Rundo Sotera, L. Venticinque and S. D'Urso, 2002. Plasmatic fatty acids of the "Sanfratellana" mares: effect of lactation. In proceedings of 53rd Annual Meeting of the EAAP, Wageningen Academic Publishers, The Netherlands, p. 114.

Doreau M., S. Boulot, D. Bauchart, J.P. Barlet and W. Martin-Rosset, 1992. Voluntary intake, milk production and plasma metabolites in nursing mares fed two different diets. J. Nutr. 122 (4): 992-999.

Muraro M.A., P.G. Giampietro and E. Galli, 2002. Soy formulas and non bovine milk. Ann. Allergy Asthma Immunol., 89 (suppl.): 97-101.

Salimei, E., F. Fantuz, G. Varisco, C. Maglieri and M. Polidori, 2005. Different fibre sources in dairy ass's diet: effects on milk yield and composition. Italian Journal of Animal Science, 4 (Suppl. 2): 430-432.

Ulbricht, T.L.V. and D.A.T. Southgate, 1991. Coronary heart disease: seven dietary factors. The Lancet 338: 985-992.

Ass' s milk nitrogen distribution: effects of different dietary fibre source

F. Fantuz[1], P. Polidori[1], C. Maglieri[2], G. Varisco[3], S. Vincenzetti[1] and E. Salimei[2]
[1]Camerino University, Via Circonvallazione 93, 62024 Matelica (MC), Italy
[2]Dept. STAAM, Molise University, Via De Sanctis, 86100 Campobasso, Italy
[3]Experimental "Zooprofilattico" Institute, Brescia, Italy

Abstract

Aiming to determine ass's milk nitrogen content and distribution and the effects of different dietary fibre sources on milk nitrogen fractions, sixteen pluriparous Martina Franca asses were used to provide milk samples. Animals were divided into two groups fed [an] isonitrogenous and isoenergetic diet including 8kg of coarse hay and 2.5kg of concentrates containing either 20% wheat bran (group A) or 20% dehydrated beet pulp. Milk samples were analysed for total nitrogen (TN), non protein nitrogen (NPN), non casein nitrogen (NCN) and urea. Among parameters of milk nitrogen content and distribution the overall average (±SD) of TN, NPN, NCN, casein N (TN-NCN), casein index (casein N/TN), and urea were respectively 241.23±36.35 mg/100g, 34.4±5.79 mg/100g, 136.95±28.49 mg/100g; 104.50±31.43 mg/100g 0.43±0.11, 34.25 mg/100g. Dietary treatment did not significantly affected the considered parameters.

Keywords: dietary fibre, ass's milk, nitrogen

Introduction

Ass's milk appear[s] to be indicated as a hypoallergenic food for infants affected by cows milk protein intolerance or multiple food intolerance (Iacono et al, 1992; Carroccio et al, 2000). In recent years different studies on ass's milk provided knowledge on milk yield and milking technique as well as milk composition such as nitrogenous fraction, lipid fraction and minerals (Fantuz et al, 2001; Doreau et al, 2002; Salimei et al, 2004; Alabiso et al, 2005; Vincenzetti et al, 2005). Nutrition represent an important factor influencing equid milk production and composition (Doreau et al, 2002) as well as the health of [the] gastrointestinal tract; in particular characteristics of the fibre fraction (soluble and insoluble fibre) can influence ceco-colic fermentations (Van Soest, 1994). As a part of a larger study on the effects of nutrition on productive and nutritional response of dairy asses, this paper reports the effect of different dietary fibre sources on ass' milk main nitrogenous components.

Material and methods

Sixteen pluriparous Martina Franca asses (125±48 days of lactation) bred in an organic farm were divided into two experimental group which were fed two isoenergetic and isonitrogenous concentrates, including either wheat bran (20% - group A) or dehydrated beet pulp (20% - group B). Asses were fed 8 kg of coarse hay and 2.5 kg of mixed feed (A or B) daily, divided into two meals. Daily dry matter intake was about 3.2% of bodyweight and was characterised by 10% crude protein and 8.5 MJ DE/kg. During the experimental period that lasted 84 d, milk samples were collected at a 3 weeks interval, using a milking machine; asses were housed with the foals that were separated from the dam 3 hours before each milking (16:00 and 11:00). Individual milk samples were analysed for total nitrogen (TN), non protein nitrogen (NPN) and non casein nitrogen (NCN) by Kjeldhal's method (A.S.P.A., 1996); casein N (TN-NCN) casein index (100 (casein N/TN)) and whey N (NCN-NPN) were then calculated. On another aliquot of individual milk samples urea (mg/100g) was determined by IR (Milkosan 605, Foss Italia).

Data were statistically analysed by analysis of variance for repeated measures also considering the covariate effect of days in milk (SAS Inc., Cary, NC USA).

Results

The overall average milk crude protein (1.56±0.50 g/100 g milk) was slightly lower then those reported by others (Salimei et al, 2004; Alabiso et al, 2005). Investigated parameters showed high variability, ranging the NPN content (*6.38) of milk from 0.16 to 0.33 g/100g and the casein content from 0.18 to 1.18 g/100g. Compared to mare's milk (Martuzzi et al, 1995; Malacarne et al, 2002), ass's milk showed a lower casein index and a higher NPN content. Our results confirm the similarity of ass's milk to human milk when compared to other dairy species. The effects of different dietary treatment on milk nitrogen distribution are summarised in Table 1: the isoenergetic and isonitrogenous replacement of 20% wheat bran with 20% dehydrated beet pulp in mixed feed did not significantly affected any of the considered parameters on milk nitrogen content and milk nitrogen distribution.

Table 1. Effects of different dietary fibre sources on ass's milk nitrogen distribution (mean±s.e.m.).

	Group A	Group B	P
Total nitrogen, mg/100g	242.05±4.52	241.56±4.34	n.s.
NPN, mg/100g	34.86±0.85	34.33±0.81	n.s.
NCN, mg/100g	135.23±4.82	138.00±4.56	n.s.
Casein N, mg/100g	106.74±4.91	103.48±4.65	n.s.
Whey N, mg/100g	103.44±4.62	105.01±4.37	n.s.
Casein index	43.81±1.89	42.44±1.79	n.s.
NPN/TN	0.14±0.03	0.14±0.03	n.s.
Urea, mg/100g	33.50±0.57	34.95±0.56	n.s.

References

Alabiso, M., G. Russo, C. Giosuè, M.L. Alicata and C. Torrisi, 2005. Donkey milk production over an entire lactation in a Sicilian farming system. In 7th Congress "New findings in equine practice", 152-158.

A.S.P.A., 1996. Metodi di analisi del latte delle principali specie di interesse zootecnico. University of Perugia Press.

Carroccio, A., F. Cavataio, G. Montaldo, D. D'amico, L. Alabrese and G. Iacono, 2000. Intolerance to hydrolised cow's milk proteins in infants: clinical characteristics and dietary treatments. Clin. Exp. Allergy, 30: 1597-1603.

Doreau, M., J.L. Gaillard, J.M. Chobert, J. Leonil, A.S. Egito and T. Haertle, 2002. Composition of mare and donkey milk fatty acids and proteins and consequences on milk utilisation, In: proceedings of 4th Congress "New findings in equine practice", 51-71.

Fantuz, F., S. Vincenzetti, P. Polidori, A. Vita and E. Salimei, 2001. Study on protein fractions of donkey milk, A.S.P.A. XIV Congress, 635-637.

Iacono, G., A. Carroccio, F. Cavataio, G. Montaldo, M. Soresi and V. Balsamo, 1992. Use of ass's milk in mutiple food allergy. J. of Pediatric Gastroenterol. And Nutr. 14: 177-181.

Malacarne, M., F. Martuzzi, A. Summer and P. Mariani, 2002. Protein and fat composition of mare's milk: some nutritional remarks with reference to human and cow's milk. Int. Dairy J. 12: 869-877.

Martuzzi, F., P. Mariani, G. Zanzucchi, A.L. Catalano, 1995. Composizione azotata e minerale e valore energetico del latte di cavalla nel corso dei primi 4 mesi di lattazione. Rivista SIDI 1: 15-93.

Salimei, E., F. Fantuz, R. Coppola, B. Chiofalo, P. Polidori and G. Varisco, 2004. Composition and characteristics of ass's milk. Animal Research, 53: 67-78.

Van Soest, P.J.1994. Nutritional ecology of the ruminants, 2nd ed. Cornell Univ. press, Ithaca, NY.

Vincenzetti, S., P. Polidori, F. Fantuz, P.L. Mariani, N. Cammertoni, A. Vita and F. Polidori, 2005. Donkey's milk caseins characterisation. Italian J. Anim. Sci. 4 (Suppl. 2): 427-429.

Machine milking of dairy asses as related to milk production and body condition

E. Salimei[1], C. Maglieri[1], M. Polidori[1], R. Socci[1], B. Chiofalo[2], M. Gambacorta[3] and G. Varisco[4]
[1]Dept. STAAM, Molise University, Via De Sanctis, 86100 Campobasso, Italy
[2]Dept. MOBIFIPA, Messina University, polo Universitario Annunziata, 98168 Messina, Italy
[3]Dept. SAVA, Molise University, Via De Sanctis, 86100 Campobasso, Italy
[4]Experimental "Zooprofilattico" Institute, Brescia, Italy

Abstract

The effects of a different machine milking management on milk yield and composition were studied on twenty pluriparous asses, bred in an organic farm. Asses were divided into two groups subjected to two consecutive milkings with a different management: 20 *vs.* 4 hours interval between the two milkings, respectively for group A and group B. Milk yield was unaffected by the different milking management nor significant effects were observed on milk protein content. Adopted milking frequencies significantly influenced both the fat content and the hygienic quality of milk. Asses' body condition score was not affected by the management of milkings.

Keywords: ass's milk, body condition score, milking management

Introduction

Clinical studies showed ass's milk as a promising hypoallergenic food for infants (Carroccio *et al.*, 2000), when appropriately adapted in chemical composition and evaluated from the hygienic point of view (Restani *et al.*, 2002). As far as the chemical composition of ass's milk is concerned, experimental data substantially confirm the compositional resemblance to human milk, even thought ass's milk is characterized by a high variability of its constituents, milk fat in particular (Salimei *et al.*, 2004). On this regard, milking seems to strongly influence milk yield and composition of *Equidae* (Doreau, 1991; Salimei *et al.*, 2004).

As a part of a larger study, the effects of a different machine milking management on milk yield and composition were investigated also considering the high degree of hygiene and safety required [for] to a hypoallergenic food for infant[s].

Materials and methods

Twenty pluriparous asses (89 ± 42 days of lactation), bred in an organic farm and machine milked in a proper [facility?] (Simoni *et al.*, 2004), were divided into two homogeneous groups (A: 382.5 ± 86 kg BW; B: 342.8 ± 55 kg BW) and subjected to two consecutive milkings with different management within 24 hours. Group A was milked at 15:00h and 11:00h of the subsequent day (20 hours interval between the two milkings) and group B was milked at 11:00h and 15:00h (4 hours interval). The animals were [fed] daily fed in [an] average 8 kg meadow hay and 2.5 kg of mixed feed, divided in two meals. Asses were stabled with their foals in two boxes provided with a wide external paddock; foals were physically separated from the dams [for] since 3 hours before each milking. The study lasted 150 days; every 28 days individual milk yield was recorded and milk hygiene and healthy status of [the] udder were monitored by total bacteria and somatic cell count (AOAC, 2000). Bulk milk samples from each group were analysed for dry matter, ash, fat, crude protein and lactose content (AOAC, 2000). Asses' body condition was monitored according to Martin Rosset (1990) every 28 d. Bulk milk data have been studied by analysis of variance; milk yield and hygiene data were statistically analysed by analysis of variance for repeated measures, considering the covariate effect of days of lactation (SAS Inc., Cary, NC USA).

Results

Asses showed a rapid adaptation to the experimental conditions and their body condition score (A: 3.50 ± 0.04; B: 3.51 ± 0.04) did not differ between the two milking strategies.

Milk yield, unaffected by the different milking strategy (A: 1365.77 ± 67.34 $mL \cdot d^{-1}$; B: 1096.68 ± 92.77 $mL \cdot d^{-1}$), was characterised by the chemical composition reported, for each group, in Table 1. Management of milking did not influence the milk dry matter, crude protein, lactose and ash content but the investigated milking intervals significantly affect the fat content of milk, result[ing]ed in a higher [content] in the 20 hours interval thesis (Table 1).

Both the milk hygiene and the healthy status of [the] udder were significantly influenced by the milking management, being [with] a lower somatic cell count observed with 20 hours interval between milkings (A: 3.82 ± 0.06 $logSCC \cdot mL^{-1}$; B: 4.01 ± 0.06 $logSCC \cdot mL^{-1}$; $P<0.05$). On the other hand, the total bacteria count of milk was lower in group B (A: 3.95 ± 0.04 log $TBC \cdot mL^{-1}$; B: 3.82 ± 0.04 log $TBC \cdot mL^{-1}$; $P<0.05$).

Results suggest that the management of milking can affect essential aspects of ass's milk as an alternative food for infancy.

Table 1. Chemical composition of bulk ass's milk (mean values ± s.e.m.).

	Group A	Group B	P
Dry matter, $g \cdot 100\ mL^{-1}$ milk	9.20 ± 0.09	9.21 ± 0.09	n.s.
Protein, $g \cdot 100\ mL^{-1}$ milk	1.58 ± 0.04	1.55 ± 0.04	n.s.
Fat, $g \cdot 100\ mL^{-1}$ milk	0.62 ± 0.05	0.41 ± 0.05	<0.05
Lactose, $g \cdot 100\ mL^{-1}$ milk	6.51 ± 0.03	6.55 ± 0.03	n.s.
Ash, $g \cdot 100\ mL^{-1}$ milk	0.42 ± 0.02	0.43 ± 0.02	n.s.

References

AOAC, 2000. Official methods of analysis of AOAC International, 17th Ed., Maryland, USA.

Carroccio, A., F. Cavataio, G. Montaldo, D. D'amico, L. Alabrese and G. Iacono, 2000. Intolerance to hydrolysed cow's milk proteins in infants: clinical characteristics and dietary treatments. Clin. Exp. Allergy, 30: 1597-1603.

Doreau, M., 1994. Le lait de jument et sa production: particularites et facteurs de variation. Lait, 74: 401-418.

Martin-Rosset, W., 1990. Bases du rationnement. In: Martin-Rosset W., L'alimentation des chevaux, Ed. INRA, Paris.

Restani, P., B. Beretta, A. Fiocchi, C. Ballabio and C.L. Galli, 2002. Cross reactivity between mammalian proteins. Ann. Allergy Asthma Immunol., 89: 11-15.

Salimei, E., A. Simoni, F. Fantuz, G. Varisco and C. Chiari, 2004. Ass's machine milking: first results on residual milk. in Proc. 6th SIDI Congress. 93-98.

Simoni, A., E. Salimei, G. Varisco, 2004. Milking parlour and routine and characteristics of ass's milk yield, a hypoallergenic food for infants. In Proc. 6th SIDI Congress. 85-91.

Behaviour and milk yield of Murgese mares subjected to machine or hand milking

M. Caroprese[1], M. Albenzio[1], A. Santillo[1], R. Marino[1], S. Pelosi[2] and F. D'Emilio
[1]Dept. PRIME, Foggia University, Via Napoli 25, 71100 Foggia, Italy
[2]CNR, ISMAR, Lesina/Foggia, Italy

Abstract

A 25-day trial was performed to assess the effects of machine and hand milking on behaviour and milk yield of Murgese mares. Milk yield and milking time were affected by milking procedure ($P < 0.05$ and $P < 0.01$, respectively). Machine milking of mares resulted in higher fat and protein content of milk ($P < 0.01$ and $P < 0.05$, respectively). Milking procedure didn't affect casein content, nitrogen fractions and somatic cell count. No differences in behavioural activities and in responses to human presence emerged. Results show that the milking procedure can affect the yield and gross composition of mare milk, without aversive consequences on the behaviour of mares.

Keywords: Murgese mares, milk, milking methods, behaviour.

Introduction

The traditional use of mare milk for human consumption was first practiced by nomadic people, it was then used for therapeutic purposes in the countries where it was produced. Currently, mares' milk, due to its nutritional characteristics, is a product of great interest not only for human consumption (children, adults, convalescent consumers), but also as a dairy product, as a therapeutic agent or in the cosmetic industry. Recently mares' milk is considered a possible substitute for cow's milk for allergic children (Malacarne *et al.*, 2002). It has been shown that the mare is hard to milk. Due to the low capacity of the udder compared to milk potential, the use of mares for milk production requires frequent milkings. For this reason, mares are milked several times a day with 2 to 3 hours intervals and the foals are allowed to suckle the mares for the rest of the day. The major problem of mare milking routine is the adaptation of mares to machine milking after foaling, but the adaptability to machine milking can be improved by the presence of the foal in front of the mother during machine milking. The success of milking procedures depends on the manageability of mares, which can be considered as the ease with which a person can impose a routine handling procedure on horse and which reflects a combination of behavioural traits including fearfulness, aggressiveness and reactivity to humans (Lansade *et al.*, 2004). The aim of the experiment was to compare the effects of machine or hand milking of Murgese mares on milk yield and composition and on mare behaviour.

Material and methods

The trial lasted 25 d and involved 8 Murgese mares, divided into two groups of 4 each, which were subjected to hand or machine milking. Milk yield and milking times were individually recorded daily. Individual milk samples were collected at d 1, 5, 10, 15, 20 and 25 of the trial and analysed for pH, fat, lactose, total protein and casein content, nitrogen fractions and somatic cell count (SCC). At d 5, 15 and 25 behavioural activities of mares were monitored using a scan sampling procedure. The behaviour of mares was video-recorded for 4 h (from 1100 to 1500) and scan samples were taken every 10min. At d 10 and 20 mares were tested for their responses to two 5 min. open field tests in the presence of a human. During the tests, the time spent in proximity to the person (within 2 m of the human stimulus), the time spent far from the person were recorded, and the number of escape attempts was calculated.

Results and discussion

Milk yield was affected by milking procedure, the machine milked mares giving higher volumes of milk than the hand milked mares ($P < 0.05$, Table 1). Milking times were shorter in the machine milking than in the hand milking (5.4 min *vs* 1.8 min, $P < 0.01$). In addition, machine milking of mares resulted in higher fat and protein content of milk ($P < 0.01$ and $P < 0.05$, respectively). Milking procedure did not affect casein content, nitrogen fractions and somatic cell count. Differences did not emerge either in mare responses to human or in anomalous behaviour, even though MM mares spent a three-fold longer time in stereotyped pacing compared to HM mares (Table2). Results show that the milking procedure has an effect on the yield and gross composition of mare milk. Machine milking resulted in an improvement of fat and protein content of milk associated with an increase in milk yield and a reduction in milking time, thus suggesting a better emptying of the mare udder compared to hand milking. In addition, the study highlighted that milking procedures did not affect the mare behavioural patterns and human-mare relationship.

Table 1. Least Square means ± SEM of milk yield, milking time, fat and protein content of milk from mares subjected to hand milking and machine milking.

	Days	HM	MM	S.E.M.	Effects		
					Treatment	Time	Treatment x Time
Milk yield, Kg	0-25	4.91 a	7.69 b	0.79	*	***	NS
Milking time, min	0-25	5.40 b	1.80 a	0.01	**	NS	NS
Fat content, %	0-25	1.06 a	1.63 b	0.09	**	NS	NS
Protein content, %	0-25	1.61 a	1.88 b	0.07	*	***	***

NS, not significant, *$P < 0.05$, **$P < 0.01$, ***$P < 0.001$. Means followed by different letters differ significantly at $P < 0.05$.

Table 2. Least Square means ± SEM of some behavioural activities and responses to human in mares subjected to hand milking and machine milking.

	HM	MM	S.E.M	Effects		
				Treatment	Time	Treatment x Time
Stereotyped pacing, s	16.66	73.87	21.82	NS	NS	NS
Crib biting, n	0.08	0.29	0.13	NS	NS	NS
Wind sucking, n	0.50	0.92	0.35	NS	NS	NS
Weaving, n	0.04	1.12	0.46	NS	NS	NS
Kicking, n	0.01	0.42	0.19	NS	NS	NS
Time spent within 2 m from human, %	21.71	22.83	8.03	NS	NS	NS
Time spent more than 5 m far from human, %	74.55	68.29	8.35	NS	NS	NS
Flight attempts, n	4.87	4.12	1.98	NS	NS	NS

NS, not significant

References

Lansade, L., M. Bertand, X. Biovin and M.F. Bouissou, 2004. Effects of handling at weaning on manageability and reactivity of foals. Appl. Anim. Behav. Sci. 87: 131-149.

Malacarne, M., F. Martuzzi, A. Summer and P. Mariani, 2002. Protein and fast composition of mare's milk: some nutritional remarks with reference to human and cow's milk. Int. Dairy J. 12: 869-877.

Part C – The foal

Physiology and metabolism in the newborn foal with reference to orphaned or sick foals

J.C. Ousey
University of Cambridge, Dept. of Veterinary Medicine Equine Fertility Unit, Mertoun Paddocks, Woodditton Road, CB8 9BH Newmarket, Suffolk, United Kingdom

Abstract

Many metabolic and endocrine changes occur in late gestation which prepare the foetus for post-natal life. In particular, functional changes to the foetal adrenal, pancreas, gastrointestinal tract and thyroid ensure that the newborn foal can maintain glucose concentrations, thermoregulate, and sustain a high rate of metabolism, utilising body energy stores until it starts to ingest milk. Healthy foals are precocious and well adapted to make these metabolic adaptations but sick foals encounter many problems. Often they cannot thermoregulate efficiently, they may have low body energy stores so that they cannot support metabolism and this may be exacerbated further by poor digestive capacity. Premature foals, in particular, have impaired endocrine functions due to immaturity of a number of organ systems leading to various metabolic and physiological problems after birth. Orphan foals that are essentially healthy may show some metabolic differences associated with artificial feeding regimes and these may persist into later life.

Keywords: foal milk intakes, sick/orphan foals, glucose, thermoregulation, energy, gastrointestinal tract

Introduction

The newborn foal is a precocious species which is capable of standing and galloping within a few hours of birth. In order to support these high energy activities, it must be born in a state of physical and behavioural maturity and have sufficient energy reserves and access to nutrients so that it can survive and thrive. The equine foetus undergoes rapid maturation during the perinatal period when many metabolic and physiological changes occur to support its transition from intra- to extra-uterine life. Diseases or other disturbances during pregnancy or birth can dramatically alter the survival chances of the newborn foal. Moreover, these adverse events may affect the foal not only during the immediate post natal period but may also continue to exert their effects into adult life. This presentation will discuss the metabolic and nutritional changes that occur in healthy foals and how these processes are disrupted in sick foals. In addition, the nutritional and metabolic demands of orphan foals will also be presented.

Physiological and metabolic development of the foetus in late gestation

Foetal metabolism is dependent mainly on maternal glucose supply and this is more important in regulating glucose homeostasis than foetal endocrine glands like the pancreas or adrenal. Foetal glucose concentrations in the horse are approximately half those of the mare (3.3 versus 6.0 mmol/l) (Silver, 1984). Foetal glucose concentrations rise in response to increases in the transplacental glucose gradient up until the active transport mechanisms become fully saturated (Fowden, 1997). Compared to carbohydrate, placental transfer of amino acids is relatively minor. There is little metabolism of fat by the foetus but the placenta is important for elongation and desaturation of essential free fatty acids (Stammers *et al.*, 1987).

Growth of the equine foetus is maximal during the last 2 - 3 months of gestation. This growth is represented primarily by a gain in body weight through accretion of muscle mass and body fat rather than growth of the linear dimensions (crown-rump length) of the foetus that peak in mid gestation (Bergin *et al.*, 1967; Platt, 1984). This high rate of body weight gain is achieved through an increase in the transfer of nutrients across the placenta partly due to a rise in uterine blood flow and partly as a result of physiological and anatomical adaptations of the placenta. First, uterine blood flow, measured by Doppler ultrasonography, doubles from about 16,000 ml/min in mid gestation to > 32,000 mls/min at term, whilst the blood flow resistance decreases (Bollwein *et al.*, 2004). Second, there is an absolute increase in the weight and surface area of the placenta and an increase in the total microscopic area of feto-maternal contact which correlates significantly with foal birth weight (Allen *et al.*, 2002; Cottrill *et al.*, 1991). The increase in placental surface area is achieved through increased branching of the terminal buds of the placental microvilli and a decrease in the diffusion distance between the maternal and foetal arteries in the final stages of gestation (Macdonald *et al.*, 2000; Samuel *et al.*, 1975). Third, the utero-placental tissues decrease their rate of glucose consumption on a weight-specific basis which enables an increase in the delivery of glucose to the foetus near to term (Fowden *et al.*, 2004).

There are a number of endocrine events that occur in late gestation which assist the foetus in its final phase of growth and prepare it for a transition from parenteral to enteral nutrition. These events are regulated by the foetal hypothalamic-pituitary-adrenal (HPA) axis which increases its activity during the last few weeks of gestation culminating in a rise in foetal cortisol over the last 2-3 days (Silver and Fowden, 1994). Cortisol has a major effect on the differenciation and maturation of many foetal tissues (Fowden, 1995). Cortisol is important for maturation of the pancreatic β cells in the foetal horse. For example, concentrations of hepatic glycogen and glucose-6-phosphatase (G-6-Pase), the enzyme responsible for mobilisation of glycogen, increase substantially between late gestation and after birth concurrent with the rise in foetal cortisol (Fowden *et al.*, 1991). Sensitivity of the pancreatic β cells, demonstrated by a glucose stimulated rise in foetal insulin, correlates positively with the pre-partum rise in foetal cortisol (Fowden *et al.*, 2005). This responsiveness is related to cortisol concentrations rather than to gestational age because basal concentrations of foetal glucose and insulin are unchanged in late gestation.

Thyroid hormones have many functions in the foal including, thermoregulation and metabolism, development of the musculoskeletal system and maturation of the respiratory and nervous system (Irvine, 1984; Irvine and Evans, 1975). Foetal concentrations of triiodothyronine (T3) and thyroxine (T4) increase gradually from mid gestation to term and are thought to be important for ossification of the skeleton and development of tendons (Allen *et al.*, 1995). In the last few days pre-partum, the increase in foetal cortisol is closely correlated with a rise in T3 suggesting that exposure to high cortisol levels is important for secretion of thyroid hormones. Foals born before the pre-natal rise in cortisol have low T3 (but not T4) concentrations, are hypothermic and have low metabolic rates compared to foals born at term (Dudan *et al.*, 1986; Irvine, 1984; Silver *et al.*, 1991).

Ingestion of amniotic fluid is important for luminal growth of the intestine in the foetus and, in other species, the pre-natal cortisol rise stimulates morphological and other changes in the gastrointestinal (GI) tract in preparation for enteral nutrition (Trahair, 1993; Trahair and Sangild, 1997). There is no direct evidence that foetal cortisol stimulates gut maturation in the horse but activity of some gut enzymes increases close to parturition (Roberts, 1975). Moreover, foals born before the rise in foetal cortisol typically cannot digest their enteral feeds and have impaired absorption of colostral antibodies, suggesting that cortisol is important for functional maturation of the GI tract.

Nutrition in the healthy newborn foal: physiological and metabolic adaptations

The foal is required to make immense physiological adjustments after delivery. It is delivered from a relatively sterile, liquid environment where it receives the majority of its nutrients parenterally, it floats in amniotic fluid which bathes its lungs, its thermal environment is regulated by the mare, and it has restricted activity. All of these change immediately after delivery as the foal enters a cooler, air breathing environment where it must support its own body mass, begin to thermoregulate, utilise its own energy reserves in order to support metabolism, and establish an enteral nutrient supply.

Behaviour

The healthy newborn foal has a suck reflex within a few minutes of birth. Even when recumbent, it will try to suck on any surface and once standing, it immediately initiates udder seeking behaviour. Usually the foal will suck successfully from the mare by 2 to 3 h after birth. The act of sucking, swallowing and recognition of the dam's udder requires neuromuscular co-ordination and activation of several cranial nerves (II, V, VII, IX-XII) (Adams and Mayhew, 1984). In addition, it requires the co-ordination of the foal's posture and balance to ensure that it remains in the correct posture whilst sucking from the mare. Therefore, any foal that has suffered neural damage, for example due to hypoxia during delivery, is unlikely to suck as proficiently as a healthy foal, and a poor or absent suck reflex is usually the first sign of ill health.

The healthy newborn foal rapidly develops a pattern of nursing behaviour. During the first week *post partum*, the foal has approximately 4 – 7 nursing bouts per hour lasting 1 -2 min for a total duration of 12 min per h when it will consume > 450 ml milk per hour (Carson and Wood-Gush, 1983; Tyler, 1972). This regular feeding pattern ensures that the foal feeds little and often and, therefore, the foal's stomach is rarely distended with milk and the GI tract is constantly digesting milk. This normal feeding pattern is usually disrupted in orphan foals which usually receive large volume feeds intermittently (see below).

Energy stores

The period between birth and when the foal first sucks from the mare is critical because the foal relies exclusively on endogenous body energy stores to fuel its high rate of metabolism (see d). The foal uses both endogenous carbohydrate (CHO) and fat until it establishes an exogenous food source (ie mare's milk). Calculation of the relative contribution of CHO and fat from the foal's non-protein respiratory quotient (RQ) over the first 24 h after birth demonstrates that, initially, the foal uses CHO when the RQ is high (Ousey *et al.*, 1991) (Table 1). By 2 to 4 h of age, the RQ decreases indicating that fat takes over as the major source of energy. Thereafter, the RQ is maintained at about 0.82 indicating a mixed contribution from CHO and fat and reflects digestion of mares' colostrum and milk. The main sources of endogenous CHO in the newborn foal are hepatic and skeletal muscle glycogen. Muscle glycogen is used *in situ* for shivering thermogenesis because there is little G-6-Pase to mobilise glycogen for general glucose utilisation (Fowden *et al.*, 1991). In contrast, the liver possesses high concentrations of G-6-Pase. However, hepatic glycogen concentrations in the newborn foal are approximately 40 mg/g wet weight which are lower than those found in other species of neonate (90 – 120 mg/g wet weight for sheep, rat and pig) and, consequently, it has been calculated that this CHO source would provide energy for < 1 h based on the foal's metabolic rate after birth (Fowden *et al.*, 1991; Ousey, 1997). Therefore, the foal relies on non-structural body fat as a secondary source of endogenous energy. In a healthy foal estimates for non-structural fat range from 1-3% which, for a well nourished foal, would provide sufficient energy to last > 24h (Meyer and Ahlswede, 1976). However, foals that have experienced nutrient restriction *in utero*, or are small for gestational age due to prematurity or other problems, are likely to have diminished endogenous energy stores at birth and this will restrict energy expenditure (see below).

Table 1. Mean energy expenditure, non-protein respiratory quotient and substrate used by 26 Thoroughbred foals during the first 24 h post partum.

Time period post partum (h)	Mean rate of expenditure (W)	Non-protein respiratory quotient	CHO used (%)	Lipid used (%)
0 - 0.5	346	0.92	74	26
0.5 – 1	327	0.87	58	42
1 – 2	279	0.81	37	63
2 – 4	227	0.77	24	76
4 – 6	186	0.86	55	45
6 – 12	210	0.80	34	66
12 – 18	209	0.82	41	59
18 - 24	223	0.80	34	66

Energy and nutrient intakes

During the first 24 h after birth, the healthy foal drinks 15% of its body mass as colostrum/milk, equivalent to approximately 8 L for a 50 kg Thoroughbred (TB) foal, of which 1-2 L is colostrum. The foal requires at least 1 litre of colostrum containing > 60 g/L of immunoglobulin to ensure that there is successful transfer of immunoglobulins (Dragoul et al - this volume). Thereafter, milk intake by the foal increases to about 23% (range 20 – 28%) of its body mass during the first week *post partum* which, for a TB foal, is equivalent to 11.6 L on day 2 and nearly 14 L by day 7 (Table 2). Mare's milk typically contains 26 g/L protein, 19 g/L fat and 61 g/L lactose and 2.4 MJ/L gross energy (Ullrey *et al.*, 1966). Further details about foal nutrient intakes are discussed elsewhere (see page x). Total milk intake by the foal continues to rise as the mare increases her milk production, peaking at about 6-8 weeks after birth when a TB mare can produce > 18 L milk / day. However, because the foal gains body weight (bwt) rapidly during the first month post partum (1-2 kg / day), its milk intake per kg bwt decreases so that by 8 weeks after birth it is < 14% bwt (Table 2). As a result of a decline in milk intake per kg bwt the foal must meet its energy demands from other food sources. A foal, even a few days old, will imitate the mare and start attempting to chew on hay, grass and concentrate feeds although it lacks the enzymes to digest these feeds until it is older (see (g)).

Table 2. Milk intakes in foals aged 0 to 3 months (Doreau and Boulot, 1989; Gibbs et al., 1982; Martin et al., 1992; Oftedal et al., 1983; Ousey et al., 1996).

Age (days)	Intake (kg milk)			Intake (% foal bwt)
	TB	Heavy	Q'Horse	
2	12			23 (20 – 28)
4	13			23 (20 – 28)
7	14	19		23 (20 – 28)
10 – 18	14 – 17		11.4	19 – 27
25 – 28	15	24	11.8	16 – 20
30 – 44	15 – 17		11.3	14 – 19
56	18	26		14
60 – 74	18		11.0	13

Mares' milk is digested efficiently by foals, leading to high rates of metabolic energy intake. Table 3 illustrates the energy partitioning for 5 healthy TB foals on days 2, 4 and 7 after birth. Gross energy (GE) intakes are high (544 and 593 kJ/kg/d) and digestive losses are minimal, so that 97 - 99% GE is available for metabolism. Based on measurements of metabolic rate, activity and air temperatures, energy expenditures for the foals aged 2 - 7 days were 307 – 319 kJ/kg/day (Table 3). Consequently, between 40 and 50% GE is retained for growth and, not surprisingly, these healthy foals gained nearly 2 kg body mass / day. However, average daily gains decrease in older foals as they start to utilize other food sources and their metabolic energy intakes decline (Pagan *et al.*, 1996).

Table 3. Energy partitioning in 5 healthy TB foals during the first week post partum.

Energy (kJ / kg / d)	Day 2	Day 4	Day 7
Milk gross energy (GE)	593	573	544
Faecal energy (FE)	2.4	9.3	15.6
Urine energy (UE)	3.2	2.7	2.5
Metabolic energy ME (as % GE)	99	98	97
Energy expenditure (NEm)	307	318	319
Energy gain (NEg)	285	246	210
Body weight (kg)	50.1	52.9	60.3

Foal metabolism

The resting metabolic rate of young animals is usually higher than that of adults due to high rates of heat loss, their higher surface area to weight ratio and lower body insulation due to less body fat and hair coat insulation (Mount, 1979). Metabolic rate in newborn foals peaks immediately after birth (Table 1) when heat losses and energy expenditure, associated with physiological and physical activities, are high. The foal's metabolic rate declines gradually over the first 6 h as its coat dries and it establishes a regular feeding pattern. The high rate of metabolism after birth, which is 2 - 3 times the resting rate, is associated with a elevated concentrations of plasma cortisol, T3 and T4 (Silver *et al.*, 1991). Cortisol stimulates protein breakdown and gluconeogenesis in the liver, whilst thyroid hormones play a major role in caloriogenesis by mobilising body fat reserves and stimulating adrenaline induced thermogenesis. The concentrations of T3 and T4 in the foal immediately after birth are much higher than in adult horses or in other newborn animals (Irvine and Evans, 1975). Clearly these high levels are important for thermogenesis, particularly shivering thermogenesis (see (e)), but they are also play an important role in post-natal adaptation of the musculoskeletal and nervous systems which are essential for behavioural adaptations after birth. Over the first month, T3 and T4 concentrations decline which may correlate with a decline in metabolic rate. However, metabolic rate has not been measured in older foals.

The foals' metabolic rate is regulated by several factors particularly thermal environment, body insulation and feeding. These relationships are shown in Figure 1. The metabolic rate of the foal increases as the environmental temperature cools below the "lower critical temperature" (Tlc) as a result of increased heat losses. Body insulation (R) will affect the slope of the increase in metabolic rate with better insulated animals having a more gradual rise than less well insulated foals. Feeding in the short term increases metabolic rate, associated with the specific dynamic action of food whilst, in the long term, increasing the plane of nutrition will increase the metabolic rate and decrease the lower critical temperature (Figure 1). These effects assume particular significance in sick foals which have low metabolic rates and poor body insulation and hence will increase Tlc. Low metabolic rates in sick foals are caused, in part, by their reduced energy intakes (see below). In animals that are

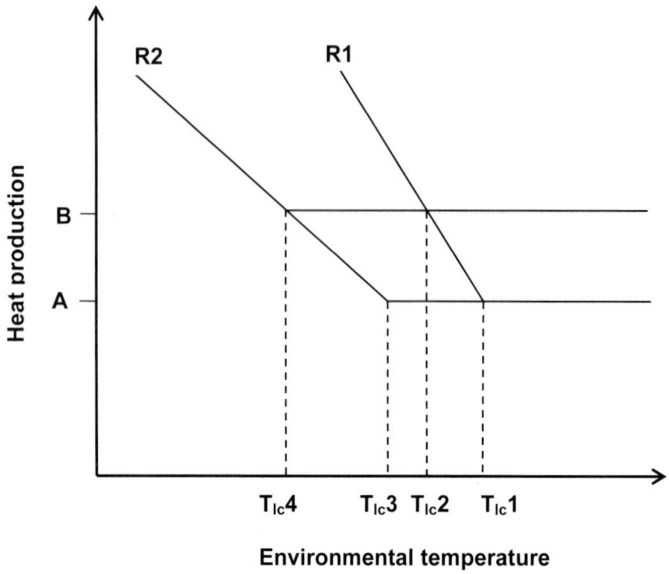

Figure 1. Diagram showing the effect of metabolic rate (A/B) and insulation (R) on the lower critical temperature (T_{lc}) (Adapted from (Mount, 1979).

starved from birth, there is no post-natal increase in metabolic rate and they are more susceptible to cold stress (Eales *et al.*, 1982; Herpin *et al.*, 1994; Vermorel *et al.*, 1989).

Thermogenesis

Precocious newborns, like the foal, have good thermoregulatory control (Alexander, 1975). The newborn TB foal has a large rise in rectal temperature of > 1 °C within 1h of birth; thereafter the temperature is relatively constant and fluctuates between 38.0 and 38.5 °C (Ousey *et al.*, 1991). Although the foal is wet at this time and is almost certainly exposed to air temperatures below Tlc, its metabolic heat production is high and exceeds heat loss. Consequently, there is heat storage in the body as the foal establishes homeothermy. This is in contrast to altricial newborn such as infants or piglets which show a decline in rectal temperature immediately after birth (Alexander, 1975). The healthy foal can maintain its rectal temperature even when exposed to air temperatures as low as 2 °C for several hours by increasing its metabolic rate to nearly 3 times the resting value (Ousey *et al.*, 1992). The Tlc for healthy pony and TB foals has been measured at approximately 20 °C and 10 °C, respectively; the lower Tlc for TB foals is attributable to their higher resting metabolic rate. At air temperatures below Tlc, the foal decreases heat losses by piloerection of its hair coat and peripheral vasoconstriction and it increasess heat production predominantly by shivering thermogenesis. Shivering is clearly visible in foals exposed to cold air temperatures and is associated with a rise in RQ indicating increased use of muscle glycogen. Wet newborn foals shiver and this probably accounts for the high utilisation of CHO at this time (see (d). Preliminary results suggest that foals do not possess brown adipose tissue (J. Ousey and M. Symonds – unpublished observations). Therefore, it appears that shivering thermogenesis is more important than non-shivering thermogenesis to increase heat production in young foals. At air temperatures above Tlc the metabolic rate is relatively constant and foals have been observed to sweat consistently when air temperatures exceed 38 °C without a concomitant increase in rectal temperature (Ousey *et al.*, 1992). These data indicate that thermal control mechanisms are well developed in foals and normally they are capable of thermoregulating effectively over a wide range of ambient temperatures without a change in body core temperature.

Pancreatic function

The healthy, mature newborn foal regulates its plasma glucose concentrations and responds to glucose challenges after birth (Fowden *et al.*, 1984). Plasma glucose concentrations rise after birth and thereafter usually remain within the normoglycaemic range (4 - 10 mmol/l). Plasma insulin concentrations correlate positively with glucose concentrations and basal concentrations do not change significantly between 1 – 10 days of age (Holdstock *et al.*, 2004). These authors demonstrated that concentrations of proinsulin, the insulin precursor molecule, increase significantly after birth which, in other species, may indicate β cell dysfunction. However, in the foal, the increasing levels probably reflect reduced clearance of proinsulin from the blood. In healthy foals, pancreatic β cells are responsive to fluctuating glucose concentrations. For example, administration of exogenous glucose causes an immediate but transient rise in glucose and insulin concentrations in foals aged 1 – 10 days of age (Fowden *et al.*, 1984; Holdstock *et al.*, 2004). However, the post prandial rise in glucose and insulin concentrations is less in foals aged 1 day compared to older foals. Moreover, their glucose clearance is reduced and insulin responses prolonged, suggesting that newborn foals may be more resistant to the hypoglycaemic effects of insulin than older foals. This could confer an advantage by helping to maintain glucose concentrations until a regular pattern of feeding is established. Alternatively, the high insulin concentrations found in colostrum may contribute to glucose homeostasis (Hess-Dudan *et al.*, 1994; Koldovsky *et al.*, 1988; Slebodzinski *et al.*, 1998).

Gastrointestinal (GI) development

The early post-natal period is a critical time when there is morphological and functional differenciation of the GI tract as the foal begins to absorb large volumes of nutrients by the enteral route for the first time. There is a marked increase in the length and diameter of the intestinal tract (increases in villus height, density, width, crypt density and depth, enterocyte differenciation and cell turnover within the GI mucosa) associated with enteral feeding and ingestion of colostrum (Trahair and Sangild, 1997; Xu, 1996). Post-natal development of the GI tract is influenced by not only luminal factors but also local and systemic factors. Mares' milk contains many factors besides macro- and micro-nutrients (Grace *et al.*, 1999; Ullrey *et al.*, 1966). It contains hormones (steroid hormones, insulin, thyroid hormones), growth factors (epidermal growth factor [EGF] and insulin like growth factors [IGFs]), enzymes (lysozyme) and bioactive factors (lactoferrin) (Schweigart, 2001; Xu, 1996). These non-nutrient factors are important for trophic development of the GI tract and they also help protect against infection and disease. High concentrations of non-nutrient factors, for example, IGF's and EGF, are found in colostrum and are important for maturation of gut enterocytes and protect against gastric ulceration (Cymbaluk and Laarveld, 1996; Hess-Dudan *et al.*, 1994; Murray *et al.*, 1992). Clearly ingestion of colostral non-nutrient factors are essential to prepare the GI tract of the newborn animal for enteral feed intake.

Feeding (volume, frequency and type) has a significant effect on GI development. Newborn animals that are deprived of enteral feeds or fed only water, have reduced weights and lengths of their GI tract compared to animals that receive milk; moreover, subsequent feeding increases these parameters (Widdowson, 1985). Similarly, growth and functional development of the GI tract is less in animals fed formula feed than those fed colostrum or milk (Mellor, 1993; Xu, 1996). Feeding, in addition to having trophic effects on the GI tract, also stimulates release of many gut hormones (Aynsley-Green, 1989). For example, gastrin produced by the antral mucosa of the stomach causes release of pepsinogen and hydrochloric acid (HCl) to promote digestion of proteins whilst pancreatic polypeptide (PP) stimulates gastric emptying and inhibits pancreatic exocrine secretions. Gut hormones have been identified in foals. Gastrin concentrations increase following feeding in foals aged 1 to 30 days, probably in response to the protein content of milk and is associated with a decline in gastric pH (Baker and Gerring, 1993; Ousey *et al.*, 1995; Smyth *et al.*, 1989). Interestingly if foals are allowed to suck freely then plasma gastrin concentrations remain high whereas foals that are muzzled after feeding show a decline in gastrin concentrations suggesting that different feeding regimes will influence gastrin secretion. Gut hormone responses differ between the first and subsequent feeds in many species including foals (Aynsley-Green, 1989; Ousey *et al.*, 1995). Following the first feed of colostrum in foals, plasma gastrin concentrations remain low. It has been suggested that this lack of gastrin response to the first feed limits the secretion of HCl and pepsinogen and allows passage of immunoglobulins through the stomach unaltered. Certainly the gastric pH of newborn foals is higher (4.1) than in older foals (2.6) (Baker and Gerring, 1993; Murray and Grodinsky, 1989). Similarly, post prandial concentrations of PP are significantly higher following the first feed than subsequent feeds and again it appears that this may promote rapid transfer of immunoglobulins through the stomach before they can be destroyed.

Several gut enzymes are present in the GI tract of the equine foetus and most increase after birth and then gradually decline or increase as the foal's diet changes with age. For example, gut activity of lactase which is essential for digestion of lactose in milk, increases at birth and then gradually declines over the next 4 years (Roberts, 1975). Some foals with diarrhoea display a lactase deficiency as demonstrated by the oral lactose test or by the hydrogen breath test (Bracher *et al.*, 1995). In contrast, the α-glucosidases (sucrase, maltase and trehalase) needed for catabolism of more complex carbohydrates have low activity at birth and increase thereafter. Consequently, foals should not be exposed to artificial diets containing complex sugars for example sucrose (table sugar) until they are older.

Orphaned foals

In this section, we shall consider nutrition in healthy, orphan foals. The primary problem with orphan foals is to supply a suitable balance of nutrients in the same quantity and feeding frequency as for foals nursing from their dams. It is difficult to replicate these conditions unless the foals are fostered on to nurse mares and usually this provides the ideal solution. However, under the correct management, orphan foals can be raised successfully to maturity.

Nutrient and energy intakes

The volume of milk intake, including nutrients and energy, of orphan foals should mimic that of mare-nursed foals as closely as possible (see section (c). Milks from other domestic animals are suitable for orphan foals, although the milk composition is different (Table 4). Cow's milk can be fed modified as 2% skimmed cows milk with 20 g dextrose added per litre of milk (Buechner-Maxwell, 2005). Cow's milk may cause diarrhoea and other GI problems whereas foals find goats' milk more palatable and have fewer digestive upsets, despite its composition being different to mares' milk (Wilson, 1987). Goats' milk can be fed unmodified but it is expensive.

Table 4. Composition of milk from different sources, including mares' milk formula.

Species	Protein (g/100 mls)	Fat (g/100 mls)	Lactose (g/100 mls)
Woman	1.1	3.8	7.6
Cow	3.3	3.7	4.8
Goat	3.8	4.4	4.9
Mare	3.3	2.9	6.9
Mare formula*	3.1	1.7	7.1

* As fed

Mares' milk replacers are probably the first choice of feed for orphan foals because they are convenient to administer although expensive. They have a similar composition to mares' milk and do not contain growth promoters or antibiotics which are often found, for example, in calf milk replacer products. Some mares' milk replacers, when reconstituted, have a higher energy content than mares' milk so that there is a risk of overfeeding and developing dietary associated orthopaedic disease. The energy content of the feed is not always stated and, therefore, it is difficult to assess accurately the foals' GE intake. Regular measurement of the foal's growth parameters (ie weight, girth, body length, hip and wither height, physis circumference, fetlock circumference) will ensure that the foal is not over- or under-fed. Growth charts, based on weight and height for different foal breeds, have been established for different geographical areas and may be used to compare orphan foal growth (eg Gro-trac™). Studies on orphan foals fed mares' milk replacer reported similar growth rates to mare nursed foals, over the long term (Cymbaluk and Laarveld, 1996; King and Nequin, 1989; Knight and Tyznik, 1985).

Recommendations about the frequency of feeds for orphan foals vary greatly. Ideally, orphan foals should be fed little and often because infrequent, high volume feeding encourages the foals to gorge themselves and can cause bloating and GI problems (Buechner-Maxwell, 2005). Some authors have found *ad libitum* feeding to be satisfactory. For example, Knight and Tyznik (1985) fed orphan foals twice a day with unlimited milk replacer and intakes appeared acceptable with no digestive disturbances reported. Cymbaluk *et al.* (1993) fed orphan foals milk replacer at 125% the recommended level and found that these foals voluntarily restricted their intake after the first week. However, in my experience and that of others (C. Turnbull, personal communication), orphan foals have a tendency to overfeed even when offered high energy, milk replacer *ad libitum*. Others reported feeding regimes of 5 to 12 feeds per day in the early stages, decreasing with post-natal age (Cymbaluk and Laarveld, 1996; King and Nequin, 1989). In my opinion, newborn orphan foals should be fed hourly for 2 days, followed by 2 to 3 hourly feeds for the first 2 weeks, decreasing the frequency gradually to about 4 feeds a day by about 8 weeks. From about 2 weeks of age, milk pellets, hay and concentrates feeds can also be offered and gradually used to replace the milk diet.

The metabolic requirements of orphan foals are different to those of mare nursed foals. Orphan foals have lower metabolic rates compared to mare nursed foals. This may make them more susceptible to energy overload, particularly if fed a high energy, formula diet. In addition, one study showed that orphan foals digested their milk formula less efficiently over the first 2-3 days compared to mare nursed foals (ME 90% versus 98%) although the orphan foals were fed a colostrum substitute (Ousey *et al.*, 1997). This effect did not persist beyond day 4 post partum. It is not clear whether this initial lack of digestibility originated exclusively from the diet or to lack of mares' colostrum. However it appears that orphan foals may take a few days to adapt to their formula diet particularly if they are not fed mares' colostrum. The lack of non-nutrient factors in formula feeds compared to mares' milk must alter digestive function as it does in other species of neonate (Koldovsky, 1994). In infants, there are significant differences in gut hormone responses between babies fed formula feeds compared to breast milk (Aynsley-Green, 1989). Foals raised on milk replacer have lower serum IGF-1 concentrations than mare nursed foals (Cymbaluk and Laarveld, 1996). Interestingly, this difference persisted up to 1 year of age despite the foals being managed similarly after weaning, suggesting that dietary manipulations may have long term consequences on physiological development.

Sick foals

Impaired foetal nutrition

Any factors that disrupt nutrient supply to the foetus will affect foetal growth and metabolism. In animals models of intra-uterine growth retardation, not only is foetal growth and the functional development of individual organ systems affected but also there are consequences for endocrine, cardiovascular and metabolic development after birth and into later life (Fowden *et al.*, 2005). Because of the diffuse nature of the equine placenta, any disturbances in placental function may limit foetal growth and alter post-natal metabolic adaptations. If the placental supply of nutrients is severely restricted then the foetus will die *in utero*; for example in twins, due to the diffuse nature of the equine epitheliochorial placenta, there is a disproportionate delivery of nutrients to the foetuses usually resulting in the death of one and hence abortion of both. Various placental disturbances can restrict foetal growth whilst foals born alive following placentitis are invariably small for gestational age (Figure 2). It is not clear whether this restriction of foetal growth occurs due to disturbances of placental blood supply, endocrine responses to hypoxia or inflammation, or activation of the foetal HPA axis which will restrict foetal growth (Fowden and Forhead, 2004; LeBlanc *et al.*, 2004). Experimental manipulations of foetal growth in horses alter the metabolic responses after birth. For example, TB foetuses carried by pony mares after embryo transfer, were low birth weight, took longer to stand and suck and showed hypercortisolaemia for 48 h after birth indicating that they were stressed *in utero* and had precocious stimulation of the HPA axis (Ousey *et al.*, 2004). In contrast, pony foals delivered from TB mares in the same study, showed exaggerated pancreatic β cell responses possibly as a consequence of enhanced delivery of nutrients *in utero* (Forhead *et al.*, 2004). Therefore, alterations in the placental supply of nutrients can influence foetal growth and alter post-natal adaptive responses.

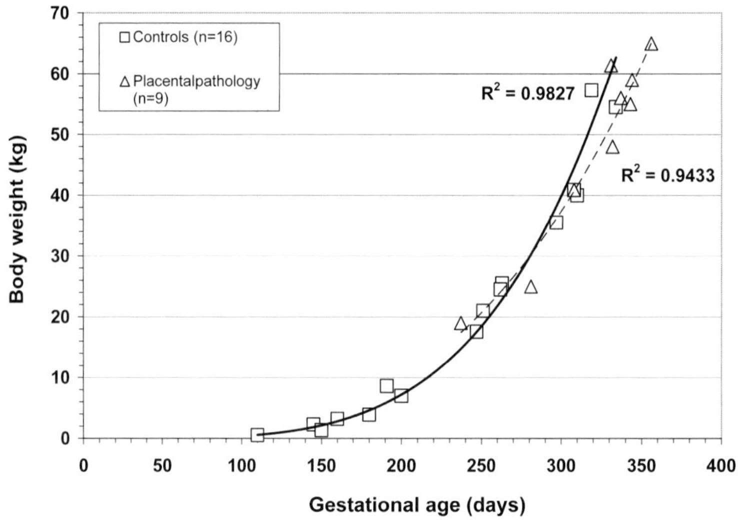

Figure 2. Foetal growth in healthy foetuses and those with placental pathology. (From Ousey, Rossdale, Sibbons – unpublished observations).

Post-natal metabolism

Sick foals show poor metabolic and adaptive responses after birth. In the case of premature foals delivered before the pre-natal rise in cortisol, this is due to inadequate functional maturation of foetal organ systems. In foals that have experienced intra-uterine growth restriction it is likely that a number of endocrine systems have been affected, as in other animals (Fowden *et al.*, 2005). This section will consider sick foals and their metabolic responses after birth.

Metabolism and thermoregulation in sick foals

In foals that are growth retarded, the normal rise in foetal body mass in late gestation is reduced and, at birth, their body weights are below the average for gestational age (Figure 2) suggesting that body muscle and fat stores are reduced. Foetal glycogen stores are also likely to be diminished because, under adverse conditions, endogenous glucose production by the foetus may contribute 50% or more to foetal and placental glucose consumption (Fowden, 1997). Premature foals show a decline in plasma glucose concentrations after birth, and many foals that are hospitalized are hypoglycaemic on admission suggesting that glycogen stores have been exhausted (Corley and Axon, 2005; Fowden *et al.*, 1984). This may be due to low enteral feed intakes, immaturity of glycogenolytic mechanisms, low hepatic glycogen reserves at birth, or, in the septic foals, endotoaxaemia which can affect gluconeogenesis (Chris Sanchez, 2005). In sick foals that have a normal body mass at birth, endogenous fat reserves should last more than 24 h, particularly if their metabolic rates are low and they are not thermally challenged. However, in growth retarded foals or foals born before term, it is likely that their body fat reserves will be quickly expended particularly in the absence of enteral feed intake. Once endogenous energy reserves are exhausted, the foal will be at risk of metabolic collapse unless exogenous energy is provided.

Sick foals are frequently unable to maintain their rectal temperature and it may fluctuate widely about the mean value suggesting they have little thermoregulatory control (Ousey *et al.*, 1997; Rossdale, 1968). Many sick foals remain hypothermic, despite active shivering thermogenesis and provision of additional warmth. Premature foals are particularly susceptible to cold stress because they have poor body insulation (short hair coat, little body fat), low metabolic rates and a high Tlc (>24 C). Sometimes their metabolic rates may be as low as 30 W/m2 (mean = 71 W/m2) compared to the mean resting value of 107 W/m2 in healthy foals exposed to the same air temperatures. Premature foals, like premature infants and lambs, are unable to increase their metabolic rate when exposed to air temperatures below Tlc and cannot maintain their rectal temperatures (Eales *et al.*, 1982; Mellor, 1993). Foals with perinatal asphyxia syndrome (PAS), or dysmature foals also have low metabolic rates (87 - 95 W/m2) but they are better able to maintain their rectal temperatures than premature foals, presumably due to greater body insulation. Damage to the central nervous system can disrupt thermoregulatory control mechanisms and hypoxia can reduce the rate of oxygen consumption. Also sedation will reduce metabolic rates, although convulsive activity will increase oxygen consumption. Low metabolic rates will increase the value of Tlc and, therefore, make sick foals more susceptible to heat losses, particularly if there is poor body insulation. This in turn will increase their nutritional and energy demands if a decline in rectal temperature is to be prevented.

Nutrient and energy intakes in sick foals

Any factor which prevents the foal sucking will limit nutrient and energy intakes and consequently restrict the foal's ability to maintain normal homeostasis and metabolism. For example, hypothermia can cause loss of the suck reflex, while limb problems may affect the foal's ability to stand and suck from the mare. If the foal's energy intake is low then energy expenditure may exceed GE intake and the foal will catabolise body tissues. A study of energy partitioning in 5 sick foals (premature, PAS) showed that they all were in negative energy balance, despite the fact that they had low rates of energy expenditure and were given combined enteral and parenteral nutrition (Table 5) (Ousey *et al.*, 1996). These data provide clear evidence of the difficulties in supplying sufficient nutrients and energy by the enteral route in sick foals and obviates the need for total parenteral nutrition to prevent catabolism of body tissues, maintain metabolism and provide sufficient energy to combat heat losses.

Table 5. Energy partitioning in 5 sick foals.

Foal	1	2	3	4	5
Condition	Premature	Premature	Premature	PAS	PAS
Age (days)	2	2	8	3	3
Body mass (kg)	38	50	21	40	55
	Energy balance (kJ/kg/d)				
Gross energy (GE)	182*§	125≠	349*≠	122*	198*§
Faecal energy (FE)	15.8	6.0	24.8	2.3	0.9
Urine energy (UE)	0.53	4.2	10.5	1.8	1.8
Metabolic energy (as % GE)	91	92	90	97	99
Energy expenditure (NEm)	Not measured	192	473	263	224
Energy gain (NEg)	Not measured	-ve	-ve	-ve	-ve

PAS = perinatal asphyxia syndrome
Energy source *Mares milk ≠ Mares milk replacer §Glucose iv.

Many conditions can disrupt the foal's ability to digest enteral feeds such as bloating, gut immaturity, sepsis, colic, meconium retention. Premature foals have poor digestion of enteral nutrients (mare's milk, milk formula) demonstrated by metabolic energy intakes of approximately 91% GE compared to the usual value of 98% for healthy foals (Table 5). In other species, a complete absence of feeding prevents the trophic effects of enteral feeds on the GI tract and diminishes the normal post prandial gut hormone responses (Aynsley-Green, 1989; Widdowson, 1985). The concept of providing extremely low volumes of milk, called "minimal enteral feeding", to sick infants receiving parenteral nutrition in order to promote gut hormone release and maintain normal morphological development of the GI tract, is an essential part of human neonatal intensive care and could be used to good effect in sick foals.

Endocrine changes in sick foals

Metabolic changes in sick foals are likely to have significant impacts on the endocrine function in neonatal foals. Premature foals have poor insulin secretion in response to exogenous glucose and wide fluctuations observed in plasma glucose concentrations demonstrating that pancreatic β-cell function is impaired. Sick foals frequently become hyperglycaemic particularly when receiving parenteral nutrition and this may due to low insulin secretion, insulin resistance or stress induced hyperglycaemia (Buechner-Maxwell, 2005). T3 concentrations are low in premature foals and account in part for their poor ability to thermoregulate after birth. T3 also influences maturation of the musculo-skeletal system, immaturity of which is a key determinant for the survival prospects of premature foals. Equally, foals that are born congenitally hypothyroid are dysmature, hypothermic and show the typical skeletal immaturity (Allen *et al.*, 1998).

Conclusions

Healthy foals show a range of physiological adaptations after birth that are necessary for the transition to extra-uterine life. Their metabolic energy requirements are high reflecting their ability, as a precocious species, to thermoregulate effectively and become physically active soon after birth. The pre-natal cortisol rise promotes maturation of various organs, in particular the adrenals, thyroids, pancreas and GI tract, all of which are essential for metabolism and homoestasis. In contrast, sick foals struggle to establish homeothermy, suffer from low metabolic rates, low energy intakes and increased heat losses which make them susceptible to hypothermia and increases their metabolic demands. Orphan foals that are healthy, need to be fed in a similar manner to mare nursed foals but they show some metabolic differences associated with artificial feeding regimes.

References

Adams, R. and I.G. Mayhew, 1984. Neurological examination of newborn foals. Equine Vet J 16: 306-312.

Alexander, G., 1975. Body temperature control in mammalian young. Br Med Bull 31: 62-68.

Allen, A.L., C.E. Doige, S.D. Haas, C.E. Card and P.B. Fretz, 1995. Concentrations of triiodothyronine and thyroxine in equine foetal serum during gestation. Biol Reprod Mono 1 1: 49-52.

Allen, A.L., P.B. Fretz, C.E. Card and C.E. Doige, 1998. The effects of partial thyroidectomy on the development of the equine foetus. Equine Vet J 30: 53-59.

Allen, W.R. et al., 2002. Influence of maternal size on placental, foetal and postnatal growth in the horse. I. Development in utero. Reproduction 123: 445-453.

Aynsley-Green, A., 1989. The endocrinology of feeding in the newborn. Baillieres Clinical Endocrinology and Metabolism 3: 837-868.

Baker, S.J. and E.L. Gerring, 1993. Gastric ph monitoring in healthy, suckling pony foals. Am J Vet Res 54: 959-964.

Bergin, W.C., H.T. Gier, R.A. Frey and G.B. Marion, 1967. Developmental horizons and measurements useful for age determination of equine embryos and foetuses. Am Assoc Equine Prac: 179-187.

Bollwein, H., F. Weber, I. Woschee and R. Stolla, 2004. Transrectal doppler sonography of uterine and umbilical blood flow during pregnancy in mares. Theriogenology 61: 499-509.

Bracher, V., J.C. Ousey, A.R. Fazeli, P.R. Murgatroyd and P.D. Rossdale, 1995. Hydrogen breath test in foals. Biol Reprod Mono 1 1: 97-105.

Buechner-Maxwell, V.A. 2005, Nutritional support for neonatal foals. Vet Clin North Am Equine Pract 21: 487-510.

Carson, K. and D.G.M. Wood-Gush, 1983. Behaviour of thoroughbred foals during nursing. Equine Vet J 15: 527-262.

Chris Sanchez, L., 2005. Equine neonatal sepsis. Vet. Clin. N. Am. Equine Pract. 21: 273-312.

Corley, K.T.T. and J.E. Axon, 2005. Resuscitation and emergency management for neonatal foals. Vet. Clin. N. Am. Equine Pract. 21: 431-455.

Cottrill, C.M. et al., 1991. The placenta as a determinant of foetal well-being in normal and abnormal equine pregnancies. J Reprod Fertil Suppl 44: 591-601.

Cymbaluk, N.F. and B. Laarveld, 1996. The ontogeny of serum insulin-like growth factor-i concentration in foals: Effects of dam parity, diet, and age at weaning. Domest Anim Endocrinol 13: 197-209.

Doreau, M. and S. Boulot, 1989. Recent knowledge on mare milk production: A review. Livestock Prod. Sci. 22: 213-235.

Dudan, F.E. et al., 1986, Circulating serum thyroxine (t_{4}), triiodothyronine (t_3) and reverse triiodothyronine (rev. T_3) in neonatal term and preterm foals. Proc Am Coll vet intern Med Forum: 881.

Eales, F.A., J.S. Gilmour, R.M. Barlow and J. Small, 1982. Causes of hypothermia in 89 lambs. Vet Rec. 6: 118-120.

Forhead, A.J., J.C. Ousey, W.R. Allen and A.L. Fowden, 2004. Postnatal insulin secretion and sensitivity after manipulation of foetal growth by embryo transfer in the horse. J Endocrinol 181: 459-467.

Fowden, A.L., 1995. Endocrine regulation of foetal growth. Reprod Fertil Dev 7: 351-363.

Fowden, A.L., 1997. Comparative aspects of foetal carbohydrate metabolism. Equine Vet J Suppl: 19-25.

Fowden, A.L. and A.J. Forhead, 2004. Endocrine mechanisms of intrauterine programming. Reproduction 127: 515-526.

Fowden, A.L., D.S. Gardner, J.C. Ousey, D.A. Giussani and A.J. Forhead, 2005. Maturation of pancreatic beta-cell function in the foetal horse during late gestation. J Endocrinol 186: 467-473.

Fowden, A.L., D.A. Giussani and A.J. Forhead, 2005. Endocrine and metabolic programming during intrauterine development. Early Hum Dev 81: 723-734.

Fowden, A.L., L. Mundy, J.C. Ousey, A. McGladdery and M. Silver, 1991. Tissue glycogen and glucose 6-phosphatase levels in foetal and newborn foals. J Reprod Fertil Suppl 44: 537-542.

Fowden, A.L., J. Ousey and A.J. Forhead, 2004. Nutritive and endocrine functions of the equine placenta. Proc. Workshop on the Equine Placenta: 36-41.

Fowden, A.L., M. Silver, L. Ellis, J. Ousey, and P.D. Rossdale, 1984. Studies on equine prematurity 3: Insulin secretion in the foal during the perinatal period. Equine Vet J 16: 286-291.

Gibbs, P.G., G.D. Potter, R.W. Blake and W.C. McMullan, 1982. Milk production of quarter horse mares during 150 days of lactation. J Anim Sci 54: 496-499.

Grace, N.D., S.G. Pearce, E.C. Firth and P.F. Fennessy, 1999. Concentrations of macro- and micro-elements in the milk of pasture-fed thoroughbred mares. Aust Vet J 77: 177-180.

Herpin, P., J. Le Dividich, D. Berthon and J.C. Hulin, 1994. Assessment of thermoregulatory and postprandial thermogenesis over the first 24 hours after birth in pigs. Exp Physiol 79: 1011-1019.

Hess-Dudan, F. et al., 1994. Immunoreactive insulin-like growth factor i and insulin in blood plasma and milk of mares and in blood plasma of foals. Equine Vet J 26: 134-139.

Holdstock, N.B., V.L. Allen, M.R. Bloomfield, C.N. Hales and A.L. Fowden, 2004. Development of insulin and proinsulin secretion in newborn pony foals. J Endocrinol 181: 469-476.

Irvine, C.H., 1984. Hypothyroidism in the foal. Equine Vet J 16: 302-306.

Irvine, C.H. and M.J. Evans, 1975. Postnatal changes in total and free thyroxine and triiodothyronine in foal serum. J Reprod Fertil Suppl: 709-715.

King, S.S. and L.G. Nequin, 1989. An artificial rearing method to produce optimm growth in orphaned foals. J. equine vet. Sci. 9: 319-322.

Knight, D.A. and W.J. Tyznik, 1985. The effect of artificial rearing on the growth of foals. J Anim Sci 60: 1-5.

Koldovsky, O., 1994. Maturative effects of hormones on the developing mammalian gastrointestinal tract. Acta Paediatr Suppl 405: 7-12.

Koldovsky, O., A. Bedrick, P. pollack, R.K. Rao and W. Thornburg, 1988. Possible physiological role in hormones and hormone-related substances present in milk. In: L. A. Hanson (ed.) Biology of human milk. Nestle nutrition workshop series No. 15. p 123-139. Vevey/Raven Press.

LeBlanc, M.M., M. Macpherson and P. Sheerin, 2004. Ascending placentitis: What we know about pathophysiology, diagnosis and treatment. Am Assoc Equine Pract 50: 127-143.

Macdonald, A.A., P. Chavatte and A.L. Fowden, 2000. Scanning electron microscopy of the microcotyledonary placenta of the horse (equus caballus) in the latter half of gestation. Placenta 21: 565-574.

Martin, R.G., N.P. McMeniman and K.F. Dowsett, 1992. Milk and water intakes of foals sucking grazing mares. Equine Vet J 24: 295-299.

Mellor, D.J., 1993. Some aspects of perinatal maturation and adaptation. Equine Vet J Suppl: 17-22.

Meyer, H. and L. Ahlswede, 1976. Uber das intrauterine wachstum und die korperzusammentragender stuten. Ubersicht. Tierernahr. 4: 263-292.

Mount, L.E., 1979. Adaptation to thermal environment: Man and his productive animals. First ed. Edward Arnold Ltd, London.

Murray, M.J. and C. Grodinsky, 1989. Regional gastric ph measurement in horses and foals. Equine Vet J. Suppl. 7: 73-76.

Murray, M.J., R.P. Schaudies and D.M. Cavey, 1992. Epidermal growth factor-like activity in mares‘ milk. Am J Vet Res 53: 1729-1731.

Oftedal, O.T., H.F. Hintz and H.F. Schryver, 1983. Lactation in the horse: Milk composition and intake by foals. J Nutr 113: 2096-2106.

Ousey, J.C., 1997. Thermoregulation and the energy requirement of the newborn foal, with reference to prematurity. Equine Vet J Suppl: 104-108.

Ousey, J.C., M. Ghatei, P.D. Rossdale and S.R. Bloom, 1995. Gut hormone responses to feeding in healthy pony foals aged 0 to 7 days. Biol Reprod Mono 1 1: 87-96.

Ousey, J.C., N. Holdstock, P.D. Rossdale and A.J. McArthur, 1996. How much energy do sick neonatal foals require compared with healthy foals? Pferdeheilkunde 12: 231-237.

Ousey, J.C., A.J. McArthur, P.R. Murgatroyd, J.H. Stewart and P.D. Rossdale, 1992. Thermoregulation and total body insulation in the neonatal foal. J therm Biol 17: 1-10.

Ousey, J.C., A.J. McArthur and P.D. Rossdale, 1991. Metabolic changes in thoroughbred and pony foals during the first 24 h post partum. J Reprod Fertil Suppl 44: 561-570.

Ousey, J.C., A.J. McArthur and P.D. Rossdale, 1997. Thermoregulation in sick foals aged less than one week. The Vet J 153: 185-196.

Ousey, J.C., S. Prandi, J. Zimmer, N. Holdstock and P.D. Rossdale, 1997. Effects of various feeding regimens on the energy balance of equine neonates. Am J Vet Res 58: 1243-1251.

Ousey, J.C. et al., 2004. Effects of manipulating intrauterine growth on post natal adrenocortical development and other parameters of maturity in neonatal foals. Equine Vet J 36: 616-621.

Pagan, J.D., S.G. Jackson and S. Caddel, 1996. A summary of growth rates of thoroughbreds in kentucky. Pferdeheilkunde 12: 285-289.

Platt, H., 1984. Growth of the equine foetus. Equine Vet J 16: 247-252.

Roberts, M.C., 1975. The development and distribution of mucosal enzymes in the small intestine of the foetus and young foal. J Reprod Fertil Suppl: 717-723.

Rossdale, P.D., 1968. Abnormal perinatal behaviour in the thoroughbred horse. Br Vet J 124: 540-553.

Samuel, C.A., W.R. Allen and D.H. Steven, 1975. Ultrastructural development of the equine placenta. J Reprod Fertil Suppl: 575-578.

Schweigart, F.J., 2001. Milk more than a nutrient: Hormones, growth factors and bioactive factors. Pferdeheilkunde 18: 665-668.

Silver, M., 1984. Some aspects of equine placental exchange and foetal physiology. Equine Vet J 16: 227-233.

Silver, M. and A.L. Fowden, 1994. Prepartum adrenocortical maturation in the foetal foal: Responses to acth. J Endocrinol 142: 417-425.

Silver, M. et al., 1991. Relationship between circulating tri-iodothyronine and cortisol in the perinatal period in the foal. J Reprod Fertil Suppl 44: 619-626.

Slebodzinski, A.B., E. Brzezinska-Slebodzinska, J. Nowak and K. Kowalska, 1998. Triiodothyronine (t3), insulin and characteristics of 5'-monodeiodinase (5'-md) in mare's milk from parturition to 21 days post-partum. Reprod Nutr Dev 38: 235-244.

Smyth, G.B., D.W. Young and J. Schumacher, 1989. Postprandial serum gastrin concentrations in normal foals. Equine Vet J 21: 285-287.

Stammers, J.P., D.P. Leadon and D. Hull, 1987. Fatty acid composition of the plasma lipids of the maternal and newborn horse. J Reprod Fertil Suppl 35: 615-622.

Trahair, J.F., 1993. Is foetal enteral nutrition important for normal gastrointestinal growth? A discussion. JPEN J Parenter Enteral Nutr 17: 82-85.

Trahair, J.F. and P.T. Sangild, 1997. Systemic and luminal influences on the perinatal development of the gut. Equine Vet J Suppl: 40 50.

Tyler, S.J., 1972. The behaviour and social organisation of new forest ponies. Anim. Behav. Monographs 5: 148-174.

Ullrey, D.E., R.D. Struthers, D.G. Hendricks and B.E. Brent, 1966. Composition of mare's milk. J Anim Sci 25: 217-222.

Vermorel, M., J. Vernet, C. Dardillat, Saido and C. Demigne, 1989. Energy metabolism and thermoregulation in the newborn calf: Variations during the first day of life and differences between breeds. Can. J. Anim. Sci. 69: 103-111.

Widdowson, E.M., 1985. Development of the digestive system: Comparative animal studies. Am J Clin Nutr 41: 384-390.

Wilson, J.H., 1987. Feeding considerations for neonatal foals. Proc. Am. Assoc. Equine Pract 33: 823-829.

Xu, R.J., 1996. Development of the newborn gi tract and its relation to colostrum/milk intake: A review. Reprod Fertil Dev 8: 35-48.

Equine colostrum production and utilisation: basic and applied aspects

C. Drogoul[1], F. Clément[2], M. Ventorp[3] and M. Orlandi[4]
[1]Milking mare experimental farm LEGTA Semur Chatillon, 21400 Chatillon sur Seine, France
[2]EPA Les haras nationaux, 61310 Le Pin au Haras, France
[3]Swedish University of Agricultural Sciences, JBT, P.O. Box 59, S-203 53 Alnarp, Sweden
[4]Dept. Animal Production, Viale delle Piagge 2, 56124 Pisa, Italy

Abstract

The failure of immune transfer through colostrums absorption is frequent and responsible for a large proportion of neonatal morbidity and mortality in new born foals. Newborn foals are born with no immune defence and protection against infections during the first 4 to 8 weeks of life must be conferred by passively transferred colostral immunoglobulins, consecutively to the ingestion and the absorption of maternal colostrum at birth. Under breeding farm conditions, failure of immune transfer through colostrum absorption is frequent. Both the foal and the dam may be involved in the failure of passive immunity transfer that can be due to poor colostrum quality, lack of colostrum ingestion or Ig intestinal absorption, or a combination of these factors. Many different factors can affect the quality of colostrums, such as time after birth, type and breed, age and rank of lactation, nutrition and body condition of mare, vaccination program, season and temperature. Even if good quality colostrum is available and ingested, impaired absorption, delayed ingestion and gut closure can cause lack of Ig intestinal absorption. Appropriate breeding practices can enhance the opportunities for the foal to get adequate immunity transfer: breeders must make sure that the foal ingests 1g of IgG per kg of bodyweight as early as possible after birth and not after 12 hours. This postulates that everything is done to improve the maternal colostrum quality, to check the quality of colostrum immediately after birth (and adequate supply is available in case of poor quality), and to make sure that foal ingests colostrum in time. But above all, it is imperative that efficient measures are taken for the breeder to be present at foaling. Looking for early colostrum losses and/or premature foaling and collecting colostrums samples to create a colostrums bank can also help to anticipate poor breeding conditions and limit FPT. Other alternatives to dam colostrum have also been tested: Bovine colostrums, Plasmatic IgG, Induced lactation of dry mare.

Keywords: colostrum, foal, passive immunity transfer

Introduction

The failure of immune transfer through colostrums absorption is frequent and responsible for a large proportion of neonatal morbidity and mortality in new born foals. The equine fetus is immunocompetent around the 7th month of pregnancy (Perryman *et al.*, 1980), but as it is not exposed to pathogenic agent before birth, no antibodies are produce by the young animal *in utero*. On the other hand, because of the epithelio-chorionic structure of the placenta of mare (Ginther, 1979), large molecules, such as immunoglobulins (Ig), can not cross the 6 layers of different tissues that separate the fetus and the mare blood capillaries. As a consequence, newborn foals are born with no immune defence (agammaglobulinemic), and protection against infections during the first 4 to 8 weeks of life must be conferred by passively transferred colostral immunoglobulins, consecutively to the ingestion and the absorption of maternal colostrum at birth (Jeffcott, 1975).

The failure of immune transfer (FPT) through colostrum absorption is frequent (Table 1) and responsible for a large proportion of neonatal morbidity and mortality in newborn foals. It represents considerable genetic and economic losses for the horse industry. Better understanding of colostral passive immunity transfer can help to decide which preventive measures could be promoted in studs to reduce the impact of its failure. Some practical solutions, issued from several clinical papers and authors' own experiments and experiences are presented and discuss.

Table 1. Incidence of failure of passive immunity transfer in stud according to literature.

IgG level in foal serum at 24 – 48 h of age				
< 2 g/l	< 4 g/l	< 8 g/l	No of foals	Author (s)
10%			87	Mc Guire et al, 1977
	18%		2 092	Perryman and McGuire, 1980
	3%		136	Morris *et al.*, 1985
	15%		48	Betsch, 1987
	17%		48	Le Blanc *et al.*, 1987
	7%	20%	419	Baldwin *et al.*, 1990
	13%		253	Koterba *et al.*, 1990
	22%		254	Guenin, 1990
	18%		1 986	Clabough *et al.*, 1991
	15%	35%	1 922	Stonehan et al, 1991
		10%	323	Raidal, 1996
	10%		10	Touboul et al, 1997
	16%	33%	88	Tyler-McGowan *et al.*, 1997
	8%		13	Chavatte et al, 1998

The colostrum and its production in mare

Colostrum secretion

Colostrum is specialized milk that contains large amount of immunoglobulins and is produced under influence of hormonal mechanisms, but the selection and concentration of the circulating blood Ig (mainly IgG in mares) by the mammary gland is unknown. IgA are produced by the mammary gland. Concentration of Ig from circulation blood is highly specific, and explains the difference in colostral IgG1/IgG2 ratio observed between colostrum and plasma. IgG receptors have been clearly identify on the basal membranes of glandular epithelial cells (Barrington *et al.*, 1997). Concentration starts during the last month of pregnancy, most of it occurring during the last two weeks, as estrogens level drops down and progesterone rises (Smith *et al.*, 1971; Jeffcott, 1974). Therefore, colostrum is fleetingly secreted at the beginning of each new lactation period. Mean colostrums production is 2.5±1,5 litres (n=27) for Saddle horse mares, (Clément *et al.*, 2000).

Colostrum composition and evaluation

Colostrum is extremely rich in protein, of which 40% are immunoglobulins (Rouse and Igram, 1970). Immunoglobulins contained in equine colostrums are mostly IgG and IgG (T), with little quantities of IgM, IgA and others associated immunoglobulins (McGuire and Crawford, 1973; Jeffcott, 1975). A total of 103±71g of IgG is secreted in average per lactation. The greater concentration has been found in the first 0.9±0.5 litres collected (Clément *et al.*, 2000).

It is commonly admitted that good quality colostrum contains not less than 60g of Ig/l, one of medium quality between 60 and 40-38 g/l and a low quality one, less than 38 g/l. These levels are in accordance with the foal protection (IgG serum concentration in foals) when the colostrums is ingested under optimal conditions (1.5 to 2 litres within 6 hours after birth). The reasons why mammary gland fails to concentrate blood immunoglobulins remains uncertain.

Variation factors of colostrum quality

Twenty-three to 32% of mares produce low quality colostrums (Higuchi *et al.*, 1989; Genin, 1990; Leblanc *et al.*, 1986; 1992). Individual variation is big (McGuire and Crawford, 1973; Rossdale and Ricketts, 1980; Leblanc et Tran, 1987; Leblanc *et al.*, 1992; Chavatte *et al.*, 1998). Many different factors can affect the quality of colostrums, such as time after birth, type and breed, age and rank of lactation, nutrition and body condition of mare, vaccination program, season and temperature.

Time after birth

According to Pearson *et al.* (1984) the IgG content of colostrums falls by 5 or 6 g every hours following the foaling (Figure 1), 6 to 8 hours after the birth, immunoglobulin concentration drastically drops down up to 80-85%. This phenomenon is not only a consequence of the emptying of the udder and the dilution or replacement of colostrum by milk secretion, but also because of the natural resorption of IgG occurring within the gland (Pearson *et al.*, 1984). As a consequence, even if the udder if not emptied, the udder no longer contains colostrum passed 24 hours after birth (Jeffcott, 1974). This is the main reason why colostrum should be artificially collected if the foal does not suck its mother within 6 hours after birth.

Type and breed

As in most domestic mammals, type and breed are known to have an influence on IgG concentration in mare. Arabian and Quarter horse mares seem to have better quality colostrum than Thoroughbreds

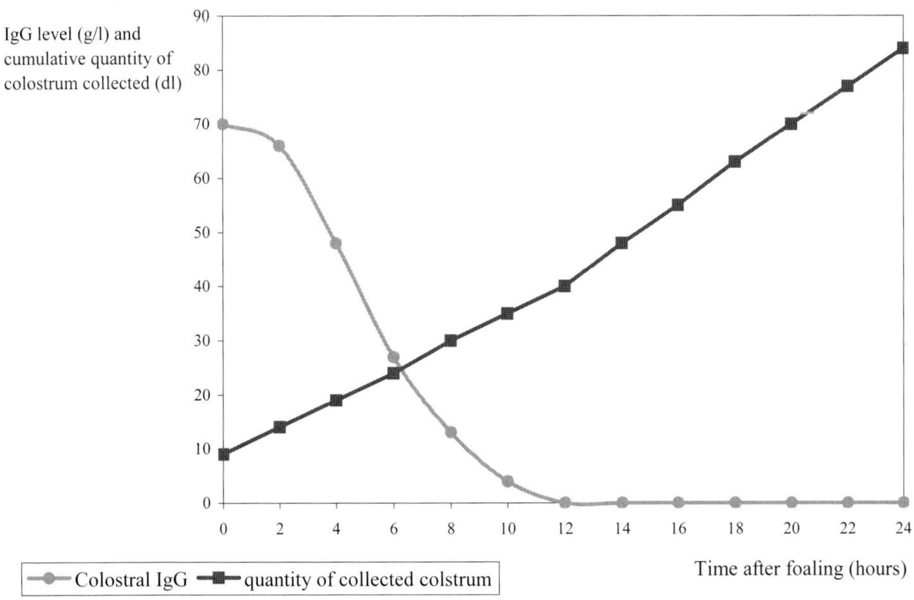

Figure 1. IgG concentration and cumulated quantity of colostrum collected every two hours during the first 24 h after foaling (according to Chavatte-Palmer et al, 1990).

and Standardbreds (trotters) (Leblanc et Tran, 1987). Heavy type mares seemed to produce slightly better colostrums than hacks (Leblanc *et al.*, 1992; Leblanc et Tran, 1987; Chavatte *et al.*, 1998).

Age and rank of lactation

Contrary with what has been observed in cows, according to Leblanc *et al.* (1992) young mares produce better colostrums than old ones (over 15 years of age).

Clément *et al.* (2000) checked the quality of colostrum in 40 mares on 58 pairs of successive foalings. The IgG levels at foaling was found slightly correlated with the IgG level at the successive foaling in the same mare ($r=0.31$, $p<0.05$), but not enough to classify mares as good or poor colostrums producers. These authors found no differences between mares according to rank of lactation, which is in accordance with Morris *et al.* (1985) results.

Nutrition and body condition of mares

Influence of nutrition is multifactorial, which render interpretation of results to be difficult. Few experiments have been carried out to measure the effect of diet on IgG production in farm animal.

Vaccination program

An experimental study, concerning vaccination against rotavirus (30 days prior foaling), has been carried out using 50 draught horse mares and their foals by Terrier-Finelle (1996). This author showed that 75% of the vaccinated mares showed seroconversion against 10% for the unvaccinated ones. The increase in antirotavirus IgG was greater ($P<0.005$) in the vaccinated group for mares sera, foals sera, colostrums and milk. A Citefoal IgG® test was performed to assess adequacy of passive transfer of immunity and gave explanation for a few abnormally low IgG rates in sera of foals born from vaccinated mares.

Season and temperature

The effect of season is controversial. Leblanc *et al.* (1992) observed that mares bred in sunny area had greater colostrum quality than those bred under humid and cold conditions. Clément *et al.* (2000) could not find any significant effect on time of the year, nor length of pregnancy.

Failure of passive immunity transfer to the newborn foal

The definition of the failure of passive immunity transfer differs according to authors (Leblanc *et al.*, 1986; Genin, 1990; Koterba, 1990a; Leblanc *et al.*, 1992; Stoneham *et al.*, 1991, Vivrette *et al.*, 1998) due to differences of breeding conditions between studies, importance of the specificity of IgG measured and tests used to measure serum Ig concentrations as they cannot be considered as equivalent (Brown, 1993). Indeed Ig (particularly IgG) gives an estimation of the potential protection of the foal against infections, as many other factors, such as IgA, Trypsine inhibitors, lactoferrin, lactoperoidase, transferring and growth factors, contained in colostrum are also involved in the foal protection (Kohn *et al.*, 1989; Berthon and Salmon, 1993, Csapo *et al.*, 1995a, Csapo *et al.*, 1995b). Apart from IgA that gives local immunity, the exact role of these other molecules is not well established. Nevertheless, it is generally agreed that a foal should present a minimum of 8g/l of serum immunoglobulin at 24 hours of life to be considers as fully protected. Between 8 and 4g/l the failure is partial (PFPT) and total below 4-2g/l and adequate treatment should then be carried out to enhance the foal protection.

Colostrum immunoglobulin transfer in newborn foal

Colostrum Ig transfer mechanisms have been well studied in rats (Silim *et al.*, 1990). Thanks to receptor mediated endocytosis mechanism in the immature epithelial fore gut cells, colostral globulins make their way towards the lymphatic system and finally the blood circulation (Jeffcott, 1973; Kruse, 1983). This phenomenon could be enhanced by an increased fluidity of intestinal cell membranes, related to longer fatty acid chain composition of the later. Duvaux-Ponter *et al.* (2004) however failed to demonstrate improvement of IgG transfer post partum by increasing the supply of fatty acid C18:3 during late pregnancy.

Genin (1990) showed that the level of IgG of the foal is correlated with the amount of IgG ingested ($r=0.31$, $n=241$, $p<0.05$), confirming that the intestinal absorption of IgG is active, but not selective. This capacity of the enterocytes to absorb large molecules is very efficient but elusive because of rapid replacement of these immature cells by proper epithelial gut cells, impermeable to Ig molecules. This "closure" phenomenon starts straight after birth. As a consequence, Ig absorption rapidly decreases: When foals are colostrum fed soon after the birth, the absorbtion of Ig is negligible at 12 to 18 hours of age, and impossible after 24 hours (Pearson *et al.*, 1984).

If the foal receives good quality colostrum within the 2 first hours after birth, IgG can be detected in its serum 4 hours later and reach its maximum level after 12-24 hours. Because of rapid catabolism of maternal immunoglobulins, this initial level drops down drastically during the first two month of life (Figure 2). In the mean times, development of the foal's own immunity system takes over. As a consequence, the IgG blood level in healthy foals is at is minimal level around 2 month of life (Jeffcott, 1974, Perryman *et al.*, 1980; Rumbaugh et Ardans, 1983) as shown Figure 2. The lesser passive transfer, the greater the endogenous synthesis; the greater passive transfer, the greater the maternal IgG catabolism. As a consequence, foals with high IgG level at 24 hours (>16 g/l) are now longer superior to those with lower level (8g/l at 24 hours) after 2 to 3 weeks of life (Touboul *et al.*, 1997, Chavatte-Palmer *et al.*, 2001) as shown Figure 3.

The absorption capacity of IgG by the foal is equal to 62.3% for healthy foals that could suck colostrum just after birth. In comparison with colostrum quality, which is very variable between

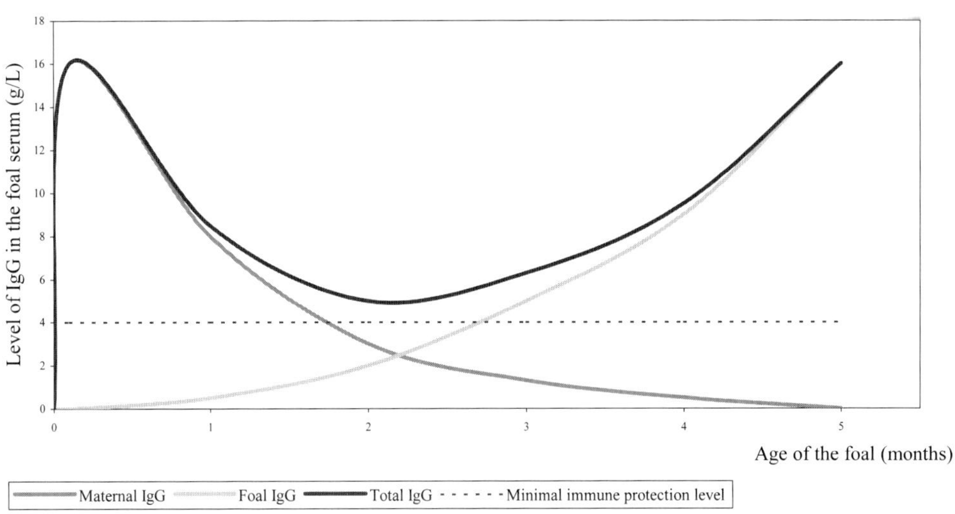

Figure 2. IgG concentration in the serum of foal during the first months of life (according to Genin, 1990 and Crawford and Perryman, 1980).

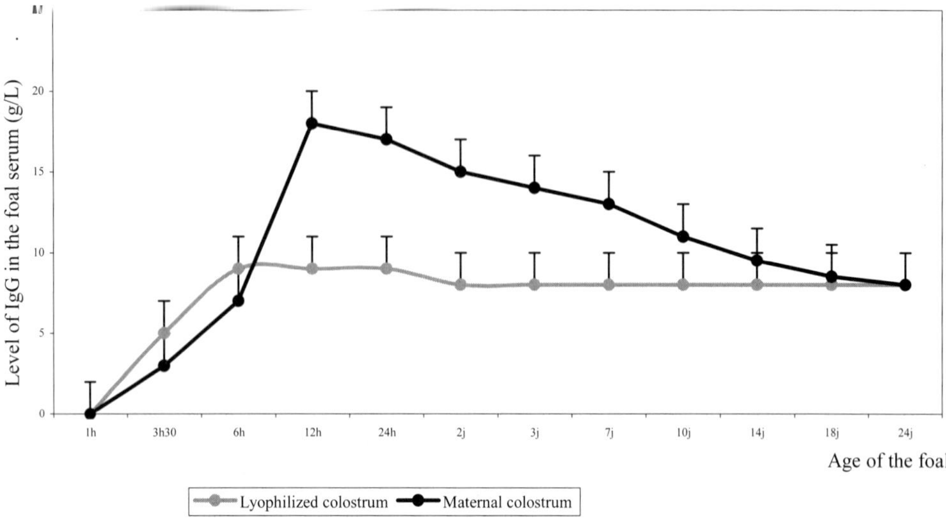

Figure 3. IgG concentration in the serum of foal receiving maternal colostrum versus lyophilized equine colostrum (according to Touboul et al, 1997).

mares, variability between foals that sucked just after birth is low (Clément *et al.*, 2002). These authors showed that the absorption capacity seems to increase as the quantity of ingested IgG increases (Figure 3), suggesting that, contrary to what has been observed in calf, no saturation of the efficiency of absorption of IgG is observed in foal.

Frequency and consequences of passive immunity transfer failure

Passive immunity transfer failure is considered to be the most important cause of *septicemia* in newborn foals. Many authors pointed out that the frequency and the gravity of infections are related to the importance of the immunoglobulin level deficiency (Jeffcott, 1972, 1974 and 1975; McGuire *et al.*, 1977; Rossdale and Ricketts, 1980; Perryman, 1981; Morris *et al.*, 1985; Genin, 1990). Under breeding farm conditions, percentages of passive immunity failure vary from 3 to 22 percent (Table 1). The chances for these foals to survive are extremely variable (0 to 80%) and rely on the quality of the breeder and veterinarian supervision, the quality of housing and microbial environment during the critical phase, i.e. until the foal's immunity system as taken over the immune protection (Baldwin *et al.*, 1991). Statistics published by the French Equine Pathology Institut of Dozulé in Normandie (Collobert-Laugier *et al.*, 1988; Chavatte and Collobert, 1994) show that half of the newborn foals (<5days of life) examined post mortem died from infection, of which 50% of them were subjected to breeding condition suggesting a possible failure of passive immunity transfer. A large farm conditions survey, conducted in France (n=254), nearly all mortality cases and most of the morbidity cases (49% versus 8%) occurred on immunodeficient foals (Table 2). Clabough *et al.* (1991) reported that Standardbred foals with less than 4 g Ig per litre at 24 – 36 hours of age (18%) were more likely (odds ratio 3.5) than foals with normal passive transfer to require medical therapy during first 3 month after parturition (total n=1 986).

Origin of passive immunity transfer failure

Both the foal and the dam may be involved in the failure of passive immunity transfer that can be due to poor colostrum quality, lack of colostrum ingestion or Ig intestinal absorption, or a combination of these factors.

Table 2. Distribution of foals according to their own history before 3 month of age and their IgG serum concentration at 24 h of life (according Genin, 1990).

		All foals	Gammaglobilin level (g/l)		
			< 4	≥4 and <8	≥8
	Dead	8% (19)	22%	5%	4%
History of foals	Infected	15% (35)	27%	14%	4%
	Healthy	77% (189)	51%	81%	92%
TOTAL		100% (243)	51	57	135

Poor quality colostrum ingestion

Morris and all, demonstrated that the IgG concentration in foals serum decreases as colostral Ig level drops. The level of IgG in the serum of foal is correlated with the level of IgG supplied by the colostrums ($r=0.3778$, $n=241$, $p<0.01$, Genin, 1990). In this survey carried on by Genin and Clément (1989) the serum levels of IgG reached by foals absorbing low quality colostrums (<55g/l of IgG), is in average two times lesser (5.87±4,01 versus 10.91±6.29) than those of foals receiving good quality colostrums (≥ 55g/l of IgG).

As it has been demonstrated for other species, in case of premature birth (<320 days of pregnancy), mammary gland has not got enough time to concentrate the immunoglobulins and therefore, colostrums available for the foal as a poor quality compared with the one he would have got if it hadn't been premature (Jeffcott, 1974; Leadon *et al.*, 1984; Leblanc and Tran, 1987).

Pre parturient lactation leading to early milk losses, some times observed in mares, can also have harmful consequences on the IgG concentration of the colostrum (Jeffcott, 1974; Morris *et al.*, 1985). According to some authors, early milk loss, observed in 16 to 22% of mares, is the main cause of passive immunity transfer failure in foals (Jeffcott, 1974; McGuire *et al.*, 1977, Rumbaugh *et al.*, 1979). The reasons of these early milk losses are unknown but it could be associated with hormonal changes, twin pregnancies, placenta infection or early placenta separation. Genin (1990) highlighted that, under farm breeding conditions, IgG concentration in foals born of mares that did not loose their milk before giving birth (n=167) was significantly greater compared with mare that had start to loose milk more than 24 h before giving birth (n=25) (10.28±6.29 g/l *versus* 5.62±4.18g/l, respectively). However, the incidence of these early losses depends on initial level of IgG, quantity and numbers of day of losses (Chavatte-Palmer *et al.*, 1999).

Impaired absorption, delayed ingestion and gut closure

Shortage and even lack of IgG intestinal absorption has been mentioned in stressed, premature foals (Rossdale and Ricketts, 1980; Koterba, 1990a).

Insufficient maturated intestinal cell may not let the IgG absorption pass into the lymphatic system in premature foals. However, this assessment has never been demonstrated. This failure of lack of maternal IgG protection of the premature foals could be the result of a rapid utilization of the absorbed IgG, as suggested by Chavatte-Palmer *et al.* (2000). On the other hand, with premature foals, the mare has not received the proper signal for colostrum production. By the time it is produced, closure has started in the foals gut, aggravating the situation.

According to McGuire *et al.* (1975), 3 to 4% of the foals present a lack of IgG intestinal absorption, even if they had received good quality colostrums. Five % of the foals that had received good quality colostrums show a failure of passive transfer (Le Blanc *et al.*, 1986; Genin, 1990; Leblanc *et al.*, 1992).

Because of the early "closure" process, delayed ingestion of colostrums is the second risk factor of failure of passive transfer in foals. Absorption at 9 hours after birth is reduced by 33%, but an adequate transfer is still possible as long as colostrums quality is good enough (Clément *et al.*, 2002). Madigan stated in 1998 that gut closure could be induced by the ingestion of nutrients more than by a delay in ingestion. This hypothesis does not appear to be confirmed for IgG, as foals receiving milk before delayed colostrum supply had better absorption efficiency compared with those receiving nothing before the ninth hour after birth (46% *versus* 39%). Moreover, suckling something seemed better than not suckling at all to prevent the lack of the suckling reflex.

Lack of colostrum ingestion

Weak foals or with legs conformation problems, that needs more time to be able to stand up after birth usually ingest less colostrum. In addition, this delays the time of ingestion, deteriorating the chances of passive immune transfer (Pearson *et al.*, 1984). Lack of suckling reflex, is rare in foals but also delays the first nursing (Rossdale, 1972).

Sometimes the dam rejects foals, especially primiparous ones. This can be due to behavioural problems or management errors (Houpt, 1984), but most of the time it is momentarily related with painful tense udder (Jeffcott, 1974) and can easily be solved by milking the mare and feed the foal this first collected colostrum by hand.

Finally, in case of death of mare at birth or if neonatal isoerythrolysis is suspected, the colostrum of the mother is not available for the foal. In these cases, unless the need of an alternative supply as been anticipated, foals will have to suffer the consequences of a lack of colostrums ingestion.

Improving breeding practices for adequate immunity transfer

In order to be adequately immunized, the breeder must make sure that the foal ingests 1g of IgG per kg of bodyweight as early as possible after birth and not after 12 hours. This postulates that everything is done to improve the maternal colostrum quality, to check the quality of colostrum immediately after birth (and adequate supply is available in case of poor quality), and to make sure that foal ingest this colostrum in time. But above all, it is imperative that efficient measures are taken for the breeder to be present at foaling.

Improving the maternal colostrum quality

Colostrum must give the newborn foal antibodies against the threatening pathogenic agents. Adapted immunoglobulins can only be secured if the mare has been exposed recently to these agents naturally or artificially through vaccination. Therefore, moving the mare at least one month before giving birth into the stud chosen for foaling reduces the stress and gives her time to produce the antibodies necessary to give the foal adapted immune protection toward its future environment (Jeffcott, 1974; Warner, 1983).

Vaccination programs carried out one month prior foaling, can increase significantly and specifically the immune quality of colostrums and milk, enhancing the immunity of foals. The impact of this practice seems to be more effective for young animals (primiparous and/or fillies) that have significantly lesser IgG concentration in sera than older ones (Terrier-Finnelle, 1996).

Assisting foaling

Most of the equine deliveries occur during the night, when assistance is difficult to provide. Besides, prevision of time of birth is also difficult to determine, as early warning signs are variable between mares. As a consequence, breeders have to sit up at mare's side and get through tiring sleepless nights. Monitoring systems (video or electronic) can relieve the person long hours watching, but none of them allows to be quit of waking up unnecessarily at nights.

Camillo *et al.* (1991 and 2000), showed that injections of micro doses of oxytocine to mares at the time were colostrum calcium concentration reached maximum levels was effective in inducing parturition within 2 hours for mares that were about to foal and that mares that did not respond to injection, would not foal during the following night. This method was considered safer than irreversible induction treatment with oxytocine (Ousey *et al.*, 1984) or prostaglandin (Ley *et al.*, 1989) as it seemed that only about to foal mares did respond to treatment, securing foetal readiness to birth and as a consequence avoiding birth of premature foals. When first published, this method seemed to give the solution to foaling assistance, and in milking mare experimental farm the protocol proposed by Camillo *et al.* (1991), has been successfully tested since 1992 on Haflinger mares (Intravenous injection of 2.5UI, 5 to 6 foals/year), allowing foaling supervision, colostrum collecting and avoiding night watch. We failed however to demonstrate the effectiveness of this protocol on our Auxois (French heavy breed) mares (intravenous oxytocine injection of 4UI, n=11 in 1992). Indeed, as confirmed on standardbreds and heavy type mares by Chavatte-Palmer *et al.*, 10 years later (2002), daily injection of low dose of oxytocine are not effective in inducing or predicting parturition in mares, as opposed to ponies. All our treated Auxois mares gave birth at unexpected time (during the night following treatment) and endured 1 to 8 hours of discomfort (colic, sweat) after each oxytocine treatment. Most of them (9/11) were giving birth to visibly suffering foals that had troubles to overcome birth (late to stand up, weakness, and even lack of suckling reflex (2/9)). This is the reason why we stopped the protocol, and set up a specific, easy and safe monitoring protocol (n=42 in 1992) that, ever since (average n=15 to 20 Auxois foals/year since 1993), allows us to assist all foaling mares that can be check for colostrum calcium concentration as advised by Ousey *et al.* (1984).

Here is the protocol set up for our Auxois mares in the milking mare experimental farm: At term, mares are kept outdoors in a small meadow enclosure under close supervision all day long (from 8am to night). Twice daily (before and after turning them out), calcium concentration in mammary gland secretion is checked, to assess readiness for birth. 1ml of colostrum is collected from one udder, diluted into 5ml of demineralised water. Test is performed using semi-quantitative calcium strips (Merckoquant® 10025, Merck Clévelot, 17 avenue de la trentaine, BP44. 77052 Chelles Cedex, France). Strips are plunge in the solution for not more than 5 seconds and result (i.e. number of zones changing from green to pink colour) is read 5 seconds later. When at least 3 zones turn pink, mares are tied in stalls, close to one another and equipped with a girth physically connected to a car horn (such equipment is cheap, easy to find and install). Under these conditions, no mare lies down at night unless she is foaling. As a consequence, we are able to assist 100% of our mares, (41 in 1991, 15 to 20 foaling/year since) with no unnecessary sleepless nights and we could reduce the mortality of foals during foaling from over 10% (field survey, Drogoul unpublished) when those Auxois mares are not assisted for foaling, to less that 1%. Nowadays, most of the breeders have successfully adopted our monitoring method, with the same reduction of birth mortality of foals. This method however is not available for mares that produce no colostrum before foaling (1/53 in 1992, none since).

Evaluating colostrum quality

Sticky and thick colostrums consistencies (rather than liquid) are better indicators of high concentration of IgG, than is colour (yellowish rather than white). However, these empirical criteria are rather subjective (Chavatte *et al.*, 1998). This is the reason why rapid, efficient and "easy to use" methods must be developed in breeding farm to evaluate the quality of colostrum. As pre-foaling samples are not reliable to give good evaluation of the colostrum's quality, sampling must be done just after foaling and before the first suck.

There is a close relationship between colostral IgG concentration and colostral specific gravity (Leblanc *et al.*, 1986; Genin, 1990, Touboul et al; 1997; Chavatte-Palmer *et al.*, 2001) which can easily been assess under farm condition using a colostrometer (Leblanc *et al.*, 1986) or a densimeter (Terrier-Finelle, 1996). In France, on the initiative of the National stud (Les Haras Nationaux), the use of the Colotest (Colotest: Les Haras nationaux, Domaine de l'Isle Braind, BP 50009 49505 Segré Cedex. Haras.angers@haras-nationaux.fr) is preferred. This sugar refractometer has been scaled for IgG concentration estimation and provide as easy, rapid and reliable estimate for colostrum quality. It has been widely spread in studs since 1999: this tool has been either sold or hired to breeders during the breeding season.

Reducing the time between birth and suckling

As mentioned before, in order to secure best condition for IgG intestinal absorption, ingestion of colostrum should happen within less than two first hours after birth. In our mare milking farm, we have experimented about colostrum bank erection. Therefore, mares have been systematically placed in a loose box and milked 1 hour after birth in presence of her foal (with an adapted cow-milking machine) and under the influence of ocytocin (intravenous injection of 40UI or 60UI for Haflinger or Auxois mares respectively) since 1992. This first maternal colostrum has been immediately bottle-fed to the foal (500 ml or 700ml for Haflinger and Auxois, respectively). Apart from usual foal care (disinfection of umbilical cord, etc), and milking procedure, dam and foal are left alone for the mare to form a good bond with her offspring. In 1992, as 41 foals were involved in a hyper-immunization program, they only received the maternal colostrum, what ever its quality was, confirming that passive IgG levels was strongly correlated with colostrums quality (Terrier-Finelle, 1996). Since 1993, all mares are still systematically milked 1 hour after giving birth, colostrums tested using a colostrometer and foals are hand fed. Depending on quality and quantity collected, this first colostrum may be completed, or mixed with stored colostrum if necessary, to secure sufficient quantity and quality to the foal for its first colostrum ingestion. To our point of view, this nursing protocol has reduced the time taken by our foals to stand up and suckle the dam unaided, especially for Auxois ones (compare with what is observed under field condition). In the meantime, no behaviour problem was noticed and no mare rejected the foal. In addition, as no foal was forced to the udder, no future behaviour problems should appear (Lansade *et al.*, 2005). Since we adopted this protocol, none of our foal contracted navel infection or arthritis, whereas, under field conditions, one third of the Auxois foals do (Retrospective field survey, Drogoul 1994, unpublished).

Usually, it is recommended to collect 200-400 ml of high quality colostrum (i.e. colostral density> 1.08 or IgG level ≥ 60g/l) within 12 hours if the dam colostral specific gravity is <1.06, with a special attention to foaling mares over 15 years of age (Leblanc *et al.*, 1992).

Anticipating poor breeding situations

All situations that generate expected transfer failure should be closely looked for and anticipated if necessary.

Looking for early colostrum losses and premature foaling

All at term mares should be closely observed for pre-parturient lactation identification. Calcium colostrum daily evaluation is of great interest as it allows this detection and in addition it gives acute information on readiness of foaling.

If a significant early colostrum loss is detected, the breeder should collect, test the quality, and deep-freeze in order to hand feed the foal after the birth (Chavatte-Palmer *et al.*, 1999).

Colostrum bank erection

Maintaining a bank of deep-frozen colostrum should be a routine practice on most studs and is a recommended breeding practice (Leblanc *et al.*, 1986; Chavatte-palmer et al, 1999). However, one must admit that if foaling is not effectively monitored, unexpected foaling or tiring sleepless nights, are not good conditions for adequate colostrum collection and storing.

Colostrum collection procedure

When colostrum is collected with a milking machine and the mare is under influence of oxytocine, the average first collected quantity varies considerably from 300 ml up to 3 litres, average collection are rarely above 1 000 ml. In this case, foal must be hand fed with some of the collected colostrum.

When mare is milked manually, quantity of colostrum collected depends also on breeder's ability, size of teats and colostrum quantity already suckled by the foal. Hand milking can take quite a long time and a lot of patience, and from our point of view, this is the main reason why too few breeders bother to store colostrum under small farms condition. In case of manual collection, it is usually recommended to collect 180-250ml of colostrum after the mare's own foal has first sucked (Leblanc *et al.*, 1986) or from just one of the two teats (Warner and Vaala, 1986) in order to left the other one to the foal. One must then make sure that the foal nurses from the remaining teat to secure adequate colostrum ingestion.

Colostrum conditioning and conservation

We recommend to split up collected samples into small plastic containers (ideally 100ml). This allows later mixtures of different origins. All samples' quality should be evaluated and containers labelled (dam, quality, date) using an adequate system that stands high humidity and low temperatures. Samples can be frozen in a domestic deep-freezer as long as temperature at –20 °C. Thawing and refreezing must be avoided, to prevent IgG spoilage. Colostrum should be used within less than 18 months (i.e. during the breeding season or the following one).

Colostrum utilization

In our mare milking experimental farm, all foals are systematically hand fed 500 to 700ml (depending of foal size) before they are allowed to suckle their mother. This quantity has been determined by experience: it corresponds to most healthy newborn foal, with good suckling behaviour, ingests when bottle-fed ad libitum during its first suckling session. It gives us the opportunity to secure a minimum of good quality colostrum to all our foals. Indeed, when first collection is too low in quantity or quality, we try to supplement the foal an adequate mixture from our colostrum bank. This is the reason why even low quality colostrum is not thrown away. These samples are used to complete high quality samples in a future mixture, especially in case of orphan foals, which need to be hand fed larger quantities of colostrum than foals allowed to suckle their mother after the first colostrum collection. When the dam's colostrum is not available (maternal death, agalactia, rejection of the foal or abnormalities such as foal neonatal maladjustment syndrome), a minimum of 0.5 to 1 liter of good quality colostrum should be hand fed (or via a nasogastric tube if necessary) to secure high serum IgG level by the foal (Crawford and Perryman, 1980). Meals of not more than 500 ml must be given every hour (Warner and Vaala, 1986). A healthy newborn foal will ingest an average of 250ml of colostrum during its first nursing session (150 to 500ml), 300ml during the second one and 350-400ml then after (Madigan, 1991). Frozen colostrum should never be boiled or micro-waved, but slowly thawed and fed at 39 °C.

Other alternatives to dam colostrum

Frozen or Lyophilized equine colostrums

Freeze-dried equine IgG as well as frozen colostral IgG are well absorbed by foals (Touboul *et al.*, 1997; Chavatte-Palmer *et al.*, 2001; Clément *et al.*, 2002). The preparation of IgG powder tested by these authors included ultra-filtration, which selected IgG and did not seem to eliminate components that are important for absorption (Csapo *et al.*, 1995a; Kohn *et al.*, 1989). The main problem is that a colostrum bank is very difficult to organize and not enough quantity of good quality colostrum can be collected to allow industrial processing and commercialization (Drogoul and Brigand, 1996).

Bovine colostrum

Some studies have tested bovine colostrum as an alternative to equine source of immunoglobulins (Genin, 1990; Leblanc, 1991; Holmes and Lunn, 1991). Indeed, bovine colostrum is easy to collect, readily available and produced in great quantities. Bovine immunoglobulins are however moderately well absorbed and rapidly catabolized and bovine IgG has a half-life of only 7.3 days (Holmes and Lunn, 1991). Most studies testing bovine colostrum pointed out a higher IgG endogenous production in bovine colostrum fed foals. The fact that bovine colostrum has no specific equine IgG is probably the main reason why bovine colostrum is not widely fed to foals.

Plasmatic IgG

Equine seric IgG transfer has also been tested in foals. Most of the studies showed that seric IgG passive transfer is poor and foal IgG seric levels hardly exceed 4g/l (Touboul *et al.*, 1997; Chavatte-Palmer *et al.*, 2001). On the other hand, the use of plasma per os as oral supplementation remains difficult as it means very large intake (6 litres per foal at least) (Chavatte-Palmer *et al.*, 1999).

Induced lactation of dry mare

Inducing lactation in nonpregnant mare could be an interesting alternative for colostrum production and raising orphan foals. It has been successfully tested by Chavatte-Palmer *et al.* (2002). Even if colostrum and milk production seams to be lesser than what could be expected postpartum, this new experiment has open interesting perspectives in the use of barren mares as foster mares for orphan foals and colostrum storing (Daels et al, 2002).

Passive immune transfer forecast

Foal serum protein fraction

A complementary study on foal serum protein evolution could be interesting as a support in immunotransfer understanding. Some researches concerning foals serum pointed out that total protein level was 3.76 g/dl, 3 h from the first suckling (Curadi *et al.*2002), according to the results obtained by Rumbaugh *et al.* (1978), to reach biggest amounts (5.76 g/dl) at 18 hours, with significative difference.

A good correlation was underlined between serum total proteins (TP) and IgG ($r=0.85$, $p<0.01$),as in previous works (Curadi and Orlandi, 1999) so that some Authors (Rumbaugh *et al.*, 1978; Tyler Mc Gowan *et al.*, 1997) suggested the possibility to forecast FPT by evaluating TP serum content, because the close correlation between TP and IgG serum amounts, moreover when IgG level reach greatest values. The same investigations (Curadi *et al.*, 2002) showed that IgG represented 5.6% of TP in the 3 h samples and 36% in the 18 h ones.

Albumin amounts were included between 2.62 g/dl and 2.77 g/dl and no significant differences were observed. α1-globulins amounts significantly increased between 3 hours and 48 hours from delivery. Trumel *et al.* (1996) indicated similar α2 and smaller α1 amounts. Not different results are indicated from the same AA for β-globulins contents. γ-globulins significantly increased betweeen 3 hours and 18-24 hours from delivery. Albumin/Globulins (A/G) ratio was 1.06 and 1.02, respectively at 18 and 24 hours, in normal foals, decreasing from 2.53 at 3 hours because of progressive γ-globulins concentration.

During this foaling season one foal died within 72 hours and showed low IgG serum levels (less than 200 mg/dl). While mare serum and colostral levels were normal, TP amounts as 3.6 g/dl and 1.42 g/dl globulin level, with a A/G altered ratio as 2.5 were observed, confirming a strong correlation between physiological serum protein amounts and adequate immunity covering.

Passive immune transfer forecast

On the basis of observations about contents of serum and colostrum Igs and serum proteins in the first period of foal life. Aim of the observations of mare's and foal's Igs and serum proteins is related to the possibility of correlation between mare's blood samples at 3, 2, 1, 0 weeks from scheduled delivery, colostrum and finally, foal's serum amounts at birth and 18-24 hours of life and verify any possible correlation with the aim to forecast a possible immunodeficiency.

In a trial performed on thoroughbreds (Orlandi and Curadi, 2005) a good correlation was noted between mare serum at delivery and 24 h p.p. colostrum IgG levels, determined by use of radial immunodiffusion. Mare serum IgA collected one week before foaling was also strictly correlated with 24 h colostrum IgA. Significative correlation was found between foal serum IgGb amount at 0 h and IgG and IgGb mare serum content collected one week before foaling. IgG foal serum amounts collected one week after birth and IgG mare serum amounts collected 2 weeks before foaling were also correlated. Concerning serum proteins, a correlation between gammaglobulins at delivery and 24h colostral IgGb was also observed.

In a previous trial performed on crossbred mares and foals (Curadi *et al.*, 2002) total proteins level showed good correlation with IgG concentration. Mares' serum and colostrum IgG were not significantly correlated. Serum IgG (T) was strictly correlated with IgG and greatest values were also observed at foaling. Significative correlation was observed between IgG and IgM. Foal serum IgG (T) was significantly correlated with IgG and showed greatest values at 18 hours. Significative correlation was found between foal serum IgG contents at 6 and 18 hours, respectively, and colostrum IgG levels at delivery.

Regarding serum proteins, foal serum α1-globulins level significantly increased between 3 and 48 hours after birth; the same was noted for γ-globulins between 3 and 24 hours. Albumin/Globulins ratio decreased during the first 24 hours, from 2.5/1 at birth until about 1/1 at 18-24 hours.

These previous researches may be useful to increase an early possibility to forecast FPT or PFPT on the basis of correlations between mare's blood and colostrum Igs and proteins amounts. More information about passive immunity transfer could get the foal able, in case of deficiency, to be fed with extra-colostrum, or later, treated with plasma transfusion.

Conclusion

It can be concluded that the enlightenment to breeders about the high incidence and high risk of passive immunisation failure by foals should be intensified. The exhortation should include following:
Let the mares be staying at the stud chosen for foaling at least one month before giving birth.
Watch mares in late pregnancy in order to discover colostrum leakage.
Supervise all foaling, without disturbing the mare.
Test all colostrums. Do use quick-test such as colostrometer and Colotest™, do not just check the colostrum colour!
If low quality colostrums or low production, feed all foals by hand good quality colostrum within 2 hours after birth, even if the foal is vital.
Secure good delivery hygiene.
Erect a colostrum bank.

Important future research and development activities are as follow:
To understand the initiation of the gut closure process in newborn foals,
To investigate causes of inability or reduced ability to absorb immunoglobulins,
To study causes of poor colostrum quality, e.g. the effect of mare nutrition,
To develop and evaluate means and technical aids giving attention to approaching birth giving,
To find key data in order to predict passive immune transfer.

References

Baldwin, J.L. et al. Prevalence (treatment days) and severity of illness in hypogammaglobulenemic and normogammaglobulinemic foals. J Am Vet Med Assoc. 198:423-428.

Baldwin, J.L., D.K. Vanderwall, W.L. Cooper and H.N. Erb, 1990. Immunoglobulin G and early survival of foals: a three years field study. Proc. of the annual convention of the American Association of Equine Practitioners 35, p.179-185

Barrington, G.M., T.E. Besser, W.C. Davis, C.C. Gay, J.J. Reeves and T.B. Mc Fadden, 1997. Expression of immunoglobulin G1 receptors by bovine mammary epithelial cells and mammary leucocytes. J. Dairy. Sci. 80: 86-93.

Berthon, P. and H. Salmon. Facteurs immunitaires des secrétions mammaires. Biologie de la lactation. Martinet, J and Houdebine, L.M. (editor); INSERM/INRA, Paris. 389-414.

Brown, C.M., 1993. Uncertainties in the significance, diagnosis and treatment of failures of passive transfer in foals. Newsletter. Int. Soc. Vet. Penn.1-2: 8-12.

Carnillo, F., P. Marmorini, S. Romagnoli, P. Cela, G. Duchamp and E. Palmer, 2000. Clinical studies on daily low dose of oxytocin in mare at term. Equine. Vet. J. 32: 307-310.

Carnillo, F., P. Marmorini, S. Romagnoli, M. Cela, S. Tamagna, G. Duchamp and E. Palmer, 1991. Essai d'induction du poulinage de jour par de faibles doses d'ocytocine. Institut du cheval (editor) Compte rendu de la 17ème journée de la recherche équine. 1991, Paris, France. 37-42.

Clabough, D.L., J.F. Levine, G.L. Grant and H.S. Conboy, 1991. Factors associated with failure of passive transfer of colostral antibodies in Standardbreds foals. J. Vet. Intern. Med. 5(6), p.335-340
Chavatte, P. and C. Colobert, 1994. Le poulain nouveau-né. Institut du cheval (editor) Compte rendu de la 20ème journée de la recherche équine. 1994, Paris, France. 124-143.
Chavatte, P., J,-F Grongnet, F. Clément, G. Arnaud and R. Cash, 1998. Taux de calcium et d'immunoglobulines dans les secrétions mammaires Institut du cheval (editor) Compte rendu de la 20ème journée de la recherche équine. Paris, France. 124-143.
Chavatte, P., F. Clément, R. Cash and J,-F Grongnet, 1998. Colostrum quality determination in the field by using a novel, practical method of refractometry. Proccedings of the 44th Annual convention of the American association of equine practioners. Baltimore, USA.44:206-208.
Chavatte-Palmer, P., G. Arnaud, C. Duvaux-Ponter, L. Brosse, S. Bougel, P. Daels, P. Guillaume, F. Clément and E. Palmer, 2002. Quantitative and qualitative assessment of milk production after pharmaceutical induction of lactation in mare. J. Vet. Intern. Med. 16: 472-477.
Chavatte-Palmer, P., C. Duvaux-Ponter, M. Piot, J-L. Maubois, J-F. Grongnet, L. Brugère and F. Clément, 2001. Absorption of IgG in the foal: efficiency of a freeze-dried colostral immunoglobulin product; Effetc of the first suckling time. 52st FEZ Meeting. Budapest, Hungry, 26-29 August.
Chavatte-Palmer, P., F. Clément and J.-M. Betsch, 1999. Failures in passive transfer of immunity in the foal. Prat. Vét. Equine. 122- 31:53-62 (133-142)
Clément, F., G. Arnaud, C. Duvaux-Pontet and P. Chavatte-Palmer, 2000. Colotest and equine colostrum. 51st FEZ Meeting. La Haye, The Netherlands, 21-24 August.
Clément, F. Duvaux-Ponter, C., G. Arnaud, M. Piot, J.L. Maubois, J.F. Grongnet, L. Bruère, M. Tournié, L. Detrimont and P. Chavatte-Palmer, 2002. Efficiency of IgG absorption in the foal. Theriogenology. 58: 805-808.
Collobert-Laugier, C., J. Vaissaire, J.-P. Gillet, E. Plateau and A. Jacquet, 1988. Causes de mortalité des poulains de 6 mois en Basse Normandie. Institut du cheval (editor) Compte rendu de la 14ème journée de la recherche équine. 1988, Paris, France. 127-141.
Crawford, T.B.and L.E. Perryman, 1980. Diagnosis and treatment of failure of passive transfer in foals. Equine Practice. 1 (2):17-23.
Csapo, J., J. Stefler, S. Makray and Z. Csapo-Kiss, 1995a. Composition of mare's colostrums and milk: fat contents, fatty acid composition and vitamin content. Int. Dairy. Journal. 5: 393-402.
Csapo, J., J. Stefler, S. Makray and Z. Csapo-Kiss, 1995b. Composition of mare's colostrums and milk: Protein contents, amino-acid composition and content of macro and micro-elements. Int. Dairy. Journal. 5: 403-415.
Curadi, M.C., D. Minori, S. Demi and M. Orlandi, 2002. Immunotransfer in the foal. Ann. Fa. Med. Vet. Pisa, 54, 127-140
Curadi, M.C. and M. Orlandi, 1999. Correlation between IgG, IgG (T), IgM, IgA mare colostrum and foal serum contents in the first hours from delivery. XII ASPA Congres: 800-802
Daels, P.F., G. Duchamp, S. Massoni and P. Chavatte, 2002. Induction of lactation in non-foaling mares and growth of foals raised by mares with induced lactation. Proceedings of th 8th ISER, Fort Collins, Colorado: 859-861.
Drogoul, C. and G. Brigand, 1996. Bilan technico-économique de la jumenterie expérimentale du GIS « lait de jument ». Institut du cheval (editor) Compte rendu de la 22ème journée de la recherche équine. Paris, France. 128-133.
Duvaux-Ponter, C., M. Tournié, L. Detrimont, F. Clément, C. Ficheux and A.A. Ponter, 2004. Effect of a supplemented rich in linolenic acid added to the diet of mares on fatty supply acid composition of mammary secretions and the acquisition of passive immunity in the foal. Animal Science. 78:399-407.
Genin, C., 1990. Le transfert de l'immunité passive chez le poulain nouveau-né. Thèse Vétérinaire. ENV de Toulouse.
Genin, C and F. Clément, 1989. Transfert de l'immunité passive chez le poulain. Institut du cheval (editor) Compte rendu de la 15ème journée de la recherche équine. 1989, Paris, France. 62-71.
Ginther, O.-J., 1979. Reproductive biology of the mare: basic and applied aspects. 0.J. Ginther, Madisson, W.I., 155-320.
Higuchi, T., M. Oikawa, H. Ohishi, H. Senba and Y. Kagaya, 1989. Field survey on unqualified colostrum in horses by latex agglutination test. Bullertin of Equine Research Institute Japan, No 26, p.69-72
Holmes, M.A. and D.P. Lunn, 1991. A study of bovine and equine immunoglobulin levels in pony foals fed bovine colostrum. Equine. Vet. J. 23 (2): 116-118.

Houpt, K.A., 1984. Foal rejection and other behavioral problems in the postpartum period. The compendium on continuing education. 3 (6):S144-S148.

Jeffcott, L.B., 1972. Passive immunity and its transfer with special reference to the horse. Biol. Rev. 47:439-464.

Jeffcott, L.B., 1973. The mechanism of transfer of maternal immunity to the foal. In proc. 3rd Conf. Equine Infectious diseases, Paris, 1972. Karger (editors), Basel, Switzerland.419-435.

Jeffcott, L.B., 1974. Some practical aspects to the transfer of passive immunity to newborn foals. Equine. Vet. J. 6 (3): 109-115.

Jeffcott, L.B., 1975. The transfer of passive immunity to the foal and its relation to immune status after birth. J. Repod. Fertil.23: 727-733.

Kruse, P.E., 1983. The importance of colostral immunoglobulin and theis absorption from intestine in the newborn farm animals. Annales de Recherches vétérinaires. 14: 349-353.

Kohn, C.W., D. Knight, W. Hueston, R. Jacobs and S.M. Reed, 1989. Colostral and serum IgG, IgA, IgM concentration in standardbred mares and their foal at parturition. J. Am. Vet. Med. Assn. 195:64-68.

Koterba, A.M., 1990a. Diagnosis and management of the normal and abnormal neonatl foal. A.M. Koterba, W.H. Drummond and P.C. Kosch (editors). Equine clinical Neonatology. Lea & Febiger, Philadelphia, USA. 3-15.

Koterba, A.M., 1990b. Nutritional support: enteral feeding. A.M. Koterba, W.H. Drummond and P.C. Kosch (editors). Equine clinical Neonatology. Lea & Febiger, Philadelphia, USA. 728-746.

Lansade L., M. Bertrand and M.F. Bouissou, 2005. Effects of neonatal handling on subsequent manageability, reactivity and learning ability of foals. Applied Animal Behaviour Science 92 (1-2), 143-158.

Leadon, D.P., L.B. Jeffcott and P.D. Rossdale, 1984. Mammary secretions in normal spontaneous and induced premature parturition in the mare. Equine. Vet. J. 16 (4): 256-259.

Leblanc, M.M., 1991. Is bovine colostrum a suitable alternative source of immunoglobulins for newborn foals? Equine. Vet. J. 23 (2): 78-80.

Leblanc, M.M. and T. Tran, 1987. Relationship among colostral electrolytes, colostral IgG concentrations and absorption of colostral IgG by foals. J. Reprod. Fert. Suppl. 35:735-736.

Leblanc, M.M., B.I. Mc Laurin and R. Boswell, 1986. Relationship among serum immunoglobulin concentration in foals, colostral specific gravity and colostral immunoglobulin concentration. J. Amer. Vet. Med. Assn. 189 (1): 57-60.

LeBlanc, M.M., T. Tran and E.L. Pritchard, 1990. Factors influencing passive transfer of immunity in foals. Proc. Int. Conf. Vet. Perinat. 2, p18

Leblanc, M.M., T. Tran, J.L. Baldwin and E.L. Pritchard, 1992. Factors that influence passive transfer of immunoglobulins in foals. J. Amer. Vet. Med. Assn. 200: 179-183.

Ley, W.B., J.L. Hoffman, T.N. Meachan, T.L. Sullivan, R.L. Kiracofe and M.L. Wilson, 1989. Day time foaling management. 2: induction of parturition. J. Equine. Vet. Sci. 9 (2): 95-99.

Madigan, J.E., 1991. Manual of equine neonatal medicine. DVM. MS; Ed (editors). Woodland lane Oak Publishing. 363 p.

Madigan, J.E., 1998. Further observations on the pathogenesis of septicemia in the neonatal foal and methods of prevention in stabled horses compared to environmental and behavioural infection. Prevention strategies utilized in wild horses. Neonatal septicemia Workshop 2. Boston, USA. 12-13.

McGuire, T.T and T.B. Crawford, 1973. Passive immunity in the foal: measurement of immunoglobulin classes and specific antibodies. Am. J. Vet. Res. 34:1299-1303.

McGuire, T.T, M.G. Poppies and K.L. Banks, 1975. Hypogammaglobulenimia predisposing in infection in foals. J. Am. Vet. Med. Assoc. 166:71-75.

McGuire, T.T, T.B. Crawford, A.L. Hallowell and L.E. Macombier, 1977. Failure of colostral immunoglobin transfer as an explanation for most infections and deaths of neonatal foals. J. A. V. M. A. 170(11): 1302-1304.

Morris, D.D., D.A. Meirs and G.S. Merrymang, 1985. Passive transfer failure in horses: incidence and causative factors on a breeding farm. Am. J. Vet. Res. 46(11): 2294-2299.

Ousey, J.C. F. Dudan and P.D. Rossdale, 1984. Preliminary studies of mammary secretion in the mare to assess foetal readiness for birth. Equine. Vet. J. 16 (4): 259-263.

Orlandi M. and M.C. Curadi, 2005. Passive immunity transfer forecast in different horse breeds. (in c.d.p.)

Pearson, R. C., A. L. Hallowell and M.B. Warwick, 1984. Times of appearance and disappearance of colostral IgG in the mare. Am. J. Vet. Res. 45: 186-190.

Perryman, L.E., 1981. Immunological management of young foals. Compend. Contin. Educ. Pract. Vet. 3(6): S223-S228.

Perryman, L.E. and T.C. McGuire, 1980. Evaluation for immune system failures in horses and ponies. J.Am. Vet. Assoc. 176, p. 1374-1377

Perryman, L.E., T.C. Mc Guire and R.L. Torbeck, 1980. Ontology of lymphocyte function in the equine fetus. Am. J. Vet. Res. 41: 1197-1200.

Raidal, S.H., 1996. The incidence and consequences of failure of passive transfer ofimmunity on a thoroughbred farm. Australian Vet. J. 73(6), p. 201-206

Rossdale, P.D., 1972. Modern concepts of neonatal disease in foals. Equine. Vet. J. 4: 117-128.

Rossdale P.D. and S.W. Ricketts, 1980. Equine stud farm medecine. Maloine (editor) Orphan foals (2nd edition). Baillière Tindall and Co. London, U.K. 563.

Rousse, B.T. and D.G. Ingram, 1970. The total protein and immunoglobulin profile of equine colostrums and milk. Immunology. 19: 901-907.

Rumbaugh et al., 1979. Field determination of the immune status of newborn foal. Equine Pract. 1 (4): 37-42.

Rumbaugh G.E., A.A. Ardans, G. Douglas and A. Trommershausen-Smith, 1978. Measurement of neonatal equine immunoglobulins for assessment of colostral immunoglobulin transfer: comparison of single radial immunodiffusion with the zinc sulfate turbidity test, serum electrophoresis, refractometry for total serum protein, and the sodium sulfite precipitation test. J. Am. Vet. Med. Ass., 172, 321-325.

Rumbaugh, G.E. and A.A. Ardans, 1983. Immunologis diseases. In current therapy in equine medecine, Robinson, N.E. (editors). W.B. Saunders Co. Philadelphia, USA. 47-54.

Silim, A., M.-R, Rekik, R.S. Roy, H. Salomon and P.-P. Pastoret, 1990. Immunité chez le fœtus et le nouveau-né. In P.-P. Pastoret, A. Govaerts, H. Bazin (editors). Immunologie animale, Médecine-Sciences Flamarion, Paris, France.

Smith, K.L., L.A, Muir and L.C. Fergusson, 1971. Selective transport of IgG into the mammary gland: role of estrogen and progesterone. J. Dairy. Sci. 54: 1886-1894.

Stoneham, S., N.J. Wingfield-Digby and S.W. Ricketts, 1991. Failure of passive transfer of colostral immunity in the foal: incidence and the effect on stud management and plasma transfusions. Vet. Reccord. 128: 416-419.

Terrier-Finelle, A., 1996. Essai d'hyperimmunisation de juments lourdes vis à vis du rotavirus. Institut du cheval (editor) Compte rendu de la 22ème journée de la recherche équine. Paris, France. 134-138.

Touboul, M., Grongnet and C. Drogoul, 1997. Intérêt de l'administration de colostrum lyophilisé ou d'un extrait de plasma sanguin pour l'acquisition de l'immunité passive par le poulain nouveau-né. Institut du cheval (editor) Compte rendu de la 23ème journée de la recherche équine. 1997, Paris, France. 107-113.

Trumel C., F. Schelcher, J.P. Braun and J.F. Guelfi, 1996. L'électrophorèse des protéines sériques; principes interprétation chez le chien, le chat et le cheval. Revue Med. Vet., 1147, 2, 123-130.

Tyler Mc Gowan, C.M., J.L. Hodgson and D.R. Hodgson, 1997. Failure of passive transfer in foals: incidence and outcome on four studs in New South Wales. Austr. Vet. J., 75: 1, 56-59.

Vivrette, S.L., K. Young, S. Manning, P. Evans and D. Cross, 1998. Efficacy of Seramune in the treatment of failure of passive transfer in foals. Proceedings of the 44th Annual convention of the American association of equine practitioners. Baltimore, USA. 44:136-137.

Warner, D.D., 1983. Equine perinatal care, Part I: Prenatal care of the dam. Compend. Contin. Educ. Pract. Vet. 5 (7): S356-S361.

Warner, D.D. and W.E. Vaala, 1986. Management of the neonatal foal. Compend. Contin. Educ. Pract. Vet. 8 (2): S81-S94.

Energy and protein requirements and feeding of the suckling foal

W. Martin-Rosset[1] *and B. Younge*[2]
[1]*INRA, Department of Animal Science, Centre of Research of Clermont-Ferrand/Theix, 63122 Saint Genes Champanelle, France*
[2]*University of Limerick, Department of Life Sciences, Equine Science, Limerick, Ireland*

Abstract

Suckling foals have a very high growth rate. Body weight doubles between birth and first month of age and at weaning body weight is five times heavier than birth weight. A curvilinear growth model (X^{3}: age in days) fits the weight-age data. Similarly, body size rises quickly with withers height reaching 80% of adult height at weaning. This dynamic rate of growth dictates the nutrient requirements of the foal. Energy and protein intakes are the primary dietary components influencing growth. Mare's milk supplies the sole source of energy and protein for the suckling foal in the first weeks of life. Daily gain of the foal is linearly related to milk, energy and protein intake up to two months of age whereas grazing time increases linearly with age and body weight between birth and weaning. Gross energy and protein intake of the foal per metabolic body weight from milk at 1, 4 and 8 weeks of age are: 1.90 - 1.42 - 1.05 MJ GE and 21g - 14g- 12 g protein, respectively. NEm for maintenance would be 200kcal/kgBW$^{0.75}$ from birth to 4 months of age. NEg / kgBW gain/ kgBW$^{0.75}$ would rise from 85 to 110 kcal. NEm % ME would rise from 56 to 69 and NEg % ME would decrease from 44 to 31 between birth and 4 months. Feeding regimes of the mare during lactation (and the last trimester of pregnancy) play an important role in the early development of the foal (0-3 months) whereas the quantity and quality of grass and concentrate have a strong influence on foal growth between 3 months of age and weaning (at 6 months). Grass intake would represent 8-10% and 50-60% of total energy requirements during these periods. Creep feed intake before weaning plays an important role in maintaining daily gain pre and post weaning. Providing quality protein in the form of essential amino acids, particularly lysine and threonine is important. Type of carbohydrates (starch or other vs. lactose) is also of importance. Forage and concentrate management systems for young growing foals vary with breed, age, growth rate and forage quality. The objective when feeding foals is to optimise feed efficiency and maintain a steady rate of growth thus minimising DOD. Ensuring access to quality protein and a well-balanced intake of energy is key to achieving this.

Keywords: foal, growth, protein, energy, requirements, feeding

Introduction

The foal is the single product of the broodmare. The foal is born either very early in winter for race horses to be ready for training at 15 months of age or in spring for sport horses which compete at a later age. Nursing foals are subjected either to a long winter feeding period and then to grazing at 2-3 months of age or to early grazing when the foals are only 1 month old. The foals of the first group are weaned in early September at 150- 160 days while the other group of foals are weaned in late September or October at 180-200 days.

Among the farm animals the horse is an early maturing species which is born after 11 months of pregnancy and a short nursing period of six months. It can be compared to cattle, another herbivore, where pregnancy and the nursing periods are both nine months in duration.

The growth and development of the foal is very early and intensive while their physiology of digestion and metabolism move from the status of monogastric to a status of herbivore. As result growth and development of the foal are strongly influenced by feeding and management.

The aim of this review is to outline growth and the effect of factors of variation, the requirements and the feeding of the foal.

Growth

Body weight

The bodyweight (BW) of foals at birth ranges from 23 to 77kg depending on breed and it ranges from 7-13 percent of adult body weight (Table 1). Adult BW varies from 180 to 1100 kg depending on breed.

Bodyweight at birth can be predicted using the following model proposed by Gütte 1972:

$$BW_f=0.45BW_m0.75$$

Where:

BW_f = Body weight of the foal
BW_m = Metabolic body weight of the mare

At one and six months of age, BW of the foal averages 18-20 and 45-50 percent of the mare's BW. BW of the foal doubles birth weight during the first month, at six months BW is five times heavier than birth weight (Figure 1).

Table 1. Birth weight as a % of adult weight for different breeds (from the review of Martin-Rosset 1983).

Breed	Birth weight as % of adult weight
Heavy breeds	7-10
Sport horses	9-10
Thoroughbreds	10
Shetland	13

Growth models have been developed to predict the BW of the foals (BW_f) from age (t).
Martin Rosset *et al.* (1986) described a curvilinear growth model in heavy breeds from birth to 200 days of age using the following equation:

$$BW_f = 68.57+2.1217t -0.0066\, t^2+0.00001t^3\ (R^2=0.95).$$

Trillaud-Geyl *et al.* (1990) developed the following growth model for sport horse breeds from birth to 180 days of age:

$$BW_f = 57.18 + 1.465t - 0.0024\, t^2\ (R^2 = 0.89).$$

Kavazis and Ott (2003) developed a model for thoroughbreds from birth to 112 days of age:

$BW_f = 1.28t + 57.82$ ($R^2 = 0.94$).

Daily gain

Average daily gain (ADG) in the foal is very high during the first two months: 1500-2000g according to breed (Figure 1). ADG is closely linked to the mare's milk yield which peaks at 2 months (see the chapter by Doreau and Martuzzi 2006,in this issue). Then ADG ranges from 700-1000g until weaning with grass increasingly becoming the main nutrient supplier.

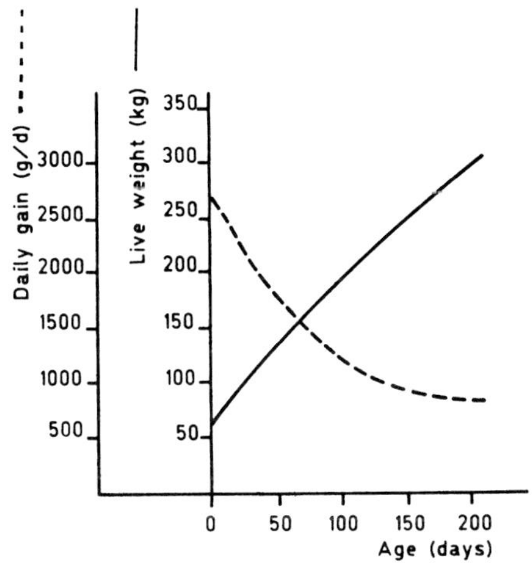

Figure 1. Live weight and daily gain in foals up to 200 days of age (from Martin-Rosset et al. 1986).

Body size

At birth withers height (HW) and thoracic perimeter (TP) in the horse accounts for 45 and 60 percent of adult values respectively (Dusek 1972) vs. 40 and 57 percent in cattle. At six months of age HW and TP reach 80 and 65 percent vs. 72 and 55 percent in cattle. Horses seem to be early maturing animals.

There is a good relationship between BW and some parameters of body size (BS). HW and TP were determined to be relevant parameters a number of years ago and different models were proposed to predict BW from these parameters (see the review of Martin-Rosset 1983). More recently however several models were suggested and these models are more specific to breed differences than the previous ones (Table 2).

Table 2. Prediction of BW of the weanling from body size parameters in horses.

Authors	Equations	Breed	Age
INRA 1990	BW = 4.5 TP – 370 ± 23	Light	6-48 months
	BW = 7.3 TP – 800 ±27	Heavy	6-30 months
ENVA 2000	BW = 0.204Age + 1.893HW+2.013TP – 333.9±16	TB, SB, SF	0-24 months
Santos *et al.* 2006	BW = 282.35TP – 190.58 ±9	Lusitanian	0- 4 months

TB: Thoroughbred; SB: Standarbred; SF: Selle Français

Factors of variation

Influence of the sex of the foal

The BW of colt foals at birth is 5 to 6 percent heavier than that of filly foals and colt foals maintain this advantage until 540 days (Hintz 1980- see review of Martin-Rosset 1983). In the thoroughbred (TB) Thompson *et al.* (1991) determined an average BW at 14 days of 81.8 kg for colts and 79.6 kg for fillies; and total weight gain through 182 days was 181.8 kg for colts and 173.5 kg for fillies. This difference would not be confirmed in heavy breeds by Martin-Rosset *et al.* (1986) and in light breeds by Trillaud-Geyl *et al.* (1990). BW of foals of heavy breeds at birth was: 65.8 ±8.8 kg for males and 66.2 ±5.8 kg for females and at weaning: 321 ±40.3 kg at 193 ±31 kg and 332.4 ±47.8 kg at 198 ±26 days respectively. BW at birth of light breeds (Selle Français, Anglo-Arab) was: 52.7 ±7.1kg for males and 51.1 ±5.9 kg for females and at weaning: 240.1 ±36.8kg for males and 233.7 ±32.4kg respectively.

The influence of sex on the evolution of body size (BS) would take place later than one year of age (Marcq *et al.* 1956, Brezsky and Tyzowsky 1964,Green 1969, Grabowsky *et al.* 1971, Heird 1973).

Influence of body weight at birth on growth

ADG of the foal from birth to weaning is significantly related to BW at birth, but the correlation is weak: $R = 0.51$; $P < 0.05$; $n = 31$ in heavy breeds (Martin-Rosset et al 1986);or in light breeds $R=0.55$ $P<0.01$; $n=94$ (Trillaud-Geyl et al 1990).

Influence of the age of the mare at foaling

BW of foals at birth is 2 to 7 kg lower in progeny from primiparous compared to multiparous mares. The BW at birth would be at maximum in progeny born from 6 – 7 year old mares (see review of Martin-Rosset 2004). ADG of foals in early lactation is on average 200g lower in progeny from primiparous mares compared to multiparous mares when both group of mares are fed the same diet *ad libitum* (Table 3).

Table 3. Comparison of ADG of progeny from primiparous (at 5 years) and multiparous (over 6 years) mares of light breed (Selle Français and Anglo Arabian: 522 ± 29 Kg BW at foaling) fed ad libitum the same hay based diet:90 percent hay-10 percent concentrate (from Doreau et al 1991).

	Primiparous	Multiparous
Body weight at foaling (kg)	510	529
Dry matter intake (week 4)		
kg/day	17.8	17.5
Kg/100kg BW	3.36	3.27
Milk yield (kg/d)	14.6	16.6
Milk output		
Fat (g/day)	239	331
Crude protein (g/day)	311	344
Lactose (g/d)	928	1057
Gross energy (MJ/day)	31.0	38.1
ADG of the foals (g/day)	1200± 177	1400± 127

There is a close relationship between milk energy output and foal weight (r= 0.74) and milk energy and foal growth during the first month (r= 0.74).

Influence of the breed

The BW of foals at birth of heavy breeds is heavier than that of light breed: 67 vs. 53 kg on average. Subsequently, ADG of the foals from birth to weaning is higher in heavy breeds than in light breeds: 1300-1600 g vs. 900 – 1100 g. ADG of the foal is linked to adult BW (see the review of Martin-Rosset 1983).

The evolution of body size (BS) is earlier in warmblood breeds than in cold bloods, namely the heavy breeds (Marcq *et al.* 1956, Heird 1973) and in the warmbloods the Arab breed is later than the TB (Grabowsky *et al.* 1971). However, the genetic effect should be weighted using the maternal BS because the genetic effect linked *sensu stricto* of the stallion would represent only 70 percent of that of the mare (Langlois 1973).

Relationships with milk intake and grazing

Daily gain of the foal is linearly related to milk intake up to two months of age whereas grazing time increases linearly with age and BW between birth and weaning (Martin-Rosset *et al.* 1978 and Doreau *et al.* 1986a). The correlation between milk intake and ADG decreases with foal age. Milk intake of the foal per kg daily gain would be: 10.6 ±0.9 and 13.7 ±1.7 for weeks 1-4 and 4-8, respectively. Models have been developed during these two periods (Doreau *et al.* 1986a):

Milk yield (kg/day) = 10.6 x ADG foal (kg/day)	R= 0.81	1st month
Milk Yield (kg/day) = 13.7 x ADG foal (kg /day)	R= 0.74	2nd month

Grazing time increases linearly with age while sucking intensity decreases (Figure 2). The number of times the foals suckles the mare can be described by the following model (where *t* =age in days) (Martin Rosset *et al.* (1978):

$y=-0.21 \log t + 56.37$ R= -0.84 n=150

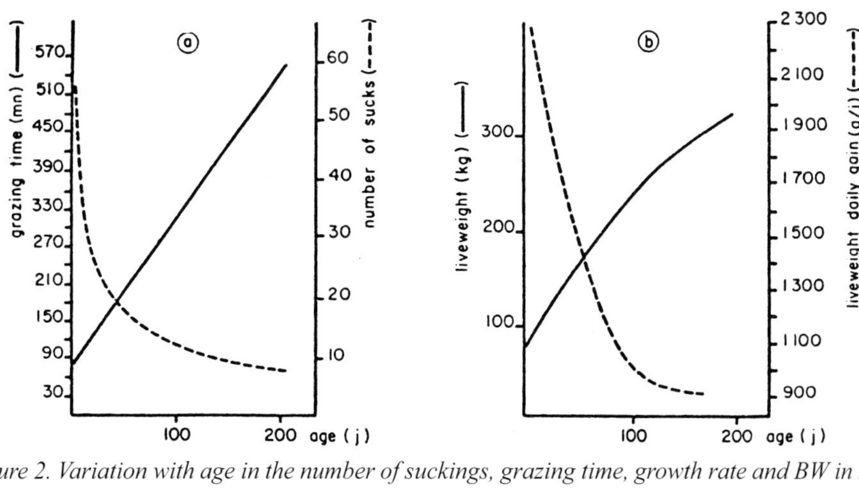

Figure 2. Variation with age in the number of suckings, grazing time, growth rate and BW in heavy foals (from Martin-Rosset et al. 1978).

The length of time the foal spends grazing can be described using the following model (Martin-Rosset et al 1978):

$$y = 2.28\,t + 69.22 \qquad R = 0.82 \quad n = 150$$

$$y = 1.79\,BW - 100.99 \qquad R = 0.85 \quad n = 150$$

As a result the foal's growth decreases curvilinearly according to the model described by Martin-Rosset *al.* 1986 due the substitution of milk by grass as a nutrient supplier (Figure 2).

Effect of date of birth relative to the date of turn out

The effect of date of foaling on BW and ADG of the foal is controversial. Hintz *et al.* 1979 and Jones and Holland 2005 reported that TB foals born in very early winter (January- March) were lighter at weaning, whereas Pagan *et al.* 1996 did not observe any difference.

Two groups of foals of heavy breeds born 15 days before: early group (EG) and after: late group (LG) turn out date was compared. BW at birth was not different: 66.3 ± 8.7 kg and 68.5 ± 7.3 kg in the EG and LG, respectively (Figure 3). ADG of the foals born in winter (EG) during the first month is high: 1800 to 1900 g, as high in winter as in early spring when the foals are at pasture. The ADG of EG is lower than ADG of foals born in spring (LG) during the first month: 1850 vs. 2000g respectively. When the BW of the two groups of the same type – age is compared, there is no difference (Table 4). This conclusion is confirmed by recent data obtained in TB's in Kentucky by Pagan 2006 (in this issue).

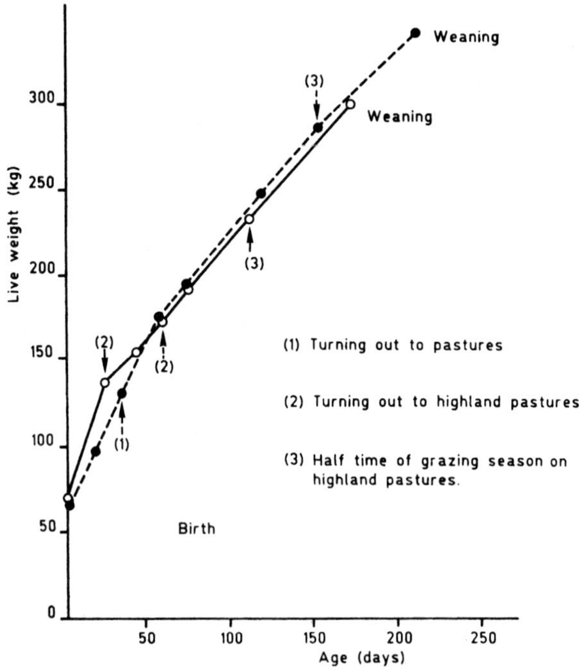

Figure 3. Variation of body weight in foals born before or after turning out (from Martin-Rosset et al. 1986).

Table 4. Body weight and average daily gain of the foal at standard ages (from Martin-Rosset et al. 1986).

	Born before turn out to pasture (n=19)	Born after turn out to pasture (n=12)
Live weight (kg)		
Birth weight	63.3±7.3	69.9±5.7
30 days	126.3±12.2	129.9±13.1
45 days	152.5±14.7	154.5±16.0
90 days	217.3±19.4	213.1±19.7
180 days	310.6±25.9	313.3*±18.4
Daily gain g/d		
0-1 months	2098±286	1999±349
0-3 months	1710±173	1591±183
1-3 months	1516±140	1388±137
3-6 months	1036±167	1117*±191
0-6 months	1373±117	1341*±97

*(n=6)

It is well established that milk yield is enhanced by an increase in energetic allowances (see the chapters Doreau and Martuzzi 2006; and Martin-Rosset *et al.* 2006b in this issue). In Spring grazing mares are fed *ad libitum,* whereas in winter mares are fed to meet their requirements only. It has been hypothesised that extra energy intake over requirements is partitioned between an increase in milk yield and BW gain of the mares (e.g. body reserves) from the work of Doreau *et al.* 1981 and 1993.

Requirements

Body composition

Body tissue composition has been determined after slaughtering by total anatomical dissection (Table 5). Between birth and six months of age the proportion of bone decreases by 13.3 points (41 percent), adipose tissue increases by 2.5 points (27 percent) whereas muscles proportion increases by 10.8 points (18 percent only). This means that the relative growth of adipose tissue to total empty BW is much higher than the relative growth of muscle and bone as it is well established after weaning. Deposition of fat is a rather early process after birth in equines.

The chemical composition of the foal at birth has been determined by chemical analysis of the total body (Table 6).

Table 5. Proportion of different tissues in empty body of the foal of heavy breeds (from Martin-Rosset 1983 and 2004).

Age Months	Body weight (kg)	p100 adult BW	Carcass weight (kg)	Bones p100	Muscles p100	Adipose p100
Foetus -8 mo	23.5	3.1	13.2	41.1	57.3	1.6
0	61.5	8.1	37.4	31.7	59.0	9.3
6	319.0	40.1	186.4	18.4	69.8	11.8

Table 6. Chemical composition of the foal at birth: per kg fresh material (Meyer and Alshwede 1976).

Water	727 g	Phosphorus	9.7 g
Calcium	18.2 g	Magnesium	0.38 g
Energy	5.48 MJ	Potassium	1.9 g
Protein	171 g	Chlorine	1.2 g
Fat	26 g	Iron	120 mg
Ash	56g	Copper	5.0 mg

The chemical composition of the foal has been determined too by Doreau *et al.* 1986 at 1– 4 – 8 weeks of age using the dilution of deuterium oxide as a marker of foal body water according to Doreau and Dussap 1980 (Table 7). The lipid content in empty body increased greatly between weeks 1 and 8 whereas the protein content remained constant.

Using the data from Meyer and Alshwede (1976) and Doreau *et al.* 1986 it is apparent that water content would decrease by 6 points (9 percent) from birth to 2 months of age, lipid content increases strongly by 6 points (345 percent) and protein content only by 2.8 points (16 percent).

Table 7. Chemical composition of empty body weight during the first weeks of age (from Doreau et al. 1986).

	Foal age (weeks)		
Week No	1	4	8
Empty LW (kg)	79.2	125.4	173.0
Empty body composition %			
Water	70.3	68.3	66.6
Lipid	5.3	6.5	9.0
Protein	19.2	19.9	19.9

Metabolism

Foal Nutrient Intake

The nutrient intake of the foal varies with the chemical composition of the milk and with the diet composition and feeding level of the mare. Doreau *et al.* (1986) examined the effect of three dietary regimes on heavy bred mares (weighing on average 800 kg) during the first two months of nursing. The diets of the mares consisted of the following: group 1a received 95% of a 2nd cut tall fescue hay and 5% concentrate (93% SBM), group 1b received 50% of the same hay and 50% concentrate (83% barley and 12% SBM) group 2 received 85% 1st cut natural grassland hay and 15% concentrate (50% barley and 45% SBM). The milk production and composition data are shown in Figure 4.

Milk yield and composition were different between the three groups. Lactose and energy intake per day increased while fat intake decreased and protein intake remained constant. On average the nutrient intake of the foals per kg BW $^{0.75}$ decreased with the week of lactation, irrespective of the mare's diet by 50.5 – 41.7 – 31.5g of lactose: 20.6 – 14.4 – 11.5g of protein; 15.4 – 9.8 – 6.0g of fat and 453 – 339 – 250 kcal of gross energy.

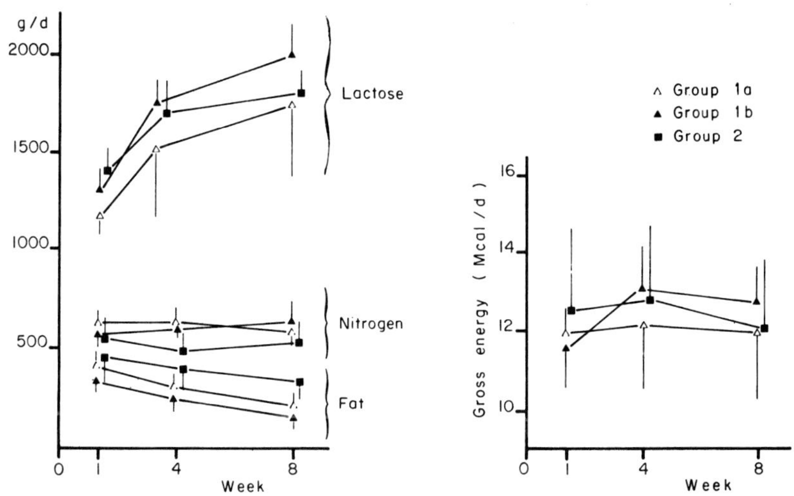

Figure 4. Quantity of foal nutrient intake (mean ±SE) (from Doreau et al 1986).

The foals intake of milk, gross energy (GE) and protein per kg daily gain (ADG) increases during the first two months of nursing (Table 8). The amount of GE and protein intake can be predicted using the following models:

GE (Mcal/day) = 5.8 x ADG R = 0.78 (1-4 weeks) P< 0.01
GE (Mcal/day) = 6.5 x ADG R = 0.68 (4-8 weeks) P< 0.01

Protein (g/day) = 258 x ADG R = 0.74 (1-4 weeks) P< 0.01
Protein g/day) = 292 x ADG R = 0.61 (4-8 weeks) P< 0.01

However, there was no correlation between ADG and milk energy/ protein ratio. The strength of the relationship decreases with age of the foal; this is likely because of the increasing proportion of maintenance requirements and due to the intake of small amounts of grass as grazing time becomes more significant at one month of age (Martin-Rosset et 1978).

Table 8. Intake in foals per kg daily gain (from Doreau et al 1986).

	Intake/kg daily gain	
Week no	1-4	4-8
Milk kg	10.6±0.9	13.7±1.7
GE Mcal	5.8±0.5	6.5±0.7
Protein g	258±27	292±34

Energy metabolism

We can gain a better understanding of foal metabolism by comparing the volume of oxygen consumed to the volume of carbon dioxide produced on a particular diet during a defined period of time. These volumes will change depending on the energy source the foal is using. Vermorel *et al.* (1987) examined heat production in young foals of heavy breed and energy balances at 83 and

132 days of age. At 83 days of age the foal was given a milk substitute only and heat production increased by 5% after each meal. The foal's respiratory quotient increased from 0.82 to 0.96 after the morning meal. At 132 days of age when hay and concentrate were added to the foals diet containing milk replacer heat production increased by 12% after the first meal and 20% after the second meal. Based on the energy balance of the foal during the different periods it can be concluded that the foal requires 2.6 Mcal NE/kg BW gain at 83 days of age with a BW of 203 kg and 3.4 Mcal NE/kg BW gain at 132 days of age and a BW 284kg. The breakdown between NE, ME and GE at both periods is shown in Table 9.

Similar NE requirements are confirmed by Ousey *et al.* (2006). Foals at 4 days of age with a BW of 52.9 kg and gaining 1.457 kg /day had an NE requirement of 2.1 Mcal/kg BW gain. Efficiency of utilization of NE for growth and maintenance for these foals are estimated and shown in the Table 9

Using the data from Vermorel *et al.* 1987 and Ousey 2006 it appears that energy requirements for maintenance from birth to 4 months of age would average 200kcal NE / Kg BW0.75 and NEm % ME would range from 56 to 69. Energy cost of one kg BW gain would rise by 161 percent from 4 days (2.1 Mcal/kg BW gain) to 132 days (3.4 Mcal/BW gain) of age which is consistent with the tremendous increase in fat content of empty BW: 345 percent and lipid retention estimated to be 184 g and 265 g at 1 and 2 months of age by Doreau *et al.* 1986. However, NEg % ME would decrease from 31 to 43. If energy cost per kg ADG is expressed in respect of metabolic weight to allow for the difference of breeds used by Vermorel *et al.* 1987 (heavy breed) and Ousey 2006 (light breed), energy cost would range from 110 (at 4 days) to 85 (at 132 days) kcal /BW0.75 / Kg BW gain. At weaning energy cost, estimated in heavy breeds is 4.4 NE Mcal/ kg BW gain using the nutritional model performed at INRA for heavy breeds from feeding experiments by Agabriel *et al.* 1984. Net energy cost Kg $BW^{0.75}$ / kg BW gain would be: 57 at 180 days. Net energy cost would vary according to a curvilinear model with daily gain as its has been stated after weaning in heavy and light breeds using the appropriate nutritional models designed for each breed by INRA (Martin-Rosset et al 1994). But the slope would be negative before weaning as ADG decrease while fat content of daily gain increase slowly whereas the slope is positive after weaning as daily gain is steadily high and fat content of daily gain increase strongly.

Table 9. Energy balance in nursing foals.

	4 days[1] 53 kg BW	83 days[2] 203kg BW	132 days[2] 284kg BW
GE (Kcal/Kg/d)	137	76	96
ME (Kcal/Kg/d)	135	65	70
ME % GE	98	86	73
NEm (Kcal/Kg/d)	76	41	48
NEm % ME	56	63	69
NEg (Kcal/Kg/d)	59	24	22
NEg % ME	44	37	31

[1]from Ousey 2006: TB breed (n=5)

[2]from Vermorel *et al.* 1987: heavy breed (n=1)

GE: Gross energy; ME: Metabolisable Energy; NE: Net Energy; m: maintenance; g: growth; d: day; BW: Body Weight

Protein metabolism

The protein content in empty body increases slightly between weeks 1 and 8 after birth: less than one point i.e. 4 percent (Table 5). However, protein retention is very high. During weeks 1-4, after birth 446 g protein would be retained per day and during weeks 4-8, foals would retain 342 g protein per day. The composition of weight gain would show a greater deposition of protein than of lipids until 8 weeks: 1-3 to 2.4 times respectively (Doreau *et al.* 1986). Therefore it could be suggested that protein supply more than energy supply would limit foal growth during the first month where protein retention is at maximum. It is clearly highlighted in experiments where the foals were fed different protein levels whereas the foals were fed to meet energy requirements (Hintz et al 1971, Borton et al 173).

Variation in energy for maintenance and growth requirements

The total energy requirements (maintenance and growth) of the foal continues to rise as BW, ADG and fat content of BW gain increases after weaning (Martin-Rosset et al 1994). We could assume the same general variation before weaning as the total energy requirement increases also (Vermorel *et al.* 1987 and Ousey 2006). However, ADG decreases by 2 times whereas: fat content of empty body BW increases by 1.7 times, fat deposition rises by 1.4 times and BW elevates by 5 times before weaning. So far energy requirements for maintenance would increase likely more than requirement for growth from birth to weaning. However we must bear in mind that protein retention is very high in the suckling foal. This process costs energy as it is well known that protein synthesis is linked to BW gain and to protein and energy allowances, both have an additive effect (Reeds and Fuller 1983). It has been shown from the data of Vermorel *et al.* 1987 and Ousey 2006 that an increase of energy cost per Kg BW gain of 1.6 Mcal NE is consistent. The absolute NE_g for growth increases by 1.7 times and the absolute NE_m for maintenance rises by 3 times between 4 and 132 days. However, the proportion of energy requirement for growth in total requirements would decrease from 43 to 31 percent as BW gain decreases with age whereas the proportion of maintenance requirement would increase from 57 to 69 percent. Corresponding to these energy requirements the nutrient intake from grass increases while that of milk decreases. From birth to three months of age and then until weaning grass intake would represent 8-10 and 50-60% of total energy intake respectively.

Energy requirements and allowances of the suckling foal

In the NRC 1989 system energy requirements for maintenance and growth of the suckling foal are calculated by using the following equation performed from experimental data obtained in yearlings (Householder *et al.* 1977; Milligan *et al.* 1985; Ott and Asquith 1986; Schryver *et al.* 1987; Scott *et al.* 1987):

$$DE\ (Mcal/day) = (maintenance\ DE) + (4.81 + 1.17\ t - 0.23\ t^{2})\ ADG$$

Where

t: age in months
maintenance DE=
DE= 1.4 + 0.03 BW (for horses 200-600 kg BW)
DE= 1.82 + 0.0383 BW – 0.000015 BW^2 (for horses greater than 600 kg BW)
ADG= Average Daily Gain (kg)

The energy requirements calculated using this model for the foal of 4 and 6 months of age is provided in Table 10.

In the GEH 1994 system energy the requirements of the suckling foal have been estimated between 3 and 6 months of age. The total requirements are broken down into maintenance and growth requirements. Maintenance requirements are calculated using daily maintenance requirement and are calculated using the following relationship:

$$DE_m = 0.6 \text{ MJ/kg BW}^{75}$$

based on Hoffman *et al.* (1967), Knox *et al.* (1970), Wooden *et al.* (1970), Argenzio and Hintz (1971), Barth *et al.* (1977). An extra 20 percent more energy is added to maintenance requirements to allow for the effect of exercise. Thus energy requirements for maintenance are 253 Mcal/kg $BW^{0.75}$.

Energy requirements for growth are calculated from the composition of BW gain (experimental data?) assuming an efficiency of DE of 60 percent established in other farm animals (Menke and Huss 1980). The total energy requirements are calculated between 3 and 6 months of age (Table 10).

No energy requirements have yet been calculated in the INRA system due to a lack of sufficient data. However, allowances have been recently determined in the scope of an experiment where two models of growth were studied from birth to one year of age (Donabedian *et al.* 2006). Energy allowances have been estimated between birth and 2 months of age using the relationship between ADG and milk yield, conducted by Doreau *et al.* 1986 and the GE content of milk determined during the experiment. The energy allowances between 3 and 6 months of age have been interpolated between those determined at 2 months of age and those calculated at 7 months of age using INRA 1990 models performed for weanlings (Martin-Rosset et al 1994). The foals energy intake were controlled until 12 months of age (Donabedian et al 2006) (Table 10).

Table 10. Energy and protein requirements at various age categories using different energy systems.

Systems	Age (months)	ADG[1] (g/d)	Energy (Mcal/d)	Protein (g/d)
NRC 1989	4	850	14.4 DE[2]	720 CP[4]
	6	650	15.0 DE	750 CP
INRA[7]	0-2	1159-1508	7.7-9.9 NE[3]	300-380 MADC[6]
INRA[7]	3-6	747-1085	9.5-12.8 NE	450-700 MADC
GEH 1994	3-6	820	15.1 DE	580 DCP[5]

[1]ADG: Average Daily Gain
[2]DE: Digestible energy
[3]NE: Net Energy (INRA 1990)
[4]CP: Crude Protein
[5]DCP: Digestible Crude protein
[6]MADC: Horse Digestible Crude Protein (Matières Azotées Digestibles Cheval, INRA 1990)
[7]Experimental data from Donabedian *et al.* 2006

Protein requirements

In the NRC system the protein requirements of the suckling foal is related to energy requirements in the weanling (Wirth *et al.* 1977;Meakim 1979; Ott and Asquith 1983) and in the yearling (Ott *et al.* 1979; Gibbs *et al.* 1987; Potter and Huchton 1975; Scott *et al.* 1987). Based on these data CP requirements were calculated to be 50g/ Mcal DE in the weanling. Using this ratio protein requirements are proposed in Table 10.

In the GEH system protein requirements of the suckling foal have been estimated between 3 and 6 months of age. The total requirements are divided between maintenance and growth requirements. Maintenance requirements are calculated using daily maintenance requirement and are calculated using the following relationship:

$DCP_m = 3g\ DCP/kg\ BW^{75}$

based on Olsson and Ruudvere 1955, Teeter *et al.* 1967 and Slade *et al.* 1975. As the protein requirements for maintenance are related to energy requirements, the protein requirements are 5.3g / kg $BW^{0.75}$ for maintenance.

Protein requirements for growth are calculated from the composition of BW gain assuming an efficiency of 65 percent for the DCP supplied by milk (0-2 months) and 35 percent for solid feed (3-6 months) established in other farm animals. The total energy requirements are calculated between 3 and 6 months of age (Table 10).

In the INRA systems no protein requirements are estimated. But protein allowances have been determined in the scope of an experiment (Donabedian *et al.* 2006). Using the same approach as for energy, protein allowances have been determined between 0 and 2 months and 3 and 6 months of age (Table 11).

Lysine, threonine and methionine content of milk is high (Table 11). Lysine would be the first limiting amino acid from the experimental data of Breuer and Golden 1971; Hintz *et al.* 1971 carried out in early weaned foals; Potter and Huchton et al 1975; Ott et al 1979, 1981 and 1986 conducted in yearlings. The lysine requirements would range 2.1- 2.3 g/Mcal DE/day (NRC 1989 and Saatamoinen and Koskinen 1993). These requirements would be supported by more recent data obtained in weanlings and yearlings (Graham *et al.* 1994; Colemenan *et al.* 1997; Staniar *et al.* 1999). Theronine would be another limiting amino acid according to the preliminary experimental data of Ott *et al.* 2001 and 0.1% per kg dry matter of concentrate supplement would be suggested. There is no experimental data for methionine. However, GEH 1994 suggest that as the optimal ratio between lysine and methionine is 1:0.6 an allowance of 0.07g/ Mcal DE/day would be relevant.

Table 11. Amino acid composition of milk and amino acid requirements at 4 months of age.

	Amino acid composition in the milk[1] g/ 16N/ kg milk (1–8 weeks)	Amino acids requirements[2] g/day at 4 months of age (500kg adult BW)
Lysine	7.95 – 8.10	30
Threonine	4.65 – 4.40	??
Methionine	2.80 – 2.85	??

[1]Doreau *et al.* 1986, 1989 and 1990
[2]NRC 1989

Allowances and feeding

Effect of milk yield or/and composition (0-2 months)

Milk composition is affected by the composition of the diet, feeding level and intake and the mare's body condition (see the chapter by Doreau and Martuzzi 2006 in this issue for extended details). Milk yield increases with dry matter intake, proportion of concentrate in the diet, feeding on *ad libitum* basis and to some extent by body condition score. Milk fat and protein concentrations are higher in mares fed a diet with a low proportion of concentrate whereas lactose concentration is higher when the diet contains a high proportion of concentrate. Protein content of milk is lower in mares fed under their requirements. Milk from overweight mares has a higher fat content than milk from thin mare: the reverse is found for protein. As a result milk output and related growth of the foals are affected by nutrient intake and body reserves of the mares.

ADG of the foal decreases by 11 percent when the crude protein allowances of the mare are restricted by 40 percent as the crude protein content and namely the protein content of the milk are reduced by 25 and 30 percent respectively. But the difference is not maintained any longer while the mares are fed the adequate nitrogen allowances (Table 12).

Table 12. Effect of protein allowances in nursing mares of heavy breeds fed isoenergetic diet on mare and foal performances (from Doreau et al., 1988).

	HL[1]	LL[2]
Number of mares	10	10
Body weight (kg) (at foaling)	743	743
Energy intake (UFC/d)	10.38	10.77
Protein intake (gMADC/d)	1291[1]	805[2]
Milk composition (g/kg)		
Crude protein	21.65**	16.69**
Non protein nitrogen x 6.38	2.41**	1.93**
Protein	19.24**	14.76**
Average daily gain of foals (g/d)		
0 – 30 d	1923	1706
0 – 160 d	1640	1631
Mare body weight		
0 – 30 d (kg/d)	- 0.213	- 0.203
Plasma urea of the mare (mg/100 ml)	41.6**	25.1**

[1]HL: 100 percent protein requirements (INRA, 1984)
[2]LL: 60 percent protein requirements (INRA, 1984)

ADG of the foal is limited by 8 to 13 percent when body condition of the mare is low at foaling, even if the mares are fed according to their requirements in early lactation. However, this limitation is not maintained as soon as the mares restore their body condition. In addition ADG of the foal at weaning shows no difference (Table 13).

Effect of grazing

ADG of foals of light breeds (Selle Français and Anglo arabian) was monitored during 10 years at the National stud in France (Trillaud-Geyl *et al.* 1990). The mares and the foals were managed according to breeding, feeding and farming system this is described in the Figure 5. All the foals were born after turn out.

ADG of the foals averaged 1046 ±129g at 181 ±21 days. ADG was 1230 ±210g from birth to 3 months and 850 ±146g between 3 and 6 months. The growth of the foals was not affected by winter feeding of the pregnant mares: hay vs. maize silage based diets supplemented adequately to meet their requirements. The ADG of the foals was influenced by the subsequent vegetative cycles of

Table 13. Effect of body reserves at foaling on weight gain of the foals (from Martin-Rosset and Doreau, 1980).

Years of experiments	1978		1979	
Mares	HL	LL	HL	LL
Level of energy intake in pregnancy[1]	100	80	100	80
Number of mares at foaling	10	7	12	12
Level of energy intake in lactation[1]	100	100	100	100
Variation of Body weight (1st month) (kg)	+ 2	+ 28	+ 24	+ 41
Foals				
Date (days)	14/4 (± 23)	12/4 (± 18)	13/4 (± 13)	17/4 (± 24)
Birth Body weight/kg	63.6 (± 5.9)	70.3 (± 7.7)	63.3 (± 5.8)	65.3 (± 5.5)
0-1 month	1991 (± 619)	1741 (± 411)	1793 (± 394)	1656 (± 345)
Growth (g/day) (Birth to Weaning)	1511 (± 186)	1539 (± 95)	1480 (± 163)	1472 (± 156)

[1]Relative to nutrient requirement (NRC, 1978)
HL: High Level
LL: Low Level

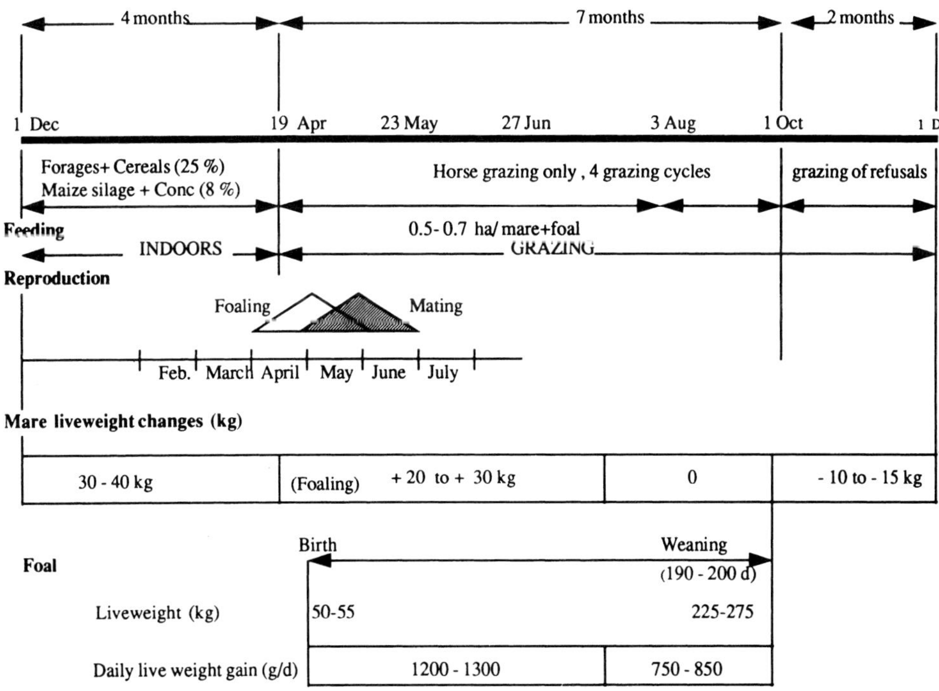

Figure 5. Management of a herd of mares of sports breeds (Selle Français and Anglo Arabian) during 10 years in grassland temperate zone (Centre West in France) (adapted by Micol and Martin-Rosset 1995 from Trillaud –Geyl et al 1990).

grazing. ADG over the four subsequent grazing cycles were: 1771 ±428g at 28 ±16 days (1st cycle); 1474 ±283g at 56 ±25 days (2nd cycle); 1228 ±204g at 93 ±25 days (3rd cycle); 1165 ±167g at 136 ±32 days (4th cycle). In spring ADG of the foals was enhanced during the first two cycles since ADG is directly related to the mare's milk yield. In addition the mare's milk yield is likely to be increased brought about by mare's increased intake of spring grass compared to the intake of mares fed at the trough.

Effect of supplementation

At approximately 10 to 12 weeks of age, the growth rate and nutrient requirement of most foals will exceed the level of energy and protein provided by both the mare's milk and grass intake. The best way to compensate for this difference is to supply creep feed. Energy source and protein quality of creep feed are critical. Few studies have compared various feed ingredients to include in creep feed for foals. ADG of the foals supplemented with milk products was 33 to 48 percent higher than with linseed meal as nitrogen retention is 10 to 22 percent higher (Table 14)

Table 14. A comparison of different feed ingredients and quantities of crude protein for creep feed use (from Hintz et al 1971).

Diet	N retained/N absorbed	ADG (g/day
10% milk products	70.8	560
20% milk products	63.8	620
15% Linseed meal	58.2	420
15% Linseed meal+0.5% lysine	68.7	580

When linseed meal was supplemented with 0.5% lysine ADG increased by 160g per day compared to linseed meal with no amino acid supplementation. The proportion of nitrogen retained was also higher on the amino acid supplemented treatment.

ADG of foals supplemented with milk products was again 27 to 46 percent higher than with soyabean meal (SBM) whatever the proportion of inclusion in the concentrate (Table 15).

Table 15. A comparison of different sources and quantities of protein on ADG and intake per Kg gain in foal s (from Borton et al 1973).

Diet	ADG (g/d)	Kg DM/kg gain
14% Soya	600	4.06
22% Soya	650	3.96
14% Skimmed milk	760	3.53
22% Skimmed milk	950	3.09

Providing the foal with its energy and protein requirements from creep feed not only prevents problems upon weaning but also aids towards preventing developmental orthopaedic disease (DOD) subsequently. DOD is increasing in both sport horses and racehorses, rapid growth rates in foals and related feed allowances and/or diet composition have been implicated (Kronefeld *et al.* 1990, Glade and Belling 1984, Savage *et al.* 1993, Jeffcott and Davies 1998, McIlwraith 2001). The early age before weaning would be a sensitive period to predispose to DOD (Dik *et al.* 1999) as the incidence of DOD considering all radiographic lesions examined by X-ray average 67 percent in the examined population of foals (Robert *et al.* 2005, Donabedian *et al.* 2006).

Donabedian *et al.* 2006 examined the effects of two balanced feeding levels on growth and some development parameters of sport horses during their first postnatal year. In this study foals were allocated to two dietary regimes; a moderate feeding level (ML) and a high feeding level (HL) (Table 16). On the ML group the foals received 100% of INRA recommendations. The foals on the HL group received 130 percent (until 2 months of age) and 150 percent (between 2 months of age and weaning and subsequently) of nutrients of the ML group. The foals were supplemented with a concentrate consisting of lactoserum, SBM, oil, other grains and minerals. ADG and HW were significantly higher for foals on the HL treatment than the foals ML during all time periods (Table 16). It was concluded from this study that plasticity of body size and bone development is under the influence of nutrient intake and that this can be related to daily gain and corresponding feed allowances. This influence might be detrimental after weaning when the foals are fed to achieve the maximum of growth and development mainly when allowances are unbalanced and/ or proportion of starch in the diet is too high.

Table 16. ADG and withers height in foals on high and medium feed intakes (from Donabedian et al. 2006).

Age months	ADG (g/d)		Withers Height (mm/d)	
	ML[1]	HL[2,3,]	ML[1]	HL[2,3]
0-2	1159±173	1508±124	0.24±0.03	0.27±0.04
3-6	747±142	1085±100	0.13±0.02	0.15±0.01
0-6	873±29	1254±25	1.58±0.07	1.90±0.07

[1]ML: 100percent of INRA 1990 recommendations
[2]HL: 130 percent of ML from 0 to 2 months of age
[3]HL: 150 percent of ML from 3 to 6 months of age

Effect of age at weaning and feeding of the foal at weaning

Two groups of foals were subjected to early (EW) or normal (NW) weaning: 4.5 vs. 6 months of age respectively. BW of the foals at 7 months of NW group was 4 percent lower than that of EW group (Figure 6). There was no difference observed for withers height. However, cannon circumference was depressed in EW group between 4.5 until 7 months (Figure 7). Medial bone density was 5 percent greater at 140 days of age ($P < 0.05$) in the NW group compared to the EW group. The difference was no longer observed after 140 days. No difference was observed in the medullary bone density between the two groups. Lateral bone density was 6 percent greater at 140 and 161 days of age in the NW group compared to the EW group ($P < 0.05$). Early weaning would limit slightly body weight and body size achieved at 7 months and ossification could be temporarily depressed before 7 months.

Supplementation of the nursing foal

Supplementation of the suckling foal depends on the goal of production i.e. race/sport horses or leisure horses. The foal devoted to be an athlete should be supplemented before weaning as the goal is to meet a high BW and BS to compete intensively at an early age. For sport horses the goal is to compete intensively for a long number of years.

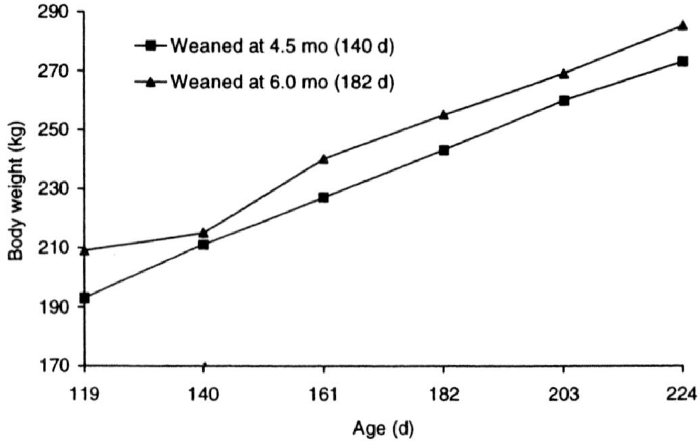

Figure 6. Comparison of BW between foals weaned at 4.5 months and 6 months of age (from Warren et al., 1998).

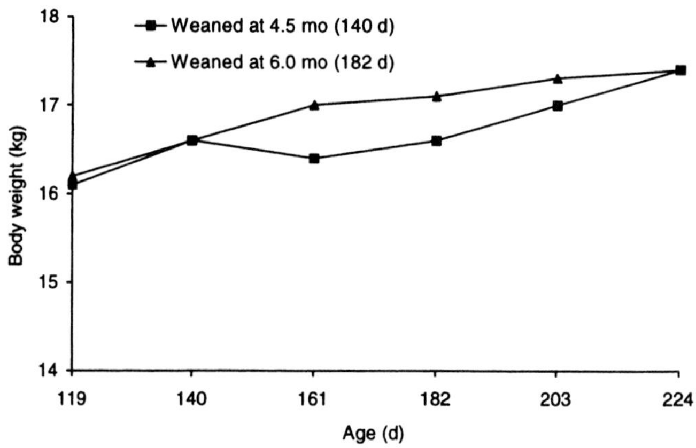

Figure 7. Comparison of cannon circumference (left MCIII) between foals weaned at 4.5 and 6 months of age (from Warren et al 1998).

Supplementation is implemented at 3 months of age when milk yield decreases and growth of the foal is increasingly dependent on solid feed, grass which should be of a high nutritive value (see the chapters by Miraglia *et al.* 2006, Pagan 2006 in this issue) or concentrates fed as creep feed. The added advantage of creep feeding is to accustom the foal to solid feed and to limit the stress effect of weaning (Mc Call *et al.* 1985; Hoffman *et al.* 1995).

Quantity, composition and nutritive value of the concentrate is of large concern when raising a healthy yearling as the suckling period is a sensitive step for preventing the occurrence of orthopaedic diseases (DOD). The occurrence of DOD is strongly related to high growth (BW and BS) and/or to an unbalanced ration (protein/energy; Ca/P; Co/Zn; Vit A/Vit D) and concentrate composition (carbohydrate: type and proportion).

Between 0.5 to 2.0 kg DM/ 100kg BW of concentrate are offered to the nursing foal depending on the age, breed: race vs. sport and the composition of the concentrate. Fat and fibre-rich feeds have several advantages to starch and sugar rich feeds. Fat and fibre-rich concentrates would limit high glycaemic peaks and related responses to insulin (and thyroxine, triiodothyronine hormones and insulin like growth factor) that would increase the risk of developing DOD (Staniar *et al.* 2001, Staniar unpublished, quoted by Harris 2005). The fat /high fibre concentrate would stimulate the immune system as the concentrations of IgA, IgG would be higher (Swanson *et al.* 2003). In addition such concentrate would help to improve behaviour conditions at weaning (Nicol et al 2005).

The total daily requirements expressed per kg DM that should be provided are: 2.90 Mcal DE and 14.5% CP; 0.6% lysine, 0.5% threonine, 0.68% calcium, 0.38% phosphorus; 0.08% magnesium; 1580 IU Vitamin A (NRC 1989, Ott 2001). The concentrate should be formulated in respect of these requirements. Energy sources should be diversified to prevent the occurrence of DOD related to excess of starch. In addition, starch from grain should be limited and fat and/or milk by products should be used (Davison et al 1989, Donabedian et al 2006)

Two groups of 20 foals were fed either a moderate (ML) or high (HL) level of allowances balanced according to INRA recommendations from birth to weaning and subjected to X-Ray examination at 5.5 months (Donabedian *et al.* 2006). HL group was supplemented from 2 months of age with 1.5kg DM of a creep feed designed specifically for this experiment. The composition of the concentrate was: 40% ultrafiltrate of lactoserum, 6.5% soya oil, 12% casein, 30% barley, 10% wheat fine, 1.5% minerals and vitamins. ADG of the HL group was much higher than of ML group (Figure 8). However there was no significant increase in lesions observed in HL Groups.

Protein sources such as milk products, soyabean meal, peanut, and sunflower cakes should be selected due to their favourable amino acid content, namely lysine, threonine and methionine.

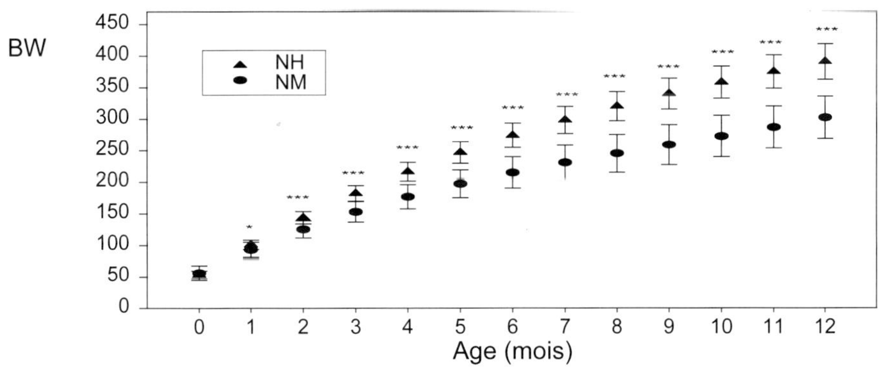

*Figure 8. Variation of body weight from birth to 12 months of age in HL and ML groups (*p<0.05, **p<0.01, ***p<0.001) (from Donabedian et al. 2006).*

Discussion and conclusion

At birth BW and BS of the foal are already very high. The foal at weaning should gain 40-45 and 60-65 percent of their total BW and BS respectively, achieved from birth to adult age. Growth of the foal is strongly related to nutrient intake. During the first two months of life, growth is linked to milk yield and related to feed allowances of the mares. Nutrient requirements of the mare and related feed allowances are up to now well known to feed adequately the mare and as a result the suckling foal. From 3 months of age requirements of the foal need to be determined more accurately as it is a critical period for physiology of digestion, metabolism, and for bone development.

Up to two months of age the main nutrient of the foal is milk lactose while cellulose and cytoplasmic carbohydrates of forage are increasingly the major nutrients up to weaning. Efficiency rates of energy supplied by glucose absorbed in the small intestine is higher than that of VFA absorbed in the large intestine. In calves of dairy breeds, the efficiency of ME utilisation for growth is very high: 0.69 and this value does not appear to vary significantly with age, BW, ADG and diet composition (Van Es 1970; Vermorel *et al.* 1974; Kirchgessner and Neese 1976). This efficiency value would be much higher than those to be determined in horse before 2 months of age. In addition foals as with young beef calves are fed with milk and grass after three months of age. Efficiencies will decrease during this second period and is likely to be related to diet composition. Hence data from cattle cannot be extrapolated to horses. The determination of the efficiency rate and the related requirements should be studied using indirect calorimetry methodology and respiratory chambers. It should be conducted with foals that are weaned before 2 weeks and fed with a diet that mimics their normal diet and feeding: milk + forage ± concentrate.

The period between 3 and 6 months is very sensitive for DOD as it is established that 67 percent of the foals exhibit potential bone lesions which regress for most of them after weaning when feeding and breeding management practices are good, optimal growth and related feed allowances are well balanced and sufficient exercise provided. Quantity and quality of grass and concentrate should be fed to manage optimal growth which facilitates the regression of potential bone lesions. Research should focus on the foal as performance, health and welfare of the yearling, namely of race breeds, is strongly linked to the nursing period.

References

Argenzio, R.A. and H.F. Hintz, 1971. Energy utilisation in the horse. Proc. Cornell Nut. Conf., 86-92.

Agabriel, J., W. Martin-Rosset and J. Robelin, 1984. Croissance et besoins du poulain. In: Le Cheval, R. Jarrige and W. Martin-Rosset (eds.) INRA Editions, 78026 Versailles. p 370-384.

Barth, K.M., J.W Williams and D.G. Brown, 1977. Digestible energy requirements of working and non-working ponies. J. Anim. Sci., 44, 585-589.

Coleman, R.J., G.W. Mathison, L. Burwash and J.D. Milligan, 1997. The effect of protein supplementation of alfalfa cubes diets on the growth of weanling horses.p 59-64. In: Proceedings.15thENPS. Symposium. Ft. Worth, TX.

Borton A., D.L. Anderson and S. Lyford, 1973. Studies of protein quality and quantity in the early weaned foal. p19-22 In: Proceedings ENPS symposium University of Florida, Gainseville, USA. 19-22.

Brzesky, E. and S. Tkurowsky, 1964. Investigations in the growth of horse. 2. The Poznan horse. Nr 22 Zootecnica Z 6 Krakowie (in polish)

Dik, K.J., E. Enzerink and P.R. van Weeren, 1999. Radiographic development of osteochondral abnormalities, in the hock and stifle of Dutch Warmblood foals, from age 1 to 11 months, Equine Vet. J. Suppl. 31 9-15.

Donabedian, M., G. Fleurance, G. Perona, C. Robert, O. Lepage, C. Trillaud-Geyl, S. Leger, A. Ricard, D. Bergero and W. Martin-Rosset, 2006. Effect of fast vs. moderate growth rate related to nutrient intake on developmental orthopaedic disease in the horse. Anim. Res. (in press).

Doreau, M. and G. Dussap, 1980. Estimation de la production laitière de la jument allaitante par marquage de l'eau corporelle du poulain. Reprod. Nutr. Dev., 20: 1883.

Doreau, M., W. Martin-Rosset and J.P. Barlet, 1981. Variations de quelques constituents plasmatiques chez la jument allaitante en fin de gestation et en début de lactation. Ann. Rech. Vét., 12, 219-225.

Doreau, M., S. Boulot, W. Martin-Rosset and J. Robelin, 1986. Relationship between nutrient intake, growth and body composition of the nursing foal. Reprod. Nutr. Develop., 26 (2B), 683-690.

Doreau, M., J.P. Bruhat and W. Martin-Rosset, 1988b. Effets du niveau des apports azotés chez la jument en début de lactation. Ann. Zootech., 37(1), 21-30.

Doreau, M., S. Boulot and W. Martin-Rosset, 1991. Effect of parity and physiological state on intake, milk production and blood parameters in lactating mares differing in body size. Anim. Prod., 53: 111-118: 992-999.

Doreau, M., S. Boulot and Y. Chilliard, 1993. Yield and composition of milk from lactating mares: effect of body condition at foaling. J. Dairy Sci., 60, 457-466.

Doreau, M. and F. Martuzzi, 2006. Milk yield of nursing and dairy mares. In proceedings 3rd Euorpean Worksho Equine Nutrition (EWEN), N. Miraglia and W. Martin-Rosset (Eds.), Campobasso 20-22 June, Italy, EAAP No 120, Wageningen Academic Publishers, The Netherlands.

Dusek, J., 1966. Notes sur le développement prenatal des chevaux (in Czech Language). Ved. Pr. Vysk. San. Chov. Keni., Slatinany, 2, 1-25.

Graham, P.M., E.A. Ott, J.H. Brendemulh and S. Tenbroeck, 1994. Effect of supplemental lysine and threonine on growth and development of yearling horses. J.Anim. Sc. 72, 380-386.

GEH, 1994. (Deutsch. Langerwirtschafts Gesellschaft) 2. Empfehlungen zur Energie und Nährstoffversorgung der Perfde. DLG. Verlage Frankfurt/Main. ISBN 3.7690.0517.1. p

Glade, M.J. and T.H. Belling 1984. Growth plate cartilage metabolism, morphology and biochemical composition in over- and underfed horses, Growth 48,473-82.

Grabowsky, J., S. Dtekens and R. Tyszkowsky, 1971. Growth and development of Pure bred Arab foals and younsters in the podlasie lowlands environment. Zesz. Nauk.Wyzsz. Szk. Rol. Szezecinie. 36. 21-40 (In polish)

Green, D.A., 1969. A review of studies on the growth rate of horses. Br. Vet. J., 117.181-191.

Gütte, J.O., 1972. Energiebedarf laktierrender Stuten, In Lenkeit, W., Breirem, K., Craseman, E., Hb. Tierrenähr. 2, 393-398, verlag Paul Parey, Berlin-Hamburg.

Harris, P.A., 2005. Hints on nutrition for optimal growth. In 1st Waltham International Breeding Symposium, P.A. Harris, S.J., Hill and L.A., Abeyasekere Eds. Newmarket, 24 June, UK, 41-50.

Heird, J.C., 1973. Growth parameters in the quarter horse. In: Proceedings 3rd ENPS symposium, Florida, Gainseville, USA, 81-92.

Hintz, H.F., H.F. Schruver and J.F. Lowe, 1971. Comparison of a blend of milk products and linseedmeal as protein suplemements for growing horses. J. Anim. Sc. 33, 1274-1277.

Hintz, H.F., R.L. Hintz and L.D. van Vleck, 1979. Growth rate of thoroughbreds. Effect of age of dam, year and month of birth and sex of foal. J. Animal Science 48, 480-487.

Hintz, H.F., 1980 Growth in the horse. In: Stud Manager's Handbook, Vol. 16, 59-66. Agriservices Foundation, Clovis, California.

Hintz, H.F., 1987. Growth and calcium metabolism in horses fed varying levels of protein. Eq. Vet. J. 19:280.

Hoffman, R.M., D.S. Kronefeld, J.L. Holland and K.M. Greiwe-Crandell, 1995. Preweaning diet and stall weaning method influences on stress responses in foals. J. Anim. Sci. 73, 2922-2930.

INRA, 1984. Tables des apports alimentaires recommandés pour lecheval. In Le Cheval. R.Jarrige and W. Martin-Rosset W.INRA, Eds. INRA Editions Versailles, 645-659.

INRA, 1990. L'alimentation des chevaux. W. Martin-Rosset Ed,. INRA Editions Paris, p 232

Jeffcott, L.B. and M.E. Davies, 1998. Copper status and skeletal development in horses: still a long way to go, Equine Vet. J. 30, 183-185.

Jones, L. and T. Hollands, 2005. Estimation of growth rates in UK thoroughbreds. Pferdeheilkunde 21, 121-123.

Kavazis, A.N. and E.D. Ott, 2003. Growth Rates in Thoroughbred Horses Raised in Florida J. Eq. Vet. Sci., Volume 23, Issue 8, August 2003, Pages 353-357

Kirchgessner, M. and K.R. Neese, 1976. Studies on the energy metabolism of the veal calf- Retention and utilization in the bipartite fattening with liquid feed.Z. Tierphysiol. Tierrenahrg. Futtermittelk., 36, 274-282.(In german)

Kronfeld, D.S., T.N. Meacham and S. Donoghue, 1990. Dietary aspects of developmental orthopedic disease in young horses, Vet. Clin. North Am. Equine Pract. 6, 451-65.

Langlois, B., 1973. Caractères quantitatifs chez le cheval. Aspects génétiques. Bull. Rech. Depart. Gene. Anim., INRA, 16, 135.

Marcq, J., Lahaye and E. Cordiez, 1956. Considérations générales sur la croissance. In: Le Cheval Tome 2, Lib Agricole La Maison Rustique, Paris, 667-679.

MCCall, C.A., G.D. Potter and J.L. Kreider, 1985. Lomotor, vocal and othe rbehavioral responses to varying methods of weaning foal. Appl. Anim. Beha. Sci. 14, 27-35.

Martin-Rosset, W. M. Doreau and J. Cloix, 1978. Etude des activités d'un troupeau de poulinières de trait et de leurs poulains au paturage. Ann. Zooetch, 27, 33-45.

Martin-Rosset, W. and M. Doreau, 1980. Effect of variations in level of feeding of heavy mares during late pregnancy. Proc. 31st Animal Meeting EAAP. Munich. Horse Commission, Session 6, p. 4.

Martin-rosset W., 1983. Revue bibliographique: Particularités de la croissance et du développement du cheval. 32, 109-130.

Martin-Rosset, W., M. Doreau and C. Espinasse, 1986. Alimentation de la jument lourde allaitante. Evolution du poids vif des juments et croissance des poulains. Ann. Zootech., 35, 21-36

Martin-Rosset, W., M. Vermorel, M. Doreau, J.L. Tisserand and J. Andrieu, 1994. The French horse feed evaluation systems and recommended allowances for energy and protein. Livest. Prod. Sci., 40, 37-56.

Martin-Rosset, W., 2004. Growth and development in the equine. In Proceedins 2nd European Workshop Equine Nutrition (EWEN) V. Julliand and W. Martin-Rosset (Eds.), Dijon, 15-17 January, France, EAAP No 114, Wageningen Academic Publishers, The Netherlands, 15-50.

Martin-Rosset, W., D. Austbo and M. Coenen, 2006b. Energy and protein requirements and allowances in lactating mares. In proceedings 3rd European Workshop Equine Nutrition (EWEN), N. Miraglia and W.Martin-Rosset Eds. Campobasso 20-22 June, Italy EAAP No 120, Wageningen Academic Publishers, The Netherlands.

Micol, D. and W. Martin-Rosset, 1995. Feeding systems for horses on high forage diets in the temperate zone. In: M. Journet, E. Grenet, M-H. Farce, M. Thériez and C. Demarquilly (Eds.). Recent developments in the Nutrition of Herbivores, 569-584. INRA Editions, Paris.

McIlwraith, C.W., 2001. Developemental otrhopedic desease (DOD) in horse- A multifactorial process. In: 17th ENPS Ssymposium, May31-June2, Lexington, Kentucky, USA, 2-23.

Meakim, D.W., 1979. Bone mineral content determination of the equine third metacarpal via radiographic photometry and the effect of dietary lysine and methionine supplementation on growth and bone development in the weanling foal. M.S. thesis, University of Florida.

Milligan, J.D., R.J. Coleman and L. Burwash, 1985. Relationship of energy intake weight gain in yearling horses. In: Proceedings. 9thENPS. Symposium East Lansing, Mich.: Michigan State University.

Menke, K.H., W. Huss, 1980. Tiernerhärung und Futtermitettelkde., Verla Eugen Ulmer, Stuttgart.

Meyer, H. and L. Ahlswede, 1976. Uber das intrauterine wachstum und die Körperzusammensetzung won Fohlen sowie den Hährstoffbedarf tragender stuten ubers; Tierernähr.,4,263-292.

Miraglia, N., M. Saastamoinen and W. Martin-Rosset, 2006. Role of pasture in mares and foals management in Europe. In: Proceedings 3rd European Workshop Equine Nutrition (EWEN), N. Miaraglia and W. Martin-Rosset (Eds.), Campobasso, 20-22 June, Italy, EAAP No, 120, Wageningen Academic Publishers, The Netherlands.

Nicol, C.J., A.J. Badnell-Waters, R. Bice, A. Kelland, A.D. Wilson and P.A. Harris, 2005. The effect of diet and weaning method on behaviour of young horse. Appl. Anim. Behav. Sc. 95:205-221

NRC, 1989. Nutrient requirements of horse, 5th rev. ed. Subcommittee on Horse Nutrition Board on Agriculture National Academey Press - Washington, DC.

Olsson, N. and A. Ruudvere, 1955. The nutrition of the horse. Nutr. Abstr. Rev. 25, 1-18.

Ott, E.A., R.L. Asquith, J.P. Feaster and F.G. Martin, 1979. Influence of protein level and quality on the growth and development of yearling foals. J. Anim. Sci.49:620.

Ott, E.A., R.L. Asquith and J.P. Feaster, 1981. Lysine supplementation of diets for yearling horses. J. Anim. Sci. 53:1496.

Ott, E.A. and R.L. Asquith, 1986. Influence of level of feeding and nutrient content of the concentrate on growth and development of yearling horses. J. Anim. Sci. 62:290.

Ott, E.D., 2001. Protein and amino acids. In: J.D., Pagan Ed. Advance in Equine Nutrition, KER, Nottingham University Press, UK, 237-246.

Ousey, J.C., 2006. Physiology and metabolism in the new born foal with reference to orphanand sick foals. In proceedings of 3rd European Workshop Equine Nutrtion (EWEN), N. Miraglia and W. Martin-Rosset Eds. Campobasso, 20-22 June, Italy, EAAP No 120. Wageningen Academic Publishers, The Netherlands.

Pagan, J.D., S.G. Jackson and S. Caddel, 1996. A summary of growth rates of thoroughbred horses in Kentucky. Pferdeheilkunde 123, 285-289.

Pagan, J.D., C.G. Brown-Douglas and S. Caddel, 2006. Body weight and condition of Kentucky Thoroughbred mares and their foals as influenced by month of foaling, season and gender. In Proceedings of 3rd European Workshop Equine Nutrition (EWEN), N. Miraglia and W. Martin-Rosset (Eds.), Campobasso, 20-22 June, Italy, EAAP No 120, Wageningen Academic Publishers, The Netherlands.

Potter, G.D. and J.D. Huchton, 1975. Growth of yearling horses fed different sources of protein with supplemental lysine. In: Proceedings. ENPS. Symposium. Pomona, California, USA.19

Saastamoinen, M,T. and E. Koskinen, 1993. Influence of quality dietary protein supplement and anabolic steroïds on muscular and skeletal growth of foals. Anim. Prod. 56, 135-144.

Reeds, P.J. and M.F. Fuller, 1983. Nutrient intake and protein turnover. Proc. Nutr. Soc. 42, 463-471.

Savage, C.J., R.N. McCarthy and L.B. Jeffcott, 1993. Effects of dietary energy and protein on induction of dyschondroplasia in foals, Equine Vet. J. Suppl. 16, 74-9.

Santos, A.S., B.C. Sousa, L.C. Leitao and V.C. Alves, 2006. The utilisation of morphometric measurements to estimate horse body weight- application to the Lusitano breed. In proceedings 3rd European Workshop Equine Nutrition (EWEN), N. Miraglia and W. Martin-Rosset (Eds.), Campobasso 20-22 June, Italy, EAAP No 120, Wageningen Academic Publishers, The Netherlands.

Schryver, H.F., D.W. Meakim, J.E. Lowe, J. Williams, L.V. Soderholm and H.F. Hintz, 1987. Growth and calcium metabolism in horses fed varying levels of protein. Eq. Vet. J. 19:280

Hintz, H.F., 1987. Growth and calcium metabolism in horses fed varying levels of protein. Eq. Vet. J. 19:280.

Scott, B.D., G.D. Potter, J.W. Evans, J.C. Reagor, W. Webb and S.P. Webb, 1987. Growth andfeed utilization by yearling horses fed added dietary fat. In: Proceedings 10^{th}ENPS Symposium. Fort Collins,: Colorado State University, USA. 101-106.

Staniar, W.B., J.A. Wilson, L.H. Lawrence, W.L. Cooper, D.S. Kronfeld and P.A. Harris, 1999. Growth of thoroughbreds fed different levels of protein and supplemented with lysine and threonine. p 88-89.In Proceedings. 16th Eq. Nutr. Physiol. Symp. Soc. Raleigh Unviversity.

Staniar,W.B., et al., 2001. Dietary fat and fibre influence plasma insulin-like growth factor: an endocrine link between diet and osteochondrosis. In Proceedings American Academy Veterinary Nutrition, Boston, Massachusetts, 13-14.

Swanson, C.A., R.M. Hoffman, D.S. Kronefeld and P.A. Harris, 2003. Effects of diets and probiotic supplementation on stress during weaning in Thoroughbred foals. In: Proceedings 18th ENPS symposium, Eas lansing, Michigan, 243.

Trillaud-Geyl, C., J. Brohier, L. de Baynast, N. Baudoin and E. Rossier, 1990. Bilan de productivité sur 10 ans d'un troupeau de jumentsde selle conduites en plein air intégral. Croissance des produits de 0 à 6 mois. World Review Anim. Prod. 25, 3, 65-70.

Van Es, A.J.H., 1970. Simulation of the growth of veals calves fed liquid milk repalcers.In Proceedins 5th Symposium Energy metabolism, Schurch, A., Wenk C., Eds. Energy metabolism of farm animal. EAAP No 13, 97-100.

Vermorel, M., J.C. Bouvier, P. Thivend and R. Toullec, 1974. Utilisation des aliments d'allaitement par le veau à l'engrais de diffèrents poids. In Proceedings 6th symposium energy metabolism, Menke, K. H., Lantzch H.J., Reichl, J.R., Eds. Energy metabolism of farm animals. EAAP No 14, 143-146

Vermorel, M., J. Vernet and W. Martin-Rosset, 1987. Donnée préliminaires sur l'évolution nycthémérale des dépenses énergétiques du jeune poulain. Reprod. Nutr. Deveop. 27, 325-326.

Warren, L.K., L.M. Lawrence, A.S. Griffin, A.L. Parker, T. Barnes and D. Wright, 1998. The effect of weaning age on foal growth and bone density. In: Advances in equine Nutrition, J.D., Pagan Ed. KER, Nottingham University Press, Nottingham, UK. 457-459.

Wirth, B.L., 1977. Cottonseed meal and lysine for weanling foals. M.S. thesis. Texas A&M University, College Station, Texas, USA.

Body weight and condition of Kentucky Thoroughbred mares and their foals as influenced by month of foaling, season, and gender

J.D. Pagan[1], C.G. Brown-Douglas[1] and S. Caddel[2]
[1]Kentucky Equine Research, Inc., 3910 Delaney Ferry Rd., Versailles, KY 40383, USA
[2]Hallway Feeds, 251 W. Loudon Avenue, Lexington, Kentucky 40508, USA

Abstract

Body weight and condition of 3909 thoroughbred mares and their foals born in central Kentucky were tracked monthly from birth through weaning. Month of birth, season, and gender affected foal growth. January, February and March foals had lower body weights than April or May foals during the first month of age. By 150 days of age, there was no difference in body weight between birth months. Colts were heavier and taller than fillies throughout the study. Winter-foaling mares showed negative daily weight change in the first month post partum compared with mares which foaled in spring. Regardless of month of birth, foals from mares that exhibited a negative energy balance post partum (losing weight or negative daily weight change) did not grow as fast as those from mares that were in a positive energy balance.

Keywords: foal growth, lactating mare, thoroughbred

Introduction

In central Kentucky Thoroughbred foals are born primarily in the winter and early spring. They typically remain with their dams for 4 to 5 months before being weaned in late summer and early fall. During these first few months, foals grow very rapidly, quadrupling their body weights by 5 months of age. During this time, foals derive the energy, protein and minerals necessary to support rapid growth from a combination of mare milk, pasture and supplemental grain. Pasture availability changes markedly between the winter and spring, so the availability of nutrients to both the lactating mare and her foal change drastically depending on the foal's month of birth.

Hintz et al (1979) reported that Canadian Thoroughbred foals born in January, February and March were smaller than foals born in April or May. These differences in weight persisted throughout all ages studied. In an earlier study from Kentucky (Pagan et al, 1996) Thoroughbred foals born in January, February and March were smaller than foals born in April and May, but these differences disappeared by 6 months of age. In the UK, Thoroughbred foals born in January were smaller than foals born in March and April (Jones and Hollands, 2005). However, month of birth did not affect growth rate up until 200 days of age. Therefore, it appears that the location as well as the season of year affects how suckling foals grow. None of these studies evaluated the effect of season on changes in body weight or body condition in the lactating mare. This paper reports on how the body weight and condition of a large number of Kentucky Thoroughbred mares and their foals are affected by month of foaling, season and gender.

Materials and method

Thoroughbred mares (n = 3909) and their foals (1958 fillies, 1951 colts) born in central Kentucky during the years 1996-2005 were weighed monthly using a portable electronic scale (Equimetrics, Inc., Redfield, Arkansas). Data were collected as part of a larger study on Thoroughbred growth and only data up until weaning are reported in this paper. Body condition score (BCS) was measured in the mares and their foals using a scoring system of 1 through 9 to estimate fat deposition and was based on the system developed by Henneke et al (1981).Wither height was also measured in the foals.

The foal population was represented by approximately 480 stallions and was raised on 50 commercial and private farms in central Kentucky. The data set consisted of foals born in January (n=354) (9.0%), February (n=998) (25.5%), March (n=1073) (27.5%), April (n=977) (25.0%) and May (n=507) (13.0%).

Average daily gain (ADG) in kg/d was calculated using the following formula.

$$ADG = \frac{\text{(body weight - previous body weight)}}{\text{(date - previous weigh date)}}$$

Mares were also categorized as being in either a positive energy balance (gaining weight, therefore positive ADG) or negative energy balance (losing weight, therefore negative ADG) post partum. All mare and foal data for the 10 seasons were initially analyzed separately, but as there were no significant differences for any parameter between the 10 seasons ($p>0.05$), data were combined for further analysis.

The data were split into foal-age categories: 1-15 days, 16-45 days (1 month), 46-75 days (2 months), 76-105 days (3 months), 106-135 days (4 months), and 136-165 days (5 months). Splits were chosen such that the relationship between foal age and foal weight was approximately linear and to ensure that the vast majority of the foals were measured only once per age category. A linear regression model with foal age or month of lactation as the explanatory variable and various response variables (foal age in days, gender, month of birth, weigh month, mare weight, and mare ADG, mare BCS and mare energy balance) was used to predict the response variable and provide a confidence interval for the mean response at a specified foal age within each foal-age category. When gender is being considered, it is included as an explanatory variable.

Results are expressed as mean and 95% confidence interval and significance is reported at the 5% level.

Results and discussion

Foals

Colts were between 1.7 and 3.0 kg heavier and 0.6 and 1.3 cm taller than fillies ($P<0.05$) throughout the study. Fillies and colts exhibited similar BCS from birth to 7 days of age ($p>0.05$); however, at 1 month of age fillies were fatter than colts ($p<0.05$) and remained so until the end of the study (Table 1 and Figure 1).

January, February and March foals had lower body weights than April or May foals during the first month of age. January and February foals remained lighter than foals born in March, April, and May until 3 months of age, and January foals remained lighter than all other foals until 4 months of age (Table 2). By 150 days of age, there was no difference in body weight between birth months.

January and February foals had lower ADG than March, April and May foals at 7 days and 1 month of age. January foals had greater ADG than all foals at 3 months of age coinciding with rapid spring pasture growth beginning in April. May foals had the lowest ADG of all foals at 3, 4 and 5 months which coincides with August, September and October when late summer pasture is losing its quality, suggesting a seasonal effect on foal ADG (Figure 2).

Table 1. Body weight, height and BCS ± 95% confidence intervals of Kentucky fillies and colts.

	Body weight (kg)			Height (cm)			BCS		
Days	Colts	Fillies	p	Colts	Fillies	p	Colts	Fillies	p
1	57.24 ± 1.04	55.12 ± 1.02	<0.05	103.20 ± 0.44	102.19 ± 0.43	<0.05	5.21 ± 0.03	5.20 ± 0.03	n/s
7	67.28 ± 0.71	65.16 ± 0.69	<0.01	105.60 ± 0.30	104.59 ± 0.29	<0.01	5.39 ± 0.02	5.38 ± 0.02	n/s
30	100.46 ± 0.61	98.75 ± 0.60	<0.01	112.98 ± 0.19	112.42 ± 0.18	<0.01	5.65 ± 0.02	5.68 ± 0.02	<0.05
60	137.81 ± 0.75	135.16 ± 0.74	<0.01	120.38 ± 0.19	119.65 ± 0.19	<0.01	5.66 ± 0.02	5.73 ± 0.02	<0.01
90	171.83 ± 0.88	168.94 ± 0.88	<0.01	126.02 ± 0.20	125.04 ± 0.20	<0.01	5.62 ± 0.02	5.71 ± 0.02	<0.01
120	202.21 ± 1.06	199.38 ± 1.04	<0.01	130.25 ± 0.21	129.54 ± 0.21	<0.01	5.56 ± 0.02	5.65 ± 0.02	<0.01
150	230.56 ± 1.61	227.59 ± 1.59	<0.01	133.90 ± 0.29	133.09 ± 0.29	<0.01	5.55 ± 0.02	5.63 ± 0.02	<0.01

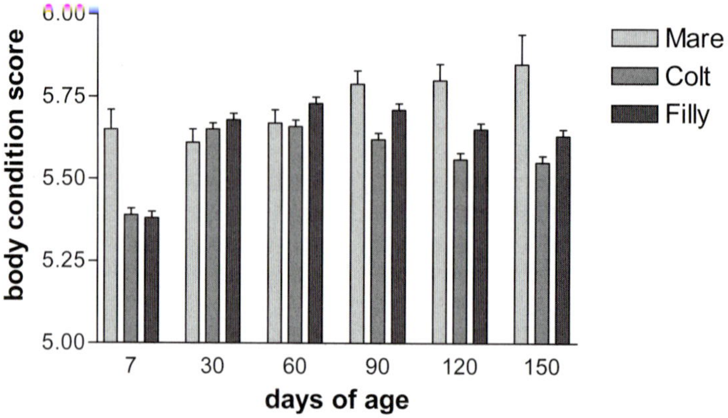

Figure 1. Body condition score ± 95% confidence intervals of Kentucky mares, fillies and colts.

Table 2. Foal body weight (kg) ± 95% confidence interval. Differing superscripts within rows indicate significant differences (P<0.05).

Days	January	February	March	April	May
1	53.69 ± 3.67[a]	54.86 ± 1.57[a]	55.21 ± 1.91[a]	57.76 ± 2.11[ab]	60.17 ± 2.60[b]
7	62.86 ± 1.99[a]	64.36 ± 0.88[a]	65.71 ± 0.84[a]	68.18 ± 1.16[b]	69.96 ± 1.43[b]
30	93.50 ± 1.37[a]	96.27 ± 0.80[b]	100.80 ± 0.78[c]	102.74 ± 0.84[d]	102.11 ± 1.18[d]
60	128.48 ± 1.75[a]	133.72 ± 1.05[b]	138.90 ± 0.96[c]	138.82 ± 0.99[c]	137.31 ± 1.62[c]
90	163.85 ± 2.24[a]	169.03 ± 1.18[b]	172.61 ± 1.12[c]	171.26 ± 1.28[bc]	170.92 ± 1.70[bc]
120	195.66 ± 2.53[a]	199.46 ± 1.31[ab]	201.98 ± 1.47[b]	202.24 ± 1.50[b]	202.55 ± 2.32[b]
150	226.00 ± 3.07[a]	228.74 ± 1.83[a]	230.63 ± 2.24[a]	230.92 ± 3.31[a]	227.11 ± 4.18[a]

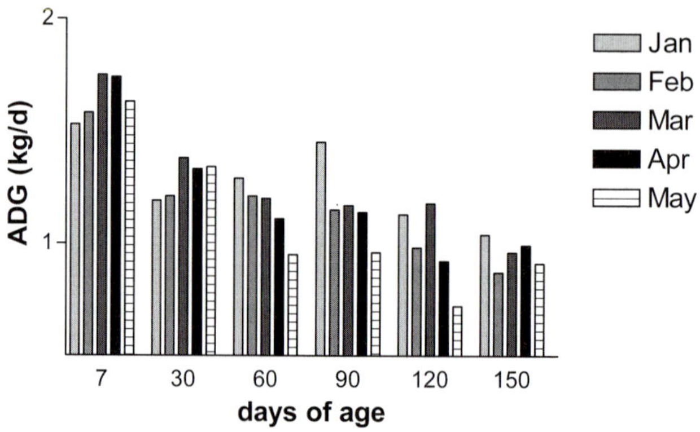

Figure 2. ADG (kg/d) of Kentucky foals separated by month of birth.

Month of birth had no effect on foal BCS at 7 days as well as 4 and 5 months of age. In all foals, BCS was lowest at 7 days and increased between 7 and 30 days. May foals had lower BCS than all other foals at 1 and 2 months of age. January and February foals had significantly greater BCS than March, April and May foals at 3 months (Table 3 and Figure 3).

Table 3. BCS (scale 1-9) ± 95% confidence interval of Kentucky foals born in January, February, March, April and May. Differing superscripts within a row indicate significant differences (P<0.05).

Days	January	February	March	April	May
7	5.39 ± 0.06[a]	5.36 ± 0.03[a]	5.39 ± 0.03[a]	5.41 ± 0.03[a]	5.37 ± 0.04[a]
30	5.68 ± 0.04[a]	5.65 ± 0.02[ab]	5.67 ± 0.02[a]	5.69 ± 0.02[a]	5.61 ± 0.03[b]
60	5.74 ± 0.04[a]	5.71 ± 0.03[a]	5.73 ± 0.02[a]	5.68 ± 0.02[b]	5.63 ± 0.03[c]
90	5.72 ± 0.05[a]	5.73 ± 0.03[a]	5.66 ± 0.02[b]	5.62 ± 0.02[b]	5.60 ± 0.04[b]
120	5.64 ± 0.04[a]	5.61 ± 0.03[a]	5.59 ± 0.02[a]	5.59 ± 0.03[a]	5.60 ± 0.05[a]
150	5.61 ± 0.04[a]	5.59 ± 0.03[a]	5.57 ± 0.03[a]	5.58 ± 0.05[a]	5.66 ± 0.07[a]

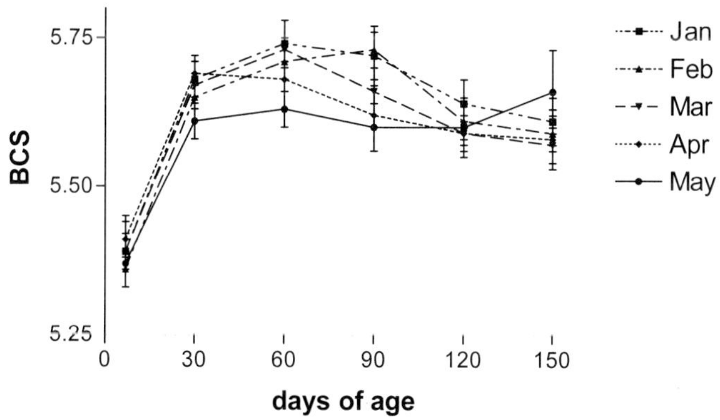

Figure 3. BCS (scale 1-9) ± 95% confidence interval of Kentucky foals separated by month of birth.

Mares

Winter-foaling mares (January and February) had lower body weights in the first 2 months post partum than mares which foaled in March, April or May. By months 4 and 5 of lactation there was no difference in mare body weight between any of the groups (Figure 4).

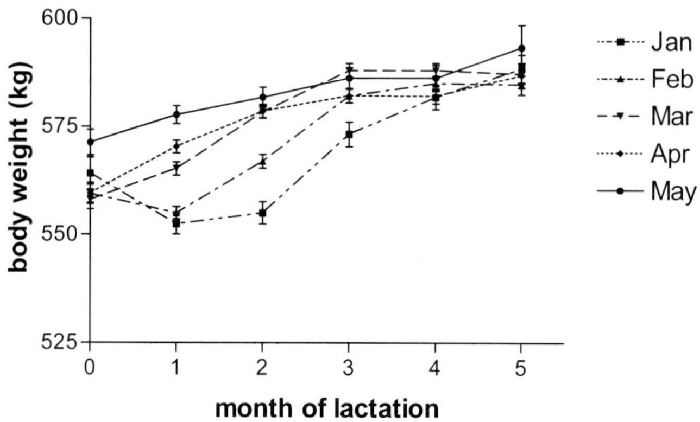

Figure 4. Mare body weight (kg) ± 95% confidence interval in relation to month of lactation.

Winter-foaling mares showed negative daily weight change in the first month post partum compared with mares which foaled in spring (March, April and May). January-foaling mares had the lowest daily weight change during month 2 and the highest daily weight change during months 4 and 5 than all other mares and during month 3 of lactation January- and February-foaling mares exhibited greater daily weight change than all other mares (Figure 5).

Mare body weight, daily weight change and BCS increased in the spring (March through June) in all mares regardless of stage of lactation (Figures 6, 7, and 8). Mares that foaled in the winter months showed a negative daily weight change during January and February which then increased to approximately 0.5 kg/d in March, where it remained positive until the completion of the study (Figure 7). Changes in mare body weight and BCS appeared to be related to seasonal and management factors. Winter mares that showed decreased body weight, negative daily weight gain and ADG after foaling are likely to spend more time indoors with restricted access to pasture until the spring.

Relationships between mare and foal data

Foal body weight was positively correlated to mare body weight ($P<0.05$), foal ADG was positively associated with mare ADG ($P<0.05$), and foal BCS was positively related to mare BCS during months 1-5. These relationships indicate that heavier mares produce heavier foals, faster-growing

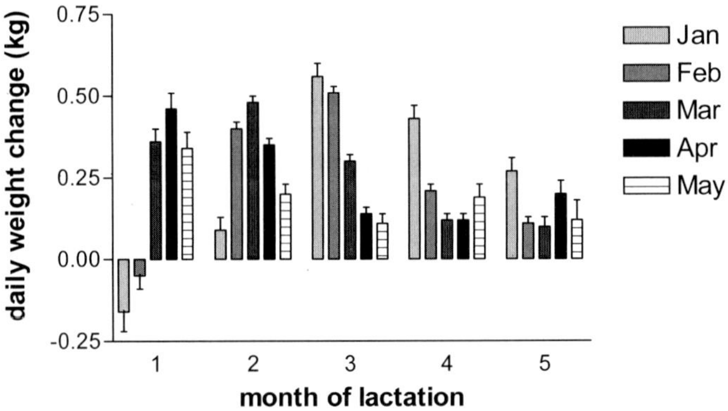

Figure 5. Daily weight change (kg/d) ± 95% confidence interval of Kentucky mares in relation to month of lactation.

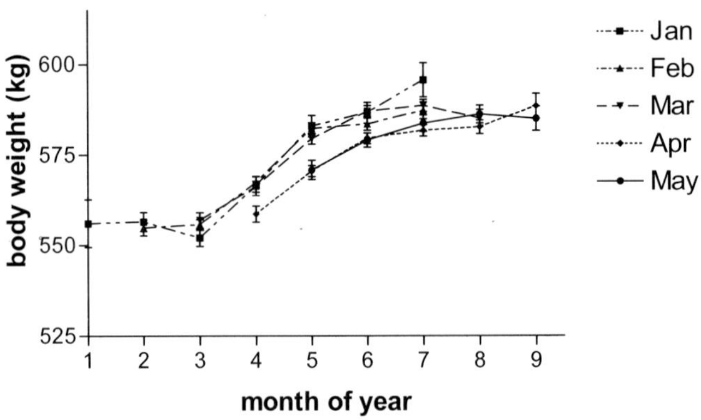

Figure 6. Body weight (kg) ± 95% confidence intervals of Kentucky mares in relation to month of the year (1, 2, 3 etc. represent January, February, March etc.).

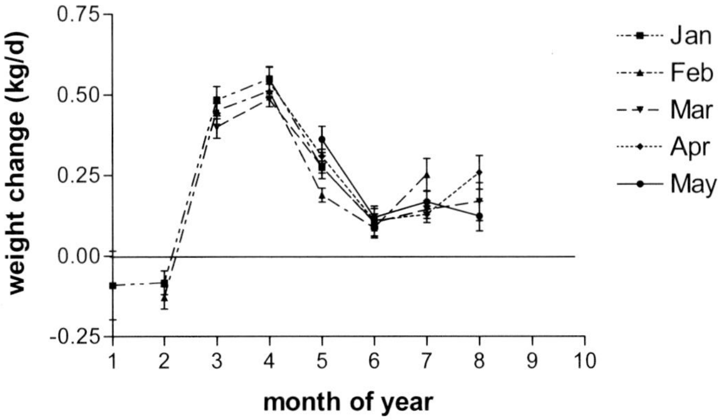

Figure 7. Daily weight change (kg/d) ± 95% confidence intervals of Kentucky mares in relation to month of the year (1, 2, 3 etc. represent January, February, March etc.).

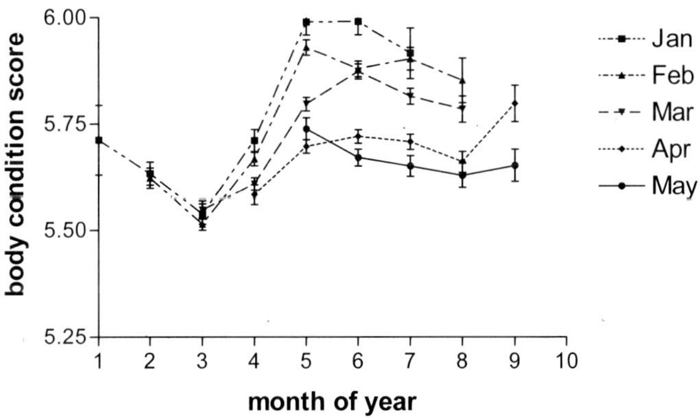

Figure 8. Body condition score (scale 1-9) ± 95% confidence intervals of Kentucky mares in relation to month of the year (1, 2, 3 etc. represent January, February, March etc.).

foals are from mares that are gaining weight, and fatter foals are produced from fatter mares. There was a positive relationship between foal BCS and mare daily weight change at 2 and 3 months (peak lactation), indicating that mares that are gaining weight during the first 3 months of lactation have fatter foals.

Regardless of month of birth, foals from mares that exhibited a negative energy balance post partum (losing weight or negative daily weight change) did not grow as fast as those from mares that were in a positive energy balance at any age ($P<0.05$).

These data clearly demonstrate that season of the year affects growth in suckling foals. Foals born in January and February were smaller at birth and grew more slowly during the first two months than foals born later in the year. January and February foaling mares tended to lose weight in early lactation, suggesting that their caloric intakes were insufficient to meet their energy requirement for early lactation. Later in lactation when there was access to adequate pasture, these early-foaling mares gained more weight and supported faster growth rates in their foals than later-foaling mares. It is unclear whether the faster growth rates in these 3-4 month-old foals were due to greater milk production, greater pasture consumption by the foals or a combination of both factors.

In Kentucky, growth rate of suckling foals was affected by birth month and season of year. Foals born in the winter grew more slowly during the first two months, but compensated by growing faster later in lactation so that the net result was that by 5 months of age there was no difference between body weights in any of the groups. This is different than in Canada (Hintz et al, 1979) where foals born early in the year remained smaller throughout their yearling year or in the UK (Jones and Hollands, 2005) where growth rate was not different between birth months for the first 200 days of age. In Canada, pasture availability in the spring may not have been enough to allow for compensatory weight gain in early-born foals. In the UK, perhaps winter pasture availability was sufficient to meet mare energy requirements and support foal growth.

References

Henneke, D.R., G.D. Potter and J.L. Kreider, 1981. A condition score relationship to body fat content of mares during gestation and lactation. In: Proc. 7th ENPS, Warrenton, Va, 105-110.

Hintz, H.F., R.L. Hintz and L.D. van Vleck, 1979. Growth rate of thoroughbreds. Effect of age of dam, year and month of birth and sex of foal. J. Animal Science 48, 480-487.

Jones, L. and T. Hollands, 2005. Estimation of growth rates in UK thoroughbreds. Pferdeheilkunde 21, 121-123.

Pagan, J.D., S.G.Jackson and S. Caddel, 1996. A summary of growth rates of thoroughbred horses in Kentucky. Pferdeheilkunde 123, 285-289.

The utilisation of morphometric measurements to estimate horse body weight: Application to the Lusitano breed

A.S. Santos[1], B.C. Sousa[1], L.C. Leitão[2] and V.C. Alves[1]
[1]CECAV, Department of Animal Science, UTAD, Apartado, 5001-909 Vila Real, Portugal
[2]Department of Animal Science, ESAC, Bencanta, Coimbra, Portugal

Abstract

The morphometric measurements – body weight (BW), withers height (WH), thoracic circumference (TC), cannon circumference (CC) and forearm circumference (FC) - were made in 13 Lusitano foals during two years, every 15 days after foaling and up to 120 days of age. Average values of measurements at birth were, 52.7±6.64 kg for BW, 100.7±0.03 cm for WH, 84.8±0.04 cm for TP, 13.3 ±0.01 cm for CC and 22.7±0.02 cm for FC. An average daily gain of 0.84 kg/d was observed during the 120 days of the study period. A strong correlation was found between BW and WH and between BW and TC, and the following regression equations were calculated: BW = 4.1646 WH – 367.64 (R^2=0.95; RSD=8.79), BW = 2.8235 TC – 190.58 (R^2=0.94; RSD=9.27). Both equations seem adequate to predict BW on suckling Lusitano foals from birth to 120 days of age.

Keywords: Lusitano breed, growth, suckling foals, body weight

Introduction

The Lusitano horse plays an important role in equine production in Portugal. According to the Portuguese Lusitano breed association, there are about 11 000 Lusitanos world wide, and its production is mainly located in Portugal (320 breeders) and Brasil (Fradinho, 2002).

The eumetric morphology of this horse and its natural versatility, combined with a gentle temperament are some of the reasons for its success as a saddle horse. The use of this horse is also well adapted to a wide range of disciplines, from dressage, driving, reining and, of course, bullfights were its use, according to many, will never be replaced.

Foal growth recommendations are based on age, body weigh (BW), mature body weight and average daily gain (NRC, 1989). In order to better obtain a correct foal growth, BW evolution should be measured. However, in the Lusitano breeding system, this practice is not widely used. This situation enhances the need for methods to easily estimate BW in growing foals. Although growth studies in the Lusitano breed are being conducted (Fradinho *et al.*, 2004) they use weaned foals and therefore, information on the evolution of growth in suckling Lusitano foals is scarce (Santos *et al.*, 2005).

The objective of this study was to utilize morphometric parameters, of Lusitano suckling foals until 120 days of age, to predict body weight.

Material and methods

Measurements were made in 13 Lusitano foals during two consecutive years. Morphometric measurements were body weight (BW), withers height (WH), thoracic circumference (TC), cannon circumference (CC) and forearm circumference (FC). Foals were measured every 15 days after foaling and up to 120 days of age. Both foals and mares were kept on pasture during the hole study period, and a supplement of 3 kg grass hay (10.8% CP) and 2 kg concentrate (14.5% CP) was given to both mare and foal twice a day, yet, no specific supplementation were made to foals. These feeding conditions are close to those observed in most of Portuguese stud farms. Average daily gain (ADG) was calculated as the ration between BW differences and animal's age:

$$ADG = \frac{Bwi - BWj}{Age_i - Age_j} \qquad (1)$$

Statistical analysis was conducted using SAS. Linear regression analysis was performeded using GLM procedure of SAS.

Results and discussion

Values for BW, WH, TC, CC, FC and ADG (average daily gain) and their evolution along the study period are shown in Table 1.

There were no differences (P>0.05) between BW of colts and fillies at birth or during the trial, nevertheless, a tendency was found for BW of colts to be higher than fillies. This is also reported by other authors (Jones and Hollands, 2005). Nevertheless, Pagan *et al.* (1998) observed a significant difference between colts and fillies using thoroughbreds.

ADG values (0.85 kg/d from birth to 120 days of age) are somewhat lower than those found by Pagan *et al.* (1998) for thoroughbreds (1.18 kg/d birth to 120 days of age). Greene *et al.* (2005), using Morgan horses found an ADG of 0.59 kg/d.

Average values at birth of WH were 100.7±0.03 cm, 84.8±0,04 cm for TC, 13.3 ±0,01 cm for CC and 22.7±0.02 cm for FC.

There were no differences for WH and TC (P>0.05) between foals and fillies. A strong correlation was found between BW and WH and between BW and TC, and the following regression equations were calculated (Figure 1):

The determination coefficient for both equations (1 and 2) is relatively high, indicating that these equations are good estimators of BW for Lusitano colts and fillies up to 4 month of age (120 days).

BW = 4.1646 WH – 367.64 (R^2=0.95; RSD=8.79) (2)
BW = 2.8235 TC – 190.58 (R^2=0.94; RSD=9.27) (3)

Table 1. Average values±sd of BW, WH, TC, CC, FC and ADG and their variation along the study period.

Age (days)	BW (kg)	ADG (kg/d)	WH (cm)	TC (cm)	CC (cm)	FC (cm)
1	52.7±6.4	---	100.7±0.03	84.8±0.04	13.3±0.01	22.7±0.02
15	68.8±8.8	1.07	106.2±0.03	93.7±0.04	13.5±0.01	28.8±0.05
30	83.4±10.7	0.97	110.2±0.04	100.2±0.06	14.0±0.01	30.2±0.03
45	95.9±12.8	0.83	113.0±0.05	104.5±0.06	14.2±0.01	32.3±0.03
60	108.3±16.5	0.83	115.8±0.05	108.3±0.07	14.9±0.01	33.3±0.03
75	119.8±17.7	0.76	119.5±0.05	112.7±0.05	15.5±0.005	33.3±0.02
90	133.4±20.1	0.91	121.5±0.05	117.3±0.05	15.8±0.005	33.5±0.02
105	141.3±20.5	0.53	122.7±0.04	118.5±0.05	16.5±0.02	33.7±0.02
120	153.1±23.0	0.79	125.3±0.05	122.0±0.07	16.5±0.01	34.7±0.03

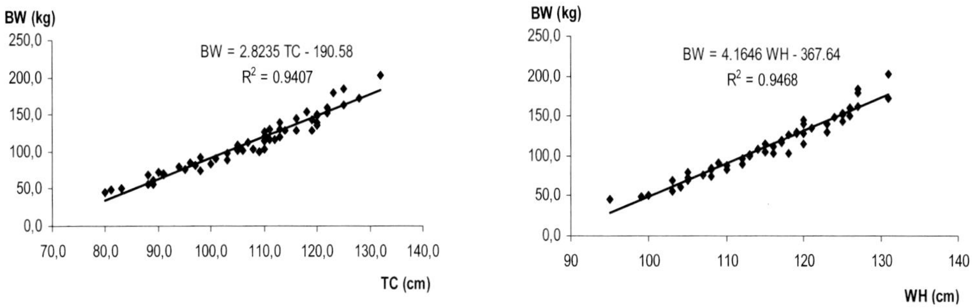

Figure 1. Linear regression between BW and WH (57 observations), and BW and TC (57 observations).

According to Martelo-Fradinho (1992) equations published for BW estimation of sadlebreds (Martin-Rosset *et al.*, 1990) don't seem very accurate for the Lusitano horse, since there are some morphological differences between breeds. This way, we can consider that the values we obtained may be used as a reference for Lusitano breed.

Values for CC and FC and their evolution as function of age are represented in Figure 2. Once again there were no differences (P>0.05) between colts and fillies.

Although no significant sexual dimorphism was found in our study, a tendency was shown for BW and WH to be higher in colts than in fillies. However, as our study was conducted with animals until 120 days of age the sexual dimorphism may not have been detected. In fact, according to Martin-Rosset (1983) the sexual dimorphism becomes obvious only when animals are 18 months old.

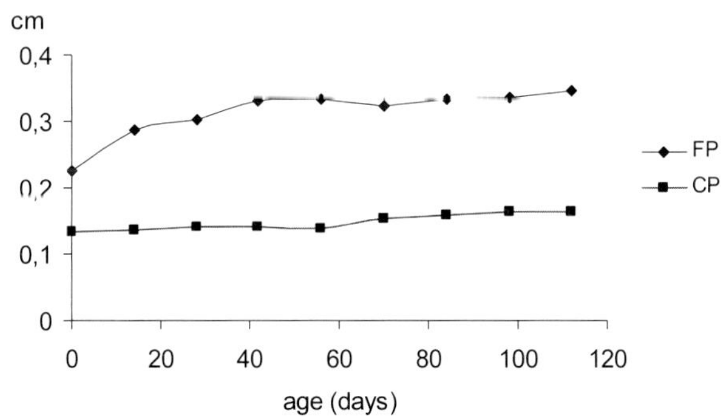

Figure 2. Evolution of cannon perimeter (CC) and forearm perimeter (FC) as a function of age during the study period.

Conclusions

The determined equations for predicting BW during the first 120 days of age can be utilized as a practical tool in the absence of weighing facilities in order to better control foals growth in stud farms.

This morphological evaluation of animals allows us to obtain a more complete report on their growth. For a more complete evaluation of the Lusitano breed growth, morphometric values of foals before weaning should be accounted. In this context, this study should serve as another tool for a complete study of the growth period in this breed, in order to help on the choice of the best possible breeding conditions or suggest new ones, especially concerning feeding supplementation to foals.

References

Fradinho, M.J.M. 2002. A influência da suplementação mineral em poldros de raça Lusitana. Tese de Mestrado. Faculdade de Medicina Veterinária. Universidade Técnica de Lisboa. Lisboa. Pp: 116.

Fradinho M.J, G. Ferreira-Dias, L. Mateus, F. Santos-Silva, R. Agrícola, M. Barbosa and J.M. Abreu, 2004. The influence of mineral supplementation on the growth of Lusitano foals. The growing horse: nutrition and prevention of growth disorders. V. Julliand and W. Martin-Rosset (eds.), EAAP publication No. 114, Wageningen Academic Publishers. 81-83.

Greene, E.A., J.R. Knapp and S.P. Davis, 2005. Predicting growth rates and mature sizes in Morgan Horses. The growing horse: nutrition and prevention of growth disorders. V. Julliand and W. Martin-Rosset (eds.), EAAP publication No. 114, Wageningen Academic Publishers. 73-74.

Jones, L. And T. Hollands, 2005. Estimation of growth rates in UK Thoroughbreds. Pferdheilkunde, 21:121-122.

Martelo-Fradinho, M.J., 1992. O cavalo de desporto em Portugal. I. Apresentação e análise de regimes alimentares praticados. II. Aspectos biométricos e ponderais avaliados em animais adultos. Relatório de Estágio do Curso de Engenheiro Agrónomo. Instituto Superior de Agronomia. Universidade Técnica de Lisboa. Lisboa. Pp: 75.

Martin-Rosset, W., 1990. L'Alimentation des chevaux. Institute National de la Recherche Agronomique, Paris, 232p.

National Research Council (NRC), 1989. Nutrient Requirements of Domestic Animals. nº 6 Nutrient Requirements of Horses, 5th revised edition. National Academy of Sciences, Washington D.C. 100 pp.

Pagan, J.D., 1998. A summary of growth rates of thoroughbreds in Kentucky. Advances in Equine Nutrition. J.D.Pagan (editor), Nottingham University Press. Thrumpton, Nottingham, UK. 449-455.

Santos, A.S, B.C. Sousa· L.C. Leitão and V.C. Alves, 2005. Crescimento de poldros de raça Lusitana até aos 120 dias de idade. In: Proceedings of the XV Animal Production Congress, I Ibero-American Animal Science Congress, Zootech I&D. Monteiro, D.O., Mena, E.G.,Sacoto, S.M. and Santos, A.S. (editors). APEZ Pub.

Passive immunity transfer forecast in different horse breeds

M. Orlandi and M.C. Curadi
Dept. Animal Production, University of Pisa, Viale delle Piagge 2, 56124 Pisa, Italy

Abstract

First trial was carried out on 11 thoroughbred mares. A correlation was noted between mare serum at delivery and 24 h colostrum IgG levels. Mare serum IgA collected one week before foaling were correlated with 24 h colostrum IgA. Significant correlation was found between foals serum IgGb amount at 0 h and IgGb mare serum content collected one week before foaling. IgG foal serum amounts collected one week after birth and IgG mare serum 2 weeks before foaling were also correlated. We noted correlation between gammaglobulins at delivery and 24h colostral IgGb. In the second trial 12 crossbred mares were examined. Total proteins (TP) mean level showed a good correlation with IgG concentration. Mare serum and mare colostrum IgG weren't correlated. Serum IgG(T) were correlated with IgG and highest values were observed at foaling as in the previous trial. Significant correlation was also observed between IgG and IgM. Foal serum IgG(T) were correlated with IgG and both showed highest values at 18 hours. Correlation was found between foal serum IgG contents at 6 and 18 hours and colostrum IgG levels at delivery. Foal serum α1-globulins level significantly increased between 3 and 48 hours from birth; the same was noted for γ-globulins between 3 and 24 hours. Albumin/Globulins ratio decreased, during the first 24 hours, from 2.5/1 at birth until about 1/1 at 18-24 hours.

Keywords: immunity transfer, newborn foal, equine

Introduction

Colostrum is the only immunoglobulins source for the newborn foal, since the diffuse epitheliochorial placenta doesn't allow the antibodies transfer during pregnancy (Steven and Samual, 1975; Perryman *et al.*, 1980). Foals are able to absorbe colostral immunoglobulins (Igs) through specialized cells lining the small intestine during the first 18-24 h after birth; after this time absorption is not possible and this could cause FPT (Failure of Passive Transfer) (Mc Guire and Crawford, 1973; Jeffcott, 1974; Morris *et al.*, 1985; Waelchli *et al.*, 1990), that is the most common cause predisposing sepsis in foal from birth to 4 weeks of age. The aim of these researches is to evaluate mare serum, colostrum and foal Igs and serum proteins concentration; if any correlations could be observed between this three classes and if it's possible to forecast foal convenient immunity transfer.

Materials and methods

Eleven thoroughbred multiparous mares in the first trial and twelve crossbred in the second one were selected for these experiments during a full breeding season. Mare's blood sample times were weekly from 3 weeks before scheduled delivery. Colostrum and milk samples (20 ml) were collected 0.1,15,30,60,90,120 days after foaling. Foals blood samples were collected within 3 hours after first suckling (0 h), after 24 h and after 1 week. Serum TP were determined by the Biuret method (Henry,1974). Colostrum TP were determined according to FIL-IDF 20B:1993 method. Serum and colostrum Igs concentrations were determined by use of single radial immunodiffusion. Main serum protein fractions, albumin, α1, α2, β and γ1 , γ2–globulins were performed with Microtech 648R. Data were expressed as mean value ± SD. MANOVA with repeated measures to evaluate differences at different collection times was performed by JMP. Data were statistically analysed about Pearson linear correlation.

Results and discussion

In the first trial good correlation was noted between mare serum at delivery and 24 h colostrum IgG levels ($r=0.82, p<0.05$). Mare serum IgA collected one week before foaling were strictly correlated with 24 h colostrum IgA ($r=0.87, p<0.05$) Significant correlation was found between foals serum IgGb amount at 0 h and IgGb mare serum content collected one week before foaling ($r=0.67, p<0.05$). IgG foal serum amounts collected one week after birth and IgG mare serum 2 weeks before foaling were also correlated ($r=0.89, p<0.05$) We noted correlation between gammaglobulins at delivery and 24h colostral IgGb ($r=0.76, p<0.05$). In the second trial total proteins level showed good correlation with IgG concentration. Mares serum and mares colostrum IgG weren't correlated. Mare's serum IgG(T) were correlated with IgG and highest values were observed at foaling as in the previous trial ($r=0.73, p<0.01$). Significant correlation was also observed between IgG and IgM. Foal serum IgG(T) were correlated with IgG and showed highest values at 18 hours ($r=0.60, p<0.01$). Significant correlation was found between foal serum IgG contents at 6 ($r=0.90, p<0.01$) and 18 hours ($r=0.88, p<0.01$) and colostrum IgG levels at delivery. Foal serum α1-globulins level significantly increased between 3 and 48 hours from birth; the same was noted for γ-globulins between 3 and 24 hours. Albumin/Globulins ratio decreased, during the first 24 hours, from 2.5/1 at birth until about 1/1 at 18-24 hours. Our results suggest that the early forecast of possible FPT,on the basis of possible correlations between mare's blood and colostrums Igs and proteins amounts can give a global information about passive immunity transfer and could get the foal able,in case of deficiency, to be fed with extra-colostrum.

References

Henry, R.J., 1974. Clinical Chemistry.Principles and technics, 2nd Ed.Harper and Rom, Maryland,USA.

Jeffcott, L.B., 1974. Studies on passive immunity in the foal. Gamma-globulin and antibody variations associated with the maternal transfer of immunity and the onset of active immunity. J. Comp. Pathol. 84, 93-101.

MC Guire, T.C. and T.B. Crawford, 1973. Passive immunity in the foal: measurement of immunoglobulin classes and specific antibody. Am. J. Vet. Res., 34, 1299-1303.

Morris, D.D., D.A. Meirs and G. Schad Merryman, 1985. Passive transfer failure in horses: incidence and causative factors on a breeding farm. Am. J. Vet. Res.,46, 2294-2299.

Perryman, L.E., T.C. MC Guire and R.L. Torbeck, 1980. Ontogeny of lymphocyte function in the equine fetus. Am. J. Vet. Res., 41, 1197-1200.

Steven, S. and C.A. Samual, 1975. Anatomy of the placental barrier in the mare. J. Reprod. Fert. Suppl., 23, 579-582.

Waelchli, R.O., M., Hässig E. Eggenberger and M. Nussbaumer, 1990. Relationships of total protein, specific gravity, viscosity, refractive index and latex agglutination to immunoglobulin G concentration in mare colostrum. Eq. Vet. J. 22: 1, 39-42.

TAHITIAN NONI™ Equine Essentials™ Regulates LPS-Induced COX-2 and cytokine expression in equine neonatal monocytes: A preliminary study

J. Xu[1], *J. Cai*[1], *R.G. Godbee*[2], *S.F. Peek*[1] *and B.J. Darien*[1]
[1]*University of Wisconsin, School of Veterinary Medicine, 2015 Linden Dr., Madison, WI. 53706-1102, USA*
[2]*University of Nevada, 1664 North. Virginia Street, Reno, NV 89557-0042, USA*

Abstract

Morinda citrifolia (NONI) has anti-inflammatory and immune enhancing effects. The objective of this study was to investigate the effects of *TAHITIAN* NONI™ Equine Essentials™ on endotoxin induced COX-2 and cytokine expression in equine monocytes from neonates during the first 60 days of life. Peripheral monocytes were collected from 4 foals aged 0, 10 and 60 days. Two foals were fed NONI for 60 days starting at 1 day after birth. LPS stimulated monocytes from NONI™ treated foal had reduced expression of COX-2, TNF-α, IL-1β, IL-8 and IL-6 compared to untreated controls. These preliminary results suggest that NONI may be a promising nutritional supplement for foals at risk from gram-negative septicaemia.

Keywords: TAHITIAN NONI™ Equine Essentials™, foal, COX-2, anti-inflammatory

Introduction

Septicemia in equine neonates and account for nearly one third of all foal mortalities. The clinical signs of septicemia result from the release of endotoxins (lipopolysaccharide, LPS), from gram-negative infections, which stimulate monocytes to express COX-2 and various cytokines.

There is a clinical need for novel anti-inflammatory therapies that are well tolerated *in vivo* without the potential side effects of NSAIDs. *TAHITIAN* NONI™® Juice is a natural herbal product made from the *Morinda citrifolia* tree, native to the South Pacific. It has a broad range of therapeutic effects including antibacterial, antiviral, anti-cancer, analgesic, anti-inflammatory, and immune enhancing effects (Liu *et al.* 2001; Wang *et al.*, 2002). It has established antioxidant (Su *et al.*, 2005), and selective cyclo-oxygenase-2 (COX-2) inhibitory activity (Su *et al.*, 2001), in human inflammatory cells. Based on these findings, we hypothesized that *TAHITIAN* NONI™ Equine Essentials™ would modulate endotoxin (lipopolysaccharide, LPS)-induced inflammatory responses in equine foal monocytes by regulating COX-2 and cytokine expression.

Materials and methods

Four neonatal foals were the subjects for the study. Adequate passive transfer (IgG >800mg/dl), was confirmed by a SNAP® Foal IgG (IDEXX Laboratories, Inc.) test at 24 hours of age. Subsequently, experimental foals (n=2) received 60ml *TAHITIAN* NONI™ Equine Essentials™ orally twice daily for 60 days. The 2 remaining foals served as aged matched controls. At days 0 (prior to receiving *TAHITIAN* NONI™ Equine Essentials™), 10 and 60 blood was obtained from the control and Noni treated foals and monocytes isolated as previously described. Monocytes from each foal were divided into an untreated control group and a group that was stimulated with LPS for 2 hours at 1000ng/ml. Total RNA was purified from equine monocytes, and 1 μg used for cDNA synthesis, using oligo (dT) and MLV reverse transcriptase. Quantitative RT-PCR analysis was performed by monitoring the real time increase in SYBR-green dye fluorescence using the iCycler iQ Real-Time PCR Detection

System. Relative mRNA levels for each cytokine were analyzed by using a comparative Ct ($2-\Delta\Delta C_T$) method with equine 18s as an internal control. Quantitative PCR analyses were performed comparing cytokine expression between Noni treated and control foals at each time point, and mathematically expressed as the relative fold increase in mRNA compared to the non-LPS treated control sample. Assays were run in parallel for each cytokine from the 3 sample time points.

Results and discussion

At day 10, *TAHITIAN* NONI™ Equine Essentials™ treated foals had a large reduction in COX-2, TNF-α (Figure 1A), IL-1β, IL-8 & IL-6 (Figure 1B), expression in LPS-stimulated monocytes of 23x, 10x, 15x, 30x and 35x, respectively, when compared to LPS-stimulated age-matched controls. Although less dramatic than day 10 results, a similar pattern was observed at day 60. *TAHITIAN* NONI™ Equine Essentials™ treated foals had a reduction in COX-2, TNF-α, IL-1β, IL-8 & IL-6 expression in LPS-stimulated monocytes of 9x, 180x, 8.5x, 22x and 35x, respectively, when compared to age-matched controls. The mean relative fold expression for all cytokines on day 0 was similar between control and NONI™ treated foals. The small number of subjects precludes statistical analyses and we realize this to be a limitation of the study.

Monocytes isolated from foals receiving *TAHITIAN* NONI™ Equine Essentials™ had markedly decreased COX-2, TNF-α, IL-1β, IL-8, and IL-6 mRNA expression following LPS stimulation when compared to moncytes from control foals. Reduction in COX-2 expression and associated pro-inflammatory mediators, most notably at 10 days of age, suggests that *TAHITIAN* NONI™ Equine Essentials™ may be a promising nutritional supplement in foals during the first weeks of life when gram-negative septicemia is the most common cause of death.

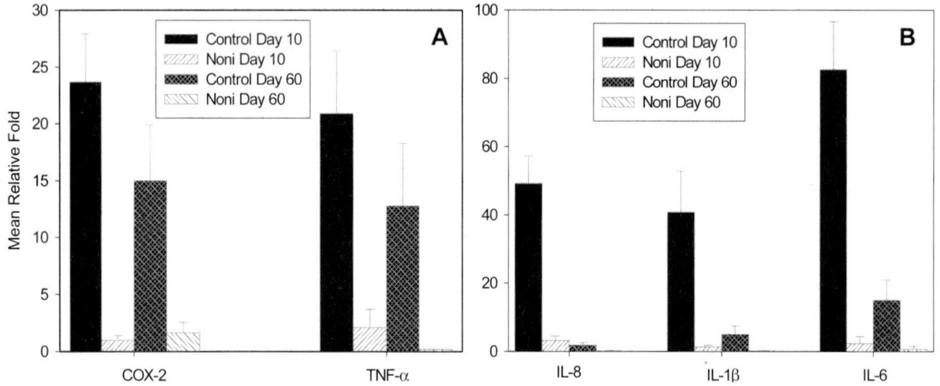

Figure 1. Mean relative fold change in COX-2, TNF-α (A) and IL-8, IL-1β and IL-6 (B) expression in LPS stimulated equine neonatal monocytes. Error bars represent sem.

References

Liu G, A. Bode, W.Y. Ma, S. Sang, C.-T. Ho and Z. Dong, 2001. Two novel glycosides from the fruits of Morrinda citrifolia (Noni) inhibit AP-1 transactivation and cell transformation in the mouse epidermal JB6 cell line. Cancer Res. 61:5749-5756.

Su B.-N., C.J. Jensen, M.-Y. Wang, J.W. Fritz and S. Jensen, 2001. A new selective COX-2 inhibitor, Morinda citrifolia (Noni). Proceedings, Eicosanoids & other bioactive lipids in cancer, inflammation and related diseases, 127pp.

Su B.-N., A.D. Pawlus, H.-A. Jung, W.J. Séller, J.L. McLaughlin and A.D. Kinghorn, 2005. Chemical constituents of the fruits of Morinda citrifolia (Noni) and their antioxidant activity. J Nat. Prod. 68:592-595.

Wang, M.-Y., B.J. West, C.J. Jensen, D. Nowicki, S. Chen, A.K. Palu and G. Anderson, 2002. Morinda citrifolia (Noni): A literature and recent advances in Noni research. Acta Pharmacol Sin 23:1127-1141.

Part D – Feeding practices and pastures management

Overview practices in the field in Europe: rationing and prevention of nutritional related problems in the mares

D. Bergero[1], M. Ventorp[2], I. Vervuert[3], N. Miraglia[4], C. Trillaud-Geyl[5] and E. Valle[1]
[1]Department of animal production, epidemiology & ecology, University of Veterinary Medicine, Via Leonardo Da Vinci 44, 10095 Grugliasco (To), Italy
[2]Department of farm buildings, Swedish University of Agricultural Sciences, Lund, Sweden
[3]Institute for Animal Nutrition, Faculty of Veterinary Medicine, University of Leipzig, Gustav Kuhn Str. 8, 04159 Leipzig, Germany
[4]Departemt of Animal, Vegetable and Environmental Sciences, Molise University, Via De Sanctis, 86100 Campobasso, Italy
[5]Les Haras Nationaux, Services Direction, Route de Troche BP N. 6, 19230 Pompadour, France

Abstract

Feeding management of the broodmares is of major concern to breed and raise adequately a foal. The nutritional requirements of the mares are 1.1 to 2.0 times maintenance higher in late pregnancy and 1.3 to 3.0 times maintenance higher in lactation. During these periods the mares gain from 5 to 15 percent of BW in pregnancy whereas milk yield ranges between 2 to 3 kg per 100 kg BW. Two questions arise in field conditions: what are the main nutritional key points to be considered, then how there are fitted in practice. Mares are bred in intensive, semi-intensive or extensive feeding and farming systems according to the goals of production. From field experience, the mares should cope with a large varieties of situations in Europe due to the types and quality of feedstuffs which are available. Situations of excess and deficiencies are routinely observed because nutritional recommendations are not well known or/and very often not well implemented by horse breeders. Some short term unbalanced rations are not too much detrimental due to body reserves of the mares and prompt supplementation. Long term unbalanced rations can predispose the mares and the foals to nutritional and pathological related problems.

Keywords: broodmares, nutrition, pregnancy, lactation, feeding practice

Introduction

In the European conditions the mares are managed in intensive, semi intensive or extensive systems devoted to produce race horses, sport horses and leisure horses respectively (Miraglia *et al.*, 2006). The reproductive cycle is usually split in reproductive season, early and late gestation, early and late lactation. (Lewis, 1995). As a result feeding allowances along the different sequences of the reproductive cycle are managed either to meet the requirements or grazing period is used to compensate winter feeding restriction according to the systems.

This review aims to describe the main feeding practices in Europe during the winter season when they are documented to highlight the main critical points which are met. Feeding the mares during the summer season is discussed elsewhere in this issue (Miraglia *et al.*, 2006).

Key nutritional points to be considered

Variation of the requirements along the reproductive cycle in the broodmares

During pregnancy and lactation, some nutritional key factors must be taken into account for optimal management: energy, protein, protein quality, calcium and phosphorous, vitamins and trace elements. The requirements increase steadily from maintenance until the 8th month of pregnancy till the parturition, and continue to rise in the first lactation period, when they reach the peak in the first month. If diets are grossly imbalanced in terms of Ca, P, energy or protein, the foal will be adversely affect at birth and reduced milk yield and infertility will ensue (see the chapters by Martin-Rosset et al., 2006a; 2006b; Doreau and Martuzzi, 2006 in this issue; Ellis *et al.*, 2006 in this issue; Frape, 2004).

The evaluation of European requirement estimation is important to improve knowledge and to propose some consideration. In Europe, a number of different systems are used to estimate the nutritional requirements of broodmares. Energy and protein requirements have been estimated in differents systems: NRC (National Research Council, 1989), GEH (Gesellschaft für Enärhungsphysiologie 1994), INRA (Institute National de la Recherche Agronomique, 1990), CVB (Central Veevoeder Bureau 2005), SCAND 2004 (Scandinavia, Austbo, 2004). So far, nutrients requirements and recommended allowances are proposed in the different systems and by the countries (Martin-Rosset *et al.*, 2006a; 2006b). This paper is focused on energy and protein requirements of 500 kg body weight (BW) mare during pregnancy and lactation; also mineral and vitamin requirements are considered, even if, most of the information are focused on the NRC and INRA recommendations.

The last trimester of pregnancy is mainly concerned as the nutrient requirements for normal conceptus growth is crucial. During these three month the mares gain from 2% to 15% of total BW according to body condition score (BCS) in early pregnancy (Martin-Rosset, 1990; Martin-Rosset et al 2006a). Until the first 8 months the mare should be fed as a mature idle, taking into due account BCS and physiological status. Nutrient allowances depend on intake capacity and body reserves of the mare throughout the breeding cycle (INRA 1990; Lewis, 1995; NRC, 1989; Frape, 2004; Martin-Rosset *et al.*, 2006a).

During the late pregnancy the energy requirements for 500 kg BW mare are 1.05 to 1.26 times maintenance higher according to the months and the recommendations proposed in the different countries. The requirements are maximum in the last months of pregnancy. But the variation according to the months are divergent between the countries (Table1).

The protein requirements of 500kg BW late pregnant mare are 1.0 to 1.79 times maintenance higher according to the month of pregnancy and the recommendations proposed in the different countries (Table 2). The protein requirements should be met as far as the effect of protein allowances is not

Table 1. Variation of daily energy requirements for 500 Kg BW mares in according to the different systems (maintenance = 100).

<table>
<tr><th></th><th>NRC
1989</th><th>GEH
1994</th><th>INRA
1990</th><th>CVB
2005</th><th>SCAND
2004</th></tr>
<tr><td>Maintenance</td><td>100</td><td>100</td><td>100</td><td>100</td><td>100</td></tr>
<tr><td>Months of pregnancy</td><td></td><td></td><td></td><td></td><td></td></tr>
<tr><td>8</td><td>-</td><td>113</td><td rowspan="2">110</td><td>105</td><td>107</td></tr>
<tr><td>9</td><td>111</td><td rowspan="2">119</td><td rowspan="2">110</td><td>113</td></tr>
<tr><td>10</td><td>113</td><td>124</td><td>118</td></tr>
<tr><td>11</td><td>120</td><td>126</td><td>126</td><td>115</td><td>125</td></tr>
</table>

Table 2. Variation of daily protein requirements for 500 Kg BW mares according to the different recommendations (maintenance =100).

<table>
<tr><th></th><th>NRC
1989</th><th>GEH
1994</th><th>INRA
1990</th><th>CVB
2005</th><th>SCAND
2004</th></tr>
<tr><td>Maintenance</td><td>100</td><td>1000</td><td>100</td><td>100</td><td>100</td></tr>
<tr><td>Pregnancy (Months)</td><td></td><td></td><td></td><td></td><td></td></tr>
<tr><td>8</td><td>-</td><td>100</td><td rowspan="2">115</td><td>116</td><td>119</td></tr>
<tr><td>9</td><td>122</td><td rowspan="2">118</td><td rowspan="2">141</td><td>139</td></tr>
<tr><td>10</td><td>124</td><td>156</td><td>152</td></tr>
<tr><td>11</td><td>132</td><td>128</td><td>164</td><td>171</td><td>179</td></tr>
</table>

yet determined (Marin-Rosset et al 2006a). The requirements are maximum during the last month. But the variation with the months is divergent between the countries.

Minerals and vitamins recommendation derive in the different systems mostly from NRC and INRA systems. Calcium requirements in pregnant mare are 1.75 to 1.85 times maintenance higher for NRC while they are 1.17 to 1.57 times maintenance higher for INRA (Table 3).The requirements are higher during the last month of pregnancy. But the variation with the months are divergent between the systems.

Phosphorus requirements are 1.86 to 2.00 times maintenance higher for NRC while they are 1.20 to 1.87 times maintenance higher for INRA (Table 4).The requirements are higher during the last month of pregnancy. But the variation with the months are divergent between the systems.

Table 3. Daily calcium requirements for 500 Kg BW pregnant mares in according to NRC 1989, INRA 1990 and proportional increase in calcium requirements (maintenance=100).

Calcium	Non lactating mare during the 8 months of pregnancy	9 month (a)	10 month (b)	11 month (c)	% (a)	% (b)	% (c)
NRC[1]	20 g	35 g	35 g	37 g	175	175	185
INRA[2]	25 g	29 g	38 g	39 g	117	153	156

Table 4. Daily phosphorus requirements for 500 Kg BW pregnant mares in according to NRC 1989, INRA 1990 and proportional increase in Phosphorus requirements (maintenance=100).

Phosphorus	Non lactating mare during the 8 months of pregnancy	9 month (a)	10 month (b)	11 month (c)	% (a)	% (b)	% (c)
NRC[1]	14 g	26 g	26 g	28 g	186	186	200
INRA[2]	15 g	18 g	26 g	28 g	120	173	187

The other critical period of breeding cycle of the broodmare is lactation (see Martin-Rosset et al., 2006b). The mare must should nurse adequately the foal and be rebred during the first month following foaling to meet an appropriate date of foaling in the next breading season, and 12 months interval between two subsequent foaling.

The energy requirements for 500 kg BW mare in lactation are 1.49 to 2.0 times maintenance higher according to the months and the recommendations proposed in the different countries (Table 5). The maximum takes place in early lactation. But the variation with month of lactation are divergent between the countries.

The protein requirements for 500 kg BW mare in lactation are 1.4 to 3.0 times maintenance higher according to the months and the recommendations proposed in the different countries (Table 6). The maximum takes place in early lactation. But the variation with month of lactation are divergent between the countries.

Calcium requirements in lactating mare are 2.80 to 1.80 times maintenance higher for NRC while they are 2.44 to 1.56 times maintenance higher for INRA (Table 7). The requirements are higher during the first months of lactation. But the variation with the months are divergent between the systems.

Table 5. Variation of the energy daily requirements for 500 Kg BW lactating mares in the first trimester of lactation across the different system (maintenance =100).

	NRC 1989	GEH 1994	INRA 1990	CVB 2005	SCAND 2004
Lactation					
1st month	173	169	212	202	200
2-3 months	173	177	182	206	204
4-6 months	149	149	162	184	182

Table 6. Variation of the protein daily requirements for 500 Kg BW lactating mares in the first trimester of lactation across the different system (maintenance =100).

	NRC 1989	GEH 1994	INRA 1990	CVB 2005	SCAND 2004
Lactation					
1st month	218	252	321	298	297
2-3 months	218	227	261	308	308
4-6 months	160	144	223	258	258

Table 7. Daily calcium requirements for 500 Kg BW lactating mares in according to NRC 1989, INRA 1990 and proportional increase in calcium requirements (maintenance=100).

Calcium	1months (a)	2 –3 months (b)	4 months to weaning (c)	% (a)	% (b)	% (c)
NRC[1]	56 g	56 g	36 g	280	280	180
INRA[2]	61 g	47 g	39 g	244	188	156

Phosphorus requirements are 2.57 to 1.57 times maintenance higher for NRC while they are 3.67 to 2.13 times maintenance higher for INRA (Table 8). The requirements are higher during the first month of lactation. But the variation with the months are divergent between the systems.

The supply of trace elements is also important either in pregnancy or during lactation even if, in the practice, we consider that lower trace elements dietary imbalances are less detrimental. Body's reserves of the mare can contribute to short term adjustment to a variety of nutritional situation. During pregnancy iodine and selenium status have considerable effect on fertility of the mare and the viability of the foal. A deficiency or excess of either iodine or selenium depresses embryonic development and resources of the foal (Frape, 2004). Copper deficiency has been implicated in equine osteochondrosis by several studies in foals. During pregnancy copper will be stored in the foetal liver and is used as Cu source during the first months of foals' life. However, in accordance with Winkelsett *et al.*, (2005) there would be no significant relation between Cu intake of the pregnant mare and osteochondrosis occurrence in the foals. Moreover selenium and vitamin E deficiency occurs in foals at birth to one month of age, as a result of inadequate selenium intake by the mare during pregnancy and lactation (Lewis, 1995) (Tables 9 and 10).

Table 8. Daily calcium requirements for 500 Kg BW lactating mares in according to NRC 1989, INRA 1990 and proportional increase in calcium requirements (maintenance=100).

Phosphorous	1months (a)	2 –3 months (b)	4 months to weaning (c)	% (a)	% (b)	% (c)
NRC[1]	36 g	36 g	22 g	257	257	157
INRA[2]	55 g	40 g	32 g	367	267	213

Table 9. Daily trace mineral requirements of broodmares in according to INRA, 1990 (mg/kg DM) and NRC 1989.

Minerals	Last trimester of pregnancy and first period of lactation INRA	Last trimester of pregnancy and first period of lactation NRC
Copper	10	10
Zinc	50	40
Selenium	0.1-0.2	0.1
Iodium	0.1-0.3	0.1-0.6
Iron	80-100	50
Cobalt	0.1	0.1

Table 10. Daily vitamin requirements of broodmares according to INRA, 1990 and NRC 1989.

Vitamins	Last trimester of pregnancy	Last trimester of pregnancy NRC	First period of lactation INRA	First period of lactation NRC
Vitamin A UI	4200	3500	3000	3000
Vitamin D UI	600	850	600	600
Vitamin E UI	11	7	80	80
Vitamin B1 mg	2.5	2.5	3	3
Vitamin B2 mg	4.2	4.2	2	2

Balance of the ration

Rations should be balanced accurately according to the main minerals and trace elements using the main following ratios between the daily nutrients allowances: N/E, Ca/P, Cu/Zn, Vit A/Vit D.

Conditions for Rationing

From a practical point of view it is not easy to implement all these recommendations namely for rationing. This is can be ascribed to the different systems utilised to evaluate and express the requirements (Martin-Rosset et al., 2006a - 2006b). The divergence between the recommendations could be due as well to the specificity of the different breeding systems and aims across Europe referring to different breeds and specializations.

Characteristics of diets and rations

An important aspect to point out for rationing field practice is the difference between requirements and feed allowances in Europe: this point needs also data about the composition of the feeds used for the broodmares, but some figures can be given at this point. The imbalance between requirements and allowances are often met in the fields (tables 11 and 12).

Diets and rations for broodmares are prepared according to the optimum nutrient intake given by the different authors (see Tables 1 to 10). However, the optimum nutrients intake can be compromised if poor quality forage is fed. In these conditions, the energy density can increase widely, because the concentrate percentage will rise (see later). This is particularly true for thoroughbred (Table 14).

In according to Harris 2001, the amount of forage and concentrate used in the field are very similar to those proposed by NRC and INRA during the last trimester of pregnancy and lactation (Martin Rosset *et al.*, 2006a - 2006b).

Table 11. Comparison of feed allowances to the requirements in pregnant mares of thoroughbred (TB), French Trotter (FT) and Selle français (SF) breeds in the area of Normandy in France (from Valette et al., 2004).

Nutrients	Requirements	Feed allowances deviation to the requirements (range)	Average deviation (%)
DM [1] kg	9.1	+ 0.8 – 1.2	+11
UFC[2]	6.3	+ 0.3 – 1.3	+10
MADC[3] g	440	+ 134 – 358	+56
Ca[4] g	39	+ 19 – 20	+50
P[4] g	25	+ 4 – 13	+34
Cu[4] mg	205	+ 23 – 51	+18
Zn[4] mg	645	+ 74 – 137	+16
Ca/P	1.6	+ 0.4 – 0.6	+31
Zn/Cu	3.1	+ 0.7 – 1.9	+42
MADC/ UFC	70	+ 10 – 32	+30

[1]DM: Dry Matter

[2]Unité Fourragère Cheval (Horse Feed Unit): requirements calculated from INRA 1990

[3]MADC: Matières Azotées Digestibles Cheval (Horse Digestible Protein): requirements calculated from INRA 1990.

[4]Minerals: requirements calculated from NRC 1989.

Table 12. Comparison of feed allowances to the requirements in lactating mares (from Valette et al., 2004).

Nutrients	Requirements	Feed allowances deviation to the requirements (range)	Average deviation (%)
DM [1] kg	12.5	+ 0.7 – 2.1	+11
UFC[2]	8.9	+ 0.5 – 2.0	+15
MADC[3] g	850	+ 224 – 495	+42
Ca[4] g	56	+ 12 – 22	+30
P[4] g	44	+ 6 – 8	+16
Cu[4] mg	205	+ 18 – 70	+21
Zn[4] mg	645	+ 88 – 153	+19
Ca/P	1.3	+ 0.3 – 0.7	+39
Zn/Cu	3.1	+ 0.3 – 1.3	+26
MADC/ UFC	97	+ 26 – 28	+28

[1]DM: Dry Matter

[2]Unité Fourragère Cheval (Horse Feed Unit): requirements calculated from INRA 1990

[3]MADC: Matières Azotées Digestibles Cheval (Horse Digestible Protein): requirements calculated from INRA 1990.

[4]Minerals: requirements calculated from NRC 1989.

Table 13. Optimum level of daily nutrient intake for Kg of DM in the last trimester of pregnancy and first period of lactation in according to INRA, 1990 and NRC 1989.

	Last trimester of pregnancy INRA 1990	First period of lactation INRA 1990	Last trimester of pregnancy NRC 1989	First period of lactation NRC 1989
Energy	0.50-0.70 UFC	0.60-0.80 UFC	2.25-2.40 Mcal DE	2.60 Mcal DE
Protein	45-70 g MADC	55-90 g MADC	10-10.6 g CP	13.2 g CP
Calcium	4.6 g	4.3 g	0.43-0.45%	0.52%
Phosphourus	3.2 g	3.7 g	0.32-0.34%	0.34%
Vitamin A	4200 UI	3500 UI	3710-3650 UI	2750 UI

DE: Digestible Energy; UFC: Horse feed unit or Unitè Fourragere Cheval; CP: Crude Protein; MADC: Matières Azotées Digestibles Cheval (Horse Digestible Crude Protein)

But intake and the proportion of concentrate are adjusted too when legumes are fed to the mares as well (Table 15) as voluntary intake of legumes is higher than that of graminea.

Nutritive value of feeds

The quality of feed used for broodmares across Europe varies widely (Table 16 and 17). In general, poor quality forages are used for the first months of pregnancy, while the best are normally used for lactation. As previously mentioned, the same forage quality can impair the forage to concentrate ratio and the protein and energy density of the diets.

Due to the fact that different nutrients increase at different rates with the pregnancy, and lactation involves even wider and sudden changes, a mere increase and subsequent decrease in the amount

Table 14. A practical guide to the amounts of forage and concentrates fed to broodmares used in UK from Harris, 2001 (modified).

Category	%BW as fed basis		
	Forage	Concentrates	Total
Mature horse at maintenance	2	0	1. 2
	1.5-1.8	0.2-0.5	2
	1.5-2	0-0.5	1.75-2
	95	5	
Mares-late gestation	1.2	0.8	2
	1.4-1.8	0.26-0.6	
	1.5-2.0	0.25-0.75	
	Non Tb 80	Non TB 20	2-2.25
	TB 40	TB 60	
Mares-early lactation	1.5	1	2.5
	1.5	1.5	1.5
	1.5-1.75	1-1.5	
	Non Tb 80	Non TB 20	1-1.5
	TB 40	TB 60	
Mares-late lactation	1.4	0.6	2
	1.5-1.75	0.75-1.0	2-2.5
	1.25-1.75	0.75-1.25	2-2.5
	Non Tb 90	Non TB 10	
	TB 50	TB 50	

Table 15. Expected feed intake and diet proportion for broodmares consuming legumes forages (alfalfa) in USA from Duren, 2001 (modified).

Category	Diet proportion forage	Diet proportion concentrates	Feed intake % of BW
9th Month	95	5	2.0-2.5
10th Month	85	15	2.0-2.5
11th Month	80	20	2.0-2.5

of maintenance feed during the late pregnancy and lactation is inadequate. The type of feed must be adapted to the development of pregnancy, physiologic status and breed. Moreover, the BCS (Body Condition Score) of the mares can be widely impaired by dietary imbalances, with subsequent negative impact on normal parturition, milk yield, fertility and the same health of the mare. The BCS is the parameter that breeders are more able to evaluate. In fact for maximum reproductive efficiency the mare prior the breeding should be moderate fleshy and be fed to maintain this weight (Lewis, 1994). The breeders are able to determine on anecdotic basis or using a proper BCS scale the mare. The BCS of broodmares is also used to adjust rationing. Thin mares are for example given 1-2 kg extra concentrate per day starting from 2-3 weeks before mating to increase fertility (flushing technique).

Table 16. Compare between average nutrient content of meadow hays referred as Good and Poor quality in France, Norway, UK. And Italy (per Kg DM).

Forages	Energy (UFC)	DCPg/kg	P g/kg	Ca g/kg
Meadow hay good quality in France [1]	0.66	58	3	6
Meadow hay pour quality in France [1]	0.46	38	2	5.5
Meadow hay good quality in Norway[2]	0.77	120	2.7	3
Meadow hay poor quality in Norway[2]	0.54	88	2.5	3
Meadow hay good quality in UK[2]	0.67	120	2.7	5.4
Meadow hay poor quality in UK[2]	0.54	80	2.3	3
Meadow hay good quality in Italy[3]	0.61	80	-	-
Meadow hay poor quality in Italy[3]	0.5	68	-	-

[1]INRA,1990
[2]Austbø, 2004
[3]Bergero *et al.*, 2004

Table17. Chemical composition and digestibility coefficients of natural meadows hays in Mediterranean countries (Corino et al., 1995 - 1996).

Hays	Natural meadws 1	Natural meadws 2	Natural meadws 3	Natural meadws 4
Chemical composition (%)				
Dry matter	91.6	93.4	96.4	96.4
Organic Matter	92.4	92.7	93.2	91.7
Ashes	7.6	7.4	6.8	8.3
Crude Protein	8.4	9.1	7.0	8.5
Crude fibre	34.2	30.2	34.0	34.0
NDF	69.8	60.1	66.2	64.7
ADF	38.1	31.3	37.2	37.5
ADL	4.6	4.2	5.9	5.2
UFC (n.)	0.5	0.6	0.5	0.5

Feeding practices and management of the mares: the European situation

Management practices and the associate nutrition planning of broodmares depend on the breed and future expected career of horses and on the expectation of the breeders: horses farming and feeding systems are determined by the objective of production and utilisation. Athlete horses include two main groups: early developing horses destined to races (thoroughbred and standardbred) and late-maturing horses (saddle horses) destined to high level equestrian competitions or to low level equestrian competitions and leisure.

In spite of the key role of nutrition for horses production, feeding and nutrition are traditionally considered a marginal aspect of the management of broodmares. Despite the research features emphasise the importance of nutrition and balanced rations, most of the horsemen continue to use traditional rations generally composed by oats and hay only or pasture (Miraglia, 2004) because the level of technical education is still low at present.

On the field the hay is generally divided in good quality or pour quality hay. Mostly, first cut meadow hay, rich in gramineae, is preferred, but alfalfa hay is nowadays also widely used, for example for Quarter horses broodmares during lactation.

If the forage contains at least 10% crude protein on DM, no supplementation of protein offered; When the hay contains less than 8% crude protein and accounts for 70% of the total diet DM a concentrate containing about 16-17% of crude protein is fed (Frape, 2004). Even if the protein requirements are satisfied, it is always important to analyse the mineral content of the diet. Generally all forage are low in phosphorous and provide insufficient calcium to meet the mares need, in particular when unbalanced concentrates are used. Mares kept during the last trimester of pregnancy and lactation are fed high-quality conserved forage, containing some 30-40% leafy clover, Lucerne or sainfoin require no other source of Ca. However not all hays have a sufficient content of calcium and contain less than 2 g/kg DM of phosphorous (Frape, 2004). For this reason it is important to use a salt balance calcium-phosphorous mineral mix.

According to the previous data, and taking into account the composition of the feedstuffs used, a theoretical composition of a premix for broodmares is proposed by INRA (Table 18).

Table 18. Theoretical composition of a premix for broodmares in according to INRA 1990.

	Daily quantities		
	50 g	100 g	150g
Magnesium %	6-8	3-4	2-3
Sodium %	10-14	5-12	3-10
Copper mg/kg	800-2000	400-1000	250-700
Zinc mg/kg	3500-10000	1750-5000	1250-3300
Cobalt mg/kg	30-50	15-25	9-16
Manganese mg/kg	0-4000	0-2000	0-1300
Vitamin A UI/kg	600000-1100000	300000-550000	200000-350000
Vitamin D UI/kg	75000-150000	370000-800000	25000-50000

Intensive system

Large breeding farms (breeding standardbred and thoroughbred) usually manage the broodmares on pasture. Commonly, when the winter is coming, they keep the barren, maiden and pregnant mares in the stable, to use a light program and providing adequate quantities of good quality food (hay and grain concentrate); in this way they regulates the ovulation by light and give a sufficient quantity of food, to provide adequate energy to maintain or improve their body condition score. In fact insufficient dietary energy or protein intake may prevent ovulation or may result in early embryonic death (Lewis, 1994).

When the mares are in the stable they are usually feed with forage and concentrate. Generally in Europe, and in particular in Italy, the 70-80% of the diet is made up of meadow sun-cured hay.

In particular the most commonly used forages are first cut meadow hay and alfalfa hay. Forages may be often dusty and mouldy with a diminished nutrient value: this condition is very variable and depend by the environmental condition during the haymaking season. For example on the field often is available poor quality hay with all the characteristic that are reported in Table 14.

Breeders feed the pregnant mares also with cereal as oat, barley and corn as single cereals or cereal mixes, but not all the breeding farm supplement the cereal mix with protein rich components (soybean, horse beans) or vitamin and mineral complexes.

Other breeding farms usually employ commercial feed formulated for the maintenance (12.5% crude protein), or for breeding (16% of crude protein).

Cereal or commercial mix may have different quality. In particular cost lowering very often involves a reduction in the quality of feedstuff used and in this situation, no vitamins and no trace elements are added. For this reason risk of deficiencies or, in turn, of excess of some nutrients are frequent. According to Harris (2001), the actual ration fed to horses will wary according to a number of factors including BCS, forage and feedstuff used, breed and other individual factors. Then, in the last trimester of pregnancy, a common diet for non thoroughbred horses might be composed of 80% of forage (hay) as fed and 20% of concentrate as fed; a diet for thoroughbreds could be composed of 40% of forages (hay) as fed and 60% of concentrate as fed. These quantities are obviously only a general indication of what happens in the field when feeding broodmares. In fact this amounts depend essentially on the BCS, managements and feedstuffs used. In field conditions, sometimes mares consume legume (alfalfa) hay and are generally fed also concentrates (Duren, 2001) (Table 11 and 12). Even if the protein requirements are satisfied, it is always important to analyse the mineral content of the diet.

When mares are bred they are kept in the stable until the echographical diagnosis. After they are brought to pastures, normally until the next autumn season. In this way they get several advantages because the grazed grass has high digestibility, requires no storage and limits labour; moreover, grazing provides exercise. However the quality of pastures is quite contrasted in different geographical areas and under different weather conditions.

Semi- intensive system

In the saddle breeding farms for high level equestrian competitions, two typologies of breeding can be practised: horses can be kept at pasture 24h/day, or more frequently only during the day. In this case it is possible to have a accurate control of the horses and the administration of concentrates is performed in box before coming out at morning and in the evening when they come back: in this way an individual feeding program can be provided, with cereals and forage. Sun-cured meadow hay is usually used, but in some cases, such as the breeding of American breeds such as Quarter horses, breeders prefer to use alfalfa hay as the feeding basis.

In the case of saddle horses for high level competitions the role of pastures is similar to that of horses destined to races.

In northern countries of Europe such as Sweden, horses may be kept in groups. In fact many of the big Swedish studs, if keeping the horses in groups, use *ad libitum* feeding of hay silage in racks or feeding tables not also for lactating mares and youngsters, but even for pregnant mares. However, when trying to ration the feed to group kept horses, including pregnant mares, restrictively, more and more breeders use feed stalls, or sometimes computer controlled concentrates and roughage feeding stations. Feed stalls are very narrow stalls (700-50 mm wide for horses, ca 1 000 mm to mares in late pregnancy), placed in a row along a feeding table or feeding alley (then have each stall a manger). In some studs the stalls have locking devices in the rear part of the stall. A few breeders, mainly at small studs, still tether group kept horses at mangers, including the pregnant mares, or are taken the horses to ordinary stalls or individual pens for feeding. Both feed stalls and feeding stations and individual pens give very good possibilities to feed the calculated feed amount. Some horse keepers are aware of measuring/weighing every meal, but mostly they do not do.

Extensive system

Mares destined to produce leisure horses are often bred outdoor all the year long. This management and feeding plans are using the exploitation of extensive surfaces in humid temperate mountainous or hilly areas and/or sometimes rangelands. The grazing season lasts 230 days and no supplementation is given to the mares during this period. Mares grazed in association or alternate with ruminants. During the winter, mares are fed either with hays or maize silages (30-35% DM content) based diets (7.4kg DM and 10.5kg DM respectively) supplemented with low or limited concentrate (2.5 or 0.9 kg DM respectively) (Trillaud-Geyl *et al.*, 1990). Foals are weaned in early fall at 237 kg BW from mares which weight 550-600 kg to allow the mares to meet their optimum BCS before the winter period where they are fed no more than the requirements and sometimes body reserves are mobilised. This system is efficient as 77 percent of the mares are fertilised but fragile as time-interval between two pregnancies averages 397 days. Indeed, the system is highly dependant of good pasture resources and climatic conditions.

Balance of the rations and related problems

Surveys in Europe

The influence of adequate rationing on the health of the mare and the foals has been studied in France and in Germany in the scope of two large surveys.

In France 28 stud farms were included in a large survey during the year 1997-1999 in the area of Normandy (Valette *et al.*, 2004). 286 mares of 3 major breeds were concerned: thoroughbred (TB), French Trotter (FT) and Selle français (SF) devoted to riding competitions. Feed allowances fed to pregnant and nursing mares were determined by time – interval sampling and control during the reproductive cycle. Feed allowances are compared to the theoretical requirements (Tables 10-11). Orthopaedic status of the foals was determined by X-Ray using the protocol designed by Denoix (Denoix *et al.*, 2000. The pregnant mares are on average slightly overfed in energy, copper and zinc: 10%-18%-16% respectively. But they are extensively overfed in protein, calcium and phosporus: 56%-50%-34% respectively. As result the main nutritional ratios are surmount by MADC/UFC (30%), Ca/P (31%), Cu/Zn (42%). It arises clearly a good relationship between excess of calcium, phosporus, copper and zinc, and related unconsistent Cu/Zn ratio with the occurrence of DOD in the foals.

The nursing mares are moderately overfed in energy, phosporus, copper and zinc: 11-16-21-19 percent respectively. So far, all the main nutritional ratios are unbalanced. There would be a strong relationship between excess of Copper and Zinc and unbalanced Cu/Zn ration with occurrence of DOD in the foals.

In Germany a similar survey was carried out during the years 2000-2001 in 83 stud farms (Winkelsett *et al.*, 2005). 629 warmblood mares were concerned. Feed allowances fed to the mares were determined by time interval sampling and control during the stable period to estimate nutrient intake. During pasture time nutrient intake by grass regarding dry matter intake (dry matter intake: 2.2% of BW) was calculated for the mares. As the foals were not fed separately from their dams during stable period and pasture time, the energy to nutrient ratio (stable ration for the mares, milk and grass) was calculated to assess the supposed nutrient intake in foals. This proceeding implied an adequate energy intake by the foals (BW development and daily BW gain). X-ray controls for osteochondrosis

(OCD) were done between the fifth and tenth month after birth. Radiographic diagnosis showed 226 foals with signs of osteochondrotic lesions. The pregnant mares generally were fed too much energy and protein but also calcium, phosphorus: 43 to 70 percent of the mares were concerned, and they were strongly restricted in copper and zinc: 48 to 63 percent of the mares; with regard to requirement during the stabled period (Table 19).

During the winter period the nursing mares would have been restricted in energy and protein: 53 to 66 percent of the mares were affected respectively and overfed of calcium, copper and zinc: 48 – 54 60 percent of the mares respectively. In summer 90 and 77 percent of the nursing mares were fed too much protein and Phosphorus respectively whereas 69 to 76 were restricted in calcium and zinc. The mares were not supplemented with compound feeds. The imbalances of broodmares nutrition did not clearly show any correlation with the development of osteochondrosis. However the nutrient supply of the broodmares and foals should be corrected by balanced diet to avoid problems.

Table 19. Deviations of nutrient intake [%] of the pregnant mare [600 kg BW] with regard to requirement during stable period [N = 298] (Winkelsett et al., 2005).

Nutrient	Deviations of nutrient intake [%] of the pregnant mare with regard to recommendation					Requirement*
	<-30	-30/-10	-10/10**	10/30	>30	
vRp	-	6.8	30.4 (627-697 g)	11.1	51.7	640 g
DE	4.7	13.5	38.5 (93-109 MJ)	37.5	5.7	101 MJ
Ca, g	4.7	1.7	32.4 (41-49 g)	18.9	42.2	45 g
P, g	1.7	24.0	3.0 (29 g)	18.6	52.7	30 g
Zn, mg	42.6	20.3	3.4 (550-562 mg)	-	33.8	600 mg
Cu, mg	35.8	12.5	11.5 (112-125 mg)	6.4	33.8	120 mg

*Requirement/day: 11th months of pregnancy, BW 600 kg

**-10/10% of requirement is estimated as adequate, in brackets nutrient intake in g, mg or MJ/day

Other concerns

Care must be taken not to get the mare too fat, for example giving too much energy with cereals. Although even severe obesity doesn't appear to affect the pregnant mare, the duration of pregnancy, placental weight or passage, or foaling, but it may decrease milk production. Also excess of thinness at foaling may decrease the production of milk and decrease the reproductive efficiency. Anyway the birth weight of the foal appears to be little affected by its dam's weight gain or loss during pregnancy, or her body weight at foaling, whether she is obese or thin (Lewis,1995). However energy is important for ovulation and embryonic development, but less for foetal growth, until the last trimester of pregnancy; an excessive energy supply may favour twins, whereas restriction prior parturition can induce premature birth, or laminitis. This severe problems can be a consequence of hindgut microflora disturbances with painful locomotion and risks for the hoof integrity. Up to 70% of grazing mares underwent at least one laminitis episode. The massive ingestion of tender grazed grass (spring rise), the huge ingestion of cereals, massive ingestion of water are the main causes related to feeding practice. Laminitis can be also a consequence of parturition, excess workload, obesity, hormonal imbalance, drugs, viral disease and stress. To avoid these problems, it is necessary to avoid excess of cereals administration, sudden dietary changes, in particular from poor to rich rationing, grazing on lush pastures during spring rise (low fiber, high protein).

Feeding broodmares low quantities of feedstuffs, during the a period of high energy requirements, as the term of pregnancy and lactation, may also result in hiperlipemia syndrome. This illness may occur also as result of inappetence or dysphagia. Hyperlipemia may occur most frequently in obese ponies during late gestation or lactation. When there is a negative energy balance the results is a peripheral body fat mobilization at rate faster than it can be utilized. This condition is also supported by peripheral insulin resistance exacerbate by pregnancy and stress. If hyperlipemia is detected at an early stage and nutritional support is adequate to meet the animal's caloric requirements with a low-fat diet, recovery will generally occur. Prevention of hyperlipemia includes guaranteeing adequate quantities of good quality feedstuffs, particularly during the later stages of pregnancy and throughout lactation especially for obese ponies (Lewis, 1994).

Conclusions

Pregnant and lactating mares have specific needs, in particular in the last three months of pregnancy and during the first month of lactation. In these periods there are some key factors: energy, proteins, minerals (calcium and phosphorous) and related vitamins (A and D), trace elements (copper zinc) and their optimal ratio. However too many often for this categories of horses the nutrition is only a marginal aspect.

The general tendency of the broodmares managements depend on the typology of horses and on the expectation of the breeders: horses farming and feeding systems are determined by the objective of production and utilisation. Nowadays in Europe too many imbalance diet are used for pregnant mares: excess in energy, protein, calcium and phosphorus are frequent especially in saddle horses. Also Zn and Cu deficit are frequently present and may predispose the foal to this deficiency.

To provide sufficient dietary energy, protein, as well other nutrients, will diminish the risk of mares' problem or foal disease such as OCD. A great effort of education should be implemented to let breeders understand the key role of a adequate nutrition of mares in general and of pregnant mares in the late stage of pregnancy in particular to secure as much as possible an interval period of one year between two subsequent foalings and an appropriate date of foaling the next following year consistent with the aim of production - race horse – Sport horses or leisure horses – horse for meat to breed and then raise healthy mare and young horses.

References

Austbo, D., 2004. Rations for intensive growth in young horses. In proceedings of 2nd European Workshop Equine Nutrition (EWEN), EAAP Nr 114, Wageningen academic publishers, The Netherlands, 137-145.

Bergero, D., N. Miraglia, C. Abba and M. Polidori, 2004. Apparent digestibility of Mediterranean forage determined by total collection of faeces and acid-insoluble ash as internal marker. Liv. Prod. Science, 85, 235-238.

Catalano, A.L. and N. Miraglia, 1986. Utilizzazione delle risorse agro-zootecniche nell'Alto Appennino Reggiano. Agricoltura e Ricerca 57/58, 27-38.

CVB, 1996. Documentatierrrapport Nr 15, Het definitieve VEP en VRE system, Centraal veevoederbureau, pp.

Corino, C., N. Miraglia and M. Polidori, 1995. In vivo digestibility of mediterranean forages employed in Italy in horse feeding. In: Proceedings 46th EAAP Annual Meeting, Praha, Czech Republic 4th – 7th September.

Corino, C., N. Miraglia and M. Polidori, 1996. Determination of organic matter digestibility and prediction of the U.F.C. value of mediterranean forages. In: proceedings 47th EAAP Annual Meeting, Lillehammer, Norway, 25th – 29th August.

CVB, 2005. Revision of CVB, 1996 (Personal communication of Blok M.).

Doreau, M. and G. Dussap, 1980. Estimation de la production laitière de la jument allaitante par marquage de l'eau corporelle du poulain. Reprod. Nutr. Dev., 20: 1883

Denoix, J.M., J.P. Valette, P. Heiles, X. Robot and L. Tavernier, 2000. Etude radiographique des affections osteoarticulaires juveniles (AOAJ) chez des chevaux de races françaises, ages de 3nas: présentation globale des résultats sur 1180 sujets. Prat. Vet. Equine., 126, 35-41.

Duren, S., 2001. Feeding practices in the united states. In Advances in equine nutrition, Ed. Nottingham University Press, UK, 547 p.

Frape, D., 2004. Equine nutrition feeding. Ed. Blackwell Publishing Ltd, 650 p.

GEH, 1994. Langerwirtschafts für Enährungphysiologie 2. Empfehlungen zur Energie und Nährstoffversorgung der Perfde. DLG. Verlage Frankfurt/Main. ISBN 3.7690.0517.1, pp.

Lewis, L.D., 1995. Equine Clinical Nutrition. In: Broodmares feeding and care, Ed. Williams and Wilkins, USA, 587 p.

Harris, P., 2001. Feeding and management practices in the UK and Germany. In: Broodmares feeding and care, Ed. Williams and Wilkins, USA, 587 p.

INRA, 1990. L'alimentation des chevaux. W. Martin-Rosset Ed,. INRA Editions Paris, 232 p.

Micol, D. and W. Martin-Rosset, 1995. Feeding systems for horses on high forage diets in the temperate zone. In proceedings of IV Intern. Symp. Nutr. Herbivores, Clermont-Ferrand, France, 11-15 September, Journet M., Grenet, E., Frarce, M.H., Theriez, M., Demarquilly, C., Eds, INRA editions, Paris, 569-584.

Martin-Rosset, W., 2001. Feeding standards for energy and protein for horse in France. In Advances in equine nutrition, Ed. Nottingham University Press, UK, 547 p.

Martin-Rosset, W., I. Vervuert and D. Austbo, 2006a. Energy and protein requirements and recommended allowances in pregnant mares. In: Proceedings of 3rd European Workshop Equine Nutrition (EWEN), Campobasso, 20-22 june, Italy, EAAP No 120, Wageningen Academic Publishers, The Netherlands.

Martin-Rosset, W., D. Austbo and M. Coenen, 2006b. Energy and protein requirements and recommended allowances in lactating mares. In: Proceedings of 3rd European Workshop Equine Nutrition (EWEN), Campobasso, 20-22 June, Italy, EAAP No 120, Wageningen Academic Publishers, The Netherlands

Miraglia, N., M. Polidori and E. Salimei, 2002. Feeding strategies, feeds and management of equines in Central-Southern Italy. EAAP annual meeting, Cairo, Egypt, Horse commission, Abstract 2.3, 251.

Miraglia, N., M. Polidori and E. Salimei, 2003. A review of feeding strategies, feeds and management of equines in Central-Southern Italy. Working animals in agriculture and transport. A collection of some current research and development observations, 103-112.

Miraglia, N., 2004. Influence of management and nutrition on growth in the young horse. In proceeding of 2nd European Workshop on Equine Nutrition (EWEN). EAAP Nr 114 Wageningen Academic Publishers, The Netherlands, 211-225.

Miraglia, N., M. Saastamoinen and W. Martin Rosset, 2006. Role of pastures in mares and foals management in Europe. In: Proceedings of 3rd European Workshop Equine Nutrition (EWEN), Campobasso, 20-22 June, Italy, EAAP No 120, Wageningen Academic Publishers, The Netherlands

NRC, 1989. Nutrient Requirements of Horses. In: Nutrient Requirements of domestic animals, 6, 5th Ed. Revised, National Academy of Sciences, Washington D.C., 100 p.

Oftedal, O.T., H.F. Hintz and H.F. Schryver, 1983. Lactation in the horse: Milk composition and intake by foals. J. Nutr. 113: 2196-2206.

Trillaud-Geyl, C., J. Brohier, L. de Baynast, N. Baudoin and E. Rossier, 1990. Bilan de productivité sur 10 ans d'un troupeau de juments de selle conduites en plein air intégral. Croissance des produits de 0 à 6 mois. World Review Anim. Prod. 25, 3, 65-70.

Valette, J.P., B.M. Paragon, G. Blanchard, C. Robert and J.M. Denoix, 2004. Feeding practices and prevention of developmental diseases. In proceedings of 2nd European Workshop Equine Nutrition (EWEN), EAAP Nr 114, Wageningen Academic Publishers, The Netherlands, 291 –302.

Winkelsett, S., I. Vervuert, M. Granel, A. Borchers and M. Coenen, 2005. Feeding practice in warmblood mares and foals and the incidence to osteochondrosis. Pferdeheilkunde, 21, 124-126.

Role of pasture in mares and foals management in Europe

N. Miraglia[1], M. Saastamoinen[2] and W. Martin-Rosset[3]
[1]Molise University, Via De Sanctis, 86100 Campobasso, Italy
[2]MTT Equine Research, Varsanojatie 63, 32100 Ypaja, Finland
[3]INRA, Department of Animal Science, Center of Research of Clermont-Ferrand/Theix, 63122 Saint Genes Champanelle, France

Abstract

The role of pastures is of high concern in horse husbandry and in nutrition planning during large part of the year. Grass production and grazing are extensively influenced by the geographical area. The overall strategy of the systems used consists generally in the synchrony of the periods of high requirements of the broodmares and their foals with the period of maximum grass production. But security scenery and surfaces particularly in case of poor climatic conditions should be included in the grazing systems too. In the Nordic countries the possibilities of grazing is limited to short summer time because of the short growth period of grass. In Central European countries the considerable grazing surfaces, generally characterized by high quality forages, permit long grazing period which supply most of the nutrients to the broodmare and their foals during lactation when the climatic condition are normal. In Southern European countries, grass production is routinely depressed by summer dryness. Whatever the zone grassland should be managed using adequate methods for maintaining and improving pastures. The broodmares with their foals are turned out to pastures as soon as possible after foaling for most of the breeds except race breeds where foaling in early winter is matched to wean the foal early in summer. Hence different grazing systems are implemented according to breeds and geographical area. But the challenge to cope with, whatever the breed, is for the mare to meet Body weight (BW) and Body Condition Score (BCS) at key periods: early lactation and drying off to nurse adequately the foal, to be rebred shortly, and restore their body reserves for winter and pregnancy periods. Dry matter intake of the mare is not a major limiting factor to meet the requirements except if the grass is of very poor quality in early lactation. But supplementation of the mare and the foals is requested to balance the diet in case of deficiencies of nutrients in the herbage or in case of grass production shortage related to poor climatic conditions. Those aims can be met if relevant husbandry systems and grazing management practices are implemented mainly by the prediction of the nutritive value of grass (and production) and harvested forages and the use of an appropriate grazing and care systems in pasture management (rotations, control of infesting plants species and parasitism in the sward, etc.).

Keywords: mares, foals, pastures, grazing practices

Introduction

In Europe horse production is generally oriented to race horses, to sport horses and to leisure horses. Little interest is given to horses destined to meat production and it is limited only to few European countries (Belgium, France, Italy, Spain) which are still breeding heavy breeds. Grass and preserved forages account for 50 to 80 percent of the feed of horses in a year. Forages can supply 40 to 70 percent of the horse's annual feed requirements. Differences can be noticed according to location and management of horse feeding areas (Miraglia et al, 2006).

The role and the exploitation of pastures in horse breeding are different; good pastures can play an important part in the management and care of horses. Pastures can be used as exercise and exhibition paddocks playing no role in the planning of nutrition; in other cases, high quality pastures are fundamental in the planning of nutrition during the largest part of the year. These pastures offer several advantages because the forage has a high digestibility, requires no storage, limits labour and provides exercise. Grazing has a large importance, because it decreases the costs of horse keeping and offers good and balanced nutrition when taking care of proper management of the pastures.

The use of pastures in horse breeding depends on the breeder's choice of production and is largely influenced by the geographical area too. Important variations depend on the duration of the grazing and growing season. The use of pastures ranges from extensive systems in rangeland or harsh conditions to the intensive use of improved pastures. In the Nordic countries the importance of high quality forages, including good pasture grass during summer, is emphasized. However, the possibilities of using grazing are limited to summer time because of the short growth period of grass, compared to Central and Southern European countries.

In Central European countries the considerable grazing surfaces, generally characterized by high quality forages, influences the nutrition planning. Concerning the Southern European countries, the pasture characteristics are affected negatively by climate and environmental factors because of considerable incidence of summer dryness. In this last case the nutritive role of pastures is limited even though it is fundamental for exercising.

In Mediterranean lands the summer dryness represents a limiting factor for cultivations and for animal productions because of a low forage production and a shortage availability of watering places. In fact, soils are often scarcely fertile, very steep and unstable; the high diffusion of clay soils influences many disorders and series of landslides, often determined by surface and deep runoff of water (Miraglia, 1989). So, the most important limiting factors are linked to the low forage production not well distributed along the year and the consequent necessity to dispose of considerable surfaces for grazing.

The aim of this paper is to compare the different characteristics of the European pastures and their role in horse husbandry. Emphasis will be given to the grazing season and to the pasture management as influenced by the length of the grazing season, the pasture types and the pasture plants. The grazing practices will be described in relation to the management and to the diets of horses at pasture.

Reproductive cycle of the brood mares, nursing the foals and grazing periods

The reproductive cycle and grazing period are specific to the different types of horses to be produced whatever the countries where they are produced and grazing should contribute to meet the production goals that are specific to the different types of horse produced. This can be achieved if the goals of production, related reproductive cycle and key parameters and periods of grazing are well defined. Then the questions which arise in each country are: which type of grass ? Which type of pasture and grazing management ? Is supplementation of the mare or/and the foal requested ?

Races horses production

Foaling takes place in winter as the yearlings are expected to race at 2 years of age (Figure 1a). As a result grazing occurs mostly during the second part of lactation. The mares are supplemented as well in summer at night in the box as in autumn and winter at through feeding. Foals are supplemented too in the early summer to be weaned no later than 160 days. The objective is to maintain the mares in good conditions during the whole reproductive cycle. Hence winter feeding period is as much important as summer grazing period. But summer period is of major concern to exercise the foal

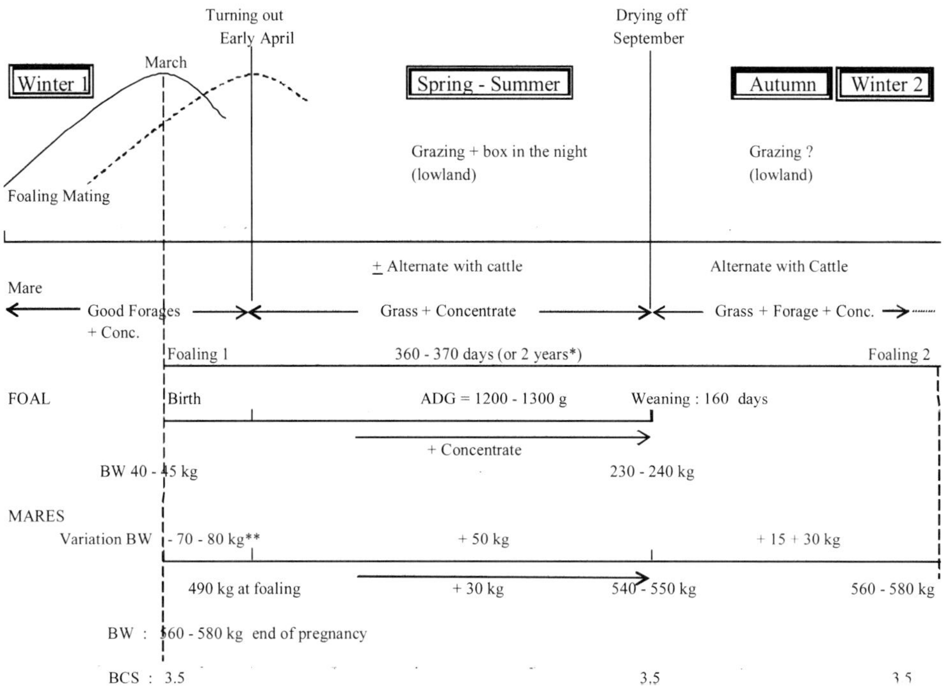

Figure 1a. Raising systems in temperate zone. Race horses = intensive system (Mare BW = 500 kg).

BW: Body Weight; BCS: Body Condition Score; ADG: Average Daily Gain

* It depends on the success of the fertilization at the appropriate date to wean the foal early in September then to prepare the early training of the yearling at 15 months of age

** Conceptus + digesta content at foaling

*** INRA-HN-IE, 1997 Scoring Scale (0 – 5)

too. Interval between two subsequent foaling is either 1 or 2 years depending on the success of fertilisation at the 1st or 2nd oestrous cycle.

Sport horses production

Foaling occurs in late winter and early spring as the young horses are devoted to compete at 4 years of age (Figure 1b). The greatest part of lactation takes place during the grazing season, namely early lactation. The mares graze lowland of medium to good quality. The mares are scarcely supplemented except in case of dry summer or/and drying area. Foals are supplemented only in the period close to weaning to be weaned at 180 days. Grazing period is of high concern to monitor body weight gain and body condition score of the mares as the growth of the foal and the foaling interval are highly dependant on the feeding level in summer.

Leisure horses production

Foaling happens in spring close to turning out as the young horses are broken in rather late: 3-4 years of age (Figure 1c). The whole lactation occurs during the grazing season. So far the mares should graze good pasture in the early lactation close to the stud farm; then extensive pasture can be grazed in the second part of lactation with moderate stocking rate. Mares and foals are not supplemented routinely. Foals are weaned at 180 – 200 days. So far grazing management is of very high concern

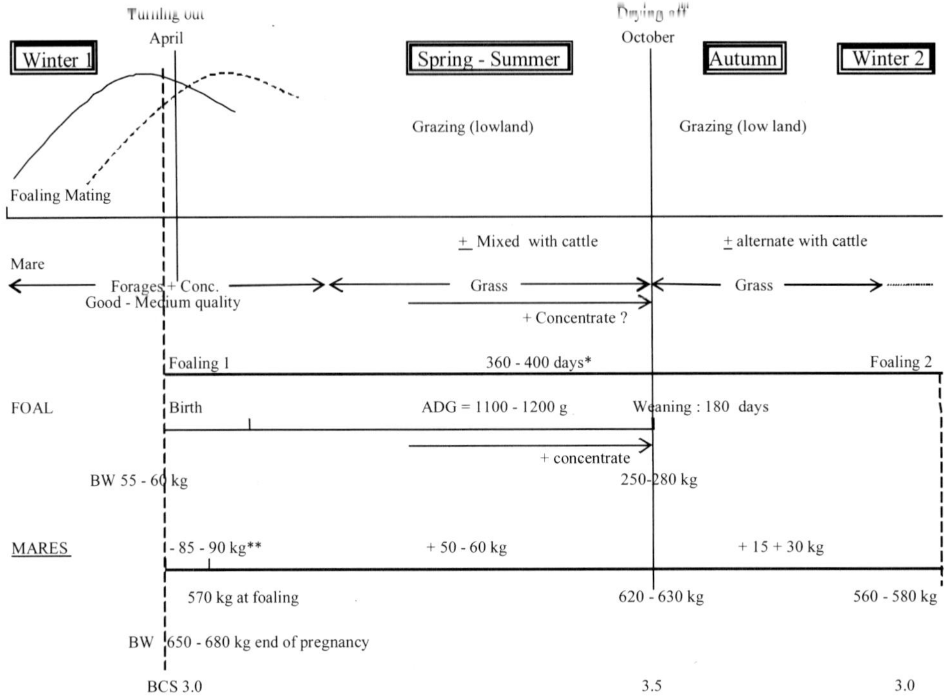

Figure 1b. Raising systems in temperate zone. Sport horses = semi-intensive system (mare BW = 550 kg).

BW: Body Weight; BCS: Body Condition Score; ADG: Average Daily Gain

* It depends on the success of the fertilization at the appropriate date to wean the foal in October

** Conceptus + digesta content at foaling

*** INRA-HN-IE, 1997 Scoring Scale (0 – 5)

for the mare and the foal to be dried off and weaned respectively at the suitable body weight and body condition score, and to meet a 12 months foaling interval, whereas the feeding level of the mare is often limited during the winter period.

Use of pastures in Europe

The models of feeding systems consist of series of driving sequences of the animals on the different areas of the farm all over the year. The strategy of the system consists generally in corresponding the periods of high requirements of animals to the periods of growing season (Moulin 1997). It must include security schemes particularly in case of climatic problems and its consequences on the availability and quality of pastures.

In humid temperate mountains and/or rangelands, husbandry systems with mares bred outdoors are usual. Horses are fed on grass close to the farms in early spring and late fall and on highlands in the summer. Different situations can be observed in Iceland for breeding Icelandic horses (Gudmunsson and Dyrmundsson 1993). Similar systems are traditionally conducted in Ireland as well for producing ponies in Connemara (Petch,1998), in UK, Finland, Norway, Iceland, Austria and in France to produce New Forest ponies, Fjord, Icelandic, Haflinger and half warmblood horses respectively, devoted to hacking and trekking in the area. In the Nordic countries horses are not routinely combined with ruminants (horse farms having other animals are rare and, if so, the animals

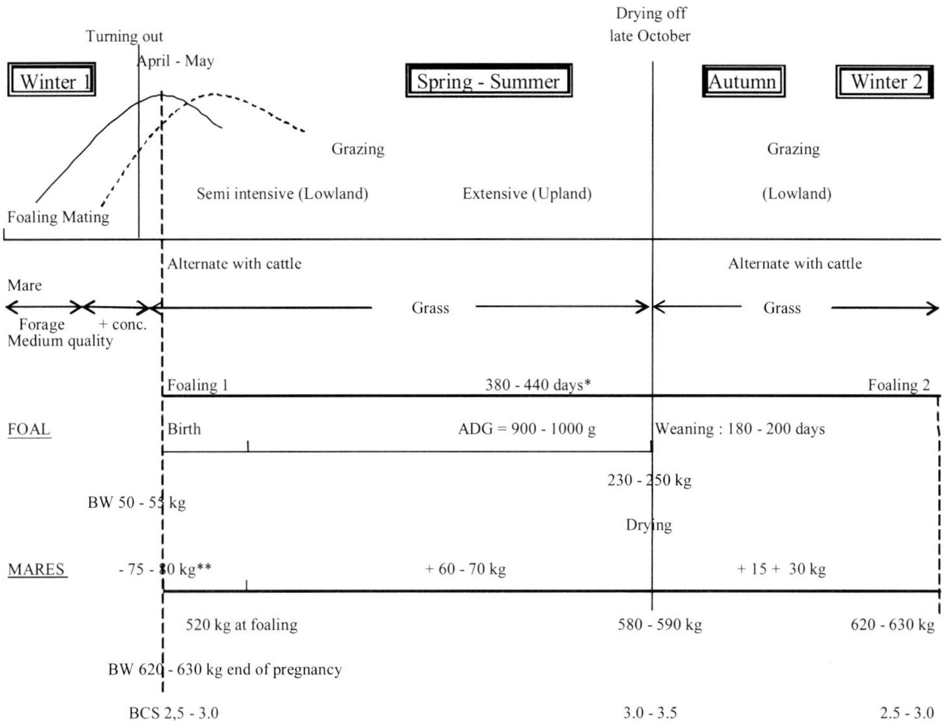

Figure 1c. Raising systems in temperate zone. Leisure horses = extensive system (mare BW = 500 kg).

BW: Body Weight; BCS: Body Condition Score; ADG: Average Daily Gain

* It depends on the success of the fertilization at the appropriate date to wean the foal in October

** Conceptus + digesta content at foaling

*** INRA-HN-IE, 1997 Scoring Scale (0 – 5)

are usually kept in separate pastures). The most common breeds are North Swedish, a cold-blooded breed in Sweden, Fjords or Dole in Norway, Finnhorses in Finland. In Central Europe horses graze mostly on rangelands during the summer season, either on their own or with beef cattle or dairy heifers mainly (Micol and Martin-Rosset, 1995; Miraglia *et al.*, 2003; Fed. Suisse d'Elevage, 2002; Roger-Lakenbrink, 1977) or with sheep (Gudmunsson and Dyrmundsson, 1993): it is the case of Franches Montagnes horses in Switzerland, Ardennes in Belgium, Comtois, Bretons and Ardennes in France. Similar systems are implemented in Italy with Pentro Horses (Miraglia *et al.*, 2001), Catria horses (La Manna *et al.*, 2002), Haflinger horses, Sanfratellano horses and Giara ponies; in Spain, in the Pyrénnées mountains with Galego horses (Santamarina, 2000), in Greece with some native ponies breeds (Zafrakas, 1995). These horses contribute significantly to pastoral management improving the sward biodiversity and the pastoral value (Loiseau and Martin-Rosset, 1985 - 1989; Miraglia *et al.*, 2001 - 2003; Gudmundsson, 1995, Fleurance et al,. 2003). Moreover, horses can also clean the land, either early or late in the grazing season, by grazing the ungrazed grass left by ruminants during the previous summer. This system is usually implemented with herds of mares of heavy breeds in France (Massif Central, Martin-Rosset and Trillaud-Geyl 1984 and Jura areas) and in Italy (Miraglia et al 2001). Ponies of light horses bred for trekking are often wintered on these land, keeping it clean and productive (Connemara in Ireland, Icelandic horses in Iceland, New Forest in UK, Fjord in Norway, heavy breeds in France and Italy).

In the lowlands of temperate zones, horses bred for sports, the so-called warm-blooded breeds (Clarke and Wallin, 1992) or for races (trotters and thoroughbreds) have been produced for many decades in different European countries. Feeding systems are based on grass, while preserved forages are extensively offered to mares and growing horses, with the use of more or less compensatory growth during the summer season (sport *vs.* race horses). Horses are routinely combined with ruminants: beef cows, heifers or steers in France (Selle Français and French trotter in Normandy), cattle and sheep in Ireland (Connemara in the West and Thoroughbreds in the South and East), dairy cows or heifers in The Netherlands (KWPN breed), in Germany (German warm bloods: Trakehners, Hannoverian, Holstein, etc.), in Switzerland (Franches-Montagnes and Swiss warm blood horses), in Belgium (Belgian warm blood), in Denmark (Danish warmblood), in Sweden (Swedish trotter and Swedish warm blood horses).

In nature conservation areas, horses are combined with cattle in order to maintain biodiversity (Loucougaray et al, 2004; Duncan, 1983 - 1992; Putnam, 1986; Putman *et al.*, 1991, Menard et al. 2002) and to preserve wild life in the territory (Duncan, 1992) and to promote socio-cultural activities in and around natural parks. In France, Camargue horses are managed with cattle destined for bull-fighting in the Camargue National Park (Duncan, 1992).

Grazing season and pasture management

Length of the grazing season

The length of the grazing season varies in different countries and different parts of each country. The Nordic countries, Finland, Sweden and Norway are quite length in their shape. In addition, the Southern parts of Sweden, Norway, Estonia and other Baltic countries on their whole, have milder climatic conditions than the southern parts of Finland. The grazing season begins usually in May in Sweden and Norway as well as in the most southern part of Finland. The length of grazing period varies according to the climatic conditions from year to year, but it usually lasts till to the end of September. In the southern parts of Sweden and Norway and in the Baltic countries the length of grazing season may be about 130 days, and in southern part of Finland about 100-120 days. In the northern parts of the Nordic countries the horses can be on pastures about 60 days during the summer. For free-ranging horses over-winter grazing might be used in Iceland (Icelandic horse) and in Estonia (Estonian native horse) in areas with very little or no snow.

In the case of Central European Countries the length of the grazing season is of 9 months, on the average. During this period low concentrate supplementation could be offered outside and should depend on the kind of horses (heavy or saddle horses) and on their use. Natural and sown swards are grazed during the grazing season (230 days) and fertilised (180 kgN/ha). Grass is plentiful until the beginning of July (beginning of the 3rd cycle) then, the production is slowed from mid-July to the end of August. During this period, other pastures (mowed or used by other animals in spring) can be used by saddle mares.

In Mediterranean Countries the length of the grazing season depends on the climatic conditions and is strictly linked to the summer dryness and to rainfall (Costantini et al, 2005). Depending on the geographical area the grazing season starts between April and May; in July, August and early September a considerable reduction of the grass production is frequent and depends also on rainfall: in fact, rainfall is extremely variable and often the rain falling in Autumn influences plant production on the following growing season (Duncan, 1992). From September till the end of October a regrowth of the grass often occurs offering the availability of fresh forages to mares and foals in the weaning period. Daily Dry matter production/ha range along the summer season and according the country and the zone in the country between 20 to 130kg in Finland (Figure 2), 20 to 70kg in Central or South part of Italy (Figures 3-4).

Pasture types and vegetation

In the Nordic countries the most common grass species of the pasture are timothy (*Phleum pratense*), creeping red fescue (*Festuca rubra L.*), meadow fescue (*Festuca pratensis Huds.*), smooth-stalked meadowgrass (*Poa pratensis L.*), perennial ryegrass (*Lolium perenne L.*) and cocksfoot (*Dactylis glomerata*). The plants are usually cultivated as mixtures, the proportions varying according to the latitude. Also red (*Trifolium pratense L.*) and white (*Trifolium repens L.*) clovers are used, especially concerning organic farming. Concerning various types of natural pastures, a large scale of species occurs (e.g. Hagman, 1994; Magnusson and Magnusson, 1990a-b).

The pastures used for horse grazing at northern latitudes are variable, ranging from cultivated pastures (artificial grassland) to natural rangelands (natural grassland). The rangelands can be divided into many categories, such as lowland and highland or wet and dry areas (Gudmundsson

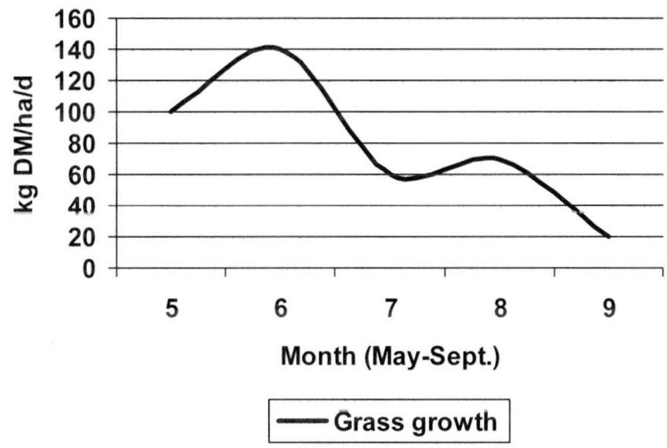

Figure 2. The average growth of pasture grass in Finland during the summer (based on the data from Agri Food Research Finland, Animal Production, 2006).
DM: Dry Matter

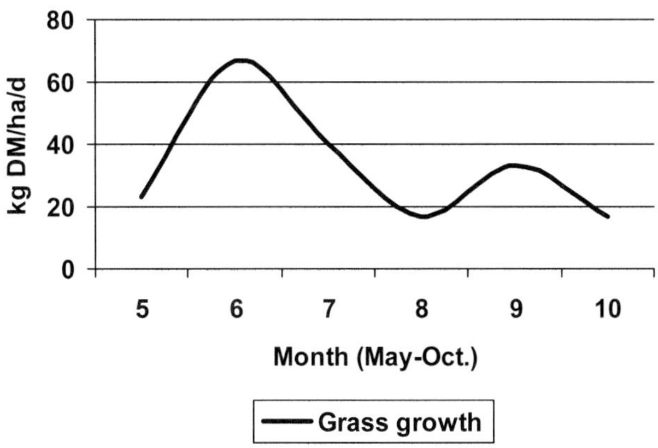

Figure 3. The average growth of pasture grass in Central Italy during the grazing period (Catalano and Miraglia, 1985).
DM: Dry Matter

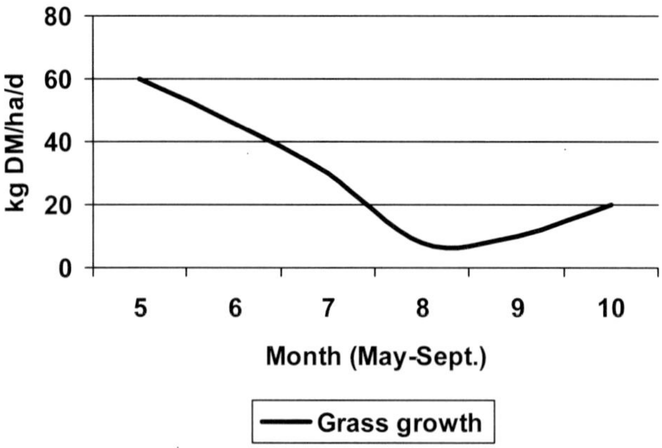

Figure 4. The average growth of pasture grass in Southern Italy during the summer (Miraglia et al., 2002).
DM: Dry Matter

and Dyrmundson, 1993). Uncultivated natural pastures are used in many countries. These pastures are e.g. wetland and old natural pastures previously grazed by cattle and now used by horses in the purpose of conservation biodiversity.

In Norway, also mountain pastures are used (Austbo *et al.*, 1993). Natural and mountain pastures offer better conditions for increased physical activity if compared to flat field pastures.
In Iceland, where horse breeding is based on pastures, both lowland and highland pastures are used. Today, horses are grazing more on drained lowland fens (Magnusson and Magnusson, 1990a).

In Sweden, there is going on an EU-project of natural rearing of show-jumping horses on natural pastures (www.hhklubben.se). The foals are exercised together with their dams utilizing the topography of the land. Management practices influence the productivity of the pasture and, consequently, milk production of mares and growth rate of horses. Austbo *et al.* (1993) reported that the growth of horses was better on lowland pastures than on mountain pastures. On the mountain pastures, energy intake might be under the requirements due to climatic conditions and increased activity caused by the varying topography.

In Finland, lower energy values were reported sometimes for natural pastures than for cultivated pastures (Hagman, 1994). In stead of that, protein content of natural grassland was as high as that of cultivated pastures' ones.

In lowland of Central European countries and in good grassland conditions the natural swards contain good graminea species and white clover. Sown pastures are generally composed by *Dactylis glomerata* and ryegrass. Natural grassland or artificial grassland are grazed by race or sport horses. A large spectrum of good graminea and significant proportion of white clover are dominant in grassland, mainly where they are well managed. Artificial grassland are most often sown with *Lolium perenne*, *Festuca arundicea or pratensis*, *Poa pratensis*, and *Dactylis glomerata* whose proportion depend on local soil and climatic conditions. The most resistant indigenous plants are bent and fescue (*Agrostis* and *Festuca).* In the uplands zone the production of grassland is largely affected by the proportion of perennial ryegrass.

In Central European countries considerable emphasis is given to the exploitation of hills and uplands. In the fall, the mares often consume refusal plants of other herbivores. In spring, they are turned out on natural lowlands, sometimes after cattle grazing. In summer, the mares graze poor upland pastures (e.g. *Nardus stricta, Festuca ovina..*), including fibrous plant species (e.g. *Vaccinium mirtillus*) in the uplands (Martin-Rosset *et al.*, 1981).In fact the vegetation of the hills and uplands covers a wide range from the sown grasslands of the uplands to the semi-natural grasslands and heaths of the hills (Bernard-Brunet and Dubost, 1979; Lienard *et al.*, 1979). Grazing can have an impact on all these different vegetation types. For instance, the semi-natural vegetation of hills and uplands of the United Kingdom is intrinsically unstable within the forest zone with a general tendency for succession to woodlands unless actively managed (Miles, 1988). Also changes in weather and in environmental factors over many years may become important in vegetation changes (Heil and Diemont, 1983). A poor climate, soils and plant species can result in a range of dry matter output between 1 and 5 t/ha in native hill swards and is highly variable (Frame *et al.*, 1985).

Pastures of Mediterranean regions are characterized by many plant species, sometimes with a high fibre percentage; gramineae and leguminosae plants are associated to many other kind of plants and to a shrubby vegetation (*nardus stricta, vaccinum myrtillus, carpinus spp.*, etc.) (Miraglia *et al.*, 2001). In these areas the diffusion of infesting vegetation occurs often with different characteristics depending on the area (wet or arid areas) (*Ranunculus spp., Taraxacum officinalis, Plantago spp., Rumex, Juncus spp.*, etc.) (Miraglia and Bocchi, 1982; Catalano and Miraglia, 1985; Miraglia, 1989, Miraglia *et al.*, 2000).

In the case of Mediterranean pastures, many studies carried out both in Central and in Southern Italy (Catalano and Miraglia, 1985-1986; Olivieri *et al.*, 1988; Catalano *et al.*, 1989; Miraglia *et al.*, 2002) showed the considerable influence of summer dryness on the dry matter production, on the nutritive value and on the quality of the forages that is often influenced by a considerable diffusion of invadent species.

Energy content of the grass is rather close between Finland, France, and Southern Italy (Table 1). But protein content is higher in Finland and Southern Italy than in France and Central Italy. The energy content of Norwegian hay is higher to that of hays harvested in UK (Table 2). In the Mediterranean zone the crude protein, cell wall content (crude fibre, ADF and ADL) and digestibility (Corino *et al.*, 1995-1996) of forages (natural meadows hays) harvested in Southern Italy (Table 3) are lower

Table 1. Average chemical composition of pasture grass in different European countries.

Origin	DM (g/kg)	CP (g/kg DM)	CF (g/kg DM)	DCP (g/kg DM)	NE (MJ/kg DM)	DE (MJ/kg DM)	Ca (g/kg DM)	P (g/kg DM)
Finland[1]	180-190	200-230	180-200	154-184	(6.5-6.9)	14.0	5.0	4.0
France[2] (lowlands)	170	131-168	244-276	83-114	7.2-7.7	12.0-12.6	6.5-7.0	3.5-4.0
France[2] (uplands)	170	111-166	223-304	67-110	6.2-8.9	10.1-12.4	7.0-8.0	2.5-3.5
Central Italy[3] (uplands)	240	145	259	98	5.8	--	--	--
Southern Italy[4] (hills)	210	210	215	149	6.6	--	--	--

[1]Finnish Feed Tables and Feeding Recommendations (www.agronet.fi/rehutaulukot 2006)

[2]French Feed Tables and Feeding Recommendations (INRA, 1984 - 1990)

[3]Catalano and Miraglia, 1986

[4]Miraglia *et al.*, 2002

DM: Dry matter; CP: Crude Protein; CF: Crude fibre; DCP: Digestible Crude Protein; NE: Net Energy; DE: Digestible Energy; Ca: Calcium; P: Phosphorous and higher respectively to other European forages harvested in France (INRA, 1984 – 1990) and in Nordic countries (Austbo, 2005).

Table 2. Comparison between average nutrient content of meadow hays referred to as "Good", "Medium" and "Poor" quality in Norway and in the UK (per kg DM)(Austbo, 2005).

Country	Quality	DE MJ	ME MJ	NE UFC	CP g	DCP g	Lysine g	Ca g	P g
N	Good	12.2	10.3	0.77	120	78	4.2	3	2.7
N	Medium	10.5	8.8	0.64	101	60	3.2	3	2.5
N	Poor	8.9	7.5	0.54	88	48	2.6	3	2.5
UK	Good	10.7	9	0.67	120	77	4.5	5.4	2.7
UK	Medium	9.5	8	0.57	107	66	3.8	4.8	2.5
UK	Poor	7.7	6.5	0.45	80	40	2.4	3	2.3

Values taken from Norwegian and UK versions of PC-Horse computer programme.
N: Norway; UK: United Kingdom; UFC: Horse Feed Unit (INRA, 1984 – 1990); DE: Digestible Energy; ME: Metabolizable Energy; NE: Net Energy; CP: Crude Protein; DCP: Digestible Crude Protein; Ca: Calcium; P: Phosphorous.

Table 3. Chemical composition and digestibility coefficients of natural meadows hays in Mediterranean countries (Corino et al., 1995 - 1996).

Hays	Natural meadows 1	Natural meadows 2	Natural meadows 3	Natural meadows 4
Chemical composition (%)				
Dry matter	91.6	93.4	96.4	96.4
Organic Matter	92.4	92.7	93.2	91.7
Ashes	7.6	7.4	6.8	8.3
Crude Protein	8.4	9.1	7.0	8.5
Crude fibre	34.2	30.2	34.0	34.0
NDF	69.8	60.1	66.2	64.7
ADF	38.1	31.3	37.2	37.5
ADL	4.6	4.2	5.9	5.2
UFC (n.)	0.5	0.6	0.5	0.5
Digestibility coefficients (%)				
Dry matter	42.3	56.4	46.7	50.5
Organic Matter	42.9	56.8	47.2	53.1
Crude Protein	47.0	57.0	47.2	51.7
Gross Energy	41.2	54.2	42.8	48.7

UFC: Horse Feed Unit (INRA 1984-1990); NDF: Neutral Detergent Fibre; ADF: Acid Detergent Fibre; ADL: Lignine.

Pasture management

A lot of studies (Archer, 1971-1973; Rogalski, 1967, 1973; 1975, 1977; Loiseau and Martin-Rosset, 1985; Miraglia 2000; Fleurance et al, 2005) have outlined the influence of alimentary behaviour, stocking rate, nutrient restitution by excreta, etc. on turf surfaces. So far horses overgraze the preferred area of the sward (so called lawns) while they are reluctant to the area contaminated with faeces (so called roughs). Pasture (and namely reseeded pasture) should not be overgrazed to the point where not enough leaf material is left to permit a correct re-growth (Cottarelli, 1989).

Pasture are fertilised namely with nitrogen, phosphorous and kalium (calcium sometimes) depending on the chemical composition of the soils and on the availability of these nutrients in the herbages determined by laboratory analysis. Two fertilisers are used: either a compound fertiliser: 20N-10P-10K, or a simple fertiliser: 33N. Compound fertiliser are selected to stimulate adequate growth and to correct any deficiencies. N fertiliser is applied to meet the demand of grazing and increase crude protein content of herbage. Chemical or organic fertiliser are used.

Pastures are sometimes aerating as horse are stepping a lot mainly in wet period. Aerating is implemented using spikes behind a tractor to break up aggregates of soil, shallow panning and surface capping. Harrowing is used in spring to encourage tilling. In fall, harrowing remove dead grass from the sward and spread droppings. Rolling is used to ensure successful reseeding. Topping is implemented to encourage growth of leafy herbage as tilling is stimulated while grasses are prevented to seed too early. Ungrazed area contaminated by faeces are controlled mainly by good grazing system (rotational *vs* continue grazing, horse mixed cattle, alternation grazing/ harvesting forage, etc.) and by harrowing to spread the droppings. Herbicides are used in extreme situation using a knapsack for spot application or weed wipers to control tall perennial weeds.

The analyse of the grass (Ca, P, Mg, Cu, Zn) is necessary to balance the mineral intake of the horses using an adequate mineral and trace elements concentrate.

Grazing systems

In lowlands rotational grazing system is often implemented for race and sport horses (Figures 1a-1b). The time of re-growth in such an intensive grazing system depends on the vegetative stage related to the seasonal period. The duration of each vegetative cycle is: 20-25 days between April and June, increasing to 30-40 days in the following months (Trillaud-Geyl et al., 1990). It is largely influenced by the summer dryness that is more or less heavy, depending on the latitude of the different European countries. In addition good silages or/and hays can be harvested in rotational grazing to feed the mares in winter (Trillaud-Geyl et al, 1990; Miraglia et al, 2000). Maximum grass production occurs from April to June (Figures 6a-6b). Good silage and hay are routinely harvested,using 30 percent of the surface, to feed the mares during the winter. (Micol and Martin-Rosset 1995). Stocking rate of broodmares range from 0.5 to 1.0 mare/ha in spring and summer respectively. Cattle are often used to monitor the refusals using steers (in TB or SB stud farms) or Beef heifers (in sport horses stud farm) in Grasslands are fertilised in March, April and May to monitor grass production and nutritive value: doses of N fertilisers which applied are very low 30 to 60 units/ha during the grazing season as breeders are afraid of too lush grass for horses (protein content or/and carbohydrates) in relation of laminitis, etc..

In lowlands continuous grazing is also implemented either in large stud farm where mixed grazing with cattle (steers, heifers) is used (Figures 1a-1b); or in small stud farms where there are only limited surface. In this last situation the mares are supplemented with forages and concentrates. Stocking rate in large stud farms range from 1.0 to 1.5 mare/ha in spring and summer respectively. N Fertilisation is very low: 15 to 30 units/ha.

In Uplands, leisure horses (or heavy breeds) are managed on extensive grassland using either rotational systems but more often continuous grazing system mixed with beef cattle (Figure 1c). Stocking rate is very low 1.5-2.0 mare/ha. The surface which is located close to the farm is only fertilised with 20 to 40 units N/ha, using often organic fertilizers to ensure a good grass production in early lactation of the mare and good nutritional condition to fertilise the mare.

Management of horses at pasture

Throughout the reproductive cycle the requirements vary strongly whatever the type of horses bred (see 2 chapters by Martin-Rosset *et al.*2006a, 2006b in this issue). The efficiency of the reproductive cycle depends on the intake capacity of forage by the mare at pasture in the different physiological status and on the quality of forages fed as in other herbivorous species (Dulphy *et al.*, 1994; Theriez *et al.*, 1994). The mare fed at through green grassland forage cut at three different vegetative stages during the first cycle is able to cover easily the requirements whatever the physiological status (Figure 5) as well as with preserved forages (see 2 chapters by Martin-Rosset *et al.*2006a, 2006b in this issue), excepted when grass is flowering for lactating mare and to some extend in late pregnant mare.

Hence the feed allowances during the summer season are either higher than the requirements in temperate zone (Figure 6a, b) and Nordic zone (Figure 2) or higher in early summer and might be lower in mid summer then again higher close to fall period in hot zone (Figures 1c, 3, 4). As a result the strategy of grazing management will differ with the type of horses bred, date of foaling, and the zone where they are raised. But, whatever the type of horses, grazing period should allow the mare to nurse adequately the foal and to meet the suitable body weight and body condition score at the key periods to fit the production goal (Figure 1).

For race horses, bred in humid lowland, the maximum of grass production occur during the second part of lactation. The Average Daily Gain (ADG) of the foals born in late March or April is higher during the first two months compared to ADG of the same range of age of the foals born in January-February because of the intake of high quality spring grass is higher than the intake of forage based diet fed in winter even supplemented with concentrate. This is the seasonal effect observed by Pagan et al (2006, see this issue) in Thoroughbred stud farm in Kentucky. But at 150 days of age BW of the foals is not significantly different as early born foals are capable, at 3 months of age, to graze

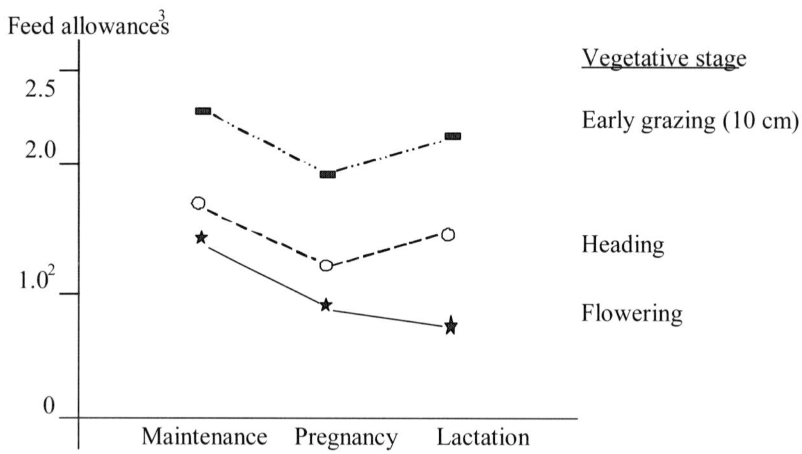

Figure 5. Energetic balance of mares according to the vegetation stage of the natural pasture[1] from INRA.

[1]Grass harvested and fed at through

[2]Maintenance requirement

[3]Feed allowances expressed as a ratio to requirements at maintenance

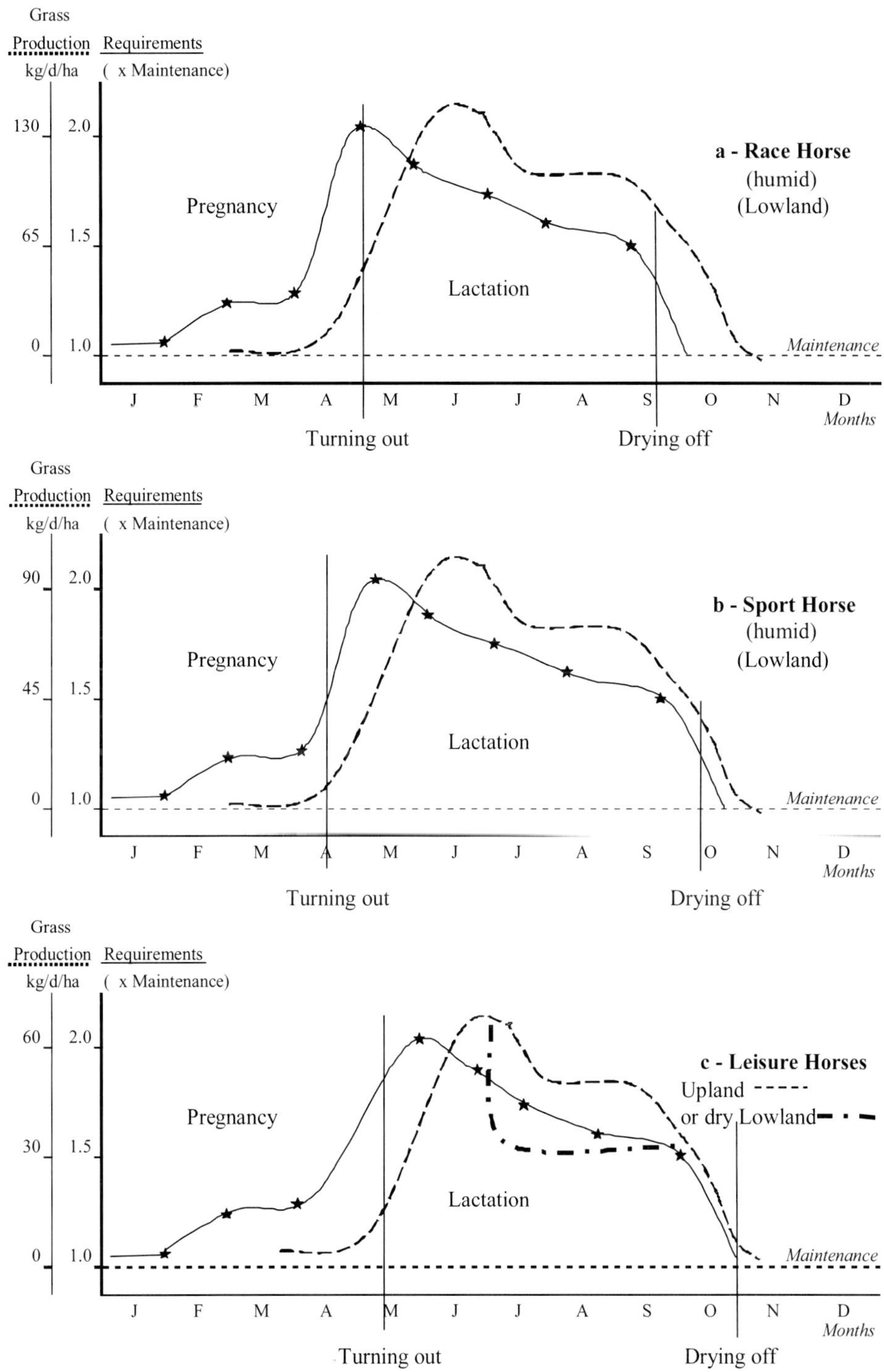

Figure 6. Variation of mares requirements and the grass production along the year in temperate zone (from INRA).

quickly high amount of good grass to achieve high ADG and compensate slower ADG during the winter. In such a system the mares maintain the optimal body condition score whatever the period of the grazing season as the mares gain BW mainly in spring and summer, but in fall after drying off if the climatic conditions would not have been good (Figure 1a).

For sport horses bred humid lowlands, the requirements of the mares and the foals are always met, except in very early lactation, if the grass production is limited by long winter or heavy rain which delay the date of turning out (Figure 6b). ADG of the foals is depending on the annual climatic condition. If these conditions are very favourable, no supplementation (except minerals and trace elements) is requested to wean the foal at 180-200days (Figure 1b).The mares meet the optimal body conditions score as she can gain BW during spring and summer, and in fall after drying off (Figure 1b).

For leisure horses bred in hilly or mountainous humid or dry zones, BW of the foals at weaning, BW and BCS of the mares at drying off and fertilisation postpartum of the mares are very linked to spring and fall grazing periods when grass production is higher than the nutritional requirements (Figures 1c- 6c). So far, a good grassland surface should be offered to the brood mares in these two periods to ensure the efficiency and perennially of this fragile system. In this system the accurate management of the mobilisation and restoration of body reserves is of major concern. It has been long time experienced with heavy breeds (Martin-Rosset and Trillaud-Geyl 1984, Micol and Martin-Rosset 1995). It requests a very accurate management of the grassland surface, as horses are often associated with cattle or more scarcely with sheep. Some competition occur between ruminants and horses, surface to be grazed or cut to harvest forage for winter feeding. A methodology to analyse, on technical and economical point of view, the strategy of the utilisation of the grassland surface has been designed in France by Moulin 1995.

Balancing pastures diets

Mares and foals are supplemented when they are facing either with deficiencies of herbage even when the climatic conditions is normal, or to cope with dryness and related abnormal grass production. In the first situation the main deficiencies are protein, minerals (calcium, phosphorus) or trace elements (copper, zinc). And the supplementation should be implemented to prevent the occurrence of physiopathologic disorders. In the other situation all the nutrients should be supplemented as the mount (and nutritive value) of grass is limited.

Calcium and phosphorus content and ratio of natural grassland in humid lowlands are often adequate: 5-8g /kgDM and 2.5-5.0 g/kgDM respectively and ratio: $1.0 < Ca/P < 2.0$. It can be more unbalanced when the proportion legumes in too low. The composition of artificial grassland seed with graminea only is much more unbalanced, namely calcium content is lower and the Ca/P ratio range between 1.0 and 1.4. Hagman (1994) reported also lower phosphorus, copper and potassium concentrations in natural grassland than in artificial grassland. Zinc content in the natural grassland was somewhat higher and that of calcium corresponded to the content in artificial grassland. The sodium content of natural grassland is even lower than in artificial grassland (Hagman, 1994).

Mineral supplement rich in calcium is recommended to be fed, because big amounts of calcium are excreted in the milk. Such a mineral concentrate usually contains also balanced amounts of other minerals. Copper and zinc are important minerals for adequate bone development. Mare's milk has rather low copper and zinc concentrations (e.g. Saastamoinen, 1990) and those minerals in the diet have also very little effect on their contents in the milk. During long hot seasons it is also recommended to feed salt. E.g. in Finland, the grass is not a sufficient source of sodium to horses and cattle. Sometimes it is also profitable to supplement the pasture grass with protein supplement to improve the amino acid composition of the feed portion. A research data (Saastamoinen and Luukkainen, unpublished) shows that a protein supplement produced a more even and balanced growth curve of the nursing foals (Figure 7). This might be due to more balanced amino acid content of the ingested feed compared to those fed with grass only.

In the case of limited administration of mineral supplements there is a possibility to have an increase in bone diseases, also depending on the mineral losses determined by diarrhoea phenomenon caused by the intake of large amounts of green grasses (mainly in spring time); in fact diarrhoea may reduce the absorptive capacity of the gut increasing the demand for minerals (Kienzle and Zorn, 2006); this situation can become worst if the *gramineneae* of the sward is high in oxalates and phytates that reduce the bioavailability of major minerals. In this case it should be better to maintain the Ca: P ratio high.

Many growth disorders arise from a fast growth before weaning. Rapid rates of body weight gain may affect growth of the epiphyseal plate, and may have a role in the onset of epiphysitis (Thompson *et al.*, 1988a). Creep-feeding may also result in accelerated growth and produce decrease in the bone quality during the first four months (Thompson *et al.*, 1988b). That is why creep-feeding has to be used accurately and with a strict monitoring of foals growth. Race horses foals (namely Thoroughbred) are mainly concerned (Figure 1a). In Northern European countries creep-feeding is not very popular, and it is used mainly only in Sweden by some breeders. In these countries a better alternative is to feed the mare to produce enough milk by taking care of the proper condition of the pasture and by supplementing the mare.

Creep-feeding can be used when introducing the foal to solid feeds before weaning, to prepare the foal for weaning and to reduce weaning stress. The foals are usually weaned at the age of 6 months, namely foals of sport breeds (Figure 1b) or later for leisure horses (Figure 1c), which means that the weaning takes place normally in the indoor feeding period. It should also keep in mind that the creep-feeds have to be well balanced to meet the nutritional requirements of foals.

When the pasture availability is scarce in quality and amounts the creep feeding technique is necessary to compensate the low milk production. Two types of management might be implemented either a supplementation of the suckling and grazing foal or early weaning. In the first situation foals are supplemented between 3 months and weaning using the creep feeding technique to balance the low milk production (Doreau *et al.*, 1986) of mares and to adjust minerals, vitamins and amino acids allowances.

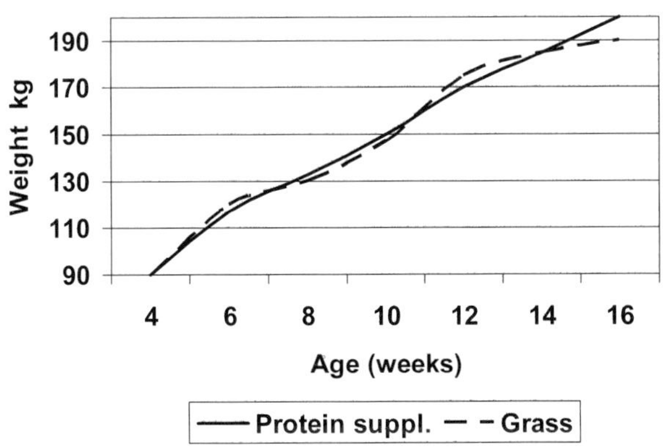

Figure 7. The effect of protein supplement on the growth of nursing foals on pasture (Saastamoinen and Luukkainen, unpublished data).

In the other situation the creep feed should support the anticipation of the weaning time, to 4 to 5 months of age, but it is established that an early weaning is detrimental to bone development wit a reduction of cannon diameter and density (Warren *et al.*, 1998).

Conclusions

Grass is the major source of nutrients to feed the broodmares and their foals along the breeding cycle. According to the type of breeds which are bred, the duration of grazing period range from 150 to 230 days. The broodmares and their foals are managed in "intensive", semi intensive or extensive systems for race, sport and leisure breeds respectively. The broodmares and their foals gain during the grazing season: 90 and 55 percent of their total BW gain for race breed respectively; 88 and 75 percent for sport breeds and 100 and 85 percent for leisure breeds.

Grass production varies much according to the country: humid or dry, and the annual climatic conditions. But whatever the breeds and the conditions for grass production the mares should gain BW in early lactation to nurse adequately the foal and to be rebred to maintain 12 months interval between two subsequent foaling. The mare should meet BW and BCS at drying off in late summer or fall to ensure good nutritional conditions to pregnancy during the winter. Dry matter intake is scarcely a limiting factor for the mare to meet their requirements. The foals should gain most of their total BW gain to be weaned in good conditions as BW at 6 months represent 45 percent of their adult BW. Hence management of the growth curve is of high concern but adequate supplementation should be adjusted according to the goal of production. So far grazing strategy is of high concern in the scope of the annual feeding planning and should be very flexible according to the zone and annual climatic conditions.

For race and most of sport horses the surface is scarcely a limiting factor. And the major problem is to prevent laminitis of the mares and to generate bone disorders in foals which grow too fast. For leisure and part of sport breeds extensive grassland are used. The major challenge is to restore body reserves of the mares in due time and to wean the foals at adequate BW and BS before the winter. Management of the growth curve of the foals is an area to be more investigated.

Grass management request increasing skills as far as the surface and quality of grass are limiting factors, mainly when the annual climatic conditions are poor. Stocking rate, fertilisation, alternation of grazing and cutting, mixing or alternation with cattle should be accurately implemented to manage adequately the grass production, grazing and parasitism. Grazing systems need further investigation either on technical or economical point of view as far as horse are herbivorous as much as ruminants and they should take part of the big challenge to use the territory and contribute to the socio economy.

References

Archer, M., 1971. Preliminary studies on the palatability of grasses legumes and herbs to horses. Vet. Res., 89, 236-240

Archer, M., 1973. The species preferences of grazing horses. J. Brit. Grassl. Soc., 28(3), 123-128.

Austbo, D., H. Gonsholt and K. Lise, 1993. Yearlings on mountain pastures in Norway. Paper. Horse breeding and production in cold climatic conditions, Iceland 1993, 6.

Austbo, D., 2005. Rations for intensive growth in young horses. In: "The growing horse: nutrition and prevention of growth disorders", EAAP Publ. N. 114, 137-145.

Bernard-Brunet, J. and M. Dubost, 1979. Gestion des ressources pastorales: nouveaux axes de recherche. In: Paturages d'altitudes et parcours méditerranéens, INRA Ed., Paris, 207-210.

Catalano, A.L., 1985. Exploitation of altitude's low productive pastures in wet areas. Proceedings 36th EAAP Annual Meeting, Halkidiki, Greece, September 30th - October 3rd, 424.

Catalano, A.L. and N. Miraglia, 1986. Utilizzazione delle risorse agro-zootecniche nell'Alto Appennino Reggiano. Agricoltura e Ricerca 57/58, 27-38.

Catalano, A.L., N. Miraglia, F. Martuzzi and P. Blanco, 1989. Utilizzazione delle risorse agro-zootecniche dell'Alto Appennino Reggiano. Rilievi agronomici e zootecnici nel secondo anno di sperimentazione. Agricoltura e Ricerca 101, 29-38.

Clarke, C. and D. Wallin, 1992. The International Warmblood Horse. The Kenilworth Press Ltd., Addington, Buckingham, 240 pp.

Corino, C., N. Miraglia and M. Polidori, 1995. In vivo digestibility of mediterranean forages employed in Italy in horse feeding. Proceedings 46th EAAP Annual Meeting, Praha, Czech Republic 4th – 7th September.

Corino, C., N. Miraglia and M. Polidori, 1996. Determination of organic matter digestibility and prediction of the U.F.C. value of mediterranean forages. Proceedings 47th EAAP Annual Meeting, Lillehammer, Norway, 25th – 29th August.

Costantini, M., N. Miraglia, M. Polidori and G. Meineri, 2005. Dry matter production and energy content of a natural pasture grazed by wild horses over a two years period, 56th Annual Meeting of EAAP, Uppsala (Sweden), June 5 – 8, 24.

Cottarelli, F., 1989. Cura agronomica del prato-pascolo per il cavallo atleta. In "Allevamento del cavallo Purosangue", ANAC Ed., Milano, 61-70.

Doreau, M., S. Boulot, W. Martin-Rosset and J. Robelin, 1986 – Relation between nutrient intake,, growth and body composition of nursing foal. Reprod. Nutr. Develop., 26(B), 683-690.

Dulphy, J.P., J.P. Jouany, W. Martin-Rosset and M. Theriez, 1994. Aptitude comparée de différentes esppèces d'herbivores domestiques à ingérer et digérer des fourrgaes distribués à l'auge. Ann. Zootech. 43, 11-32.

Duncan, P., 1983. Determinants of the use of habitat by horses in a Mediterranean wetland. Journ. Anim. Ecology, 52, 93-109.

Duncan, P., 1992. Horses and grasses: the nutritional ecology of Equids and their impact on the Camargue. Springer-Verlag Ed., New York, 287 pp.

Féderation Suisse d'élevage du cheval de la race des Franches Montagnes, 2002. Rapport Annuaire Avenches.

Fleurance, G., P. Duncan, D. Durant and G. Loucougaray, 2003. Impact of horses on pastures in the Atlantic marshes of France and consequences for management. Paper. 54th Annual Meeting of EAAP, 21.

Fleurance, G., P. Duncan, H. Fritz, J. Cabaret and I.J. Gordon, 2005. Importance of nutritional and anti-parasite strategies in the foraging decisions of horses: an experimental test. Oikos, 110, 602-612.

Frame, J., P. Newbold and J.M.M. Munro, 1985. Herbage production from the hills and uplands. In: Hill and upland livestock production. British Society of Animal Production, 10, 9-38.

Gundmunsson, O., 1995. Growth performances of horses grazing lowlands mire at different grazing pressure under cold climatic conditions. In proceedings: IV Intern. Symp. Nutr. Herbivores. Clermont-Ferrand, France, September, 11-15.

Gudmundson, O. and O.R. Dyrmundson, 1993. Horse grazing under cold and wet conditions: a review. Paper. Horse breeding and production in cold climatic conditions, Iceland 1993 13.

Hagman, I., 1994. Grazing of young horses on natural pastures (in Swedish). BSci thesis. Turku Polytechnic. pp.35.

Heil, G. and W.H. Diemont, 1983. Raised nutrient levels change heathland into grassland. Vegetatio, 53, 113-120.

Kienzle, E. and N. Zorn, 2006. Bioavailability of minerals in the horse. In: "Horse health nutrition – Proceedings of the 3rd European Equine health and nutrition conference", Gent, March 17-18, 27-36.

INRA, 1984. Le Cheval. Reproduction, sélection, alimentation, exploitation, Jarrige, R. and Martin-Rosset, W. (eds),, Paris, 600 pp.

INRA, 1990. L'alimentation des chevaux. Martin-Rosset, W. (ed). INRA Paris, 232pp.

La Manna, V., A. Rosati, M. Ferretti, S. Rossetti and C. Renieri, 2002. Indagini demografiche e genetiche sulla razza equina del Catria. In proceedings: 4th Convegno Nuove acquisizioni in materia di Ippologia, Campobasso, Itlay, 11-13 July, 27-33.

Lienard, G., C. Beranger, M. Theriez and W. Martin-Rosset, 1979. Choix des systèmes d'exploitation et des animaux utilisateurs des surfaces peu productives. In: Paturages d'altitudes et parcours méditerranéens, INRA Ed., Paris, 493-518.

Loiseau, P. and W. Martin-Rosset, 1985. Utilisation des paturages pauvres en moyenne montagne humide par le cheval. In proceedings: EAAP annual meeting Halkidiki, Greece, September 30-October3.

Loiseau, P. and W. Martin-Rosset, 1989. Evolution à long terme d'une lande de montagne paturée par des bovins et des chevaux. II. Production fourragère. Agronomie, 9, 161-169.

Loucougaray, G., A. Bonis and J.B. Bouzillé, 2004. Effects of grazing by horses and/or cattle on the diversity of coastal grasslands in western France. Biological Conservation, 116, 59-71.

Magnusson B. and S. Magnusson, 1990a. Studies in the grazing of drained lowland fen in Iceland I. The responses of vegetation to livestock grazing. Icel. Agr. Sci. 4, 87-108.

Magnusson, B. and S. Magnusson, 1990b. Studies in the grazing of drained lowland fen in Iceland II. Plant preferences of horses during summer. Icel. Agr. Sci. 4, 109-124.

Martin-Rosset, W. and C. Trillaud-Geyl, 1984. Exploitation des troupeaux de juments lourdes allaitantes. In: Jarrige, R. and Martin-Rosset, W. (eds.), Le Cheval. Reproduction, sélection, alimentation, exploitation, 563-570. INRA, Paris.

Martin-Rosset, W., P. Loiseau and G. Molénat, 1981. Utilisation des pâturages pauvres par le cheval. Bulletin Technique d'Information n° spécial Cheval 362-363, 587-608.

Martin-Rosset, W., I. Vervuert and D. Austbo, 2006. Energy and protein requirements and allowances in pregnant mares. In: proceedings of 3rd European Workshop Equine Nutrition (EWEN); N. Miraglia and W. Martin-Rosset (eds.), Campobasso (I), June 20-22; EAAP no. 120, Wageningen Academic Publishers, The Netherlands.

Martin-Rosset, W., D. Austbo and M. Coenen, 2006. Energy and protein requirements and allowances in lactating mares. In: proceedings of 3rd European Workshop Equine Nutrition (EWEN); N. Miraglia and W. Martin-Rosset (eds.), Campobasso (I), June 20-22; EAAP no. 120, Wageningen Academic Publishers, The Netherlands.

Micol, D. and W. Martin-Rosset, 1995. Feeding systems for horses on high forage diets in the temperate zone. In: Journet, M., Grenet, E., Farce, M-H., Thériez, M., Demarquilly, C. (eds). Recent developments in the Nutrition of Herbivores, 569-584. INRA Editions, Paris.

Miles, J., 1988. Vegetation and soil change in the uplands. In: Biological change in the uplands. Blackwell Scientific Publications, Oxford, 55-70.

Miraglia, N., 1989. Erbe infestanti o invadenti. In: Allevamento del cavallo purosangue. ANAC Ed., Milano, 71-75.

Miraglia, N. and A. Bocchi, 1982 – Significato e valore di alcune comuni infestanti nei prati- pascoli italiani. Il purosangue in Italia, 83, 365-369.

Miraglia, N., D. Bergero and D. Gagliardi, 2000 – Il Cavallo atleta: gestione e miglioramento delle prestazioni. Edagricole Ed., Bologna, 400 p.

Miraglia, N., M. Polidori, F. Lucchese and E. Pietrolà, 2001. Exploitation of low productive areas by wild horses: zootechnical and environmental factors. In proceedings: 52nd EAAP annual meeting, Budapest, Hungary, Horse commission, Session 2, Abstract H2. 9, 326.

Miraglia, N., M. Polidori and E. Salimei, 2003. A review on feeding strategies, feeds and management of equines in Central-Southern Italy. In: "Working animals in agriculture and transport", EAAP technical series N. 6, 103–112.

Miraglia, N., D. Burger, M. Kapron, J. Flanagan, B. Langlois and W. Martin-Rosset, 2006. Local animal resources and products in sustainable development: role and potential of equids. In: Livestock farming systems «Product quality based on local resources leading to improved sustainability», EAAP publication no. 118, 217-233.

Moulin, C., 1997. Le pâturage du cheval: questions techniques posées par les pratiques d'éleveurs. Fourrages, 149, 37-54.

Olivieri, O., N. Miraglia, P. Pollidori and V. Barbieri, 1988. L'allevamento del cavallo per il recupero delle aree marginali. Economia Montana, 5, 33-38.

Pagan, J.D., 2006. Body weight and condition of Kentucky Thoroughbred mares and their foals as influenced by month of foaling, season, and gender. In: proceedings of 3rd European Workshop Equine Nutrition (EWEN); N.Miraglia and W. Martin-Rosset eds. Campobasso (I), June 20-22; EAAP publication no. 120, Wageningen Academic Publishers, The Netherlands.

Petch, E., 1998. Connemara Pony Breeders' Society 1923-1998. Published by the Connemara Pony Breeders' Society, Clifden, Co. Galway, Ireland.

Putman, R.J., 1986. Grazing in temperate ecosystems: large herbivores and the ecology of the New Forest. London & Sydney Ed.

Putman, R.J., A.D. Fowler and S. Tout, 1991. Pattern of the use of ancient grassland by cattle and horses and effects on vegetational composition and structure. Biological conservation, 56, 329-347.
Rogalski, M., 1967. Action des chevaux sur leur paturage. Rocz. Nauk Roln, 71 (B4), 72.
Rogalski, M., 1973. Comportement du poulain en paturage. Przeglad, Hodowlany, 41, 5.
Rogalski, M., 1975. Effect des conditions climatiques sur le comportement des chevaux au paturage. Rocz. Nauk Roln, 97, 7-16.
Rogalski, M., 1977. Behaviour of animals kept on pastures. Thesis Roc. Ahad. Rokn., Poznan, 78, 1- 41.
Roger-Lakenbrink, I., 1997. Freiberger, Zug Ed., 13-18.
Saastamoinen M., 1990. Factors affecting growth and development of foals and young horses. Acta Agric. Scand. 40, 387-396.
Santamarina, G., 2000. O cavalego do Monte. In Proceedings: Jornadas de equinicultura, Via Real, Portugal, March2-3.
Thériez, M., M. Petit and W. Martin-Rosset, 1994. Caractéristiques de la conduite des troupeaux allaitants en zones difficiles. Ann. Zootechn. 43, 33-47.
Thompson, K.N., S.G. Jackson and J.R. Rooney, 1988a. The effect of above average weight gains on the incidence of radiographic bone aberrations and epiphysitis in growing horses. Equine Vet. Sci. 8, 383-385.
Thompson, K.N., J.P. Baker and S.G. Jackson, 1988b. The influence of supplemental feed on growth and bone development of nursing foals. J. Anim. Sci. 66, 1692-1696.
Trillaud-Geyl, C., J. Brohier, L. de Baynast, N. Baudoin, E. Rossier and O. Lapierre, 1990. Bilan de productivité sur 10 ans d'un troupeau de juments de selle conduites en plein air intégral. Croissance des produits de 0 à 6 mois. World Review of Animal Production, 25(3), 65-70.
Warren, L.K., L.M. Lawrence, A.S. Griffin, A.L.Parker, T. Barnes and D. Wright, 1998. The effect of weaning age on foal growth and bone density. Proceedings 1st Kentucky Equine Conf., Lexington (USA), 457-460.
Zafrakas, A.M., 1995. Role of native breeds of horses in Greece. In: "Animal production and roural tourism in Mediterranean regions", Proceedings of international Symposium on Animal Production and rural Tourism in Mediterranean regions, EAAP Publ. N. 74, 43-46.

Relationships between the management and health of pastures and mares and foals: A U.S. perspective

W. Burton Staniar
Virginia Polytechnic Institute and State University, Middleburg Agricultural Research and Extension Center, Middleburg, Virginia 20117, USA

Abstract

Forages are an important resource to the equine industry in the United States. Nearly 77% of equine operations that used pasture for at least 3 months in the Southern United States stated that pasture provided at least 90% of the total roughage intake (NAHMS, 1998). The breeding industry is heavily represented in this group as broodmares and foals are often maintained on pasture. The focus of this paper is on the Mid-Atlantic region which acts as home, as well as a migratory route for many horses on the East coast. The horse evolved as a grazing species in North America, but current management practices have moved the horse to an environment that is more constrained in terms of space and nutrient availability. Horses are now maintained on relatively small improved pastures with man-made concentrates making up for pasture nutrient and energy deficiencies. Management strategies vary depending on the objectives of those raising the horses, but usually are focused on health and athletic performance. The challenge to those raising horses on pasture is to maintain not only the health of their animals, but also the land and plants that are a part of that system. Equine health issues that have been indirectly connected with horses kept on pasture in the Mid-Atlantic region include excessive weight gain, laminitis, colic, developmental orthopedic disease, and laminitis. Current research is examining ways to avoid these health concerns while at the same time taking advantage of the benefits pasture can offer the horse as a source of nutrients and energy, an area to exercise, and an environment where natural equine behavior is exhibited.

Keywords: pasture, horses, growth, health, management

Introduction

The horse evolved as a grazing/browsing species, and until its extinction in North America in the late Pleistocene or early Holocene period utilized the plants growing on the extensive rangelands as a source of nutrients and energy (Evans *et al.*, 1990). Horses likely returned to North America along with other livestock brought by Spanish missions in the early 1600's. In a way, the horse was returning home, to an environment that it had evolved in over 55 to 60 million years. At the time, North America had vast rangelands of what might be considered today, low quality forages. With sufficient time spent grazing, and available acreage, the horse was able to meet its nutrient and energy requirements. Today, both grazing time and available acreage are often limiting factors, leading to the need for supplemental feed formulated to compensate for nutrient and energy deficiencies or imbalances.

Adjectives found in the literature used to describe the quantity of research data available describing the relationship between the horse and pasture include "scarcity", "paucity", or "lack of" (Hoskin and Gee, 2004). As an optimist, this represents a clear opportunity to study a complex and potentially rewarding series of physiologic mechanisms that describe the relationship between the land, plant, and animal. In 1949, Mr. and Mrs. Paul Mellon made a gift of 420 acres of farmland to the Virginia Polytechnic Institute and State University and also provided financial support to help establish the Virginia Forage Research Station, now the Middleburg Agricultural Research and Extension (MARE) Center. Mr. Mellon envisioned forage systems that would promote animal productivity and, at the same time, maintain the integrity and fertility of the soils/livestock and the land in harmony. This philosophy has been maintained as an integral component of the equine research that has been carried out at the MARE Center over the last 15 years. It is also a mindset that is still in need of strengthening for those managing land, pasture and horses elsewhere in the United States.

The continental United States is comprised of at least 12 climate zones, representing a wide variety of pasture and environmental conditions for horses. This paper focuses on the Mid-Atlantic region. The "Middle Atlantic" colonies of the original thirteen were considered to be New York, Pennsylvania, New Jersey and Delaware. We also include the District of Columbia, Maryland, Virginia, and West Virginia. The "Mid-Atlantic" is the area east of the Appalachian Mountains. Climate zones in this region range from Zone 4 (average annual minimum temperature range, -29 to -34 °C) in northern New York State to Zone 8 (-7 to -12 °C) south of Norfolk, Virginia. Environmental and pasture data from the Mid-Atlantic region may be applicable to Illinois, Indiana, Ohio, Kentucky, and Missouri.

Objectives of raising horses on pasture

In order to understand the role that pastures play in keeping broodmares and foals, one must first explore the owners' objectives. A diverse segment of the equine industry is represented within the Mid-Atlantic region. This results in a range of objectives that are probably more variable than nutritionists' estimates of pasture intake. Generally though, those raising horses have the objective to produce healthy, athletic animals. If these basic objectives are met, than many others, like sale price or performance, are likely to follow. Pastures provide several important resources that can help to meet the above objectives. Pasture is a source of nutrients and energy, a space for exercise, and a place where horses can exhibit their natural behaviors. Horse owners' use of pasture can be placed on a scale from those that do not allow, or have access to pasture, or those that keep their broodmares and foal on pasture at all times. The MARE Center is an example of the latter. The role that pastures play in meeting horse owners' objectives has changed for some in the Mid-Atlantic region, where the availability and cost of pasture has changed considerably (Figure 1). This emphasizes the important influence economics can have on the role that pastures play. Figure 1 is indicative of one of the reasons that the role pastures play in the Mid-Atlantic region is changing considerably.

Pasture Species

The Mid-Atlantic region is in a climactic transition area between cool and subtropical zones (Ball *et al.*, 1998). This means that a wide variety of plant species can grow, and is also a reason that this region of the United States is well suited to the pasture needs of broodmares and foals. Most successful pastures have a varied botanical composition, with a combination of grasses and legumes, as well as cool and warm season species. In this way the seasonal fluctuations in nutrients are reduced and the quality of the pasture is not dependent on any one species.

Grasses

Grasses make up the majority of plant species in horse pastures. Pastures in the Mid-Atlantic region are likely to have mixtures of cool and warm season grasses. In northern areas the cool season species will make up the majority. To maintain warm season species, a separate pasture will be established to reduce competition with cool season species. Some of the more common grasses are timothy, orchardgrass, ryegrass, Kentucky bluegrass, tall fescue, bermudagrass and bahiagrass. Warm season grasses make most of their growth during the summer when the average daily temperatures ranges from 16 - 24 °C, whilst the cool seasons grow most rapidly in the spring and fall in a temperature

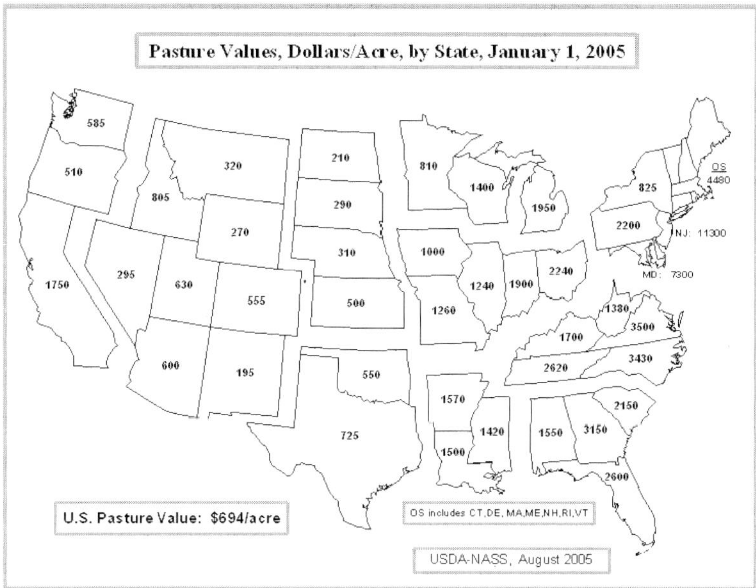

Figure 1. Monetary value of pasture land in the United States according to the 2002 national census of agriculture.

range of 7 - 16 °C. Seasonal fluctuations in nutrient content are a partial result of the botanical composition of the pasture and the periods when these different grasses are growing.

Kentucky Bluegrass (Poa pratensis)

Kentucky bluegrass, a cool season grass, is a valuable component in a pasture mix. Its characteristics of forming a dense sod and tolerating close grazing make it a useful and popular addition to pasture mixtures utilized in this region. In addition, horses find Kentucky bluegrass highly palatable. A disadvantage of this species is that its yield is relatively low. This problem is often overcome by mixing with other better yielding grasses and legumes.

Orchardgrass (Dactylis glomerata)

Orchardgrass, a bunch-type cool season grass, is growing in popularity for use in both pasture and hay mixtures. It is more tolerant of shade and direct sun, drought and heat than Kentucky bluegrass or timothy. Its growing characteristics make it well suited to mixtures with legumes such as alfalfa or clover. It does not tolerate heavy grazing and requires careful management.

Tall Fescue (Festuca arundinacea)

Tall fescue, a cool season sod forming grass, is common as both a source of pasture and hay. Tall fescue is very well adapted to the middle and southern regions of the Mid-Atlantic area. Tall fescue is relatively drought and pest resistant and often out-competes other cool season grasses. This grass stores considerable nutrients and energy in its leaf material and hence can be stockpiled to improve late fall grazing. Some of tall fescue's improved survival characteristics are a result of its symbiotic relationship with an endophytic fungus. The fungus produces alkaloids that, when ingested by broodmares, can cause health complications in late pregnancy (Hall, 1994).

Timothy (Phleum pretense)

Timothy, a bunch-type cool season grass, is well suited to the more northern environments of the Mid-Atlantic region, such as New York, New Jersey, and Pennsylvania. While it is used some for pasture, it is more traditionally grown as hay for horses. Timothy seems to be a preferred choice of hay, but the reasons for this preference may not extend beyond traditional feeding practices.

Bahiagrass (Paspalum notatum)

Bahiagrass, a warm season sod forming grass, is mainly seen in southern regions of the Mid-Atlantic area. Bahiagrass is more tolerant of the sandier soils in this region and is used both for pasture and hay production.

Bermudagrass (Cynodon dactylon)

Bermudagrass, a warm season sod forming grass, is popular into areas of northern Virginia. Some varieties are somewhat cold-adapted allowing it to be used in this region. Bermudagrass is utilized to extend nutrient availability into the summer months.

Legumes

Legumes are mixed with grasses to provide several important benefits to meeting the management objectives of both the pasture and broodmares and foals. First, legumes have different seasonal patterns of growth and nutrient production compared to grasses (Figure 2). By utilizing a mixture of grasses and legumes the overall annual fluctuations of nutrients can be reduced. This can help

Table 1. Nutrient composition on a dry matter basis of general legume and grass pasture (data from Dairy One n ~ 70 – 4000) and mixed grass/legume pasture sampled at the MARE Center over the past 10 years.

Nutrient	Legume pasture Mean	Grass pasture Mean	MARE Center Pasture Mean
Crude protein, %	26.8	15.3	18.3
Crude fat, %	3.9	3.7	3.3
Acid detergent fiber, %	24.6	35.6	32.4
Neutral detergent fiber, %	32.5	58.8	57.5
Starch, %	4.6	3.5	2.5
Sugar, %	10.2	10.2	9.5
Ca, %	1.2	0.5	0.5
P, %	0.4	0.3	0.3
Mg, %	0.3	0.2	0.2
K, %	2.8	2.1	2.4
Na, %	0.2	0.1	0.01
Fe, mg/kg	275	371	525
Zn, mg/kg	40.8	27.5	26.1
Cu, mg/kg	9.1	9.5	7.1
Mn, mg/kg	58.5	83.9	62.1
S, %	0.3	0.2	0.2
Cl, ion %	1.2	0.8	0.9

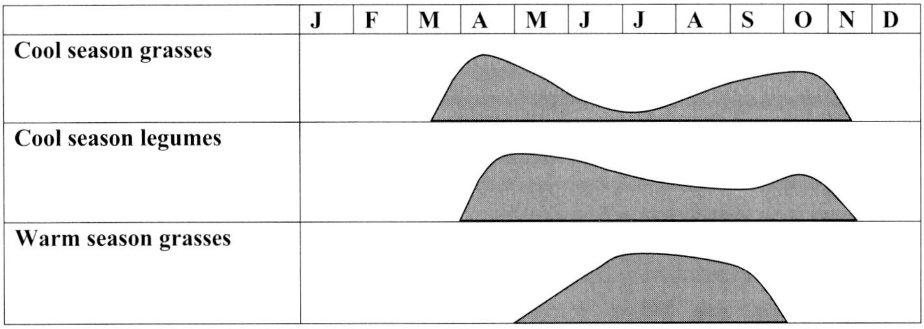

Figure 2. Generalized annual patterns of forage availability for grasses and legumes. Illustrates how mixtures of varieties can be utilized to reduce seasonal fluctuations in nutrient availability from any single variety.

reduce connected physiologic responses in the horses, such as slow or rapid growth, changes in body condition, or gastrointestinal problems associated with changes in rapidly fermented carbohydrates (Hudson *et al.*, 2001). Second, bacteria that live symbiotically in the legumes roots are able to convert atmospheric nitrogen into nitrogen available to other plants in the pasture. This process reduces the amount of nitrogen fertilizer needed to maintain the pasture.

Alfalfa (Medicago sativa)

Alfalfa, a cool season legume, is mainly used for hay production, but certain strains are also suitable as a component in a pasture mix. Alfalfa mixed with other cool season grasses can extend the nutrient productivity of a pasture into warmer months because it continues to grow into the early and mid-summer.

White or Ladino Clover (Trifolium repens)

There are a number of varieties of this popular cool season legume included in horse pastures in the Mid-Atlantic region. Ladino is characterized by taller leaf stems and larger leaves, with the potential for a greater yield than more common varieties. Ladino is more difficult to sustain than the more common white or Dutch clover which has smaller leaf stems and leaves. These smaller white clovers persist better, and are more tolerant of heavy grazing.

Red Clover (Trifolium pratense)

Red clover, a cool season legume, shows considerable growth during spring months and is often seen in horse pastures. It is not as common as varieties of white clover because it is not as tolerant of grazing pressure or winter kill. In addition, a toxin (slaframine) produced by a fungus that grows on red clover is responsible for an over production of saliva in horses grazing on infected fields. While not a direct health threat, this condition is enough of a concern that red clover is not a preferred legume species for horse pastures.

Pasture management

When horses were grazing range and pasturelands in western North America, there were no farm managers "maintaining" that grazing land. However today, a common misconception is that pasture is an easy to maintain, inexpensive source of nutrients and energy. The difference is that more horses are being kept on smaller acreage. Objectives need to be focused not only on the health of the horse, but also the plants and land utilized to support it. Successful pasture management requires a considerable knowledge of plant biology, as well as an input of labor and money. This being recognized, maintaining pasture as a part of an overall management scheme is likely to benefit animal health, reducing veterinary, feed and labor costs.

Land

While the health of the land is as important as the plants and horses, it is the component that is most likely neglected in most management schemes in the United States. Managing the land requires attention to soil nutrients, pH, and physical characteristics. Nitrogen, phosphorus, and potassium are monitored and maintained through a regular fertilization program. An added benefit of including legumes in a pasture is the contribution of nitrogen from rhizobial fixation, reducing the need to fertilize with exogenous nitrogen. Including clover in a pasture mix for this reason is a regular practice in this region of the United States. This is important in relation to concerns about the potential negative influence of excessive fertilization on both the land and water. Monitoring pH is critical to maintain soil microbe and plant health. Many nutrients become unavailable and root growth is inhibited at pH's below 6.0 (Teustch and Fike, 2005).

Physical characteristics of the soil are important in relation to soil erosion, water run-off, and water availability for seedlings. Two management strategies that are commonly utilized to address some of these issues are no-till seeding and soil aeration. No-till seeding of pastures has grown in popularity as an environmentally friendly and effective tool in pasture renovation. No-till seeding has benefits that include a reduction in ruts and gullies formed due to plowing, reduction of water run-off, conservation of both water and soil, and reduced labor and time expense. Soil aeration is meant to reduce soil compaction and improve porosity and soil structure. Research studying the benefits of soil aeration generally show minimal benefits (Shah *et al.*, 2004). At the MARE Center aeration is mainly used to reduce soil compaction prior to a full renovation.

Grazing

Grazing management balances the objectives of utilizing available forage while maintaining the quality of the pasture. To approach this balance several strategies are used:

- New seedlings and very young growth are not grazed. New seedlings do not have well established root systems that are easily damaged and grazing young plants early in the growing season goes against the maintenance of the pasture.
- Recommended pasture stocking rates are approximately 0.8 hectares of pasture to meet the grazing and exercise needs of each mature horse. In the Mid-Atlantic area this recommendation becomes harder and harder to follow because of decreasing availability of pasture acreage. Illustrating the decrease in pasture availability in the Mid-Atlantic area is the 4% decrease in land used for pasture in Virginia between 1997 and 2002 compared to only a 0.4% decrease for the entire United States (USDA-NASS, 2004b, a).
- Rotational grazing has been a successful technique for achieving a balance in grazing management. It allows grazing of pasture when nutrients and energy are likely to be high, but also allows for resting pasture sufficiently between periods of grazing. Common recommendations depending on the botanical composition are to graze pasture to between 7 and 12 cm, move the animals and allow the pasture to recover to 25 to 40 cm before returning animals. In reality, the physical layout of pastures and the labor and attention required for a successful rotational grazing program are often reasons for failure.
- The use of a dry lot or sacrifice paddock is another strategy aimed at preserving the quality of pastures when acreage is limited. During poor weather conditions or during rest periods for the pasture, horses can be kept in these sacrifice paddocks and fed hay.

While these management techniques are relatively easy to implement and are taken advantage of on larger equine operations, the majority of smaller equine operations in this region do not have a grazing management protocol.

Mare and foal management

Synchrony with Physiology

Reproduction and growth, two critical periods for survival in the horse, are synchronized with seasonal patterns. This is a multi-layered effect in that the horse's metabolism is affected by changes in day length, temperature, and nutrient and energy availability (Cubitt, 2004; Wesson and Ginther, 1982). At the Middleburg Agricultural Research and Extension Center (Middleburg AREC) seasonal patterns are incorporated into the management of broodmares and growing stock. Mares are bred and foals are born when forage nutrient and energy concentrations are at their highest at this point. This helps to maintain the body condition of broodmares for improved reproductive efficiency, provide for the increased energy and nutrient requirements of early lactation, and supply foals with a highly digestible forage source. Breeding management programs that begin in January and February are unable to take advantage of natural forage sources, and hence must compensate by feeding concentrate and hay, increasing feed and labor costs, as well as risks associated with grain feeding (Kronfeld and Harris, 2003).

Forage rises to a second nutrient and energy peak in November from a low in July. Foals are weaned at six months of age in October and November to take advantage of forage availability and quality to help maintain condition and growth during a stressful period. Mares in the second trimester that have been weaned from their foals can also take advantage of the pasture to improve condition prior to the hardest months of winter and the extra energy and nutrient demands of the third trimester. Management strategies that wean in mid-summer are maintaining weanlings on pasture at one of the lowest points in pasture quality.

Pasture supplements

To meet the objectives of owners keeping horses under typical pasture conditions in this region, it is often necessary to supplement the nutrients and energy available from the pasture. This relatively straightforward strategy is complicated by the need to understand pasture botanical and biochemical variation with time, quantify pasture intake, and understand the nutrient and energy requirements of the horse. A research goal at the MARE Center has been to develop a novel and versatile multi-fiber supplement for broodmares and foals maintained on pasture. This required investigation of the possible sources of variation to allow for optimal feed formulation (Hoffman and Kronfeld, 1999).

Plant variation

The living plant and, on a larger scale, the pasture is constantly changing. One approach in characterizing changes in the pasture is to examine them on different time scales. On one end of this scale are studies that examine hourly changes in nutrients such as carbohydrate content (Longland *et al.*, 1999). These changes occur due to changes in light, temperature and humidity influencing plant metabolism. Data that provides a clearer description of these short term changes has important implications for horses kept on pastures in which these biochemical changes are likely to have an impact on health. An example would be the modification of grazing management to avoid periods when sugars and starches are at their highest in an attempt to avoid laminitis (Byrd and Staniar, 2005). Annual changes in the nutrient and energy content (Figure 3) characterize the pasture on a

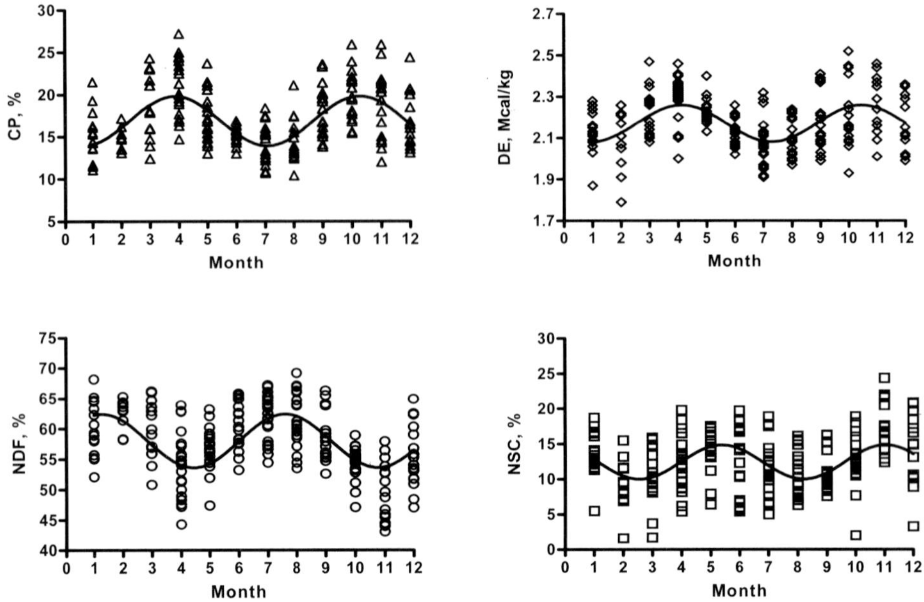

Figure 3. Seasonal fluctuations in nutritive value of pasture in Virginia represented by a sine wave. (CP (R^2 = 0.34), DE (R^2 = 0.23), NDF (R^2 = 0.34), NSC (R^2 = 0.15)) (Cubitt et al., 2005).

different timescale (Cubitt *et al.*, 2004; Kronfeld *et al.*, 1996). Nutrient and energy fluctuations in this time frame are due to biochemical changes in the individual plants as well as changes in the botanical makeup of the pasture related to seasonal patterns in the environment (Ball *et al.*, 1998). In the Mid-Atlantic region, the objective of having Thoroughbred broodmares foal as close to January 1st as possible runs in opposition to nutrient and energy availability in the pasture. During this time of year, pastures are high in neutral detergent fiber (NDF) while digestible energy (DE) and crude protein (CP) are low. In order to meet the requirements of mares in early lactation and rapidly growing foals, supplementation with quality hay as well as concentrate is important under these winter environmental conditions (Cubitt *et al.*, 2005). The "real world" implementation can be seen in the management of broodmares at the MARE Center. There the management strategy is more closely aligned with climatic and pasture seasonal patterns. Mares are bred over a 10 wk period from April 15th to June 22nd, and approximately 95% of the foals over the last 14 years have been born in April and May of the following year. This strategy takes advantage of the peak in DE and CP in April and May. In Figure 4, mean body weights of growing Thoroughbreds at the MARE Center are compared with Thoroughbreds raised in Canada and Kentucky. The higher rate of early growth seen in the MARE Center foals may be in part due to the environment that they are born into. Average daily gain (ADG) for all the groups in Figure 4 slows between 200 and 300 days of age as daylength shortens and pasture quality decreases. Current research on growth and pasture at the MARE Center is working to characterize the mechanisms via which the changes in both occur and how they relate to one another. The implications of this research will be the development of management practices that are more effective in supporting optimal growth due to a clearer understanding of the relationship between the pasture and horse.

Pasture intake

An important factor in optimizing production of young horses is the understanding of nutrient and energy supply to the broodmare and growing foal. A number of studies indicate that the nutrient

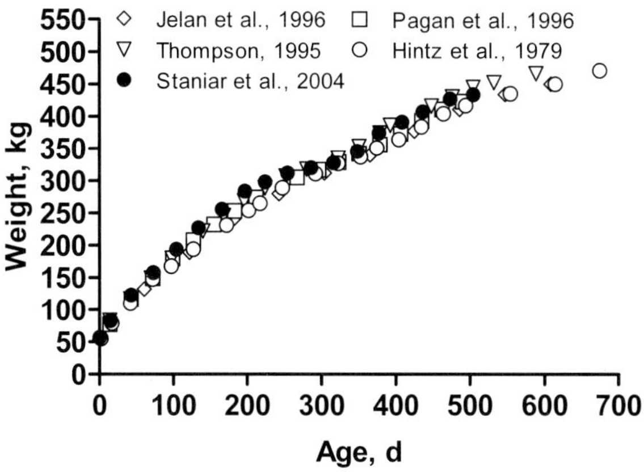

Figure 4. Mean monthly weights of Thoroughbred foals raised at the MARE Center compared with previously published data.

and energy supply from the pasture is often less than optimal for growth and reproduction (Cubitt *et al.*, 2004; Cubitt *et al.*, 2005; Griewe-Crandell *et al.*, 1992; Kronfeld *et al.*, 1996). A fundamental difficulty in connecting the nutrient and energy composition of the pasture with the requirements of the horses is establishing the quantity of pasture intake.

Numerous techniques have been utilized to try to accurately estimate pasture intake in horses and other livestock species (Gordon, 1995; Holland *et al.*, 1998; Ordakowski *et al.*, 2001). The most rudimentary and yet often used method of estimating pasture intake is by subtracting the DE provided by supplement and hay from the total DE requirements (NRC, 1989). The inadequacy of this technique becomes clear when pasture intake estimates are negative for horses that are observed grazing. Other techniques include the use of markers such as chromium sesquioxide and odd and even-chain alkanes (Holland *et al.*, 1998; Ordakowski *et al.*, 2001). Estimates of the dry matter intake of horses on pasture range from 1.5 to 3.3% of body weight, but data for growing foals and broodmares in various stages of gestation and lactation is lacking (Cuddeford, 2002). Considerable work remains to be done characterizing how horses change their intake of pasture under different physiologic conditions and when fed different amounts of concentrate.

Feed formulation via sensitivity analysis

Sensitivity analysis is a method of feed formulation that has been proposed to take into account the variability in factors that parameterize the optimal concentrations of nutrients and energy in the diet (Hoffman and Kronfeld, 1999). The objective to using sensitivity analysis in the formulation of feeds that complement pasture is to take into account known sources of variation and determine target ranges for nutrients in the diet (Kronfeld, 2001). The sources of variation include pasture intake and pasture nutrient and energy content. An example of the result of this formulation technique is a feed that is appropriate for a region where the ranges in pasture nutrient and energy content have been determined. Formulating feeds for the pasture kept horse would be improved by taking into account the variability that is a part of the real world, and facilitates the design of feeds that are more flexible to a changing environment. For a more in depth discussion of sensitivity analysis please see either reference cited in this section.

Challenges to raising horses on pasture

Raising horses on pasture presents several difficulties that must be overcome in management. These include the physical safety of the animals, the labor and attention involved in managing the pastures, and attention to botanical factors that will influence equine health.

Carbohydrates

Carbohydrate fractions in the forage offered to horses are receiving a considerable amount of research attention. This is due to the role hydrolyzable and rapidly fermentable carbohydrates play in various metabolic and digestive disturbances, examples of which include equine polysaccharide storage myopathy, laminitis, and colic (Watts and Chatterton, 2004). Metabolic disturbances occur as a result of abnormal patterns of glucose absorption, directly or indirectly influencing a number of other factors that include insulin, insulin-like growth factor I as well as other food signals and hormones ultimately affecting the metabolism of individual cells. Digestive disturbances result from the accumulation of lactic acid produced by those carbohydrates that are rapidly fermented in the equine hindgut. The lactic acid results in a significant lowering of cecal pH, lysis of bacteria, and release of endotoxin (Clarke *et al.*, 1990).

A survey of equine practitioners showed that 83% felt laminitis, over other equine health issues including colic, was in need of future research, emphasizing the importance of this health issue to the equine community (AAEP, 2003). Due to the fact that fructans in pasture and hay has been hypothesized to play a significant role in the etiology of laminitis, it is likely that forage producers will have to become more aware of carbohydrate fractions that may be affecting their equine customers (Longland and Cairns, 2000). Fructans are a storage form of the sucrose formed as the primary product of photosynthesis. A number of environmental and maturity factors will affect fructan production in the plant, resulting in significant changes in fructan content in only a few hours. Fructans are not well hydrolyzed in the small intestine, but are rapidly fermented upon reaching the hindgut. For these two reasons, a horse grazing pasture or being fed a new batch of hay can be exposed to a relatively rapid change in the proportion of rapidly fermentable carbohydrates. This can result in the cascade of events leading to the lysis of a portion of the bacterial population and the release of toxins initiating diet-induced laminitis.

Carbohydrates that are hydrolyzed, such as some di- and oligosaccharides and starches, inevitably lead to increases in plasma glucose. Laminitis has a second causative mechanism that may be a result of insulin resistance. Forage carbohydrates may not be the primary causative factor, but animals that are already at risk for health risks associated with insulin resistance, may see them manifested at times of year when the hydrolyzable carbohydrates increase in pasture. A classic example of this is laminitis observed in ponies with too much exposure to spring pasture (Coffman and Colles, 1983). Researchers at the Middleburg AREC are currently working with a group of ponies to try to better understand how carbohydrates in spring pasture growth may aggravate the genetic predisposition to insulin resistance.

Chemical Hazards

Chemical hazards to the horse associated with forages come in two general categories. Mycotoxins are toxins produced by fungi that live in symbiotic or parasitic relationships with the plant, and less frequently, the forage itself will produce a toxin such as prussic acid. Both of these plant hazards will typically be manifested during particular times of year when toxic substances may accumulate in the plants due to environmental conditions.

A well known example of a mycotoxin related to pasture in the United States is that produced by the endophyte that lives in a symbiotic relationship with tall fescue. It has been estimated that approximately 688,000 horses in the United States have access to tall fescue in either pasture or hay (Hoveland, 1993). Tall fescue is well suited to many of the climates in the United States resulting in its presence in 14.2 million hectares (Blodgett, 2001). The endophyte that lives in a symbiotic relationship with the grass is *neotyphodium coenophialum*. This endophyte produces multiple chemicals that are toxic to insects and herbivores. The group of toxins that are detrimental to the horse are the ergot alkaloids. The alkaloids produced by the endophyte infected tall fescue appear to have their main effect via the alkaloids function as dopamine agonists (Blodgett, 2001). Binding to lactotrophs in the anterior pituitary results in decreased production of prolactin. This then has broad acting effects on reproductive, vascular, immune, and gastrointestinal function. The negative health effects are seen mainly in broodmares that have grazed endophyte infected pasture between 30 to 90 days prior to parturition (Cross *et al.*, 1995). These effects may include agalactia, lowered circulating progesterone during late pregnancy, prolonged gestation, and foal loss. Horses seem to recover relatively quickly upon removal from infected fescue, and may return to normal within 2 to 3 weeks (McCann *et al.*, 1992). Due to the broad reaching health risks associated with endophyte infected tall fescue, there is considerable pressure to develop new pasture management strategies to reduce equine exposure.

From a pasture management perspective, the difficulty is the often ubiquitous nature of tall fescue, particularly in the more southern areas of the Mid-Atlantic region. Tall fescue is a well adapted and competitive species, and it thrives under conditions that are difficult for many other species. Its nutrient and energy profile would make it an excellent choice for many horse pastures in this region. Demonstrable negative effects in horses other than broodmares are relatively limited (Aiken *et al.*, 1993). For managers that want maximal reduction of risk, a complete pasture renovation is often the solution, with an economic impact that has been estimated at approximately $200 per acre (Ivy *et al.*, 2000). A more economical solution that is often selected is removal of broodmares from tall fescue pastures 60-90 days prior to parturition. While this solution is usually successful in avoiding negative health effects, it is difficult to establish whether it is 100% effective.

Certain forages, such as sudangrass, sorghums, and johnsongrass can accumulate toxic concentrations of prussic acid (a form of cyanide) that can cause death in horses. Cyanide interferes with the oxygen carrying ability of the horse's red blood cells. Factors that are associated with the risk of prussic acid poisoning are the proportion of the prussic acid producing plant available, the stage of plant maturity, and environmental stresses on the plant that result in prussic acid accumulation in the leaves or shoots, which are most attractive for the selectively grazing horse. Horse owners need to be aware of these plants both in their pastures as well as in hay. While these plants are not dangerous all the time, equine breeding operations have established pasture management strategies that work to remove them from equine fields and along fence rows.

Nutrient management

Nutrient management is still a foreign term to many in the equine industry in the United States. With decreasing acreage available and the number of horses increasing attention to nutrient/waste management has grown. The equine impact is likely to be relatively small compared to other more intensively farmed livestock, as well as the human impact. Having said this, it is estimated that the approximately 9.2 million horses in the United States produce 81 million tons of manure per year, containing 671 million kg of nitrogen and 97 million kg of phosphorus (ASAE, 2005). A number of recent studies have begun to examine nitrogen and phosphorus excretion from the horse with potential implications on nutrient management plans for the horse (Lawrence *et al.*, 2003; van Doorn *et al.*, 2004). At this year's Mid- Atlantic Nutrition Conference one of the speakers will address manure management from a nutritional perspective (Warren, 2006). Numerous racetracks in the United States have installed biofermentation facilities to make better use of the manure they produce. Some larger equine operations in Kentucky have purchased equipment to compost their manure so that it can be more effectively used to enhance the land and pasture.

Conclusions

Agriculture and humans' relationship with the land is changing. The horse represents an opportunity to maintain the important connection between the two. In the United States, particularly the Mid-Atlantic region the role that pastures play in broodmare and foal management remains in question. This is because the cost of land is steadily increasing to the point where it is no longer economically feasible to maintain horses on that land. Slowing population or economic growth is not the role most equine scientists would chose, but instead facilitating the continued health of the horse as well as the pasture by better understanding the physiologic mechanisms that link the two. This means developing supplements that are more appropriate for growing horses kept at pasture, establishing new management protocols for horses that may be prone to laminitis, and developing proactive nutritional strategies that make changes to the diets of growing horses in anticipation of changes in growth, not in response to them.

References

AAEP, 2003. Membership equine research study. www.aaep.org/phfs/research_study_final.pdf (accessed 03/10/04)

Aiken, G.E., D.I. Bransby and C.A. McCall, 1993. Growth of yearling horses compared to steers on high- and lowendophyte infected tall fescue. J. Equine Vet. Sci. 13: 26-28.

ASAE, 2005. Manure production and characteristics. ASAE Standard D384.2, American Society of Agricultural and Biological Engineers, St. Joseph, MI.

Ball, D.M., C.S. Hoveland and G.D. Lacefield, 1998. Southern forages. 2nd Edition ed. Williams Printing Company, Atlanta, GA.

Blodgett, D.J. 2001, Fescue toxicosis. Vet. Clin. N. Am. 17: 567-577.

Byrd, B. M. and W.B. Staniar, 2005. Avoidance of equine laminits through management of risk factors in pastures. In: Proceedings of the 3rd Mid-Atlantic Nutrition Conference, Timonium, MD. p 161-170.

Clarke, L.L., M.C. Roberts and R.A. Argenzio, 1990. Feeding and digestive problems in horses. Vet. Clin. N. Am. Equine Pract. 6: 433-450.

Coffman, J.R. and C.M. Colles, 1983. Insulin tolerance in laminitic ponies. Can. J. Comp. Med. 47: 347-351.

Cross, D.L., L.M. Redmond and J.R. Strickland, 1995. Equine fescue toxicosis: Signs and solutions. J. Anim. Sci. 73: 899-908.

Cubitt, T.A. 2004, Endocrine patterns associated with reproductive development in growing thoroughbreds. MS thesis, Virginia Polytechnic Institute and State University, Blacksburg, VA.

Cubitt, T.A., W.B. Staniar and D.S. Kronfeld, 2004. Environmental factors and nutrient composition of pasture in northern virginia. J. Anim. Sci. 82 (Suppl. 1): 96.

Cubitt, T.A., W.B. Staniar, D.S. Kronfeld, B.M. Byrd and P.A. Harris, 2005. Environmental effects on nutritive value of equine pastures. Pferdeheilkunde 21: 13-14.

Cuddeford, D., 2002. Equine nutrition: Some unique features, functions, and frailties of the digestive system of the horse. In: P.C. Garnsworthy, D.J.A. Cole and J. Wiseman (eds.) Recent advances in animal nutrition. p 269-318. Nottingham University Press, Nottingham, UK.

Evans, J.W., A. Borton, H.F. Hintz and L.D. Van Vleck, 1990. The horse. 2nd Edition ed. W. H. Freeman and Company, New York.

Gordon, I. J., 1995. Animal-based techniques for grazing ecology research. Small Ruminant Research 16: 203-214.

Griewe-Crandell, K.M., G.A. Morrow and D.S. Kronfeld, 1992. Phosphorus and selenium depletion in thoroughbred mares and weanlings. Pferdeheilkunde 12: 96-98.

Hall, M.H., 1994. Tall fescue. Agronomy Facts 28, Pennsylvania State University, University Park, PA.

Hintz, H.F., R.L. Hintz and L.D. Vleck, 1979. Growth rate of thoroughbreds: Effect of age of dam, year and month of birth, and sex of foal. J. Anim. Sci. 48: 480-487.

Hoffman, R.M. and D.S. Kronfeld, 1999. Nutrient requirements for grazing horses: Development of an optimal pasture supplement. In: P. C. Garnsworthy and J. Wiseman (eds.) Recent advances in animal nutrition. p 19-35. Nottingham University Press, Nottingham, U.K.

Holland, J.L., D.S. Kronfeld, D. Sklan and P.A. Harris, 1998. Calculation of fecal kinetics in horses fed hay or hay and concentrate. J. Anim. Sci. 76: 1937-1944.

Hoskin, S.O. and E.K. Gee, 2004. Feeding value of pastures for horses. New Zealand Veterinary Journal 52: 332-341.

Hoveland, C.S., 1993. Importance and economiv significance of the acremonium endophytes to performance of animals and grass plants. Agriculture, Ecosystems, and Environment 44: 3-12.

Hudson, J.M., N.D. Cohen, P.G. Gibbs and J.A. Thompson, 2001. Feeding practices associated with colic in horses. J. Am. Vet. Med. Assoc. 219: 1419-1425.

Ivy, R.L., G.B. Triplett, M.L. Broome, D.R. Reynolds, D.J. Lang, J.L. Howell and K.M. Bloodworth, 2000. Means of renovation of stands of toxic endophyte tall fescue In: Proceedings of the Tall Fescue Toxicosis Workshop, Chapel Hill, TN. p 19.

Jelan, Z.A., L.B. Jeffcott, N. Lundeheim and M. Osborne, 1996. Growth rates in thoroughbred foals. Pferdeheilkunde 12: 291-295.

Kronfeld, D.S, 2001. A practical method for ration evaluation and diet formulation: An introduction to sensitivity analysis. In: J. D. Pagan and R. J. Geor (eds.) Advances in equine nutrition ii. p 1-12. Nottingham University Press, Nottingham, UK.

Kronfeld, D.S., W.L. Cooper, K.M. Crandell, L.A. Gay, R.M. Hoffman, J.L. Holland, J.A. Wilson, D. Sklan and P. Harris, 1996. Supplementation of pasture for growth. Pferdeheilkunde 12: 317-319.

Kronfeld, D.S. and P.A. Harris, 2003. Equine grain-associated disorders. Compend. Contin. Educ. Pract. 25: 974-983.

Lawrence, L.M., J. Bicudo, J. Davis and E. Wheeler, 2003. Relationships between intake and excretion for nitrogen and phosphorus in horses. In: Proceedings of the 18th Equine Nutriyion and Physiology Society Symposium, East Lansing, MI. p 306-307.

Longland, A.C. and A.J. Cairns, 2000. Fructans and their implications in the aetiology of laminitis. In: Third International Conference on Feeding Horses, Perth

Longland, A.C., A.J. Cairns and M.O. Humphreys, 1999. Seasonal and diurnal changes in fructan concentration in lolium perenne: Implications for the grazing management of equine predisposed to laminitis. In: Proceedings of the 16th Equine Nutrition and Physiology Society Symposium, Raleigh, NC. p 258-259.

McCann, J.S., A.B. Caudle, F.N. Thompson, J.A. Stuedemann, G.I. Heusner and D.L. Thompson, 1992. Influence of endophyte-infected tall fescue on serum prolactin and progesterone in gravid mares. J. Anim. Sci. 70: 217-223.

NAHMS, 1998. Equine '98 study: Part iv: Reference of health mangement for horses and highlighted diseases, 1998, USDA:APHIS, Fort Collins, CO.

NRC. 1989. Nutrient requirements of horses (5th ed.). National Academy Press, Washington, DC.

Ordakowski, A.L., D.S. Kronfeld, J.L. Holland, B.J. Hargreaves, L.S. Gay, P.A. Harris, H. Dove and D. Sklan, 2001. Alkanes as internal markers to estimate digestibility of hay or hay plus concentrate diets in horses. J. Anim. Sci. 79: 1516-1522.

Pagan, J.D., S.G. Jackson and S. Caddel, 1996. A summary of growth rates of thoroughbreds in kentucky. Pferdeheilkunde 12: 285-289.

Shah, S.B., J.L. Miller and T.J. Basden, 2004. Mechanical aeration and liquid dairy manure application impacts on grassland runoff water quality and yield. Transactions of the American Society of Agricultural Engineers 47: 777-788.

Staniar, W.B., D.S. Kronfeld, K.H. Treiber, R.K. Splan and P.A. Harris, 2004. Growth rate consists of baseline and systematic deviation components in thoroughbreds. J. Anim. Sci. 82: 1007-1015.

Teustch, C.D. and J.H. Fike, 2005. Virginia's horse pastures: Forage establishment. Extension publication 418-103, Virginia Polytechnic Institute and State University, Blacksburg, VA.

Thompson, K.N, 1995. Skeletal growth rates of weanling and yearling thoroughbred horses. J. Anim. Sci. 73: 2513-2517.

USDA-NASS, 2004a. 2002 census of agriculture. AC-02-A-46.

USDA-NASS, 2004b. 2002 census of agriculture. AC-02-A-51.
Van Doorn, D.A., H. Everts, H. Wouterse and A.C. Beynen, 2004. The apparent digestibility of phytate phosphorus and the influence of supplemental phytase in horses. J. Anim. Sci. 82: 1756-1763.
Warren, L.K., 2006, From oats to road apples: Modifying horse manure through nutrition. In: Proceeding of the 4th Mid-Atlantic Nutrition Conference, Timonium, MD
Watts, K.A. and N.J. Chatterton, 2004. A review of factors affecting carbohydrate levels in forage. J. Equine Vet. Sci. 24: 84-86.
Wesson, J.A. and O.J. Ginther, 1982. Influence of photoperiod on puberty in the female pony. Reprod. Fert. Suppl. 32: 269-274.

Part E – Nutrition and reproductive performances

Effects of nutrition level in mares' ovarian activity and in equines' puberty

D. Guillaume[1], *J. Salazar-Ortiz*[1] *and W. Martin-Rosset*[2]
[1]*UMR 6175, INRA/CNRS, Université F. Rabelais of Tours-Haras Nationaux, Centre of research of Tours, 37380 Nouzilly, France*
[2]*INRA, Department of Animal Science, Research Centre of Clermont-Ferrand/Theix, 63122 Saint Genes Champanelle, France*

Abstract

The aim of the present review is to outline the main effects of nutrition level on horses' reproduction before fertilisation. In adult mares the nutrition level modulates reproduction physiology by influencing on the duration of winter ovarian inactivity and on mares' follicular growth during the breeding season. As in other species the nutrition level also affects on males and females puberty. Mares present a winter ovarian inactivity, which takes place from fall to spring. This winter inactivity is synchronised by the photoperiod, which is mediated by melatonin to the GnRH neuron through an unknown pathway. 50 percent of fat mares which have not nursed a foal during the previous summer continue to cycle all along the year whereas the other have a very short inactivity and miss only 1 or 2 cycles. Conversely restricted mares systematically exhibit long winter inactivity and only have few sexual cycles during summer. Increasing the feeding level in the early autumn cannot reactivate the cyclicity. When cyclicity is established in spring, a lot of differences are found on follicular growth and plasma sexual hormone concentrations between well fed and restricted mares. In fat mares, follicular growth of follicles smaller than 25 mm is more intense than in restricted mares. As a result in well fed mares: the length of the follicular phase is shorter and the ovarian hormone plasma concentrations are higher. These high levels of ovarian hormone act on the gonadotrophin plasma concentrations. After ovulation, the plateau of plasma progesterone concentrations is lowest in the restricted group. As in other species, puberty occurs when the foal meet 90 percent of its adult body size. Puberty would occur between 12 and 15 months but a great variability is observed between 8 to 30 months. Well-fed foals would be potentially pubescent younger than it is classically described, but their puberty is delayed until their first breeding season. The restricted foals have to wait till their second breeding season. This hypothesis would be confirmed by our data especially for male. In horses the neuro-endocrine mechanisms implemented by the strong influence of nutrition on reproduction is poorly investigated. The main hormones probably involved in this influence are the GH-IGFs-insulin systems and leptin. The thyroid hormones cannot be excluded. These effects focus on the hypothalamus and the main implicated neuromediators would be neuropeptide-Y and orexin.

Keywords: equines, nutrition, seasonal ovarian inactivity, oestrus cycle, puberty, hormones

Interaction between nutrition level and season of reproduction

Introduction

Mares are seasonal poly-oestrous species. The breeding season occurs and ends in spring then in fall when the daylight, temperature and availability of feed allowances rise then decrease respectively. The natural breeding season is approximately focused on the longest day of the year, the 20th June and lasts from April to September, in the northern hemisphere (Hughes *et al,* 1975) whereas grazing season takes place from April to October. As a result a maximum of births occur at the end of May. For wild mares living in this zone, this event constitutes a tremendous adaptation. This adaptation should be overcome by problems the breeders who manage to get the mare pregnant as soon as possible in the year. January the 1st is the official birthday of foals stated by the regulations of many breeding associations in the northern hemisphere. Subsequently the dates of the official breeding season are from February to June. It results that all the foals born during the same season have the same age (Ginther, 1992). So far the breeders should mate the mares as early as possible in the year to get an age advantage over the foals born later in the year (Langlois and Blouin 1996, 1997, 1998). This breeding challenge requests to develop methods for induction of an early onset of the breeding season in mares. Indeed the numbers of usable cycles and the odds to be pregnant at the end of the year are of major concern when the mares can be matted soon in the year (Langlois and Blouin 2004).

Since the first investigations of Burkhardt (1947) and Nishikawa (1959) on the effect of artificial light on ovarian activity and one year later the discovery of melatonin by Albert (1958) and its chemical formulation by Learner *et al* (1959), the important role of this pineal hormone in the photoperiod effects on equine reproduction began to be investigated in the eighties. More recently, the discovery of leptin, identified and cloned by Zhang *et al* in 1994, had induced a lot of experimental work on this physiological role. This hormone secreted by the adipose tissue seems to be the key mediator between nutrition and reproduction. In equine species, Fitzgerald and McManus (2000) published the first study on this topic, using a commercial assay kit of this hormone. Melatonin and leptin have this common point that their neuro-endocrine pathway is up to now completely unknown. Photoperiod, feed allowances and their interactions seem to have different effects on winter ovarian inactivity. This review attempts to highlight this interaction using recent data obtained in our group and published in the literature. The implications to advance the onset of cyclic reproductive activity in the early spring, is discusses with regard to treatment strategies.

Effects of Photoperiod and melatonin on winter inactivity

The photostimulation of anoestrus mares

The photoperiod is independent on the weather and so it is the more stable parameter from one year to the other. Under temperate zones a lot of animals and plants have chosen this parameter to adapt their physiology to the season. An anovulatory phase takes place in fall when the length of the day is decreasing whereas ovulatory phase arises when the length of the day is rising in spring.

It is well accepted that in the horses, photoperiod is the most important external factor that influences the circannual endogenous reproductive rhythm in the horses (Ginther, 1992). Additional light exposure during winter and early spring stimulates ovarian activity in anoestrous mares and is commonly used to advance the onset of the breeding season (Burkhardt, 1947).

A lot of experiments have implemented different light treatments, beginning around the winter solstice, on mares previously chosen to be in ovarian inactivity. These experiments have clearly indicated that the length of the light phase efficient to advance the first ovulation of the year is 14.5 h under our temperate latitude. Using this light treatment, the first ovulation of the years occurs around 2 months before the control groups subjected to natural photoperiod. The same effect is obtained with 1 or 2 h of light flash during a long night, 9.5 to 10 hours after the abrupt beginning of darkness (Palmer and Driancourt, 1981; Palmer *et al,* 1982; Malinowski *et al,* 1985). Some conditions have been recently specified to implement this treatment (Guillaume *et al,*2000). A light intensity of 10 lux is sufficient to advance the first ovulation, and the light-treatment beginning around the winter solstice can be stopped 35 days after, when the natural photoperiod is short, without adverse effect on the treatment (Figure 1). The effects of this light treatment are not dramatically disrupted by some perturbation of the light dark cycle induced by some breakdowns of the clock which monitors the

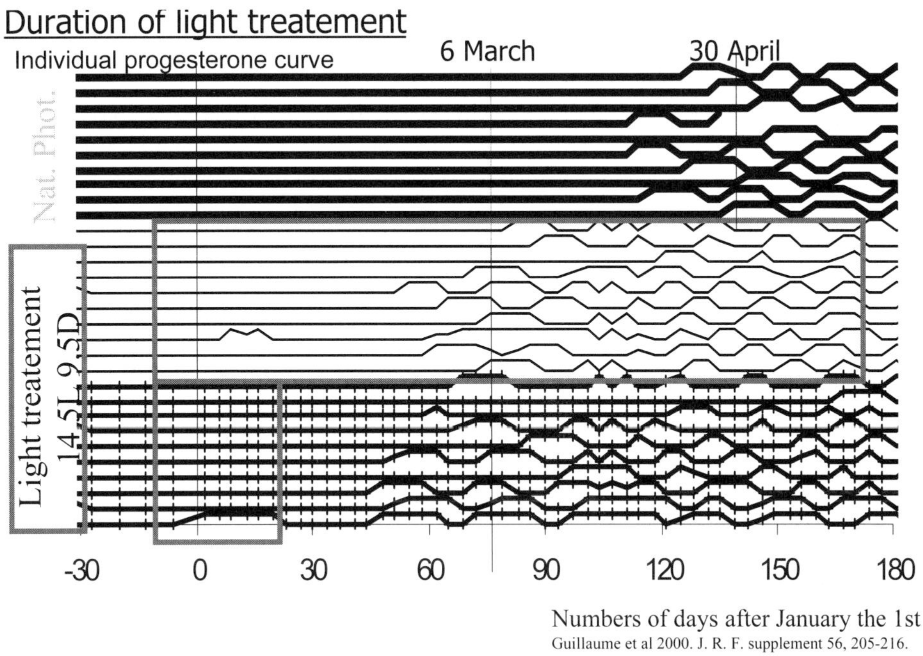

Figure 1. Photostimulation and winter anoestrus (Individual progesterone curve in each mare for the 3 groups kept under natural photoperiod or under artificial long days [14.5L:9.5D] after winter solstice. The rectangle in bold line represents the duration of light treatment. The dates on the top of the graph are the arithmetical means of the first ovulation date of mares in each group).

light. (Legros *et al,*2004, Guillaume *et al,*2006). The light treatment performed during the anoestrus of mares in good body condition is very secure.

The role of melatonin

The role of melatonin on the seasonal variations of reproduction has been strongly investigated in a lot of other species (Malpaux *et al* 1999). The pineal gland is involved in the control mechanism of seasonal reproduction and conveys the photoperiodic signals registered by the eyes to endocrine signals. In mares, elevated plasma melatonin concentrations are strongly associated with the dark phase. Melatonin secretion increases at the beginning of the dark phase and decreases rapidly at the end of the night. The secretion of melatonin is proportional to the duration of the night (Guillaume *et al,*1995). A short exposure to light during the dark phase results in an immediate decrease in melatonin concentrations; the return to dark-phase is followed by a new increase in melatonin concentrations (Guillaume et al 2000).

The role of melatonin in the regulation of mares' cyclicity was demonstrated by Guillaume and Palmer (1991), who reported that exogenous melatonin, administered 4 hours before the beginning of short nights (14.5L:9.5D), prevents the stimulatory effect of long days. Similarly, mares in seasonal anoestrus subjected to artificial photoperiod (14.5L:9.5D), do not respond to these stimulatory photoperiod when melatonin is administered every 2 hours, during a 12-hours period, that includes the 9.5-hour dark period (Guillaume and Palmer 1992). In these mares, the high levels of exogenous melatonin mask the onset of darkness, marked by an increase in melatonin secretion, and the onset of daylight, marked by a decrease in melatonin secretion. Seasonal reproduction in horses is affected as well as by a daily melatonin administration as a permanent melatonin application. Melatonin implants, inserted near the shortest day of the year, suppress the stimulating effect of long days, but do not prevent the occurrence of cyclic ovarian activity (Guillaume *et al* 1995).

Although, the effect of photoperiod is well documented, the site of action of melatonin has not been studied in horses. We know from studies in other species, that melatonin does not influence GnRH-secretion directly, but acts through a complex network of interneurons involving a number of different neurotransmitters. Its target sites appear to be located within the hypothalamus (Malpaux *et al,* 1993). In horses, specific melatonin binding was found in the pars tuberalis, in the median eminence and in the suprachiasmatic nucleus (Stankov *et al,* 1991).

The nocturnal plasmatic melatonin concentration appears to be unrelated to the reproductive status, and some mares, showing no cyclicity in winter do not exhibit a rise in plasma melatonin during darkness. Plasma melatonin concentrations are sometimes difficult to distinguish at the beginning of the dark phase and can even be absent during the entire dark period (Fitzgerald and Schmidt, 1995; Guillaume *et al,*2006). This very low or absence of melatonin concentrations in peripheral blood cannot be interpreted as a lack of physiological effect of this hormone in equine. In sheep, melatonin concentrations are many-fold higher in the third ventricle than in peripheral blood (Skinner and Malpaux, 1999) and in this species, the route of melatonin to this specific site of action in the mediobasal hypothalamus (Malpaux *et al,* 1993) can be the blood or the cerebrospinal fluid through the third ventricle (Tricoire *et al,* 2003). These observations suggest that, in equine species, the main route of melatonin to the reproduction axis is not the general blood circulation but probably the cerebrospinal fluid, through the third ventricle and circulating melatonin concentrations are a poor reflection of efficient melatonin secretion.

Evidence for an endogenous circannual rhythm of reproduction in mares

In ewes, Karsch *et al* (1989) provided clear evidence for the existence of an endogenous circannual reproductive cycle. Ovariectomized, estrogens-implanted ewes maintained in constant light conditions for 5 years, maintain circannual changes in LH and prolactin secretion. However, the period of elevated LH levels, representative of the breeding season, differs among individuals, reflecting the lack of synchronising environmental factors. The seasonal reproductive pattern is the result of a circannual endogenous rhythm that is synchronised by external environmental factors, which the main one is photoperiod.

In horses, available data indicate that the annual reproductive rhythm has a strong endogenous component. The first direct evidence for the existence of an endogenous circannual rhythm was given by the removal of the pineal gland or the cervical superior ganglion (Sharp *et al,* 1979; Grubaugh *et al,* 1982). In the 2 cases, the lesions did not resulted in the disappearance of seasonal reproductive activity. In pinealectomized mares, placed under extended photoperiod, the onset of reproductive activity was not advanced by artificial photoperiod and these mares resumed cyclic ovarian activity significantly later than controls, during the second season after surgery.

Another evidence for the existence of an annual endogenous rhythm is the variation of ovarian activity in mares kept under constant photoperiod or constant melatonin level during several seasons. Mares, maintained under constant long day photoperiod (16 hours), beginning at the summer solstice, enter into anoestrus and mares maintained under short days photoperiod (8.5h light) beginning at the winter solstice resume cyclic ovarian activity (Kooistra and Ginther, 1975; Palmer and Driancourt, 1981; Palmer *et al,* 1982; Scraba and Ginther, 1985). This is interpreded as an inability to continue to respond to the current type of photoperiod and is described as a refractory state. For this reason, mares kept under 16L:8D starting in winter (Palmer *et al,* 1982) or summer (Kooistra and Ginther, 1975; Scraba and Ginther, 1985), still return to winter anoestrous.

Melatonin implants, inserted near the summer solstice, on adults draught mares a few days before the birth of their foal (very fat at this moment), not induce or advance the beginning of winter inactivity but advance the ovulatory season of the following year (Guillaume *et al,* 1995). The likely explanation for this observation is a sequence of an early short-day perception, caused by the continuous high melatonin concentrations, followed by an early onset of the refractory state caused by continuous elevated levels of melatonin. In the same experiment, the same melatonin treatment applied to adults mares, which had not nursed a foal during summer, does not induced winter inactivity and these treated mares had permanent reproduction. These previous results were verified by Fitzgerald and McManus (2000) and Peltier *et al* (1998). Under this refractory state, the annual reproductive cycle is phase advanced which is characterized by an earlier occurrence of the ovulatory season on the next year. On another hand, the same melatonin treatment, applied on young haflinger mares (1.5 years old), induced an advance of 2 months of the beginning of winter inactivity but the advance of its end was only of one month and appears to be not significant (Guillaume *et al,* 1995). At this age, at the moment of their melatonin implantation, these young haflinger mares had not finished their growth. These differences between young and adult mares can be interpreted consecutively to the recent results on body score and winter inactivity (see below). These observations support the concept that photoperiod and rhythm of melatonin secretion drive the endogenous circannual rhythm but do not influence directly reproductive activity. This settlement of a photo refractoriness states against the constant photoperiod or constant melatonin level highlights the existence of an endogenous rhythm (endogenous calendar). It seems that this endogenous circannual rhythm can be monitored by photoperiod transmitted by melatonin just a few month in advance.

When one mare presents permanent reproduction, without winter inactivity, it does not mean that this mare has no circannual rhythm but only that this rhythm is not extrapolated on its cyclicity. Some other environmental factors are necessary to highlight this annual rhythm.

Effect of nutrition and body condition on winter inactivity

Effects on the end of winter inactivity

Several authors suspected the effects of nutrition and body condition on the resumption of winter inactivity. Van Niekerk and Van Heerden (1972) showed that mares, which are supplemented diet with concentrates, ovulate earlier after winter anoestrus than control mares without supplementation. Ginther (1974) also noted that the anovulatory period is shorter in mares, which gain weight during early spring. McDaniel *et al,* (1979) reported an additive effect of nutritional supplementation and artificially extended photoperiod on the onset of reproductive activity. Henneke *et al* (1984) observed that the average date of the first ovulation was significantly latter in mares with body condition score less than 5.0 (scale from 1, poor to 9, extremely fat) compared to mares with body condition score above 5.0. The interaction between energy intake and body condition in the reproductive performance of non-pregnant mares was evaluated by Kubiak *et al* (1987). A high-energy intake shortens the interval to the first ovulation in transitional mares with a low level of body fat but does not have any effect in mares in moderate or fat body condition. Mares with a body fat content greater than 15% had a shorter interval to the first ovulation compared to those with a body fat content lower than 15%. The authors suggest that non-lactating mares should be brought into the breeding season with a body fat content above 15% e.g. a body condition score above 5.0 and then maintained in a positive energy balance to obtain an earlier onset of ovulation. The quality of dietary proteins influence the onset of the breeding season. Mares fed with a high-quality protein diet exhibit increased FSH secretion and ovulated approximately 2-3 weeks earlier than mares fed low-quality protein diet (Van Niekerk and Van Niekerk, 1997). The stimulatory effect of pasture grazing on the time of first ovulation has also been reported. First ovulation occurs over a large period of time in Thoroughbred mares that are housed inside at night and are allowed to eat grass on pasture for 4-6 hours per day, whereas pony mares that are kept in concrete yards during winter ovulate in synchrony after they are turned out to lush spring grass (Allen, 1987). Carnevale and Ginther (1997) demonstrated the beneficial effect of pasturing on the onset of cyclic ovarian activity. Anoestrous mares pastured on green grass from early May ovulate sooner than mares housed on dry lot and fed hay. It is possible that the earlier onset of anoestrus in young mares (Ginther, 1992) and the high incidence of anoestrus in lactating mares (Palmer and Driancourt, 1983) are related to nutritional factors.

In a 10-year survey of breeding records in a thoroughbred farm in Australia, Guerin and Wang (1994) reported significant differences between years for the time of the first ovulation. The authors concluded that the onset of reproductive activity was closely related to minimum and maximum environmental temperatures. Field data for thoroughbred mares in the United Kingdom suggest that the spring transition is slowed by cold weather (Allen, 1987). Thus, it appears that under similar conditions of photoperiod, nutrition, management system and temperature play a role in the timing of the circannual reproductive rhythm. The mechanism of the effect of temperature is completely unknown. But, the lack of energy supplementation or/and body reserves to meet the extra energy cost due to thermoregulation would be responsible. (See chapter by Martin-Rosset et al in this issue).

Effect on the beginning and duration of winter inactivity

In our laboratory (Guillaume et al, 2002), some recent data indicate the important role of nutrition and body condition on the onset of anoestrus in mares. In a more recent experiment, the influence of feed allowances on the annual rhythm of reproduction was studied in adult ponies and the changes in the plasma melatonin, insulin, GH and glucose daily patterns were determined to identify a possible signal between nutritional status and ovulatory activity (Salazard-Ortiz and Guillaume *et al,* 2005). The mares were randomly assigned in 3 groups: well feed group (WF), variable group (V) and restricted group (R) referring to INRA 1990 recommendations. A special attention was paid to the R mares, to keep them healthy but very thin all along the experiment, which lasted 3 years. The group V was fed to mimic the seasonal variations of the available forage resources in natural foraging system under temperate latitudes, but with an important out of phase with these natural variations with the aim to advance the ovulatory activity. In the R group, the winter ovarian inactivity was systematically advanced, longer and ends later than in the WF group (Figure 2). During the 3 years of the study, in the WF group, 5 mares never present any ovulatory inactivity, 2 mares systematically have a short inactivity and the 2 last mares have a short inactivity for 2 successive winters. The high level of feed allowances doubles the number of cycles in comparison with the low level. The occurrence or the lack and the duration of ovulatory inactivity were repeatable in adult mares fed with a constant and high feeding level. These results support those of Fitzgerald *et al'* (2000), which observed a tendency of adult mares with a higher percent of body fat and a higher concentration of plasma leptin to exhibit a continuous cyclicity. These results are comparable with those obtained in cows (Bossis *et al,* 1999). The V group present an intermediate body weight between the R and WF groups. In the V group, despite an important increase of body condition score during the late fall and winter no difference was observed in the end of winter inactivity. In this group, 2 mares never present winter inactivity. The lack in the response to the change of feeding level is contradictory with studies previously mentioned (Van Niekerk and Van Herden, 1972, Ginther, 1974, Mac Daniel *et al,* 1979, Allen, 1987, Carnevale and Ginther, 1997). But these studies are likely confusing the global effect of breeding system and the temporary effect of feeding level. In the 3 groups, The observation of Nagy *et al* (1998): "later is the last ovulation of the year, earlier is the first ovulation of the following year" is clearly supported by our data.

In our experiment, GH concentrations were higher in R and V groups than in WF and were correlated with the body condition score. The IGF-I level was reduced by about 50% in the R group comparing with the WF group. In horses, the plasmatic rates of leptin are correlated with the body condition

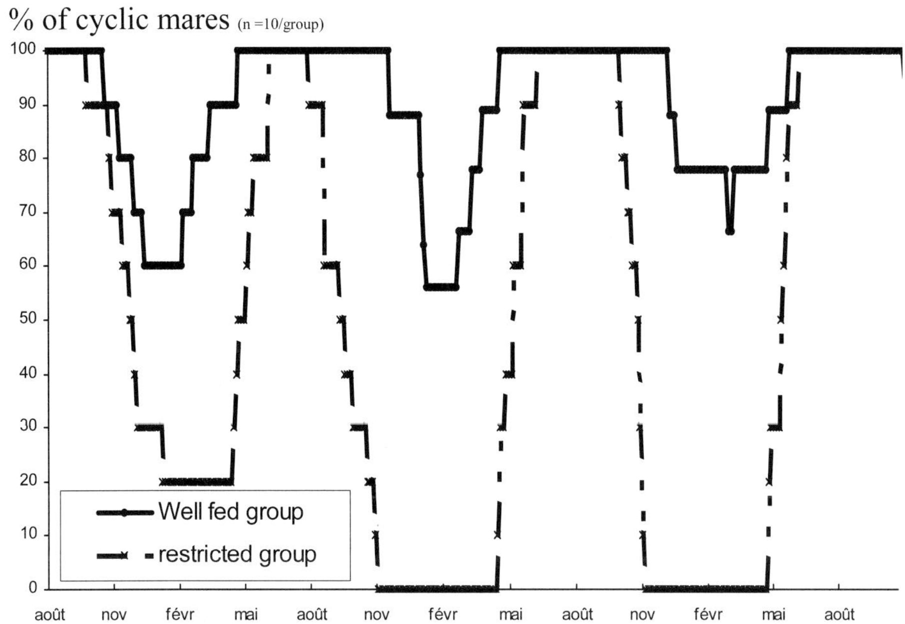

Figure 2. Variation of the proportion of cyclic mares in the restricted and the well fed groups (referring to INRA 1990 Requirements for all the nutrients) (Adapted from Salazard-Ortiz and Guillaume, 2004).

score (r = 0,64 p<0,0001, Buff *et al,* 2002). So far, in our experiment we can assume than leptin level is higher in the WF group than in the 2 other ones. Important postprandial peaks of glucose and insulin were observed in the WF group and the V group fed as the WF group. But these postprandial peaks completely disappeared in the R group and in the V group fed as the R groups.

Conclusion on interaction between feeding level and season of reproduction

The ovulatory activity of the mare fits a sinusoïdal curve (Figure3). During spring and summer the ovulatory activity represents the visible part of the annual endogenous rhythm. The spring-summer

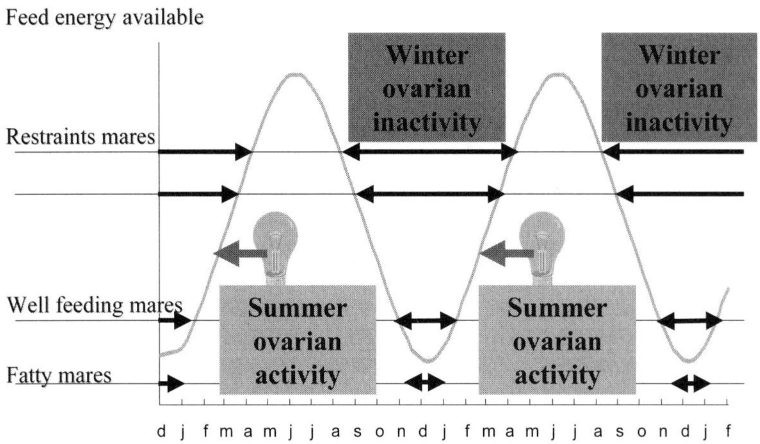

Figure 3. Interaction between feeding level and season of reproduction.

ovulatory activity is regulated by the photoperiod, mediated by melatonin. The highest feeding level is important, the highest the phase of the ovulatory activity is long. The period when the feeding level should be adjusted to reduce the length of winter inactivity is still to be defined; but it is likely during the previous season to winter. The peripheral hormones indicating the optimal nutritional status to be met for optimising reproduction is no yet defined but leptin should be the more interesting candidate.

Effects of nutrition level on cycle endocrinology and follicular growth aspect

Introduction

In mares, the inter-ovulatory interval is around 22-25 days. The folliculogenesis is usually divided in two periods: the basal follicular growth and the terminal follicular growth. The basal follicular growth is defined as the growth of follicles from the primordial stage up to the preantral stage corresponding to a follicle diameter of 0.2-0.4 mm (Driancourt *et al,* 1984). The terminal follicular growth occurs in a "wave-like pattern" in mares (Sirois *et al* 1989). In mares, usually one wave emerges at each cycle, which conducts to only one ovulatory follicle (Ginther, 1992).

The follicular wave is characterized by a succession of events: recruitment, selection (or deviation) and dominance (Hogden, 1982). In mares, a cohort of 10 mm-diameter follicles that become gonadotrophin-dependent defines a follicular wave. Inside a wave, the selection begins at the end of this common growth phase, 6 or 7 days before ovulation for the mare (Ginther *et al,* 2003; Ginther, 1992; Gastal *et al,* 1997). Routinely the largest follicle becomes the dominant one and continues to grow, whereas the subordinate follicles regress by atresia. As ovulation approaches, significant changes occur in the dominant follicle, which becomes the preovulatory follicle, with a diameter around 40 mm (Ginther, 1992; Pierson and Ginther, 1985). At ovulation, the follicular wall is disrupted and the follicle evacuates the ovocyte and the follicular fluid and turn into the corpus luteum, secreting progesterone.

The gonadotropins, are the major hormones controlling follicular growth. Some ovarian factors such as inhibins, activins or steroids and some peripheral factors such as insulin or insulin-like growth factors (IGFs) are also involved in folliculogenesis at different levels of regulation. In Equine, estrone represents the principal estrogens. Estrogens are responsible for enhancing LH secretion via a positive feedback and also induce sexual behaviour.

The initiation of the development of the ovarian follicles occurs through an unknown control mechanism in which gonadotrophins may not be involved (sheep: Campbell *et al,* 2000; mice: Kumar *et al,* 1997; for review: Knight *et al,* 2001). The terminal follicular growth is clearly dependent on the pituitary gonadotrophins. The circulating FSH increases in mares after the largest follicle reaches about 13 mm in diameter (Bergfelt and Ginther, 1993a; Gastal *et al* 1997). The increase in FSH could be the stimulus that triggers recruitment of the cohort of follicles (mare: Ginther and Bergfelt, 1993a; cattle: Turzillo *et al,* 1990). Recruitment is also characterized by an increase in sensitivity to FSH of the granulosa cells.

The selection process may involve two different mechanisms. When the follicles reach 30 mm of diameter, a depression of FSH occurs. This decrease is induced by the negative feedback of estradiol and inhibins ((Gastal *et al,* 1997 Gastal *et al,* 1999; Donadeu and Ginther, 2001, 2004). Thus, small follicles, which do not express enough FSH receptors, stop their growth, due to their inability to use FSH. The future dominant follicle which is less dependent of FSH for its growth, becomes LH-dependent. The future dominant follicle may be able to increase its responsiveness to the increased concentrations of LH. Estradiol, IGFs, activins and inhibins are apparently involved in this process (mare: Donadeu and Ginther, 2002), promoting the expression of LH receptors on the granulosa cells of the future dominant follicle (rat: Bao *et al,* 2000). The dominant follicle of the mare still produces higher concentrations of estradiol and inhibins (Donadeu and Ginther, 2001). From a specific concentration, the circulating concentrations of estradiol cause a positive feedback on the hypothalamus and thus, on the pituitary, resulting in a surge in LH responsible for ovulation.

The IGF system

The Insulin-like Growth Factors, IGF-I and IGF-II, their receptors and their 6 different binding proteins (IGFBP) and the IGFBPs proteases constitute the IGF system, which is very conserved in all mammalian species. Growth Hormone (GH) stimulates IGFs production in the liver and this production is probably and indirectly regulated by leptin. It seems that this growth factors system is the main factor implicated in the effects of nutrition level on follicular growth.

IGFs and IGFBPs are mainly produce in the liver but other tissues including the ovary are also able to produce them (mares: Davidson *et al,* 2002; for review: Spicer and Echternkamp, 1995). The 6 different IGFBPs specifically bind IGF-I and IGF-II and so suppress the IGFs availability. The IGFBP-3 constitutes a trimeric complex in association with IGF-I or IGF-II and an acid-labile subunit, which weighted 150 kDa. IGF-I and IGF-II have had a molecular weight of approximately 7.5 kDa. Their structures are closely related to that of the insulin and the proinsulin. The liver is the major source of IGF-I and IGF-II. Granulosa and theca of equine growing follicles also synthesize IGF-I (Watson *et al,* 2004). IGFs are present in all biological fluids but essentially in the plasma (for review: Humbel *et al,* 1990). Under normal conditions, free IGF-I accounts only for 1% of the total amount of the circulating growth factors. Indeed, 90% of the circulating IGF-I are complexed with IGFBP-3 (Hodgkinson *et al,* 1989).

There are 2 types of IGFs receptors. The first type of receptor is closely related to that of the insulin receptor and it is more specific of IGF-I. The second type of the receptor is specific of the complex IGF-II/mannose-6-phosphate (IGF-II/M-6-P). In vivo, it does not bind insulin and binds IGF-I with very low affinity. Both receptors are expressed in various tissues and cell lines, including ovarian granulosa and theca cells of healthy follicles in sheep and in cattle (LeRoith *et al,* 1995; for review: Mazerbourg *et al* 2003).

The IGF-I and IGF-II and their binding proteins are involved in regulating proliferation and/or differentiation in diverse cell types. IGF-I and IGF-II form inactive complexes when bound to IGFBPs, which modulate the IGFs bioavailability and control the IGF accessibility to the receptors. IGFBPs also regulate the transfer of IGFs between the intra and the extravascular space (for review: Zofkova, 2003). IGF-I and IGF-II play a role in stimulating differentiation or proliferation of the ovarian granulosa and thecal cells during follicular development. IGF-I promotes the formation of the theca interna and is responsible for the formation of the antrum (for review: Spicer and Echternkamp, 1995; Mazerbourg *et al,* 2003). Thus, IGF-I is a promoter of the follicular growth. IGF-I amplifies the FSH action at the level of granulosa cells and the LH action in theca-interstitial cells (DeMoura *et al,* 1997). In mice and cattle, IGF-I plays an important role in increasing the sensitivity of small antral follicles to gonadotropins. This suggests that IGF-I acts in the transition from the gonadotropin independent to the gonadotropin dependent follicular stage (for review: Mazerbourg *et al,* 2003) and is able to amplify the effect of gonadotropins on the ovary. In equine, as in other species, IGF-I promotes the ovarian steroidogenesis (Ginther *et al,* 2001). However, IGF-I necessarily acts in a synergistic manner with gonadotropins in both theca and granulosa cells (rat: Magoffin *et al,* 1993). In ovaries, by binding to IGFs, IGFBPs inactivates their effects and inhibit follicular steroidogenesis, in particular estradiol synthesis (mares: Gérard and Monget, 1998).

Generally, in farm animals, concentrations of IGF-I in follicular fluid are equal or lower to those observed in plasma (for review: Spicer and Echternkamp, 1995). In most mammals the concentration of IGF-I in follicular fluid does not differ with follicular size. In some species, FSH, LH and estradiol increase the production of IGF-I by granulosa cells (rat: DeMoura *et al,* 1997; cattle: Ginther *et al* 2001). This amplifying property of IGF-I, coupled with its selective expression in healthy (but not atretic) follicles may underlie the ability of IGF-I to initiate and/or maintain the process of follicular selection (DeMoura *et al,* 1997). In farm animals, concentrations of IGF-II in follicular fluid are equal or lower than in plasma (for review: Spicer and Echternkamp, 1995) and do not vary significantly during follicular growth (mare: Bridges *et al,* 2002).

Equine serum and follicular fluid contain IGFBP-2 (35 kDa), the native form of IGFBP-3 (42-44 kDa) and the "large complex" form of IGFBP-3 (150 kDa), IGFBP-4 (24 kDa) and IGFBP- 5 (28-32 kDa). However, the 150 kDa-IGFBP-3 is clearly more abundant in serum whereas the 42-44-kDa-IGFBP-3 is the major form in follicular fluid (mare: Gérard and Monget, 1998).

The concentrations of IGFBPs in follicular fluid dramatically change during folliculogenesis, compared to those of IGF-I and IGF-II. In mares, follicular fluid levels of IGFBP-2, IGFBP-4, and IGFBP-5 decrease during follicular growth but increase during atresia. Only IGFBP-3 remains constant during follicular growth (mare: Gérard and Monget, 1998; Bridges *et al,* 2002). Changes in intrafollicular IGFBP proteolytic activity and mRNA expression are responsible for these changes in follicular fluid concentrations (mare: Monget *et al,* 2002; Watson *et al,* 2004). Recently, Mazerbourg *et al,* (2001) and Gérard *et al,* (2004) have shown that the decrease in IGFBP-2 and IGFBP-4 is essentially due to an increase in proteolytic cleavage by an intrafollicular enzyme: the "Pregnancy-Associated Plasma Protein-A" (PAPP-A) in mares. IGFs bioavailability due to the large changes in IGFBPs, rather than IGFs concentrations, dramatically changes during growth and atresia of ovarian follicles (Ginther *et al,* 2004).

Effects of nutrition on the different phases of œstrus cycle of the mares

The effects of nutrition on follicle development have been largely studied, particularly in cattle. For example, short-term changes in nutrition have been shown to influence small antral follicles recruitment, without affecting circulating concentrations of FSH (cattle: Gutierrez *et al,* 1997; Armstrong *et al,* 2001; mares: Salazar-Ortiz *et al* 2004). Negative energy balance has also been negatively correlated with the growth rate of the dominant follicle and its diameter (cattle: Bossis *et al,* 1999; Armstrong *et al,* 2001, mare: Gastal *et al,* 2000). In case of a severe undernutrition, the ability of the dominant follicle to ovulate can be compromised (cattle: Mackey *et al,* 1999). During lactation, the negative energy balance is a major parameter for decreasing follicular growth (cattle: for review, Butler, 2000; mare: Godoi *et al,* 2002).

A negative energy balance is also associated with a decrease in the number of follicles entering the terminal stages, leading to a decrease in ovulation rate and in the frequency of pulses of GnRH and LH (pig: Cox *et al,* 1987). Eventually, the low rate of secretion of LH can block the final maturation, the steroids synthesis and ovulation of dominant follicles (for review: Monget and Martin, 1997).

Changes in metabolic hormones are involved in the alteration of ovarian activity induced by the negative energy balance. A decrease in gonadotropins secretion, circulating levels of insulin, IGF-I, leptin and glucose but also an increase in circulating concentrations of GH are usually associated with a negative energy balance (for reviews: Monget and Martin, 1997, cattle: Diskin *et al,* 2003). The secretion of insulin is accurately regulated by glucose availability. In addition to its role in carbohydrate metabolism, insulin also serves as a metabolic signal influencing LH release by the anterior pituitary gland and has been shown to play a role in regulating ovarian responsiveness to gonadotropins (for review: Monget and Martin, 1997). Dietary restriction and negative energy balance reduce circulating concentrations of insulin and decrease the LH pulse frequency (cattle: for review, Gong *et al,* 2002).

GH receptors may be found in many reproductive tissues such as hypothalamus, pituitary and ovarian follicle, suggesting the implication of this hormone in the reproductive function. The main effects of GH on reproduction appear to be operated through its regulatory effects on hepatic IGF-I synthesis and secretion. Dietary restriction has been shown to increase blood concentrations of GH in cattle (for review, cattle: Diskin *et al,* 2003).

However, correlations between intrafollicular IGF-I concentrations and nutrition remain unclear: it seems that nutritional status may influence the relationship between ovarian and systemic levels of IGF-I depending on the type of dietary restriction (for review: Spicer and Echternkamp, 1995).

Dietary restriction also affects circulating IGFBPs, increasing the concentrations of IGFBP-1 and IGFBP-2 and decreasing the concentration of IGFBP-3 (for review: Martin et Monget, 1997), which are believed to alter the bioavailability and the half-life of the IGFs. Altogether, studies strongly suggest that those nutritional effects on ovarian activity are at least partially mediated via the IGF system.

Leptin is well known as a modulator of feeding behaviour and high plasma concentrations are known to suppress appetite. Leptin is a 16-kDa protein produced by adipose tissues. This hormone may be a signal between body condition and hypothalamus. Circulating leptin levels are directly proportional to the adipose tissue mass, reflecting adipose reserve (mare: Gentry *et al,* 2002; Buff *et al,* 2002). Leptin is also known as a regulator of reproductive function. It stimulates LH secretion at the pituitary level (rat: Nagatani *et al,* 1998) but reduces the synergism between FSH and IGF-I on estradiol production in granulosa cells (rat: Zachow *et al,* 1997).

The impact of the feeding level on follicular growth and on associated endocrine parameters (LH, FSH, estrogens, progesterone, GH, insulin, IGFs and IGFBPs) was also studied during 3 successive breeding season in WF and R groups designed previously (Salazar-Ortiz *et al* 2004).

During the first breeding season of the study, follicular growth was monitored during 2 cycles in each mare after a prostaglandin injection. The interval from prostaglandin injection to ovulation was shorter in the WF group than in the R group (9.2 ± 0,6 *vs* 11.6 ± 0.5 days respectively). The total volume of follicles was higher in the WF group than in the R group. No difference was shown in preovulatory follicles diameter (38 ± 1 mm). A tendency to have more double ovulations in the WF group (4 cycles with a double ovulation / 16 observed cycles) than in the R groups (0/14) is observed. The plasma LH during ovulatory surge (7 ± 1.2 *vs* 4.7 ± 0.52 ng/ml) and total estrogens levels 2 days before ovulation (2.3 ± 0.3 *vs* 1.2 ± 0.2 ng/ml) are higher in the WF group than in the R group, respectively. No difference was shown on plasma circulating levels of FSH and progesterone slope after ovulation. The IGF-I concentration was two folds higher in WF group compared to R group (on the day before the ovulation: 178 ± 39 ng/ml *vs* 75 ± 15 ng/ml). During winter and spring, before the follicular growth monitoring; blood samples were collected every hour, for 2 periods of 24 h, for GH and insulin assays. Mean plasma concentrations of GH in the 1st period were 0.66 ± 0.11 and 2.59 ± 0.34 ng/ml in the WF and R group, respectively. On the 2nd period, the concentrations were 0.32 ± 0.06 and 1.75 ± 0.25 ng/ml in the WF and R group, respectively. The differences in plasma GH concentration support the IGF-I discrepancy (Salazar-Ortiz *et al,* 2004, 2005). In the WF group an very important postprandial pic of insulin was observed and not in the R group.

During the second breeding season, mares did not receive any prostaglandin injection and follicular growth was monitored during 2 successive cycles. This long-term restricted feeding level dramatically modified the follicular development and serum levels of reproductive hormones. The total activity of the 2 ovaries of each mare was estimated by the sum of the volume of all the follicles, which are supposed to be a sphere (Figure 4). The WF group would exhibit more double ovulation than the R group (2 cycles with a double ovulations / 18 observed cycles *vs* 0/19 cycles) In this experiment, the difference on the follicular growth between the 2 groups was not confirmed by an effect on plasma estrogens concentrations or plasma LH concentrations. For progesterone profile only the plateau is lower in the R group in compared to the WF group (11 ng/ml *vs* 15 ng/ml); the duration and the slope after the ovulation were similar in the two groups.

Assuming that the difference on follicular growth between WF and R mares could be attributed to the involvement of the IGF-system; a last experiment was carried out during the third breeding season, the variations of IGF-I and IGF–II, IGFBPs, GH, insulin, LH, FSH, estrogens and progesterone in blood and in follicular fluid with the feeding level were determined (Guillaume et al unpublished).

Follicular development was daily scanned and follicular fluid of preovulatory follicles was collected by ultrasound-guided follicular aspiration. Blood samples were collected daily. Plasma and follicular fluid samples were assayed for IGF-I, IGF-II, GH, insulin, LH, FSH and progesterone with validated radioimmunoassay and IGFBPs with Western ligand blotting.

The number of total follicles in the R group was 53% lower than in the WF group. In plasma, as in follicular fluid, insulin concentrations decreased in the R group and this difference was more important in the follicular fluid. Concentrations of IGF-I were lower in the R group than in the WF

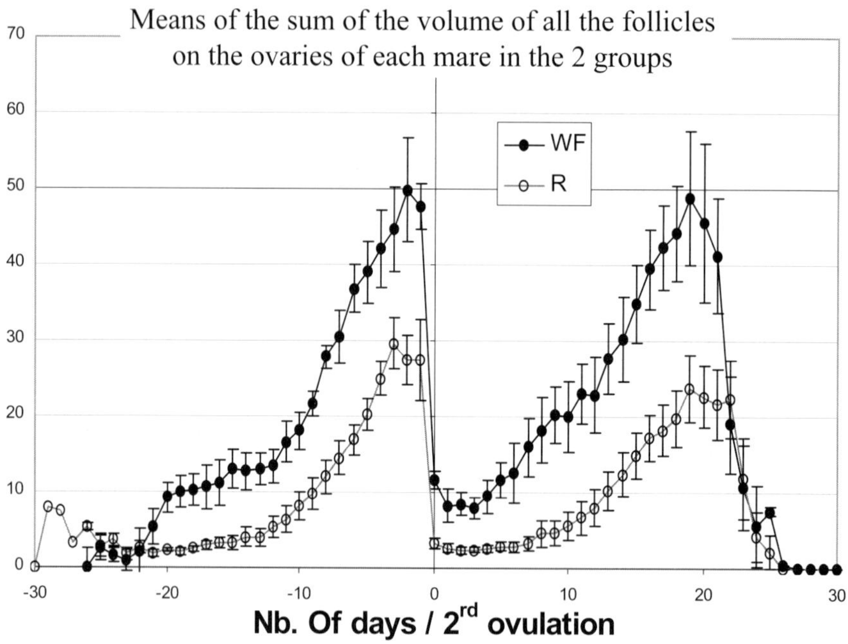

Figure 4. Variation of follicle growth in restricted and well fed groups (Variation of the sum of the volume of each follicle on the 2 ovaries of the mares in the "well fed" and "restricted" groups, during 2 successive cycles, from a 1st ovulation to the 3rd ovulation; the 2sd ovulation is the time origin) (Salazar-Ortiz et al., 2004).

group and it was the contrary for IGF-II. The IGFBP-2/ IGFBP-3 ratio was higher in the plasma of the R group than in the plasma of the WF group but it was not the case in the follicular fluid in which the level were similar. Only intrafollicular concentrations of insulin were largely decreased. Interestingly, in WF animals, the intrafollicular concentrations of insulin were strikingly higher than those of the plasma.

Overall, chronic restricted feeding in mares affects recruitment and selection process of ovarian folliculogenesis by the decrease in insulin concentrations and in the bioavailability of the IGFs in plasma. In contrast, chronic restricted feeding has no impact on the intrafollicular bioavailability of the IGFs at the preovulatory stage. Therefore, chronic restricted feeding does not affect dominance of the follicle in mares.

During the 1st and 2nd breeding seasons a tendency to have more double ovulation was observed in WF mares. This effect was described too in a 10 years retrospective study on our experimental herd (Briant, 2004). On 5335 cycles monitored in 262 Welsh pony mares, the percentage of double ovulation was estimated at 5.9%. The heritability of this phenomenon is low 0.06. During the 10 years of the study, a change (sweet corns, oat and alfalfa pellets to commercial pellets) and a restriction of feed allowances were related to decrease the percentage of double ovulation. In pony mares this percentage is low compared to values observed in saddle mares (11.9% Saltiel *et al,* 1982; 27.3% Henry *et al,* 1982). It is possible that on saddle mares the effect of the feed allowances on percentage of double ovulations is more important than in pony mares.

Effect of nutrition on the oestrous cycle of the broodmare

Few experiments have been carried out mainly in mares of heavy breeds as there are bred in extensive systems similarly to beef cattle with the alternation of winter restriction and summer overfeeding (Martin-Rosset and Trillaud–Geyl 1984)

Twenty eight mares, in good condition at the beginning of the 2 successive trials, weighing 786 kg after foaling and matched in two groups were fed either a "High Level" of energy (HL) or a "Low Level" (LL) in the 10th and 11th months of pregnancy. The LL group was fed at 80 percent and the HL group at 100 percent of the energy requirements of INRA 1984. For all the other nutrients, their requirements were estimated according to INRA 1984 recommendations. In the first month of lactation and before turning out to pasture the mare were fed according to the requirements of INRA 1984 for lactating mares (e.g. 100 percent). The trials took place during 2 subsequent years but the same animals were not always involved. Mean variation in body weight of the mares in the two trials was low, at the end of pregnancy: + 7.5 kg and – 6 kg in HL and LL group respectively. At the end of the 1st month of lactation HL and LL groups gained: 18 and 35 kg respectively. No significant effect was measured with the mare as regards of ovarian activity, and the time-interval between two subsequent foaling and associate factors (Table 1). A moderate restriction in energy intake in late pregnancy would not affect the cyclicity and reproductive performance of the mares when they are in good body condition score at 9th of pregnancy (BCS=3 according to INRA–HN-IE 1997 scale: 0 to 5), and when the mares are fed according to their requirements in early lactation.

In a other experiment two groups of mares were fed either 100 percent (HL) or 60 percent (LL) of protein requirements according to INRA 1984 recommendations in early lactation (45 days) whereas they were fed 100 percent of the other nutrients. No significant effect on cyclicity and reproductive performance were found (Table 2). These data are consistent with those of Webb et al 1979 and Gill et al 1985. Hence reproduction is not affected by a limitation of protein allowances in early lactation of broodmares well fed according to their requirements in pregnancy and in good body conditions at foaling (BCS=3 according to INRA-HN-IE 1997 scale and INRA recommendations 1990).

Table 1. Effect of a moderate energy restriction in late pregnancy on reproductive performance of mares of heavy breeds (from Martin-Rosset and Doreau 1984; and Martin-Rosset et al, unpublished, personal communication).

Trials		I		II	
Energy levels		HL	LL	HL	LL
Number of animals		14	14	14	13
Duration (days)		58	65	84	78
Daily nutrients intake	– Energy: NE (UFC)	7.0	5.6	6.8	5.4
	– Protein: MADC (g)	570	548	601	631
Body Weight variation (kg) Measured		+7	+6	+8	-12
Number of mares at foaling		14	14	14	13
Date of birth (days)		14/4±23	13/4±18	13/4±13	17/4±24
Reproductive performance:					
Oestrous cycle within 0-35 days					
Number of mares with oestrous		14	12	14	12
Intervals between parturition and the					
	– 1st day of oestrous (days)	7±1	7±1	7±1	7±0
	– Last day of oestrous (days)	19±8	16±4	18±4	15±3
Fertilisation	– 1st oestrous	11	8	11	8
	– 2nd oestrous	2	2	2	2
	– 3rd oestrous	0	2	0	0
Pregnancy	– at 45th day	13	10	13	10
	– at 85th day	13	10	13	10
Intervals (days) between	– foaling and fertilisation	20±8	27±7	21±8	16±6
	– 2 subsequent foaling dates	363±8	364±14	363±10	358±15

Table 2. Effect of protein allowances in nursing mares of heavy breeds fed isoenergetic diet on reproductive performance (from Doreau et al 1988).

Groups	HL	LL
Number of mares	10	10
Body weight (kg)	753	753
UFC[1]/d	10.4	10.8
MADC[2] g/d	1291	805
Mare body weight change (kg/d)	0.213 ± 0.903	-0.203 ± 0.586
Foal ADG[3] g/d (0-30d)	1923 ± 364	1706 ± 226
Time between foaling and first heat (d)	13.5 ± 6.4	11.5 ± 3.6
Time between foaling and fertilization (d)	25.0 ± 14.8	18.5 ± 7.5
Mare plasma Urea (mg/100ml)	41.6 ± 4.5	25.1 ± 4.0

[1]UFC: Horse Feed Unit (INRA 1984-1990)

[2]MADC: Horse Digestible Crude Protein (INRA 1984- 1990)

[3]ADG; Average Daily Gain

Conclusion on the effect feeding level on follicular growth and fertility

In conclusion, in fat mares the follicular growth is more active than in thin mares particularly at its beginning. This difference affects the plasma endocrine level (LH FSH estrogens progesterone). But it is difficult to evaluate if these effects can compromise the fertility of each cycle. Each cycle conduced to an ovulation for all the different feeding level studied. In fat mares, the risk of double ovulation seems to be important and needs a gestation diagnostic in case of twins. In thin mares, the low number of cycles might be a limiting factor of reproductive performance.

Effect of nutrition level on puberty

In Equines, the growing horses meet 60 and 90% of his adult body weight and height at withers at one year of age respectively (Martin-Rosset 2004).At this age bone development is far advanced whereas adipose tissue development arises. As in other mammalian species, puberty occurs in equines at 12-15 months (Table 3). But there is a great individual variability of the age of puberty.

Studies of puberty in horses is of poor interests for managing horse reproduction, because males and females are generally matted, for the first time, several years after their puberty, except for breeds which are kept under extensive conditions (Martin-Rosset and Trillaud-Geyl 1984).

In a first experiment, 2 groups of fillies of heavy breeds were fed either 100 or 77 percent of INRA (1990) requirements from 6 to 24 months of age (Table 4). The first cycle of well-fed (WF) fillies occurred, during the first breeding season following the weaning, 20 days earlier (not significant difference) whereas their body weight was 8.5 percent heavier than in restricted (R) fillies. During the second breeding season the first cycle occurred only 2 days earlier whereas body weight was still 8.8 percent heavier in well fed than in restricted fillies. A grooming stallion matted all the fillies. The number of well-fed fillies, which were fertilised during all this breeding season, was 19 percent higher than that of restricted fillies whereas their body weight was still 8.8 percent higher. So far, feeding level might influence the occurrence of the first cycle at 12 months of age but not at 24

Table 3. Age of the puberty in Equine species foal by different authors.

Authors		Race/birth	Criteria (progesterone: P4, spermatozoa: spz)	Moment or age of the puberty in months
Skelton et al, 1991	♀	Australian Stock Horses	P4 increasing	13.1 n = 4
Wesson and Ginther 1980	♀	Pony mares	P4 increasing	End of May
		born in April		13.5 n = 6
		born in June-Sept		11.2 n = 5
Nogueira et al, 1997	♀	Thoroughbred horses	P4 increasing	14.2 ± 1 n = 4
Camillo et al, 2002	♀	Haflinger	P4 increasing	n = 8
		born in winter		14.0
		born in spring		11.9
Guillaume 1995 (com.per.)	♀	Welsh ponies	P4 increasing	9.6 ± 0.2 n= 7
		born in autumn		22.0 n = 1
Naden et al, 1990	♂	Quarter Horses	$50 \cdot 10^6$ spz/ejaculate	From 12.9 to 22.3 n=15
Melo et al, 1998	♂	Pantaniero Horses	End of infantile period	14.4 n = 26
Skinner and Bowen 1968	♂	Welsh ponies	Spz apparitions	From 11.5 to 14.5 n = 4

Table 4. Influence of feeding level from 6 to 24 months of age in fillies of heavy breeds on reproductive performance (Martin-Rosset et al unpublished).

Feeding level:		WF	R
Percent INRA requirements[1]		100	77
Number of animals		26	27
Age,	Date of birth (±days)	15/4 ± 22	15/4 ± 21
Body weight (kg)	BW at 6 months (% adult BW)[2]	332.1 ± 25.9 (45.8%)	319.6 ± 28.4 (45.5%)
	Age at weaning (days)	197 ± 27	195 ± 28
	BW at 12 months	446.7 ± 39.1***	408.7 ± 29.0
	(% adult BW)[2]	(63.5%)	(58.1%)
	BW at 24 months	604.4 ± 44.1***	553.3 ± 41.9
	(% adult BW)[2]	(86.0%)	(78.7%)
Reproduction:	Cyclicity (progesterone)		
1st breeding season:	1st cycle Date (± days)	28/5±29	16/6±20
	Age (month, days)	13 mo 27±43	14 mo 21±31
	BW (kg) (% adult BW)[2]	454.0 ± 31.0** (64.8%)	418.1 ± 32.3 (59.5%)
2nd breeding season:	1st cycle Date (± days)	20/4±10	22/4±12
	Age (month, days)	24 mo 5±17	24 mo 12±18
	BW (kg) (% adult BW)[2]	602.7 ± 33.5** (85.7%)	553.9 ± 35.6 (78.8%)
Fertilisation	Percent	85.3	66.6
	Age (months, days)[3]	25 mo 18±28	25 mo 6±32
	BW (kg) (% adult BW)[2 3]	612.3 ± 48.5** (87.1%)	566.0 ± 26.3 (80.5%)
	Number of cycle for fertilisation[3]	1.4±0.6	1.2±0.4

* P< 0.05 ** P< 0.01 *** P< 0.001

[1]INRA 1984 requirements: 100 percent: optimum growth, 77 percent: moderate growth

[2]Adult body weight: 703 kg

[3]For pregnant fillies only

months of age even body weight is significantly affected. But fertilisation rate at 24 months of age is affected by feeding level and related body weight met at this period.

In equine (Nogueria *et al,* 1997) as in humans (Nicolino and Forest 2001), when puberty occurs, a short increase in growth rate is observed and then is followed by a quick termination of growth. This interaction between growth and puberty implicates the sexual steroids. A lot of studies carried out to manage the growth in humans, have well highlighted theses implications. Conjugated estrogens are used in growth-suppressant therapies for tall adolescent girls since 1956 (Barnard *et al,* 2002). Weise *et al,* (2001) have demonstrated that estrogens induce and accelerate growth plate senescence in juvenile ovariectomized female rabbits. In the case of patients with early puberty, a GnRH agonist therapy is successfully used, to overcome the subnormal growth rate (Lampit *et al,* 2002). In Equine, the same therapy using GnRH antagonist can be also envisaged because it was tested successfully to suppress ovarian activity (Guillaume *et al,* 2004). Estrogens can inhibit normal bone elongation in growing rats by reducing the number of proliferating chondrocytes in the growth plate and accelerating apoptosis in differentiated chondrocytes (Sibonga 2002). The action of estrogens (particularly the total oestrogen extracted from pregnant mares), in elderly patient with osteoporosis, which increase the osteoblastes growth, is well known. This interaction between puberty and bone growth relaunches the study of puberty in equine species: an advanced puberty would be suspected to fix the osteochondrotic lesions which are frequent in athlete horses and maximal around 8 months (Barneveld and Van Weeren 1999, Donabedian *et al* 2006) and to reduce the chance of a natural reparation of these lesions.

The great variability observed in the occurrence of puberty is likely due to winter reproduction inactivity, which prevents the apparition of puberty, whereas the young horse is potentially pubescent. This effect is even more important if the feed allowance is reduced. The main different situations may be met as followed:

- A foal born in fall and very well fed has a very quick growth and will be pubescent at the first breeding season, between 8 and 12 months.
- Another foal born in spring and very well fed will potentially be pubescent at about 8 month of age in winter, but during the winter inactivity phase. So far puberty will take place only the following breeding season and then the young horse will be pubescent at 14 months of age only.
- A restricted foal born in spring will be potentially pubescent during its second or third winters during the inactivity phase. It will be pubescent only the following breeding at about 36 months of age.

A recent experiment was carried out jointly by INRA and Haras Nationaux (French National Stud) to determine the influence of nutrition on the date of puberty. 23 foals of French Saddle Horses and Anglo Arabian horses, born in spring, were fed 2 feeding levels according to INRA 1990 to monitor from birth to 30months of age a moderate growth (MG) and high growth (HG). MG group was fed 100 percent of INRA recommendations, while the HG group was fed between 130 to 150 percent according to the period: before and after the weaning (Donabedian et al 2006, Fleurance *et al,* 2006). Body weight (BW) was determined every 2 weeks to monitor accurately growth using INRA 1990 nutritional models (Martin-Rosset et al 1994). Plasma samples were collected: monthly during the first year of life and weekly until the puberty or 30 months. Assays of progesterone on fillies and testosterone on male foals were carried out in order to determine the age of puberty. A female was considered pubescent when her concentrations of progesterone exceeded 1 ng/ml. A male was considered pubescent when his concentrations of testosterone exceeded 0.5 ng/ml (winter low level of testosterone for adult stallion giving a normal ejaculate in our assay) in for 4 consecutive blood samples. Total estrogens, LH and GH were also assayed with validated and specific RIA. The growth curves were established using the Gompertz's model ($BW=BW0*(1-exp(-A_2*t)$.

Body weight was significantly higher for HG than for MG from 2 to 30 months of age. This difference was confirmed by the eGH rates, which was higher (p=0,0002) in MG than HG group.

For the 6 fillies of the HG group, the puberty occurred at about 12 months of age. For the fillies of the MG group, the puberty occurred from May to June of their first breeding season at 13.6 months for 4 of them, whereas the puberty was not observed during the 1st breeding season in the 2 others fillies. One of them had its puberty in April of his 2nd breeding season at 23 months, The last one was discarded due to a fracture at a front leg.

The testosterone rates of the male between 6 months and 2 years were higher for the HG than for the MG (0,42 ± 0,02 ng/ml vs. 0,23 ± 0,02 ng/ml p<0,0001 for HG and MG groups respectively). This difference was still important during their first sexual season, between 11 months and 19 months (0,38 ± 0,02 ng/ml vs. 0,17 ± 0,01 ng/ml p<0,0001 for HG and MG groups respectively). The puberty was delayed in all the young males of the MG group for one year due to the season effect. For one male of the MG group, the puberty was never observed during the experiment and was probably delayed to the next breeding season when he was 3 years old (for the data analysis it is the end of the experience, which was considered). The puberty occurred at 17 months and 25 months for the HG and MG groups respectively. Variation in testosterone, total estrogens and LH of one typical stallion in each group are given in the Figure 5. The criteria chosen for testosterone concentration in male to assess the age of puberty seems to be consistent between all the other sexual assayed hormones: oestrogen increased at the same moment as testosterone does, while LH decreases.

Unfortunately for females, the age of puberty does not appear different between the groups; whereas the effect of growth rate on the age of puberty of the male, is significant (Table 5).

It clearly demonstrates the existence of an interaction between the growths rate and related feeding allowances, and season of reproduction. The increases of testosterone and estrogens concentration

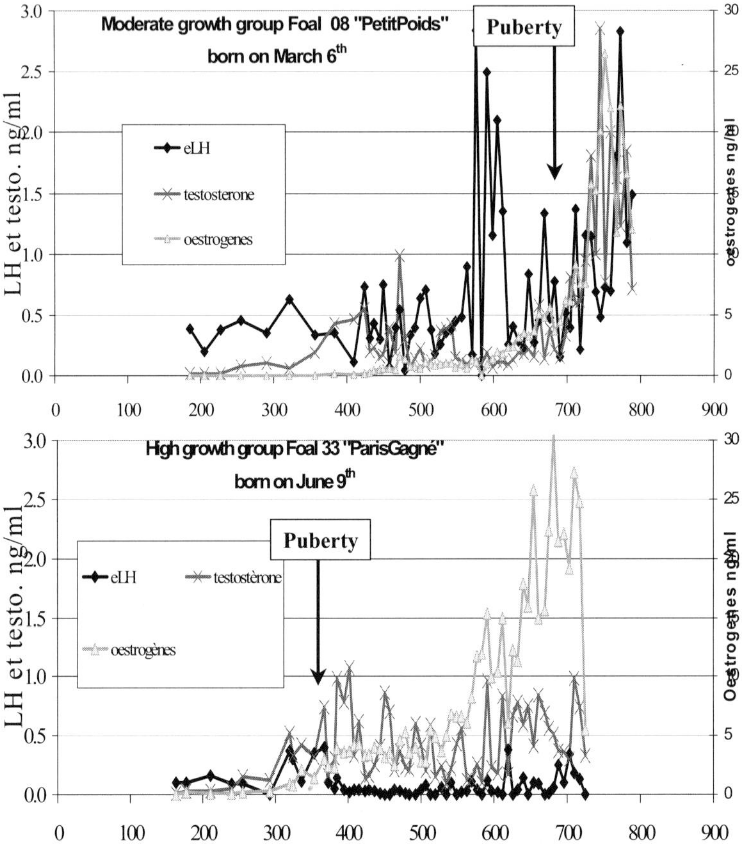

Figure 5. Variation with age of LH, Testosterone and total estrogens plasma concentration in young males well fed (foal Nr 33) or restricted (foal Nr 08).

Table 5. Influence of feeding level on puberty of fillies or stallions of saddle breed (Guillaume et al 2006).

Feeding level and sexes:	HL ♂		LL ♂	HL ♀		LL ♀
Date of the puberty	23 Nov.		14 May	4 May		31 July
Age of the puberty (days ± SEM)	507 ± 64	P=0.001	754 ± 30	393 ± 11	P=0.09	472 ± 57

are approximately synchronous in the two groups. But the estrogens concentration increased slowly during the first sexual season in the IG group. It is likely because in equines, Leydig and Sertoli cells have the P_{450}-aromatase transforming androgens in estrogens (Sipahutar *et al,* 2003) and because tissue transformations during the puberty are progressive (Clemmons *et al,* 1995; Staub *et al,* 2002).

Discussion and conclusion

The reproductive performance is highly affected by the interactions of the nutrition level fed to the mares and the season of the reproduction. Well fed mares can offer yearly until 14 cycles which is of great interest to foal early in the year then to raise a young horse devoted to be an athlete, namely race horses, or/and to wean in good condition a foal dedicated to be a sport horses (see the chapters by Younge and Martin-Rosset, Pagan *et al* and by Falaschini *et al* in this issue). Restricted mares only exhibit about 4 cycles during the summer, which is of poor interest even for the production of late horses oriented to leisure. The opportunity for the mare to be fertilised is reduced. The foaling date is far too late in respect of the period of maximum grass production, to wean at low cost the foal at a good body weight and size (see the chapters by Younge and Martin-Rosset, Miraglia *et al* in this issue). The nutritional status of the mares related to the nutrition level is of major concern, namely the energetic body reserves (see the chapters by Martin-Rosset *et al* in this issue). The body reserves are estimated using body condition score (BCS) methods. The mares should meet optimum BCS at key periods to maximise reproductive performance: interval foaling-first oestrous, interval foaling-fertilisation, interval between two subsequent foaling, date of fertilisation according to the type of production. Optimum BCS should be met at least at weaning and foaling as defined by Martin-Rosset *et al* in this issue. So far the mares which are in poor conditions at these key periods should be supplemented at least 3 months before and 2 months after foaling to meet a minimum BCS and be fertilised. It should be reminded that energy intake of the mares is always splitted up to cover the requirements for maintenance and production (conceptus growth or milk yield) and for restoration of body reserves whereas body reserves contribute always to milk synthesis whatever the level of body reserves of the mares at foaling. The effects of protein allowances and quality should be considered as well, but it needs additional investigation.

The mechanisms, which are involved in the influence of the nutrition level and related body reserves on the oestrus cycle and follicle growth, are not yet all elucidated in the Equines. But follicular growth and follicles recruitment would be stimulated by a high feeding level or/and a good BCS. Hormonal response would take place before ovulation. An increase in gonadotropins secretion, circulating levels of insulin, IGF-1, leptin and silmutaneously an increase in circulating concentration of GH would be associated with a low feeding level. But the correlation between IGF-1 concentrations and nutritional status should be clarified. Leptin would be a major candidate to explain the interaction between the changes between metabolic hormones and the alteration of endocrinology of the ovarian cycle. The impact of these interactions on the fertility of each cycle should be clarified even the influence seems to be limited at present in adult mares. Ellis et al in this issue discusses the effects on the global fertility.

References

Albert, C., 1958. Melatonin: the first hormone isolated from the pineal body. Farmaco [Prat]. Aug; 13(8): 604-605.

Allen, W.R., 1987. Endogenous hormonal control of the mare's oestrus cycle. Proceedings of the Bain-Fallon Memorial Lectures. 2-13.

Armstrong, D.G., T.G. McEvoy, G. Baxter, J.J. Robinson, C.O. Hogg, K.J. Woad, R. Webb and K.D. Sinclair, 2001. Effect of dietary energy and protein on bovine follicular dynamics and embryo production in vitro: Associations with the ovarian insulin-like growth factor system. Biol. Reprod. 64: 1624–1632.

Bao, B., N. Kumar, R.M. Karp, H.A. Garverick and K. Sundaram, 2000. Estrogen receptor-beta expression in relation to the expression of luteinizing hormone receptor and cytochrome P450 enzymes in rat ovarian follicles. Biol. Reprod. 63: 1747-1755.
Barnard, N.D., A.R. Scialli and S. Bobela, 2002. The current use of estrogens for growth-suppressant therapy in adolescent girls. J. Pediatr. Adolesc. Gynecol. 15: 23-6.
Barneveld, A. and P.R. Van Weeren, 1999. Conclusions regarding the influence of exercise on the development of the equine musculoskeletal system with special reference to osteochondrosis. Equine Vet J Suppl. 31: 112-9.
Bergfelt, D.R. and O.J. Ginther, 1993. Synchronous fluctuations of LH and FSH in plasma samples collected daily during the estrous cycle in mares. Theriogenology. 40: 1137-1146.
Bossis, I., R.P. Wettemann, S.D. Welty, J. Vizcarra and L.J. Spicer, 2000. Nutritionally induced anovulation in beef Heifers: ovarian and endocrine function during realimentation and resumption of ovulation. Biol Reprod 62: 1436-44.
Bossis, I., R.P. Wettemann, S.D. Welty, J.A. Vizcarra, L.J. Spicer and M.G. Diskin, 1999. Nutritionally induced anovulation in beef heifers: ovarian and endocrine function preceding cessation of ovulation. J. Anim. Sci. 77: 1536–1546.
Briant, C., 2004. Stimulation ovarienne de la ponette Welsh en vue de la production d'embryons Limites physiologiques et techniques. Thèse pour obtenir le grade de docteur de l'université de Tours, discipline: Science de la vie. 2 juillet.
Bridges, T.S., T.R. Davidson, C.S. Chamberlain, R.D. Geisert and L.J. Spicer, 2002. Changes in follicular fluid steroids, insulin-like growth factors (IGF) and IGF-binding protein concentration, and proteolytic activity during equine follicular development. J Anim Sci. 80: 179–190.
Buff, P.R., A.C. Dodds, C.D. Morrison, N.C. Whitley, E.L. McFadin, J.A. Daniel, J. Djiane and D.H. Keisler, 2002. Leptin in horses: tissue localisation and relationship between peripheral concentrations of leptin and body condition. J.Anim. Sci 80: 2943-2948.
Burkhardt, 1947. Transition from anestrus in the mare and the effects of artificial lighting Journal of Agricultural Science 37: 64-68.
Buttler, W.R., 2000. Nutritional interactions with reproductive performance in dairy cattle. Anim. Reprod. Sci. 60-61: 449-457.
Camillo, F., I. Vannozzi, A. Rota, D. Panzani, A. Illuzy and D. Guillaume, 2002. Age at puberty, cyclicity, clinical response to PGF2α, hCG and GnRH and embryo recovery rate in yearling mares. 8th International Symposium on Equine Reproduction, Colorado USA. Theriogenology 6642: 627-630.
Campbell, B.K., E.E. Telfer, R. Webb and D.T. Baird, 2000. Ovarian autografts in sheep as a model for studying folliculogenesis. Mol. Cel. Endocrinol. 163: 131-139.
Carnevale, E.M. and O.J. Ginther, 1997. Age and pasture effects on vernal transition in mares Theriogenology. 47: 1009-1018.
Clemmons, A.J., D.L Thompson Jr. and L. Johnson, 1995. Local initiation of spermatogenesis in the horse. Biol. Reprod. 52: 1258-1267.
Cox, N.M., M.J. Stuart, T.G. Althen, W.A. Bennett and H.W. Miller, 1987. Enhancement of ovulation rate in gilts by increasing dietary energy and administering insulin during follicular growth. J. Anim. Sci. 64: 507-516.
DeMoura, M.D., D. Choi, E.I. Adashi and D.W. Payne, 1997. Insulin-Like Growth Factor-I-mediated amplification of follicle-stimulating hormone-supported progesterone accumulation by cultured rat granulosa cells: enhancement of steroidogenic enzyme activity and expression. Biol. Reprod. 56: 946-953.
Donabedian, M., C. Robert, G. Fleurance, G. Perona, C. Trillaud-Geyl, O. Lepage, D. Bergero, S. Léger and W. Martin-Rosset, 2006. Effets de deux modèles nutritionnels sur le statut osteoarticulaire du cheval de sport au cours de la première année postnatale. In 32ème Journée de la Recherche Equine, 1 mars, Paris, Editions Les Haras Nationaux 16 rue Claude Bernard 75231 Paris Cedex; 95-104
Donabedian, M., G. Fleurance, G. Perona, C. Robert, O. Lepage, C. Trillaud-Geyl, S. Leger, A. Ricard, D. Bergero and W. Martin-Rosset, 2006. Effect of fast vs moderate growth related to nutrient intake on developmental orthopedic disease in the horse. Anim. Res. (in press).
Donadeu, F.X. and O.J. Ginther, 2001. Effect of number and diameter of follicles on plasma concentrations of inhibin and FSH in mares. Reproduction. 121: 897-903.

Donadeu, F.X. and O.J., Ginther 2004. Interrelationships of estradiol, inhibin and gonadotropins during follicle deviation in pony mares. Theriogenology. 61: 1395-1405.
Doreau, M., J.P. Bruhat and W. Martin-Rosset, 1988. Effets du niveau des apports azotés chez la jument en début de lactation. Ann. Zootech., 37, 21-30.
Driancourt, M.A. and E. Palmer, 1984. Time of ovarian follicular recruitment in cyclic pony mares. Theriogenology. 21: 591-600.
Fitzgerald, B.P. and C.J. McManus, 2000. Photoperiodic versus metabolic signals as determinants of seasonal anestrus in the mare. Biol. Reprod. 63: 335-40.
Fitzgerald, B.P. and M.J. Schmidt, 1995. Absence of an association between melatonin and reproductive activity in mares during the nonbreeding season. Biol. Reprod. Mono. 1: 425-434.
Fleurance, G., M. Donabédian, G. Perona, C. Trillaud-Geyl, S. Léger, C. Robert, D. Bergero, O. Lepage and W. Martin-Rosset, 2006. Effet de deux modèles nutritionnels sur la croissance et le développement au cours de la première année postnatale du cheval de sport. 32ème Journée de la Recherche Equine, 1 mars, Paris, édition: Les Haras Nationaux 16 rue Claude Bernard 75231 Paris Cedex; 69-81.
Foster, D.L. and D.H. Olster, 1985. Effect of restricted nutrition on puberty in the lam: patterns of tonic luteininizing hormone (LH) and competency of the LH surge system. Endocrinology 116: 375-381.
Foster, D.L. and S. Nagatani, 1999. Physiological perspectives on leptin as a regulator of reproduction: role in timing puberty. Biol. Reprod. 60: 205-215.
Gastal, E.L., M.O. Gastal, D.R. Bergfelt and O.J. Ginther, 1997. Role of diameter differences among follicles in selection of a future dominant follicle in mares. Biol Reprod. 57: 1320-1327.
Gastal, E.L., M.O. Gastal, M.C. Wiltbank and O.J. Ginther, 1999. Follicle deviation and intrafollicular and systemic estradiol concentrations in mares. Biol Reprod. 61: 31-39.
Gastal, M.O., E.L. Gastal, V. Spinelli and O.J. Ginther, 2000. Body condition diameter of the ovulatory follicle in mares. 33st meeting of Society for the study of reproduction. Madison, Wisconsin, USA.
Gentry, L.R., D.L. Thompson, G.T. Gentry, K.A. Davis, R.A. Godke and J.A. Cartmill, 2002. The relationship between body condition, leptin, and reproductive and hormonal characteristics of mares during the seasonal anovulatory period. J. Anim. Sci. 80: 2695-2703.
Gérard, N. and P. Monget, 1998. Intrafollicular insulin-like growth factor-binding protein levels in equine ovarian follicles during preovulatory maturation and regression. Biol. Reprod. 58: 1508-1514.
Gérard, N., T. Delpuech, C. Oxvig, M.T. Overgaard and P. Monget, 2004. Proteolytic degradation of IGF-binding protein (IGFBP)-2 in equine ovarian follicles: involvement of pregnancy-associated plasma protein A (PAPP-A) and association with dominant but not subordinated follicles. J Endocrinol. 182: 457-466.
Gill, R.J., G.D. Potter, J.L. Kreider, G.T. Shelling, W.L. Jenkins and K.K. Hines, 1985. Nitrogen status and postpartum LH levels of mares fed varying levels of protein. In proceedings of the 19th Equine Nutrition and Physiology Symposium. Michigan, US, 23-25 May, 84-89.
Ginther, O.J. and D.R. Bergfelt, 1993. Growth of small follicles and concentrations of FSH during the equine oestrous cycle. J. Reprod. Fertil. 99: 105-111.
Ginther, O.J., 1974. Occurrence of anestrous, estrus, diestrus and ovulation over a twelve-month period in mares American Journal of Veterinary Research. 35: 1173-1179.
Ginther, O.J., 1993. Reproductive biology of the mare; basic and applied aspects. Ed. Library of Congress Catalog Cross plains Equiservices Publishing, 2nd ed.
Ginther, O.J., M.A. Beg, D.R. Bergfelt, F.X. Donadeu and K. Kot, 2001. Follicle selection in monovular species. Biol. Reprod. 65: 638-647.
Ginther, O.J., M.A. Beg, F.X. Donadeu and D.R. Bergfelt, 2003. Mechanism of follicle deviation in monovular species. Anim. Reprod. Sci. 78: 239-257.
Ginther, O.J., E.L. Gastal and M.A. Beg, 2004. Critical role of insulin-like growth factor system in follicle selection and dominance in mares. Biol. Reprod. 70: 1374-1379.
Godoi, D.B., E.L. Gastal and M.O. Gastal, 2002. A comparative study of follicular dynamics between lactating and non-lactating mares: effect of the body condition. Theriogenology. 58: 553-556.
Gong, J.G., 2002. Influence of metabolic hormones and nutrition on ovarian follicle development in cattle: practical implications. Dom. Anim Endocr. 23: 229-241.

Grubaugh, W.R., D.C. Sharp, L.A. Berglund, K.J. McDowell, D.M. Kilmer, L.S. Peck and K.W. Seamans, 1982. Effects of pinealectomy in pony mares. Journal of Reproduction and Fertility Suppl. 32: 293-295.

Guerin, M.V. and X.J. Wang, 1994. Environmental temperature has an influence on timing of the first ovulation of seasonal estrus in the mare. Theriogenology. 42: 1053-1060.

Guillaume, D. and E. Palmer, 1991. Effect of oral melatonin on the date of the first ovulation after ovarian inactivity in mares under artificial photoperiod Journal of Reproduction and Fertility Suppl. 44: 249-257.

Guillaume, D. and E. Palmer, 1992. Lumière, mélatonine et reproduction chez la jument. Annales de Zootechnie 41; 263-269.

Guillaume, D., G. Arnaud, F. Camillo, G. Duchamp and E. Palmer, 1995. Effects of melatonin implants on reproductive status of mares. Biology of Reproduction Monograph 1: 435-442.

Guillaume, D, B. Bruneau and C. Briant, 2002. Comparison of the effects of two GnRH antagonists on LH and FSH secretion, follicular growth and ovulation in the mare. Reprod. Nutr. Dev. 42:251-64.

Guillaume, D., G. Duchamp, P. Nagy and E. Palmer, 2000. Approach of the minimum lighting conditions for photostimulating mares in winter inactivity. Journal of Reproduction and Fertility suppl. 56: 205-216.

Guillaume, D., G. Duchamp, J. Salazar-Ortiz and P. Nagy, 2002. Nutrition influences the winter ovarian inactivity in mares. 8th International Symposium on Equine Reproduction, Colorado USA. Theriogenology. 6642: 593-597.

Guillaume, D., F. Regnier, F. Arnaud, J.L. Larry, D. Chesnau and B. Malpaux, 2006. Effet d'un éclairement permanent sur la reprise de l'activité sexuelle chez la jument. 32ème journée d'étude sur les équidés, 1er mars 2006, Paris. ed. Les Haras Nationaux. 33-38

Guillaume, D., G. Fleurance, D. Donabédian, C. Robert, G. Arnaud, M. Leveau, D. Chesneau, M. Ottogalli, J. Schneider and W. Martin-Rosset, 2006. Effets de deux modèles nutritionnels depuis la naissance sur l'âge d'apparition de la puberté chez le cheval de sport. In 32eme Journée Recherche Equine, Paris 1er Mars, Editions Haras Nationaux, 95-104

Guillaume, D., L. Zarazaga, B. Malpaux and P. Chemineau, 2006. Variability of plasma melatonin level in pony mares (Equus caballus), comparison with the hybrid: mules and with jennies (Equus asinus). Accepted for publication in Reprod. Nutr. Dev.

Guillaume, D., P. Nagy, G. Duchamp and E. Palmer, 2000. Approach of the minimum lighting conditions to photostimulate mares in winter inactivity. Journal of reproduction and fertility supplement 56: 205-216.

Guillaume, D., N. Rio and P.L. Toutain, 1995. Kinetic studies and production rate of melatonin in pony mares. American Journal of Physiology 268; R1236-1241.

Gutiérrez, C.G., J. Oldham, T.A. Bramley, J.G. Gong, B.K. Campbell and R. Webb, 1997. The recruitment of ovarian follicles is enhanced by increase dietary intake in heifers. J Anim Sci. 75: 1876-1884.

Henneke, D.R., G.D. Potter and J.L. Kreider, 1984. Body condition during pregnancy and lactation and reproductive efficiency of mares. Theriogenology. 21 897-909.

Henry, B.A., J.W. Goding, A.J. Tilbrook, F.R. Dunshea, D. Blache and I.J. Clarke, 2004. Leptin-mediated effects of undernutrition or fasting on luteinizing hormone and growth hormone secretion in ovariectomized ewes depend on the duration of metabolic perturbation. J Neuroendocrinol. 16: 244-255.

Hodgkinson, S.C., L. Moore, J.R. Napier, S.R. Davis, J.J. Bass and P.D. Gluckman, 1989. Characterization of insulin-like growth factor binding proteins in ovine tissue fuids. J. Endocrinol. 120: 429–438.

Hogden, G.D., 1982. The dominant ovarian follicle. Fertil Steril. 38: 281-300.

INRA, 1984. Le cheval. R.Jarrige and W.Martin-Rosset eds. INRA Editions, Versailles.

INRA, 1990. Alimentation des chevaux. W. Martin-Rosset (Ed), Editions INRA Publications, Route de St Cyr, 78000 Versailles

INRA, HN, IE, 1997. Notation de l'état corporel des chevaux de selle et de sport. Guide pratique. Institut Elevage ed. Paris.

Hughes, J.P., G.H. Stabenfeldt and J.W. Evans, 1975. The oestrous cycle of the mare Journal of Reproduction and Fertility Suppl. 23: 161-166.

Humbel, R.E., 1990. Insulin-like growth factor I and II. Eur J Biochem. 190: 445-462.

Karsch, F.J., J.E. Robinson, C.J.I. Woodfill and M.B. Brown, 1989. Circannual cycles of luteinizing hormone and prolactin secretion in ewes during prolonged exposure to a fixed photoperiod: Evidence for an endogenous reproductive rhythm. Biology of Reproduction. 41: 1034-1046.

Knight, P.G. and C. Glister, 2001. Potential local regulatory of inhibins, activins and follistatin in the ovary. Reproduction. 121: 503-512.

Kooistra, L.H and O.J. Ginther, 1975. Effect of photoperiod on reproductive activity and hair in mares. American Journal of Veterinary Research. 36: 1413-1419.

Kubiak, J.R., B.H. Crawford, E.L. Squires, R.H. Wrigley and G.M. Ward, 1987. The influence of energy intake and percentage body fat on the reproductive performance of nonpregnant mare Theriogenology. 28: 587-598.

Kumar, T.R., Y. Wang, N. Lu and M.M. Matzuk, 1997. Follicle Stimulating Hormone is required for ovarian follicle maturation but not male fertility. Nat. Genet. 15: 201-204.

Lampit, M., A. Golander, H. Guttmann and Z. Hochberg, 2002. Estrogen mini-dose replacement during GnRH agonist therapy in central precocious puberty: a pilot study. Journal of Clinical Endocrinolgy Metabolism 87: 687-690.

Langlois, B. and C. Blouin, 1996. Effect of a horse's month of birth on its future performances Proceedings of the 47th Annual Meeting of the European Association for Animal Production.

Langlois, B. and C. Blouin, 2004. Statistical analysis of some factors affecting the number of horse birth in France. Reproduction Nutrition Development 44: 583-596.

Legros, C., J. Salazar-Ortis and D. Guillaume, 2003. Photostimulation de la jument: la technique supporte-t-elle des accidents durant l'éclairement ? 29ème Journée de la Recherche Equine. 26 février, Paris édition: Les Haras Nationaux 16 rue Claude Bernard 75231 Paris Cedex; 1-10.

Lerner, A.B., J.D. Case and R.V. Heinzelman, 1959. Journal of American Chemistry society 81 6084

Lerner, A.B., J.D. Case, W. Mori and M.R. Wright, 1959. Melatonin in peripheral nerve. Nature. 27: 1818-1821.

LeRoith, D., H. Werner, D. Beitner-Johnson and C.L. Roberts, 1995. Molecular and cellular aspects of the Insulin-like growth factor I receptor. Endocrine Reviews. 16: 143-163.

Mackey, D.R., J.M. Sreenan, J.F. Roche and M.G. Diskin, 1999. Effect of acute nutritional restriction on incidence of anovulation and periovulatory estradiol and gonadotropin concentrations in beef heifers. Biol Reprod. 61: 1601-1607.

Magoffin, D.A. and Weitsman, 1993. Insulin-like growth factor-I stimulates the expression of 3β-hydroxysteroid dehydrogenase messenger ribonucleic acid in ovarian theca-interstitial cells. Biol Reprod. 48: 1166-1173.

Malinowski, K., A.L. Johnson and C.G. Scanes, 1985. Effects of interrupted photoperiods on the induction of ovulation in anestrous mares Journal of Animal Science 61 951.

Malpaux, B., J.C. Thiéry and P. Chemineau, 1999. Melatonin and the seasonal control of reproduction. Reproduction Nutrition Development. 39 355-366.

Malpaux, B., A. Daveau, F. Maurice, V. Gayard and J.C. Thiery, 1993. Short days effects of melatonin on LH secretion in the ewe: evidence for central sites of action in the mediobasal hypothalamus. Biol. Reprod. 48: 752 760.

Mazerbourg, S., C.A. Bondy, J. Zhou and P. Monget, 2003. The insulin-like growth factor system: a key determinant in the growth and selection of ovarian follicles? A comparative species study. Reprod. Dom. Anim. 38: 247-258.

Maretin-Rosset, W. and C. Trillaud-Geyl, 1984. Exploitation des troupeaux de juments lourdes allaitantes. In Le Cheval, R. Jarrige and W. Martin-Rosset Eds. INRA Editions, Route de St Cyr, 78026 Versailles, France. 540-554.

Martin-Rosset, W., 2004. Growth and development in the equine. In Proceeding of 2nd European Workshop Equine Nutrition (EWEN), V Julliand and W Martin-Rosset (Eds.), EAAP Nr 114, Wageningen Academic Publishers, The Netherlands. 15-50.

Martin-Rosset, W., M. Vermorel, M. Doreau, V. Tisserand and J. Andrieu, 1994. The French horse feed evaluation systems and recommended allowances for energy and protein. Livest. Prod. Sci., 40: 37-56.

Mazerbourg, S., M.T. Overgaard, C. Oxvig, M. Christiansen, C.A. Conover, I. Laurendeau, M. Vidaud, G. Tosser-Klopp, J. Zapf and P. Monget, 2001. Pregnancy-associated plasma protein-A (PAPP-A) in ovine, bovine, porcine, and equine ovarian follicles: involvement in IGF binding protein-4 proteolytic degradation and mRNA expression during follicular development. Endocrinology. 142: 5243-5253.

McDaniel, J.B., J.L. Kreider and D.M. Thrasher, 1979. The influence of artificial light and a nutritional supplement on the onset of the breeding season in mares. Journal of Animal Science Supplement. 1: 141-145.

McManus, C.J. and B.P. Fitzgerald, 2000. Effects of a single day of feed restriction on changes in serum leptin, gonadotropins, prolactin, and metabolites in aged and young mares. Domest Anim Endocrinol. 19: 1-13.

Melo, M.I.V., J.R.B. Sereno, M. Henry and G.D. Cassali, 1998. Peripuberal sexual deveopment of Pantaneiro stallions. Theriogenology. 50: 727-737.

Monget, P. and G.B. Martin, 1997. Involvement of insulin-like growth gactors in the interations between nutrition and reproduction in female mammals. Human. Reprod. Suppl. 1: 33-52.

Monget, P., S. Fabre, P. Mulsant, F. Lecerf, J.M. Elsen, S. Mazerbourg, C. Pisselet and D. Monniaux, 2002. Regulation of ovarian folliculogenesis by IGF and BMP system in domestic animals. Domestic Animal Endocrinol. 23: 139-154.

Naden, J, R.P. Amann and E.L. Squires, 1990, Testicular growth, hormone concentrations, seminal characteristics and sexual behaviour in stallions. Journal of Reproduction and Fertility 88: 167-176.

Nagatani, S., P. Guthikonda, R.C. Thompson, H. Tsukamura, K.I. Maeda and D.L. Foster, 1998. Evidence for GnRH regulation by leptin: leptin administration prevents reduced pulsatile LH secretion during fasting. Neuroendocrinology. 67: 370-376.

Nagy, P., Gy. Huszenicza, J. Juhasz, L. Solti and M. Kulcsar, 1998. Diagnostic problems associated with ovarian activity in barren and postpartum mares early in the breeding season Reproduction in Domestic Animals 33 187-192.

Nicolino, M. and M.G. Forest, 2001 La puberté in La reproduction chez les Mammiféres et l'homme. Chap. 29 654-679. Thibault C. and Levasseur MC. INRA editions Ellipse Edition Marketing S.A. 32 rue Bargue 75740 Pari cedex15 France.

Nishikawa, Y., 1959. Studies on reproduction in horses. Jap. Racing Ass., Shiba Tamuracho Minatokou, Tokio.

Nogueira, G.P., R.C. Barnabe and I.T.N. Verreschi, 1997. Puberty and Growth rate in Thoroughtbred Fillies. Theriogenology 48: 581-588.

Palmer, E. and M.A. Driancourt, 1981. Photoperiodic stimulation of the winter aneostrous mare: what is a long day? In Photoperiodism and reproduction in vertebrates (International Colloquium No 6) pp 65-82 Eds R Ortavant, J Pelletier and J-P Ravault. Intitut National de la Recherche Agronomique, Versailles (France).

Palmer, E. and M.A. Driancourt, 1983. Some interactions of season of foaling, photoperiod and ovarian activity in the equine Livestock Production Sciences 10: 197-210.

Palmer, E. and D. Guillaume, 1992. Photoperiodism in the equine species -- what is a long night? Animal Reproduction Science 28: 21-30.

Palmer, E, M.A. Driancourtand and R. Ortavant, 1982. Photoperiodic stimulation of the mare during winter anoestrus Journal of Reproduction and Fertility 32: 275-282.

Peltier, M.R., G. Robinson and D.C. Sharp, 1998. Effects of melatonin implants in pony mares. 2. Long-term effects. Theriogenology. 49: 1125-42.

Pierson, R.A. and O.J. Ginther, 1985. Ultrasonic evaluation of the preovulatory follicle in the mare. Theriogenology 1985. 24: 359-368.

Salazar-Ortiz, J. and D. Guillaume, 2005. La date de la première ovulation annuelle de la jument, peut-elle être avancée en agissant sur la ration alimentaire à partir de l'automne ? 31ème Journée de la Recherche Equine, 2 mars, Paris, édition: Les Haras Nationaux 16 rue Claude Bernard 75231 Paris Cedex; 69-81.

Salazar-Ortiz, J., E. Audouin, T. Delpuech, P. Monget and D. Guillaume, 2004 Effet du niveau d'alimentation sur la croissance folliculaire et certains taux hormonaux plasmatiques de la jument. 30ème Journée de la Recherche Equine, 3 mars, Paris, édition: Les Haras Nationaux 16 rue Claude Bernard 75231 Paris Cedex. 15-27.

Saltiel, A., A. Calderron, N. Garcia and D.P. Hurley, 1982. Ovarian activity in the mare between latitude 15° and 22°N Journal of Reproduction and Fertility Suppl. 32: 261-267.

Scraba, S.T. and O.J. Ginther, 1985. Effects of lighting programs on onset of the ovulatory season in mares. Theriogenology. 24: 667-679.

Sharp, D.C., M.W. Vernon and M.T. Zavy, 1979. Alterations of seasonal reproductive patterns in mares following superior cervical ganglionectomy. Journal of Reproduction and Fertility Supplement 27: 87-93.

Sibonga, J.D, U. Sommer and R.T. Turner, 2002. Evidence that 2-methoxyestradiol suppresses proliferation and accelerates apoptosis in normal rat growth plate chondrocytes. J. Cancer. Res. Clin. Oncol. 128: 477-483.

Sipahutar, H., P. Soudaine, S. Moslemi, B. Plainfossé and G.E. Séralini, 2003. Immunolocalisation of aromatase in Stallion leydig Cells and seminiferous tubules. Journales of Histochemistry 51: 311-318.

Sirois, J., B.A. Ball and J.E. Fortune, 1989. Patterns of growth and regression of ovarian follicles during the estrous cycle and after hemiovariectomy in mares. Equine Vet J. suppl. 8: 43-48.

Skelton, K.V., K.F. Dowsett and N.P. McMeniman, 1991. Ovarian activity in fillies treated with anabolic steroids prior to the onset of puberty. Journal of Reproduction and Fertility Supplement 44: 351-356.

Skinner, D.C. and B. Malpaux, 1999. High melatonin concentrations in the third ventricular cerebrospinal fluid are not due to galen vein blood recirculating through the choroid plexus. Endocrinology. 140: 4399-4405.

Skinner, J.D. and J. Bowen, 1968. Puberty in the Welsh Stallion Journal of Reproduction and Fertility 16: 133-135.

Spicer, L.J. and S.E. Echternkamp, 1995. The ovarian insulin and insulin-like growth factor system with an emphasis on domestic animals. Dom. Anim. Endocrinol. 12: 223–245.

Stankov, B.,B. Cozzi, V. Lucini, P. Fumagalli, F. Scaglione and F. Fraschini, 1991. Characterization and mapping of melatonin receptors in the brain of three mammalian species: rabbit, horse and sheep. Neuroendocrinology. 53: 214-221.

Staub, C., N.L. Heninger, C.L. Donnelly, D.W. Forrest, T.L. Blanchard, C.C. Love, D.D. Varner and L. Johnson, 2002. Apoptosis during the initiation of equine spermatogenesis. Theriogenology. 58: 367-371.

Tricoire, H., M. Moller, P. Chemineau and B. Malpaux, 2003. Origin of cerebrospinal fluid melatonin and possible function in the integration of photoperiod. Reprod. Suppl. 61: 311-321.

Turzillo, A.M. and J.E. Fortune, 1990. Suppression of the secondary FSH surge with bovine follicular fluid is associated with delayed ovarian follicular development in heifers. J. Reprod. Fertil. 89: 643-653.

Van Niekerk, C.H. and J.S. Van Heerden, 1972. Nutrition and ovarian activity of mares early in the breeding season Journal of the South African Veterinary Medical Association. 43: 351-360.

Van Niekerk, F.E. and C.H. Van Niekerk, 1997. The effect of dietary protein on reproduction in the mare. III. Ovarian and uterine changes during the anovulatory season, transitional and ovulatory periods in the non-pregnant mare. Journal of the South African Veterinary Medical Association. 68: 86-92.

Watson, E.D., S.E. Bae, R. Thomassen, S.R.M. Tomson and K. Woad, 2004. Armstrong DG. Insulin-like growth factors-I and -II and insulin-like growth factor-binding protein-2 in dominant equine follicles during sping transition and the ovulatory season. Reproduction. 128: 321-329.

Webb, G.W., G.D. Potter and D.G. Meadows, 1979. Effect of nitrogen status on reproductive performance in the mare. Proceedings of the 6th Equine Nutrition Physiology Symposium. Texas, US, 17-19 May, 20-23.

Weise, M., S. De-Levi, K.M. Barnes, R.I. Gafni, V. Abad and J. Baron, 2001 Effects of estrogen on growth plate senescence and epiphyseal fusion. Proc Natl Acad Sci USA. 98: 6871-6876.

Wesson, J.A. and O.J. Ginther, 1981. Puberty in the female Pony: Reproduction behavior, ovulation and plasma gonadotrophin concentrations. Biology of Reproduction. 24: 977-986.

Zachow, R.J. and D.A. Magoffin, 1997. Direct intraovarian effects of leptin: impairment of the synergistic action of insulin-like growth factor-I on Follicle-Stimulating Hormone dependent estradiol-17 beta production by rat ovarian granulosa cells. Endocrinology. 138: 847-850.

Zhang, Y, R. Proenca, M. Maffei, M. Barone, L. Leopold and J.M. Friedman, 1994. Positional cloning of mouse obese gene and its human homologue. Nature 372; 425-432.

Zofkova, I., 2003. Pathophysiological and clinical importance of insulin-like growth factor-I with respect to bone metabolism. Physiol. Res. 52: 657-679.

Nutrition and equine fertility

A.D. Ellis[1], M. Boekhoff[2], L. Bailoni[3] and R. Mantovani[3]
[1]Nottingham Trent University, Brackenhurst, Southwell NG25 0QG, United Kingdom
[2]Animal Science Group, Wageningen University Research, Lelystad, The Netherlands
[3]Department of Animal Science, University of Padova, Italy

Abstract

Advice on feeding broodmares before and during conception is often based on general assumptions passed on within the industry. This review aimed to give an overview of scientific evidence currently available on fertility in mares in relation to nutritional factors. Certainly the current understanding of the fertility cycle highlights several areas which may be affected by nutrition. The amount and sometimes level of the literature found was inadequate and much of the research stemmed from before 1990. Research did highlight that there is a basis for feeding mares at increasing energy levels prior to conception (this may support the argument for spring grass increasing fertility) and that provision of good quality proteins and adequate levels of minerals and vitamins should be ensured. This will also decrease the risk of early embryo loss. In conjunction with these findings a correct body condition score should always be aimed at. There is no evidence for reduced fertility in obese mares. Finally, particularly as the feeding of ensiled forages increases in Europe, forages should be analysed for mould and toxin contamination regularly as some of these have been proven to reduce fertility in mares and to increase the risk of resorption. Literature relating to fertility and nutrition in stallions is even scarcer, and in most cases evaluates the effects of moderate changes in feeding availability rather than severe malnutrition or deficiency of specific nutrients. On the other hand, feeding candidate stallions during growth or adult males during the reproductive season has only minor implications, due to the mild higher requirements in respect of maintenance. Attempts have been made in analysing the relationship between feeding and semen quality, but results, often derived from other species, have produced conflicting evidence of a positive connection between nutrition and fertility. This may be due to the fact that in stallions sperm output is in most cases larger than required and therefore sub-fertility is often due to genetics rather than nutrition. As for the mare, the effect of toxin contamination and its relationship with fertility may also need to be explored futher with regards to stallion fertility.

Keywords: nutrition, fertility, mare, stallion

Introduction

Conception rates may be influenced by age, parity, physiological condition, hormone metabolism, sperm quality, disease, trauma, genetics and environmental factors such as nutrition, stabling and exercise. However, this wide range of additional factors does not mean that nutrition should be disregarded as it is one aspect of horse management which can easily be optimised. Nutrition is one of the contributing environmental factors to mare and stallion fertility, the significance of which is generally unknown.

This paper aims to review current knowledge on equine fertility in relation to nutrition. It will be divided into two sections – Section 1 relating to current knowledge on nutrition and mare fertility and Section 2 relating to current knowledge on nutrition and stallion fertility.

The mare

Current feeding advise to mare owners is theoretically based on physiological nutrient requirements according to growth of foetus and milk yield while in practice it is often based on 'common knowledge' and assumptions made by practitioners. At that level an interesting amount of 'concepts and ideas' are passed on in relation to mare fertility, which have not been systematically examined in the past. Amongst these the following theories are repeatedly proclaimed:

- mares conceive better when in a rising plane of nutrition;
- obesity reduces conception rates;
- a protein/mineral supplement will increase conception rates;
- vitamin C stimulates fertility;
- spring grass stimulates fertility;

Fertility cycle

The mare's oestrus cycle is seasonal with the fertile period normally commencing in early spring and ending in early autumn. Under natural circumstances mares are infertile (anoestrus) during the winter. During the fertile period around 12 oestrus cycles are completed, each lasting around 21 days within which the mare is sexually receptive for four to five days. The transition between oestrus and an-oestrus (spring and autumn) is linked to wide-ranging physiological changes, which are regulated through the endocrine system.

Endocrine control is facilitated by the felopian tubes, the uterus and three endocrine glands located in the brain (hypothalamus, anterior pituitary, epyphysis). The pineal gland plays a role in registration of daylength. As day length changes the activity of the hypothalamus and anterior pituitary changes. Lack of day light leads to the production of the hormone melatonin by the pineal gland. Melatonin together with prolactine influence the function of the hypothalamus-pituitary-ovary axis. Melatonin reduces the activity of the hypothalamus and the pituitary and thus as day length shortens the higher levels of melatonine lead to reduction and eventual ending of fertility (anoestrus) (Kilmer *et al.*, 1982). As day length increases the pineal gland produces less melatonin and the hypothalamus and anterior pituitary become more active. The hypothalamus starts to produce gonadotrophin releasing hormone (GnRH), which stimulates the production of follicle stimulating hormone (FSH) and the lutenising hormone (LH) in the pituitary. These latter two hormones (FSH, LH) influence the activity of the ovaries.

The commencement of the oestrus period in spring has been directly related to increased day length and exposure to UV rays and to an increased plane of nutrition. Direct relationships between nutritional factors and the fertility cycle have been established in other species. In sheep the infusion of dextrose-amino acid mixtures led to increased Lutenising Hormone (LH) activity (similar to that seen due to increasing plane of nutrition and day length). In cattle the role played by micronutrients such as molybdenum, acting as an LH inhibitor and thus delaying puberty has been highlighted (Robinson *et al.*, 2006). Thus nutrition, in particular feeding level and micronutrient balance, may play an important factor in the onset of puberty and early fertility of young mares.

Nutrition in relation to puberty, endocrine factors and early embryonic death or resorption are discussed in more detail else where (Guillaume *et al.*, 2005).

Energy balance

Energy itself is not a nutrient but is a measure of the potential nutrient value for maintenance of body condition supplied by horse feed. As mentioned earlier the mare's condition is generally perceived to have an influence on fertility. As such a rising plane if nutrition during conception is said to be advantageous and at the same time it is often assumed that fat mares are less fertile. The following paragraphs try to look at the scientific evidence behind these beliefs.

A limited amount of research into nutritional factors on mare's fertility can be found and much of this is not recent. Several authors have concluded that bad body condition due to a lack of energy intake does lead to incomplete ripening of follicles, delayed onset of oestrus cycles in spring, irregular oestrus cycles and reduced conception rates (Van Niekerk and Van Heerden, 1972; Belonje and Niekerk, 1975; Henneke *et al.*, 1984 and Gill *et al.*, 1983). There are marked changes in carbohydrate metabolism and in pancreatic β-cell function during pregnancy in the mare (Fowden *et al.*, 1984). The mare develops increased β-cell sensitivity to glucose with increased degradation of insulin which can enhance the resistance to insulin to enhance glucose uptake and utilisation for a stable glucose supply to the placenta and the foetus. In humans this mechanism has been describes as 'facilitated anabolism'. Fowden *et al.* (1984) concluded that the mare may be in diabetogenic stress during pregnancy and this may explain how nutritional mismanagement during early stages of pregnancy could lead to increased rates of embryonic death or/and resorption.

During the foaling heat and the first heat thereafter the mare produces the greatest amount of milk and a short term negative energy balance may occur. The nutrient requirements are at their highest levels during this period (Ellis, 2001; Ginther, 1992). Henneke *et al.* (1981, 1984) showed that the risk of embryo resorption can be considerably reduced in mares which are fed at higher energy levels during late pregnancy and early lactation. Thus a negative energy balance must be avoided during this period for optimum fertility. Energy balance will be discussed in more detail in the following chapter.

In an experiment with 32 lactating Quarter mares, mares with a body condition score (BCS) of less than 4 (on a scale from BCS 0 - starving to 10 - obese), fed on a low energy diet during pregnancy and lactation (low-low), had delayed oestrus cycles after parturition (Henneke *et al.*, 1981). However, mares fed the high levels pre and post parturition (High-High) with a condition score of 7.6 did not show any signs of reduced fertility (Table 1).

A larger field study looking a 927 mares and correlating pregnancy rate and number of cycles to conception with body fat and condition scores further confirms this result (Henneke *et al.*, 1984).

Table 1. Effect of energy (DE, MJ) and protein intakes (CP, kg) pre partum and post partum on fertility parameters in 32 mares (Source: adapted from Henneke et al., 1981).

	Parturition	Mean energy and protein intake per horse				Days to ovulation		Days to pregnancy	
		Pregnancy		Lactation		First	Second	63	105
Energy Feeding level	Body score	DE (MJ)	CP (kg)	DE (MJ)	CP (kg)				
High-High	7.6	135	1.3	159	1.7	12.7	32.8	8/8	8/8
High-Low		135	1.3	113	1.4	13.2	37.2	7/8	8/8
Low-High	3.6	65	0.8	209	2.3	13.2	37.3	5/5[1]	5/5
Low-Low		65	0.8	135	1.7	16.8	45.8	4/8	1/4

[1]The authors gave no explanation as to what happened to the three mares missing from this group

Breeding efficiency was enhanced in mares with a body condition of good (Score 5) and above at the beginning of spring compared to mares below a score of 5.0 ($p<0.05$). More recently Cavinder *et al.* (2005) also found that there was no difference in mean time to ovulation and in conception rates between 12 mares on a 'fat' condition score (score 7.2 ± 0.1) produced by over feeding during gestation and 12 mares on a moderate condition score (5.4± 0.01).

Unfortunately in both the experimental study and the field study above the effect of energy level cannot be distinguished from protein levels. Nevertheless, these experiments also confirm results from an earlier study by Belonje and Van Niekerk (1975). These authors compared oestrus cycles in mares left out all year round without additional feeding and a group of mares left out with additional feeding. The additionally fed mares received 11 kg of Lucerne and 2.7 kg of concentrate feed during the winter. The fed mares showed mild signs of oestrus throughout the winter and resumed full oestrus cycles much earlier in the spring. The mares, which were not fed additional feed in the winter, did not show big differences in body condition but their oestrus cycle was delayed in spring.

In two experiments by INRA (1984), 28 mares per trial (786 kg after foaling, not all the same animals per trial) were fed either a high energy level (HL 100% UFC requirement) or low energy level (LL 80% UFC requirement) diet during the 10th and 11th months of pregnancy while protein, mineral and vitamins were fed at 100% of INRA (1984) recommendations. After parturition both groups were once again fed at 100% requirement level (INRA, 1984). The trials took place over two subsequent years. Mean variation in live weight of the same of the two trials were low in late pregnancy (+ 7.5 kg and –6 kg with HL and LL group respectively). At the end of the 1st month of lactation HL and LL groups gained 18 and 35 kg respectively. No significant effect of diet before parturition was found for ovarian activity, fertility, pregnancy, mortality rates of the foals and and associate factors (Table 2).

More recently, Guillaume *et al.* (2002) fed 10 pony mares 53% of energy requirements while a second group of 10 mares acted as control on 100% of the recommended requirements. Mares on low energy intake stopped ovulating much earlier in autumn and resumed oestrus cycles much later in spring ($p<0.01$). These pony mares showed a much lower body condition score than the control group.

Table 2. Effect of moderate energy restriction in late pregnancy on reproductive performance of mares of heavy breeds (Source: Martin-Rosset and Doreau, 1984 and Martin-Rosset et al., unpublished, personal communication).

Trial	I		II	
	HL	LL	HL	LL
Number of mares	14	14	14	13
Energy: NE (UFC)	7.0	5.6	6.8	5.4
Protein: MADC (g)	570	548	601	631
Body Weight variation (kg)	+7	+6	+8	-12
Date of birth (days)	14/4±23	13/4±18	13/4±13	17/4±24
Mortality of foals	0	1	0	1
Fertility Results				
Oestrous cycle within 0-35 days	14	12	14	12
Fertilisation on 1st oestrus	11	8	11	8
Pregnancy at 45th day	13	10	13	10
Interval parturition to pregnancy	20±8	27±7	21±8	16±6

Around 15 to 40 days after ovulation is the most critical period during which embryo death and resorption can occur (Van Niekerk, 1965a; Belonje and Van Niekerk, 1972; Ginther, 1993 and Allen, 2001). Van Niekerk (1965a) reported increased resorption of embryos after 25 days following ovulation in mares held on low energy intake during and after conception. In contrast, mares, which were on a low energy level until 18 days after ovulation but then fed additional feed showed no increase in embryo death or resorption. These results were confirmed in more recent studies which showed that low energy intake in spring can lead to an increased chance of resorption during first weeks of pregnancy (Van Nierkerk *et al.*, 1997a, 1998a).

When introducing 74 hour fasting periods in mares, prolactine concentrations were significantly reduced (Sticker *et al.*, 1995). In 12 thin mares (BCS 3-3.5) a significant reduction in IGF-1, leptin, prolactine and LH was measured in comparison to 12 fat mares (BCS 7-7.5; Gentry *et al.*, 2002). Leptin concentrations in blood have been used in other mammals to measure body fat content (Houseknecht *et al.*, 1998). Low body fat stores and leptin concentrations in blood have been highlighted as possible indicators for feeding related changes in reproductive metabolism (Henneke *et al.*, 1984; Fitzgerald and McManus, 2000 and Guillaume, 2002). Leptin acts as a signal in relation to the function of the hypothalamus but further research is necessary to confirm this hypothesis.

Only one study contradicting the above evidence was found. Banach and Evans (1981a) reduced energy intake of 13 Quarter horse mares to 55% of the recommended levels (NRC, 1978) during the last 90 days of pregnancy. There was no effect of this on days to parturition or condition of foals at birth, but mares did have a reduced body condition to a control group (13 horses). Six of these mares where then fed 75% of the recommended NRC (1978) levels during lactation for 25 days. In comparison to the control group (fed 100% of requirements) these mares did not show a delay in return to pregnancy. It may be possible that 75% of requirements for 25 days were still adequate and number of horses within the experiment were too small.

In general it can be concluded that mares with long term energy intakes below requirements will show reduced periods of fertility and the chance of embryo death and resorption will increase.

In contrast none of the studies which fed higher than recommended energy levels or used mares in fat body condition showed that there was a negative effect on oestrus cycle or conception rates or increased risk for embryonic death or resorption (Gentry *et al.*, 2002; Guilaume, 2000; Van Niekerk, 1997c, Van Niekerk and Van Niekerk, 1998a; Meyer and Stadermann, 1991; Henneke *et al.*, 1984; Banach and Evans, 1981a and b). Henneke *et al.* (1984) showed that there was no detrimental effect on fertility in mares of fat body condition and concluded that initial body fat at the beginning of the season may enhance fertility. Morris *et al.* (1987) points out that even mares in above normal body condition can be at risk of reduced fertility and embryo resorption when the energy level in the diet is suddenly reduced.

Therefore, the popular belief that obesity my reduce fertility in mares cannot be underpinned by scientific evidence.

Protein

Protein nutrition and in particular the supply of essential amino acids play an important role in the endocrine reproductive metabolism. A literature review, however, highlights that there is very limited scientific research in this area (Ellis, 2002; Van Niekerk and Van Niekerk, 1998 a-c, Doreau *et al.*, 1988). The above described experiment by Henneke *et al.* (1981) highlighted the possibility that protein rather than energy could have been the limiting factor.

In an experiment by Doreau *et al.* (1988), 20 heavy mares were split into two groups of 10 and fed either a high (HH) or low (LL = 62% of HH) protein level while on an isoenergetic diet. Reproductive performance measures (see Table 3) showed that there was no significant differences at this level of protein reduction in diet.

Van Niekerk (1997, 1998a-c) equally divided 62 Thoroughbred and Arab mares (36 non-pregnant, non-lactating and 24 pregnant) into 4 diet groups. The research was carried out on a stud farm in South Africa. All mares were fed energy and mineral and vitamin requirements according to NRC (1989) recommendations. Diets varied in protein content (Table 4) and protein quality (Table 5).

Table 3. Effect of protein allowances on reproductive performance in nursing mares of heavy breeds fed an isoenergetic diet (Source: adapted from Doreau et al., 1988).

	HL	LL
Number of mares	10	10
Body weight (kg)	743	743
UFC/d	10.38	10.77
Mare – change in bodyweight	-0.21 ± 0.9	-0.20 ± 0.6
Time between foaling to first heat	13.5 ± 6.4	11.5 ± 3.6
Time between foaling and fertilization	25.0 ± 14.8	18.5 ± 7.5

Tabel 4. Mean daily intake of crude protein (g) for non-pregnant mares (Source: Van Niekerk, 1997).

Period	Diet 1	Diet 2	Diet 3	Diet 4	NRC (1989)
1 (july-sep: anoestrus pregnant)	806	1130	934	1258	656 (non pregnant)
2 (oct.-dec: breeding season)	714	1374	842	1502	801
3 (jan.-march)	676	1174	804	1302	801
4 (april-june)	706	1350	834	1478	815
5 (july-sep.)	782 (1066)[1]	1598 (1882)	910 (1194)	1726 (2010)	866
Mean	737	1325	865	1435	

[1]values in brackets: increased protein intake during the last trimester of pregnancy

Tabel 5. Amino acid composition (g/day) supplied by each diet (Source: Van Niekerk, 1997).

Amino Acids	Diet 1	Diet 2	Diet 3	Diet 4
Threonine[1]	0.32	0.70	0.42	0.82
Methionine[1]	0.12	0.14	0.18	0.22
Iso-leucine	0.41	0.87	0.52	1.02
Leucine	0.77	1.46	0.82	1.55
Lysine[1]	0.59	1.06	0.78	1.33
Arginine	0.67	1.37	0.71	1.46
Total essential (g/day)	1.0	1.9	1.4	2.4

[1]counted as essential Amino Acids in horses

Results showed a significant difference in number and development of follicles according to diets. Van Niekerk and Van Niekerk (1998b) linked this to the ratio of essential to non-essential amino acids, with a high intake (Diet 4) leading to increased ovarian activity and increased follicular development (size) early in the season. Mean occurrence of embryonic death or resorption in groups on diets 2 to 4 was 7.3%. Mares on diet 1 had a delayed onset of first ovulation in spring compared to the other mares. Within the group of mares which was pregnant from the start of the study on diet 1 (low in lysine) a loss in body weight of around 25 kg per mare was recorded despite adequate energy levels in the diet. Furthermore, an occurrence of embryonic death or abortion occurred in 37% of these mares during the next breeding cycle (period 2). This is probably due to the high increase in protein requirements during the last trimester of pregnancy and during early lactation and may indicate that energy and protein balance alone are less vital than an adequate supply of essential amino acids.

Although clinical in vivo research in this area is scarce the above results support the general assumption that a protein supplement high in essential amino acids given prior and during the conception period may be beneficial.

Minerals

Once again scientific research relating to mineral nutrition and fertility in mares is scarce. Generally assumptions from extensive research in other species (often farm animals) are made. Specific research into the effect of Calcium, Phosphorus, Magnesium and Sodium supply from feed on fertility of mares could not be found. In cattle several reports state that an excess intake of Potassium leads to fertility problems (Dohms, 2002). Finkler-Schade (2000) reports that many hoses on good quality pasture in Germany will be taking in levels of Potassium high above requirements but no reports into possible effects on fertility have been published.

Monroe *et al.* (1988) supplied an artifical substitution for Selenium to eight out of 16 pregnant mares in the last timester of pregnancy and during early lactation. Blood serum values of Selenium were not increased in the supplemented group and there was not difference in ovarian activity or time to oestrus and pregnancy rates. Selenium metabolims is linked to Vitamin E metabolism and if Vitamin E is not sufficiently present in the diet the Selenium requirements will increase (Schöntaler; 1998).

Iodine is an important building block of the hormone thyroxine and thus has the potential to intefere with endocrine regulation of the fertility cycle. Meyer and Staderman (1991) report that the requirements of iodine hardly increase for pregnant mares (to 1-2mg/day) but no recent literature of idodine excess or deficiency in relation to fertility could be found. Ekmann (1970) reported that a shortage of iodine in the diet of mares leads to irregular oestrus cycles and infertility. Excess iodine intake has been blamed for abortion and embrionic death in a gorup of mares which received 40 mg Iodine/day form their diet (Drew and Williams, 1975). Feeding supplements containing sea algae may lead to an excess intake of iodine. Despite plenty of research into effects of iodine excess and deficiency on growth rates, musco-skeletal development and health in horses and other species there is a lack of publications relating to fertility. The same is also true for the micro minerals of copper and zinc.

Some limited research into the effect of mixed mineral supplements on fertility has been carried out. Ott *et al.* (1994) pooled results from a series of experiments (some first reported in 1981) which looked at the relationship between mineral supplements and serum concentrations of minerals in pregnant mares, their fertility after foaling and mineral concentrations (Cu and Zn) in the uterus (Table 6). There were no significant differences between the three treatments, but sample groups per treatment were small (Table 7). Mineral supplementation did lead to a reduction in oestrus cycles to pregnancy, however the conception rate (per covering) was higher in mares which were

Table 6. Summary overview of the experiments by Ott. et al. (1994).

	Experiment 1 and 2	Experiment 2 and 3
Horses	18 TB and Quarter horses	24 TB and Quarter horses
Status	pregnant	pregnant
Begin	56 days pre partum	84 days pre partum
Energy and protein levels	According to NRC (1972) and condition score	According to NRC (1989) and condition score
Treatment	3 Groups (n=6)	3 Groups (n=8)
Supplements used	A: low mineral soja-placebo plus vitamins[1] B: supplement of anorganic minerals plus vitamins[1] C: supplement of anorganic minerals plus vitamins[1] plus protein bound (organic) minerals	

[1] Vitamins added to concentrate feed (IU/kg) Vit A, 6600; Vit. D., 660; Vit. E., 22; TB=Thouroughbred;

Tabel 7. Overview of mineral intake and mean results (Ott et al., 1981, 1994).

Minerals	Concentrate feed (mg/kg)	Supplemented (mg/day)		
		A	B	C
Ca	4600			
Ph	5100			
Fe	228	7.5	165	165
Zn	47	1.6	70	70
Cu	8.3	0.4	58	58
Mn	39	0.6	11	11
Co			1.4	1.4
Iodine			4.1	4.1
Fertility results:				
Mean oestrus cycles to pregnancy		1.95 ± 0.2	1.56 ± 0.2	1.25 ± 0.2
Conception Rate %		69.2	57.1	61.5
Uterine biopsy results:				
Cu concentrations (mg/kg)		46.6 ± 6	48.1 ± 8	56 ± 6
Zn concentrations (mg/kg)		138 ± 15	140 ± 24	160 ± 24

not supplemented, possibly due to less occurrence of resorptions on the second heat after foaling. The zinc and copper values from the post-foaling uterine biopsy were slightly higher in the group supplemented with the inorganic and organic Mineral supplement (group C), possibly indicating better absorption of organic minerals (Ott *et al.*, 1994).

Lindner *et al.* (1993) supplemented 12 out of 24 pregnant mares shortly before parturition with 200mg Zinc, 60mg Copper, 160mg Manganese and 10mg Magnesium per day. Post partum progesterone levels in the blood, maturation of follicles (4 mares per group only) and first ovulation were recorded. These authors concluded that feeding a mineral supplement led to a faster development of follicles by the second oestrus cycle (Table 8). This may be due to the fact that mares only received the mineral supplement shortly before parturition and thus the mineral metabolism may also take some time

Tabel 8. Follicle development (+/- s.d.) in supplemented and non-supplemented mares (Lindner et al., 1993).

	N	Duration to 1st Corpus Luteum *post partum* (days)	Duration to 2nd Corpus Luteum *post partum* (days)
Supplemented	4	10.0 ± 4.32	7.50 ± 2.8
Control	4	11.0 ± 4.16	10.0 ± 2.6

to adjust to new dietary levels (Lindner *et al.*, 1993). Further research with larger groups would be necessary to confirm this hypothesis.

There is currently very little evidence that a mineral supplement will improve fertility but some evidence that a deficiency in certain minerals may impair fertility and in these situations a supplement given in conjunction with a good quality protein supplement may be beneficial.

Vitamines

Vitamin A has been identified in many species as playing an important role in relation to fertility. The pro-vitamin β-carotene is taken in with food and then absorbed and metabolised into Vitamin A. A shortage of Vitamin A has been linked to infertility in farm animals and even when no shortage seems to be present additional feeding of β-carotene has led to increased fertility (Schams *et al.*, 1977). Deficiencies have been associated with cysts forming along the fallopian tubes, sub-optimal luteal function and reduced fertility in cattle (Seitardis, 1963; Lotthammer and Ahlswede, 1977; Anwandter, 1974 and Cooke and Comben, 1978). Due to these previous reports a general assumption has been made that β-carotene supplementation could increase fertility in mares (Meyer, 1995).

Bondi and Skan (1984) highlight that β-carotene is only absorbed and converted into Vitamin A at 33% efficiency. The plasma values for β-carotene are much increased when the pro-vitamin is ingested with grass, indicating that there is an associative effect between nutrients. Fats in the diet may influence the absorption of β carotene as this is a fat soluble vitamin. Ashworth and Antipatis (2001) linked higher Vitamin A levels in the blood to a decreased risk of embryonic death and resorption, although this author highlights that most equine diets contain adequate levels of Vitamin A and reports of deficiencies are rare. Additional supplementation with β-carotene in winter stabled horses has been reported as increasing conception rates (Ahlswede and Konermann, 1980; Ferraro and Cote, 1984; Van der Holst *et al.*, 1984). Ferraro and Cote (1984) reported stronger oestrus behaviour and earlier oestrus cycles in spring and Klemt (1986) reported that supplemented mares had more regular oestrus cycles than unsupplemented mares.

However, several studies report no additional benefit from β–carotene supplementation. Eitzer and Rapp (1986) fed 12 out of 24 mares a β-carotene supplement and found no difference between fertility parameters. Whether unsupplemented mares had a deficiency, however, does not become clear. In a study by Watson *et al.* (1996) 13 mares received a hay diet only (low in β-carotene). Seven of the mares were supplemented with β-carotene but once again no difference in fertility parameters could be seen (Table 9).

There is some contradictory evidence of the beneficial effects of feeding additional β-carotene but it can certainly be concluded that a deficiency of β-carotene would have a detrimental effect on fertility.

Tabel 9. Effect of feeding additional β-carotene on fertility parameters of 13 mares (± s.d.) (Watson et al., 1996).

	Supplemented β-caroteen[1] (n=7)	Hay only (n=6)
Duration of first oestrus signs (days)	5.5 ± 1.7	5.4 ± 0.4
Time between ovulation (days)	21.6 ± 1.9	22.4 ± 1.8
Diameter of follicles on day of ovulation (mm)	41.3 ± 3.4	40.3 ± 3.8
Progesteron concentrations during di-oestrus (ng/ml)	8.6 ± 3.8	8.6 ± 3.8

[1] 1.8 mg/kg bodyweight/day

Research into the influence of folic acid, vitamin E and vitamin D on the fertility of the mare is not currently available. Folic acid requirements are stated to increase during pregnancy (Frape, 1998; Ginther, 1992).

Phytohormones

Finally it is worth mentioning the effect of phyto-hormones (iso-flavins) ingested during grazing on fertility in mares. Cholesterol is the basic and major component for the endogenous synthesis of steroidal hormones like testosterone, estradiol and progesterone. Some chemical substances in plants can inhibit the cholesterol production and can thus be considered as endocrine disruptors and these have been isolated as possible contraceptives in humans (Schwarz *et al.*, 2005; Setchell and Cassidy, 1999). Once again there is no research currently available linking these substances to infertility in mares but a change of pasture may need to be considered when unexplained fertility occurs.

Contamination of feedstuffs with mycotoxines

Recent research has also identified food contamination with mycotoxins as possible causes for abortion, resorption and infertility (McCann *et al.*, 1992). Mycotoxins are fungal metabolites which can be toxic to humans and animals. They are particularly produced in anaerobic conditions and may be taken in via contaminated food. Forage which has developed mouldy patches should therefore be avoided. Mycotoxins are absorbed into the bloodstream from the digestive tract through passive transport across the mucosa and are then broken down through biotransformation in the liver into secondary substances (Hussein *et al.*, 2001). These secondary metabolites are expelled via the urine, although some cannot be excreted and remain in the body. There are several types of mycotoxins, of which Zeraleones produced by the *fusarium species* are known to be harmful to mammals by interfering with oestrogen metabolism. Zeraleones bind to oestrogen receptors intefering with the metabolic control of the oestrus cycle. One of the metabolites of Zeraleones, zeranol, has also been used as an anabolic growth enhancer in pigs and cattle (Fitzpatrik et al, 1989). Another mycotoxin, ergot alkaloid, has been identified as leading to resorption and abortion in farm animals and horses (CVB, 2003). Abortion in particular occurs because this mycotoxin leads to the narrowing of bloodvessels supplying the placenta and the ambilical cord.

Mould contaminated food has been directly linked to infertility, abnormal pregnancies (early or late parturition), dismature and weak foals and abortions (Monroe *et al.*, 1988; Putnam, 1991 and Cross *et al.*, 1994). McCann *et al.* (1992) studied the effect of feeding tall fescue grass and hay contaminated with the endophyte *Acremonium coenophialum* (producing the mycotoxin sterigmatocystine) in 30 three year old pregnant mares over a period of three years. They showed that the prolactin metabolism was significantly affected ($p<0.01$) and that progesteron concentrations in the blood were abnormally reduced ($p < 0.05$). Three weeks after the contaminated hay was removed values returned to normal.

Dutton (1996) described the danger of Fusarium infections in feed stuffs. The moulds occur particularly in grains and in the USA maize contamination has let to toxic conditions in farm animals and horses. In horses fumosines are the cause of equine leucoencephalomalacia, but links with fertility in mares have not been made so far.

Conclusion: The mare

Advice on feeding broodmares before and during conception is often based on general assumptions passed on within the industry. This study aimed to give an overview of scientific evidence currently available on fertility in mares in relation to nutritional factors. Certainly the current understanding of the fertility cycle highlights several areas which may be affected by nutrition. The amount and sometimes level of the literature found was inadequate and much of the research stemmed from before 1990. Research did highlight that there is a basis for feeding mares at increasing energy levels prior to conception (this may support the argument for spring grass) and that provision of good quality proteins and adequate levels of minerals and vitamins should be ensured. In conjunction with these findings a correct body condition score should always be aimed at. There is no evidence for reduced fertility in obese mares. Finally, particularly as the feeding of ensiled forages increases in Europe, forages should be analysed for mould and toxin contamination regularly.

Stallion fertility

Stallion fertility is usually identified by the quality of semen and the sexual behaviour (libido) of a given animal (Magistrini *et al.*, 1996); however, both these aspects do not reflect necessarily the breeding ability of a stallion, since its breeding soundness is not strictly correlated with the number of pregnant mares per season (Dowsett and Pattie, 1982; Palmer and Fauquenot, 1984; Jasko *et al.*, 1990). Despite the need for a better evaluation of the breeding capacity of a stallion over more reproductive seasons, the starting point to evaluate the breeding reliability of a male is mainly linked to the semen characteristics of the animal. Within this evaluation two main aspects are related to stallion fertility, i.e. the sexual maturity and the sperm production ability; both these factors are mainly under the endocrine control and, therefore, interactions between nutrition and a normal endocrine function could interfere with a normal fertility in the stallion, particularly with regard to the quality of semen.

Sexual maturity

The sexual maturity, i.e. the time of maximum reproductive capacity, is the result of a specific anatomic, endocrine and behavioural process that starts during the foetal life and ends when the stallion is about five years of age (Johnson *et al.*, 1991). However, the lack of data regarding the development of a gametogenic activity in the foal, leads to the use of data from other mammals, particularly from cattle, to explain the development of a reproductive ability and the endocrine events involved in the onset of puberty. For example, the increase in the circulating gonadotrophins and sexual steroids (testosterone, estrogens) could be dated in bulls at about 6 months of age (Amann *et al.*, 1986; McCarthy *et al.*, 1979; Naden *et al.*, 1990) and, according to Amann (1993b), also in the foal the infantile stage could end in a pre-pubertal stage at ≥6 months, depending on breed and season of birth. At this stage the new endocrine framework leads to the differentiation of Sertoli cells, increases in the number of Leydig cells and to the beginning of testosterone secretion. Close to puberty, spermatogenesis starts and the stallion acquires the ability of a successful reproductive activity. However, these end points do not reflect the beginning of a sexual maturity, which occurs

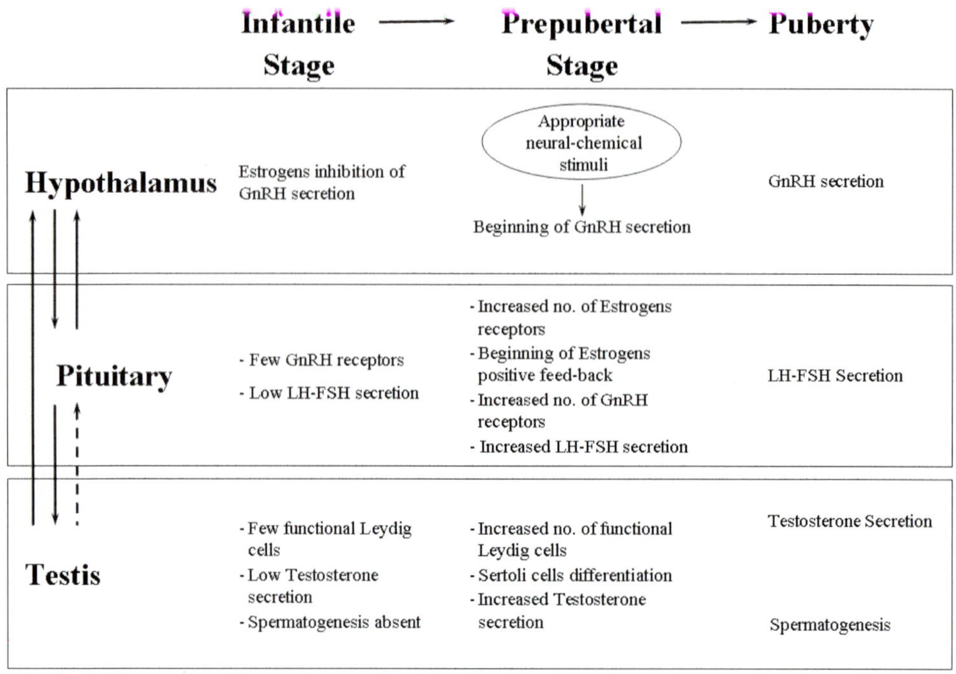

Figure 1. Hypothesised endocrine events involved in puberty (From Marinelli and Bono, 1999).

2 to 4 years later than puberty for the stallion.Figure one hypothesises the possible endocrine events involved in the acquisition of puberty, although the process is still not well known (Amann, 1993b; Marinelli and Bono, 1999).

Following the puberty, which most likely occurs between 14 to 24 months of age (Marinelli and Bono, 1999), the post pubertal phase is associated with an enhanced interrelationship within the hypothalamus-pituitary axis and testis, leading to an increased spermatozoa production (Amann, 1993b). However, it has been demonstrated that only at about 4-5 years of age a stallion reaches its maximum reproductive capacity, when the anatomical development is completed (Amann, 1993a) and the spermatogenesis is at its most efficient stage (Pickett, 1993; Table 8). It is therefore essential to avoid too precocious exploitation of young stallions or a limited use of older animals (Marinelli and Bono, 1999).

An efficient production of semen from sexual mature stallions depends on the testicular development and in particular on the number of Sertoli cells, whose number do not change after puberty (De Kretser and Kerr, 1988; Hochereau de Reviers *et al.*, 1987; Setchell, 1978). Although the number of Sertoli cells are under the control of genetic factors (Russel and Peterson, 1984), it is nevertheless important to avoid any possible negative effect on their proliferation up to puberty in order to obtain a complete sexual maturity in the male. A correct control of environmental, pharmacological and toxicological factors in the foal and in the young stallion are then essential for a regular testicular development and differentiation (Hagenas *et al.*, 1978; Williams and Foster, 1988).

Sexual maturity and nutrition

It is well known that normal growth is essential to ensure a correct development and structural soundness which are correlated with a normal gametogenic activity and fertility in the stallion

Table 10. Effect of age on sexual maturity of stallions (adapted from Amann, 1993a and from Pickett, 1993).

	Age of the stallions (*)	
	2-3 yrs	4-6 yrs
Testicular weight:		
• parenchyma (g)	105	146
• tunica albuginea (g)	12	15
Mean scrotal width (mm)	96	100
Parenchymal composition:		
• Leydig cells (%)	6	12
• other interstitial cells (%)	22	16
Seminal characteristics:		
• gel free semen volume (ml)	14.2	26.2
• total spermatozoa (10^9)	1.8	3.6
• spermatozoa concentration (10^6/ml)	120.4	160.9
• motility (%)	55	63
Daily sperm output (10^9/testis)	1.3	2.7

*Data in different column were statistically different ($P<0.05$)

(NRC, 1989; Martin-Rosset, 1990; Lewis, 1996). Under normal environmental condition it seems that no limiting factors exist for a correct growth and development of a young stallion promoting an average sexual maturity and fertility. However, correct feeding management is essential to cover animal nutritional requirements in relation to its age, weight, adult body weight and planned average daily gain (NRC, 1989; Martin-Rosset, 1990; Lewis, 1996).

Malnutrition in other species does not seem to impair fertility but there is no research to verify this in stallions,. Ghafoorunissa (1989) showed that feeding rats at 60 and 80% of voluntary intake had an effect on body weight gain but did not change epididymal sperm count, relative weights of reproductive organs and fertility measured as no. of pregnant females. Furthermore, severely restricted feeding programs during growth in male guinea-pigs showed continued maintenance of spermatogenesis, despite a delayed sexual maturity and generally lower blood testosterone level, indicating that testicular development is more affected by age rather than nutrition (Slob *et al.*, 1979). However, feed deprivation during dam gestation in mice could play a negative effect on reproduction of male offspring, higher than the effect on female offspring (Meikle and Westberg, 2001). Indeed, male offspring of food deprived dams had smaller preputial glands and seminal vesicles, were about 50% less frequently dominant and were less attractive to oestrous of females in comparison to male offspring from normally fed mothers. This negative testosterone-mediated effect in males could result, at the end, in a loss of competition in intrasexual encounters, reducing survivorship. Therefore, it could be of interest only within a wild or feral group of animals, rather than in a domesticated population.

In another study in sheep, undernutrition during gestation could modify male foetus development, depending on the timing of malnutrition. Rae *et al.* (2002) have found that foetal mass could be significantly reduced after 110 days of gestation in undernourished sheep (50% of requirement) without any effect on testes mass and testosterone secretion. However, no significant effect were found when undernutrition lasted up to 65 days of gestation or was alternated with a normal feeding plan. Indeed, the only reported effect of malnutrition in sheep is a delay in the puberty and a lighter body weight (Robinson, 1996).

Instead of general malnutrition there could be a greater effect of certain specific nutrient deficiencies on puberty and sexual maturity. For instance, Zinc deficiency has been investigated as a possible source of impaired fertility in males. Zinc is involved in several enzymatic reactions as a component of many metallo-enzymes (Smith and Akinbamijo, 2000). These enzymes are mostly associated with carbohydrate metabolism, protein synthesis and nucleic acid metabolism, and they are therefore essential in the gonads, where an active mitosis process takes place. For these reasons, zinc deficiency has been reported as a possible source of impaired spermatogenesis in adults, but it also could be negatively implicated in development of primary and secondary sex organs in male (Underwood, 1981). Pitts *et al.* (1966) have found that a zinc deficient diet given to Holstein bull-calves from 8 to 21 weeks of age produced a reduction in the testicular size; however, the effect of the low level deficiency were not permanent, since it was reversed by increasing dietary zinc supplementation when animals were 64 weeks old.

Among other possible negative effects of nutrition, toxic substances can have a negative effect on sexual function when contamination occurs during the prenatal or infantile stage. Recently, Veeramachaneni *et al.* (2006) have shown in Dutch-belted rabbits that the fungicide Vinclozolin given during gestation and up to 4 weeks after parturition had a negative effect on copulatory ability, FSH secretion and spermatogenesis of offspring with additional higher incidence of degenerative changes in seminiferous tubules.

In summary, although there is no specific evidence for horses, it could be speculated that malnutrition could affect the onset of puberty, delay the time at which sexual maturity is reached and negatively affect semen characteristics in this species. However, the sometimes temporary reported effect of malnutrition and, in some cases, its reversibility leads to the conclusion that such an incorrect feeding management in foals, yearlings and long yearlings, has no great long term effect on sexual ability of young stallions. However, more problems could arise from an incorrect growth in an opposite sense or from management practices such as the attempts to discourage masturbation (spontaneous erection and penile movements) because unaesthetic in show situations. In the latter case, McDonnell and Hinze (2005) have shown that aversive conditioning of masturbation caused significant modification of sexual behaviour and decreased seminal characteristics.

In terms of unbalanced nutrition and, particularly, an excess of feeding in foals and yearlings, its negative effect is more related to a variety of possible developmental orthopaedic diseases (DOD) rather than a direct effect on reproduction. Although the optimum growth rate and energy intake have not been established, high intake of soluble carbohydrates have been associated with DOD (NRC, 1989, Ellis, 2005)

Sperm production in the adult stallion

The reproductive activity of the adult stallion is, as that of mare, under the main control of the season. Although semen production and collection can be performed all rear round, seasonal influences on sexual behaviour and on both spermatozoa and seminal plasma characteristics have been reported (Johnson and Thompson, 1983; Johnson and Thompson, 1987; Pickett *et al.*, 1970; Pickett *et al.*, 1976). The positive effect of photoperiod, although not demonstrated on stallions as in mares, seems the key event that regulates the sperm production and output (Pickett, 1993). Indeed, a reduction in the FSH, LH and Testosterone concentrations in blood has been reported for the winter season in stallions, together with a reduction in testicular size. On the other hand, an enhancement on the frequency of GnRH pulse has been reported approaching the reproductive season, thus increasing the gonadotrophin release by the pituitary (Johnson and Thompson, 1983; Thompson *et al.*, 1985; Thompson *et al.*, 1986, Nett, 1993). However, the reproductive activity of the male is not only under the control of FHS, LH and Testosterone. Indeed, many other chemical mediators, endocrine and paracrine factors are involved in regulating the reproductive activity and, therefore, play an important role in the male fertility (Amann, 1993b; Carreau, 1996; Skinner, 1991; Spiteri-Grech and Nieschlag, 1993, Roser, 2001). Moreover, other hormones such as prolactine, growth hormone and insulin seem to exert testicular effects (Matsumoto, 1989; Weinbauer and Nieschlag, 1995; Huhtaniemi and Toppari, 1995). Therefore, an intricate network of cellular interactions is involved in regulating spermatogenesis in the male (Roser, 2001), and season, age and exploitation of the stallion could interfere with a regular and normal spermatozoa production, affecting sometimes the fertility and the sexual behaviour of the male (Pickett et al, 1976).

Sperm production and nutrition in the adult

Feeding stallions for a normal sperm production and quality is not too specialised. Indeed, both NRC (1989) and INRA (Martin-Rosset, 1990) suggest moderate requirements during the reproductive season, on average 25% higher than requirements for maintenance, i.e. outside of the breeding season (Table 11). This equates to a similar feeding level as that recommended for geldings and mares in light work (NRC, 1989).

The only exception between the two systems, despite the expression of energy (digestible vs. net energy=equine forage units) and protein (crude vs. digestible protein), is mainly in the much higher protein requirement indicated by the French system in stallions during the breeding season. Energy, calcium and phosphorus supplementation due to the breeding activity are enhanced within a similar range comparing the two systems. On the other hand, Lewis (1996) has pointed out that the increase requirements for breeding are small, since they are due to a physical activity linked to a higher pacing and nervousness. Indeed, compared to sports horses which can require up to twofold the energy for maintenance, stallions during the breeding season have moderate requirements. To avoid weight loss during the reproductive season, due mostly to reduced appetite, it appears important the quality of food, particularly its palatability and the energy density.

In relation to the quality of feed it has been demonstrate by Nadal *et al.*(1997) that prolactin level, insulin and circulating glucose are stimulated differently in stallions fed with pellet feed rather than corn or chopped alfalfa. Particularly, chopped alfalfa produced a prolactin response not followed by an enhanced insulin and glucose response as for corn or pellet feed. In human and laboratory animals a possible negative effect of prolactin on sexual behaviour has been demonstrated (Sobrinho, 1993;

Table 11. NRC (1989) and INRA (Martin-Rosset, 1990) requirement for stallions.

	Maintenance (M)	Breeding season (B)	Difference (B-M/M)
NRC:			
• Digestible energy (Mcal/d)	16.4	20.5	25.0%
• Crude Protein (g/d)	656	820	25.0%
• Calcium (g/d)	20	25	25.0%
• Phosphorus (g/d)	14	18	28.6%
INRA:			
• Net energy (UFC/d)	5.8	7.3	25.9%
• MAD* (g/d)	400	550	37.5%
• Calcium (g/d)	25	30	20.0%
• Phosphorus (g/d)	15	18	20.0%

*Digestible protein (*matiéres azotées digestibles*)

Carrani *et al.*, 1996), highlighting for the necessity for further studies on the relationship between quality of feeding and reproduction in stallions.

Studies on Simmental and Hereford beef bulls have shown that neither high energy levels nor low energy feeding for 200 days modified serving capacity and semen morphology in young animals (Pruitt and Corah, 1985). However, Coulter *et al.* (1997 and 1987) have indicated a better reproductive potential from a moderate energy diet given to beef or beef cross bulls after weaning, with an increased testicular tone, reduced temperature testicular gradient, better motility and less defective cells than those on a high energy diet (Table 12).

Reviewing the effects of nutrition on boars, bulls and rams, Brown (1994) has reported that dietary restriction of energy and protein affected adult males less than in young males, and that only severe malnutrition could result in permanent damage in gonadal and neural tissue. Restricted feed intake could reduce both androgens and semen quality but the re-feeding at normal level restored reproductive functions.

A multitude of studies performed in sheep and ram by Australian authors showed that instead of feed energy or protein levels, the influence of nutrition on reproduction processes would be mediated via effects of dietary constituents on the hypothalamic-pituitary axis and, in some cases, by direct effect of single constituent on testis. (Blache *et al.*, 2002; Blache *et al.*, 2000; Hotzel *et al.*, 1997; Walkden–Brown *et al.*, 1994). Particularly, glucose did not seem directly involved in stimulating endocrine responses in sheep (Blache *et al.*, 2002), while fatty acid administration seemed to stimulate GnRH release by the pituitary, acting subsequently at testicular level in rams increasing testicular size (Blache *et al.*, 2002; Blache *et al.*, 2000; Boukhliq and Martin, 1997; Boukhliq *et al.*, 1997). However, all these studies did not demonstrate a significant effect of diet on seminal characteristics of rams and bucks, but only the possible modulation of seasonal activity in sheep and goat males.

Table 12. Effects of different energy levels in feeding bulls for 168 d after weaning (adapted from Coulter et al. 1997).

	Energy level of the diet		P
	Moderate	High	
Scrotal circumference (cm)	31.1±0.2	32.2±0.3	<0.05
Testicular tone (mm of displacement)	19.6±0.1	19.4±0.1	<0.05
Scrotal surface temperature gradient (°C)	3.9±0.1	3.4±0.1	<0.02
Progressive Motile Sperms (%)	53.4±2.1	44.5±2.4	<0.01
Normal Cells (%)	68.8±2.1	62.5±2.5	<0.01

Sperm production and micronutrients

Many important functions can be ascribed to micronutrients, such as intracellular detoxification of free radicals, synthesis of steroids and hormones, metabolism of carbohydrates, protein and nucleic acids. They are therefore essential for spermatogenesis and for sexual behaviour and libido in males (Smith and Akinbanijo, 2000).

Vitamin A in livestock is converted from its inactive form: beta-carotene or provitamin A. This vitamin is involved in spermatogenesis and it may play a very important role in conditioning the quality of semen. A positive effect of β-carotene on spermatogenesis and therefore on the quality of sperm ejaculated has been reported in bulls from Weiss (1975), and from Klug *et al.* (1976) that indicated an improvement of sperm motility and a reduction in the number of abnormal spermatozoa. However, on stallions Ralston *et al.* (1986) have not identified any beneficial effect of vitamin A supplementation given for 3 month during the reproductive season to stallions both in terms of spermatozoa motility and scrotal width. These differences between species could be due to different sperm concentration and motility between bulls and stallions, and due to the lower variability in stallion semen but also due to the different control groups used. Contro bulls used by the German study had low β-carotene in the diet, while control stallions used by Ralston *et al.* (1986) where probably in a normal level of β-carotene; thus the absence of beneficial effect on stallion reproduction could be interpreted as a consequence of no beneficial effect of a higher than normal dose of vitamin A.

With regard to Vitamin C or Ascorbic Acid, a possible positive role of this substance on semen by acting as an antioxidant has been hypothesised. However, in the past contradictory results have been found on fertility of stallions for this vitamin (NRC, 1989; Ralston et al, 1988). In spite of this, a recent survey on humans has pointed out that vitamin C intake was associated with a higher total sperm count and percentage of progressive motile spermatozoa, although surprisingly no dose related relationship between semen quality and vitamin C intake could be determined (Eskenazi *et al.*, 2005).

Particular attention among micronutrients has been placed on vitamin E, alone or in relationship with selenium. Smith and Akinbamijo (2000) have reported for both micronutrients an antioxidant effect and, therefore, a role of cell protection from peroxides formed from fatty acids. While vitamin E should be involved in a specific antioxidant effect at membrane level, selenium effect is directly associated with antioxidant destruction it is a component of the glutathione peroxidase, i.e. preventing radicals from attaching to cell membranes (Smith and Akinbamijo, 2000). In male reproduction there are findings in pigs and humans that indicate a positive role of vitamin E and/or selenium on fertility. Particularly, Liu *et al.* (1982) reported reduction in testicular size and spermatogenesis, with reduced sperm motility in boars due to Vitamin E deficiency. Subsequently, Marin-Guzman *et al.* (1997) confirmed these findings, pointing out that a prolonged absence in boars of vitamin E or selenium decreased sperm motility and increased abnormal spermatozoa. Moreover, they indicated a greater detrimental effect of selenium deficiency (60.4 vs. 87.9% motility and 24.2 vs. 61.9% normal sperm) rather than vitamin E deficiency (72.5 vs. 75.8% motility and 41.4 vs. 44.8% normal sperm). This was seen not only in sperm quality but also in terms of fertilised gilts, the number of which was significantly higher with selenium supplementation was given in comparison with vitamin E supplementation (Table 13).

However, in men, Eskenazi *et al.* (2005), have reported a significant improvement of motility and motile sperms concentration in high vitamin E fed subjects, postulating that healthy diets with supplements of antioxidant may enhance semen quality and fertility.

Among micronutrients, also L-carnitine, a vitamin-like compound synthesised in liver, kidney and brain from essential amino acids as lysine and methionine, has been hypothesised to play an important role in fertility. Indeed, it has been found in seminal plasma and spermatozoa, and its known involvement in cellular energy metabolism has suggested investigations on possible relationship between L-carnitine supplementation and seminal characteristics. However, Kozink *et al.* (2004) have not found any beneficial effect of L-carnitine supplementation on boars at a dose of 500 mg/d on a 5 months period. In this study no positive effect was seen on semen volume, sperm concentration, total spermatozoa and sperm motility. On the other hand, Stradaioli *et al.* (2004) indicated a positive effect of 20 g/d of L-carnitine administration for 60 days in oligoasthenospermic stallions in comparison to normal stallions. Normal stallions did definitely not show any particular enhancement of progressive motility after 30 or 60 days from L-carnitine supplementation (Table 14), while oligoasthenospermic stallions showed a significant increase of motility, that was almost twofold after 60 days (Table 14).

Table 13. Effects of dietary selenium and vitamin E on fertility of boars (adapted from Marin-Guzman et al. 1997).

	Se (ppm)			Vitamin E, IU/kg		
	0.0	0.5	P	0	220	P
Sperm concentration (10^6/ml)	290	253	n.s.	238	306	n.s.
Total sperm (10^9)	43.5	38.9	n.s.	38.0	44.2	n.s.
GSH-Px activity:						
• sperm (units/ml)	579	977	<0.01	753	804	n.s.
• seminal plasma (units/ml)	12.3	37.3	<0.01	26.9	23.0	n.s.
α-Tocopherol:						
• sperm (μg/ml)	0.412	0.349	n.s.	0.167	0.595	<0.05
• seminal plasma (μg/ml)	0	0	n.s.	0	0	n.s.
Sperm motility (%)	60.4	87.9	<0.01	72.5	75.8	n.s.
Normal sperm (%)	24.2	61.9	<0.01	41.4	44.8	n.s.
Fertilization rate on gilts (%)	73.4	98.5	<0.05	89.1	82.7	n.s.

The positive effect on motility was also accompanied by an increased percentage of morphologically normal spermatozoa in supplemented oligoasthenospermic stallions (Table 14).

Reviewing important micronutrients for feeding stallions, copper, molybdenum and zinc have also received attention as possible substances that can play an active role in fertility. Zinc and its possible role has been discussed above. In regard to copper and molybdenum, literature is scarce for stallions. Nevertheless, reproductive disorders have been reported for these interrelated micronutrients in bulls by Thomas and Moss (1951), who found negative effects of high molybdenum concentrations (which inhibit copper metabolism), on sexual behaviour and spermatogenesis. However, reproductive disorders due to these micronutrients are after all scarce and related to grazing deficiency (Smith and Akinbamijo, 2000). Therefore, in stallions which are not turned out to pasture for long periods care must be taken as to an adequate supply of these micronutrients (NRC, 1998; Lewis, 1996).

Table 14. Seminal characteristics evaluated at 0, 30 and 60 days from oral L-carnitine administration in stallion of different fertility (from Stradaioli et al. 2004).

	Normal fertility stallions			Oligoasthenospermic stallions		
	d 0	d 30	d 60	d 0	d 30	d 60
Gel-free volume (ml)	56.8	80.5	68.7	81.5	50.0	45.6
Sperm concentration (10^6/ml)	191.8	143.3	205.5	51.8	53.9	63.7
Total sperm concentration (10^9)	9.1	9.5	11.8	3.5	2.6	3.2
Progressive motility (%)	59.9	62.3	62.8	26.8	39.1[a]	48.8[b]
Morphologically normal unstained (%)	58.0	61.4	60.5	35.9	40.0[a]	50.3[b]
Total live abnormal spermatozoa (%)	18.8	19.0	17.2	22.0	21.8	23.1

[a, b] indicates significant differences within group of stallions at different time,

Sperm production ability and other nutritional factors

Among other nutrients that could be reviewed in literature used in stallion feeding, positive effect of live yeast has been reported on feeding digestibility and seminal characteristics in Italian saddle stallions (Anglo-Arabo-Sarda breed). Two months after the end of a live yeast administration lasting 90 days, stallion exhibited a better progressive motile concentration and an increased percentage of live spermatozoa (Rassu *et al.*, 1999).

Feeding stallions with decosahexanoic acid (DHA), a long-chain polyunsaturated fatty acid (omega 3 series) with hypothesised positive effect on sperm membrane, Brinsjko et al, (2005) have reported no beneficial effects of 14 weeks of supplementation on sperm motion characteristics, total and progressive motility after 24 hrs of cooled storage or after freezing and thawing of semen.

As described above (mare fertility) mycotoxins (i.e. zearalenone) have received attention by researchers as possible source of impaired fertility in mammals (Adams *et al.*, 1993). However, no studies have been carried out on males investigating possible negative effects on fertility. At present only studies on light mares have been performed, but neither effects on pregnancy, nor on newborns have been investigated (Raymond *et al.*, 2003).

Finally, pesticide have been investigated mostly in men, where no particular risk effect has been reported on spermatozoa concentration, morphology and motility (Juhler et al, 1999).

Conclusion - The stallion

Literature regarding the relationship between nutrition and fertility in stallions is generally scarce and sometimes conclusions on possible negative effects of feeding are derivates from other species. Much work has been done in cattle, swine, sheep and goat, rather than in the horse. On the other hand, this ranking reflects the relative low interest in horse reproduction when compared with species that have a greater economical magnitude as food producing livestock. Moreover, much research has examined the effects of mild to moderate changes in food availability on the activity of reproductive axis. Indeed, only prolonged or severe undernutrition and/or single high deficiency could be related to reproductive hormone suppression, with accompanying decreases in fertility. The sensitivity of the reproductive axis to severe malnutrition would be advantageous when energy is a limiting factor and energy could be saved avoiding reproduction. This postulate is even more important for females than for males, where reproduction has a very low requirement in comparison with pregnancy and/or lactation (Cameron, 1996). Moderate or mild underfeeding has been demonstrated to be of less magnitude on male reproduction and in many cases can be reverted with an adequate feeding regime. Therefore, effects of nutrition on stallion fertility mostly relate to a reduction in semen quality rather than semen quantity (Pickett and Shiner, 1994). On the other hand it has to be pointed out that normal sperm output in stallions is larger than that required, thus the mean sperm concentration used per insemination dose is much higher than the suggested minimum (Pickett *et al.*, 1976; Mantovani *et al.*, 2002). Moreover, sub-fertility in stallions, even though not scientifically proven, is related by most practitioners more to genetic causes rather than to wrong feeding practices. As for the mare, the effect of toxin contamination and its relationship with fertility may also need to be explored further with regards to stallion fertility.

References

Adams, R.S., B.K. Kephart, V.A. Ishler, L.J. Hutchinson, G.W. Roth, 1993. Mold and mycotoxin problems in livestock feeding. College of Agricultural Science, Pennsylvania State University, PA.

Ahlswede, L. and H. Konermann, 1980. Experiences with oral and parenteral administration of β-carotene in the horse. Praktische Tierarzt 68: 56-60.

Allen, W.R., 1980. Hormonal Control of early pregnancy. Vetenary Clinics of North America: Large Animal Practice, Vol 2., 2: 291-302.

Allen, W.R., 2001. Luteal deficiency and embryo mortality in the mare. Reprod Domest Anim. 36 (3-4): 121-31.

Amann, R.P., M.E. Wise, J.D. Glass and T.M. Nett, 1986. Prepubertal changes in the hypothalamic-pituitary axis of Holstein bulls. Biol. Reprod. 34: 71-80.

Amann, R.P., 1993a. Functional anatomy of the adult male. In: Equine Reproduction, A.O. McKinnon and J.L. Voss (editors), Lea & Febiger, Philadelphia, 645-657.

Amann, R.P., 1993b. Physiology and endocrinology. In: Equine Reproduction, A.O. McKinnon and J.L. Voss (editors), Lea & Febiger, Philadelphia, 658-685.

Anwandter, Q.C.G., 1974. Progesteron- und β-Carotin-Gehalt des Bovinen Corpus Luteum wahrend der verschiedenen Phasen des Sexualzyklus in Abhangigkeit von der Jahreszeit. Dissertation, Tierarztl. Hochschule, Hannover

Ashworth, C.J. and C. Antipatis, 2001. Micronutrient programming of development throughout gestation. Reproduction. 122(4): 527-535.

Banach, M.A. and J.W. Evans, 1981a. The effects of energy intake during gestation and lactation on reproductive performances in mares. Proceedings of the Western Section of the American Society of Animal Sciences, Vancouver, British Columbia, 23-25 June 1981, 32: 264-267.

Banach, M.A. and J.W. Evans, 1981b. Effect of inadequate energy during gestation and lactation on the estrous cycle and the conception rates of mares and on their foal weights. Proc. 7th Equine nutri. Phys. Symp. P 97.

Belonje, P.C. and C.H van Niekerk, 1975. A review of the influence of nutrition upon the oestrus cycle and early pregnancy in the mare. J. Reprod. Fert., Suppl. 23: 167-169.

Blache, D., C.L. Adam and G.B. Martin, 2002. The mature male sheep: a model to study the effects of nutrition on the reproductive axis. Reprod. Suppl. 59: 219-233.

Blache, D., L.M. Chagas, M.A. Blackberry, P.E. Vercoe and G.B. Martin, 2000. Metabolic factors affecting the reproductive axis in male sheep. J. Reprod. Fertil. 120: 1-11.

Bondi, A and D. Skan, 1984. Vitamin A and carotene in animal nutrition. Progess in food and nutrition Sci. 8: 165-191.

Boukhliq, R. and G.B. Martin, 1997. Administration of fatty acids and gonadotrophin secretion in the mature ram. Anim. Reprod. Sci. 49 (2-3): 143-159.

Boukhliq, R., C.L. White, M.A. Blackberry and P.J. Murray, 1997. Role of glucose, fatty acids and protein in regulation of testicular growth and secretion of gonadotrophin, prolactin, somatotrophin and insulin in the mature ram. Reprod. Fertil. Dev. 9 (5): 515-524.

Bridges, T.S., T.R. Davidson, C.S. Chamberlain, R.D. Geisert and L.J. Spicer, 2002. Changes in follicular fluid steroids, insulin-like growth factors, IGF and IGF-binding protein concentration and proteolytic activity during equine follicular development. J. Anim. Sci. 80: 179-190.

Brinsko, S.P., D.D. Varner, C.C. Love, T.L. Blanchard, B.C. Day, M.E. Wilson, 2005. Effect of feeding a DHA-enriched nutriceutical on the quality of fresh, cooled and frozen stallion semen. Theriogenology 63: 1519–1527.

Brown, B.W. 1994. A review of nutritional influences on reproduction in boars, bulls and rams. Reprod. Nutr. Dev. 34 (2): 89-114.

Cameron, J.L. 1996. Regulation of reproductive hormone secretion in primates by short-term changes in nutrition. J. Reprod. Fertil., Reviews of reproduction. 1: 117-126.

Carrani, C., A.R.M. Granata, M. Faustini Fustini and P. Marrana, 1996. Prolactin and testosterone: their role in male sexual function. Int. J. Androl. 19: 48-54.

Carreau, S., 1996. Paracrine control of human Leydig cell and Sertoli cell functions. Folia. Histochem. Cytobiol. 34 (3-4): 111-119.

Cooke, B.C. and N. Comben, 1978. A study of the relationship between β-carotene and fertility problems in dairy cows. Anim. Prod. Abstr. 26: 356-357.

Coulter, G.H., R.B. Cook and J.P. Kastelic, 1997. Effects of dietary energy on scrotal surface temperature, seminal quality, and sperm production in young beef bulls. J. Anim. Sci. 75: 1048-1052.

Coulter, G.H., T.D. Carruthers, R.P. Amann and G.C. Kozub, 1987. Testicular development, daily sperm production and epididymal sperm reserves in 15-month-old Angus and Hereford bulls: Effects of bull strain plus dietary energy. J. Anim. Sci. 64: 254-262.
Cross, D.L., L.M. Redmond and J.R. Strickland, 1994. Equine Fescue Toxicosis: signs and solutions. J. Anim. Sci. 73: 988-908.
CVB, 2003. Mycotoxine. [Review into the occurrence and dedection of mycotoxins in animal feed; Review on the effect of mycotoxins on single stomached agricultural animals] Kwaliteitsreeks nr. 88 and 89. Productschap Diervoeder, Den Haag.
Davies Morel, M.C.G., 1993. Equine reproductive physiology, breeding and stud management. Farming Press.
De Kretser, D.M. and J.B. Kerr, 1988. The cytology of the testis. In: The Physiology of Reproduction, E. Knobil and J. Neill (editors), Raven Press, New York, 837-932.
Dohms, T., 2002. Einfluss von genetischen und umweltbedingten Faktoren auf die Fruchtbarkeit von Stuten und Hengsten. Wissenschaftliche Publikation 25. FN-Verlag der Dt. Reiterlichen Vereinigung, Warendorf.
Doreau, M., J.P. Bruhat and W. Martin-Rosset, 1988. Effets du niveau des apports azotés chez la jument en début de lactation, Ann. Zootech., 37, 21-30
Dowsett, K.F. and W.A. Pattie, 1982. Characteristics and fertility of stallion semen. J. Reprod. Fert., Suppl. 32: 1-8.
Drew, B. and J. Williams, 1975. The effect of excess dietary iodine on pregnant mares and foals. The Vetenary Record, August 2: 93-94.
Dutton, M.F., 1996. Fumonisins, mycotoxins of increasing importance: Their nature and their effects. Pharmacol. Ther. 70 (2): 137-161.
Eitzer, O. and H.J. Rapp, 1985. Oral use of synthetic β-carotene in breeding mares. Praktische Tierarzt 66: 123-126.
Ekmann, L., 1970. Klinisch chemische Diagnostik von Schilddrusenstorungen un der Veterinarmedizin. Wien, Tierarztl. Wschr. 57: 286-292.
Ellis, A.D., 2005. The potential impact of nutrition on bone growth in horses, In: Julliand and Martin-Rosset, eds. 2005.The growing horse: nutrition and prevention of growth disorders, Second European Conference on Equine Nutrition, ENESAD, Dijon, France, EAAP publication No. 114, p 257-272, Wageningen Academic Publishers
Ellis, A.D., 2002. Protein and essential amino acid requirements in the horse. Intern rapport VPA-02-31. Research Institute for Animal Husbandry, Wageningen University, the Netherlands. 36p.
Ellis, A.D., 2001. Merries voeren veulens. Voeding in relatie tot osteochondrose. Praktijkonderzoek Veehouderij, Wageningen UR, 55p.
Eskenazi, B., S.A. Kidd, A.R. Marks, E. Sloter, G. Block and A.J. Wyrobek, 2005. Antioxidant intake is associated with semen quality in healthy men. Human Reprod. 20 (4): 1006-1012
Ferraro, J. and J.F. Cote, 1984. Broodmare management techniques improve conception rates. Standardbred 12: 56-58.
Finkler-Schade, C., 2000. So wird-bzw bleibt ihre Stute tragend. Der Hannoveraner 6, 00, 74-77.
Fitzgerald, B.P. and C.J. McManus, 2000. Photoperiodic versus metabolic signals as determinants of seasonal anestrus in the mare. Biol Reprod. 63(1): 335-340.
Fitzpatrik, D.W., C.A. Picken, L.C. Murphy and M.M Buhr, 1989. Measurement of the relative binding affinity of zearalenone, alpha-zearalenol and beta-zearalenol for uterine and oviduct estrogen receptors in swine, rats and chickens: an indicator of estrogenic potencies. Comp. Biochem. Physiol. C, 94 (2), 691-694.
Fowden, A.L., R.S. Comline and M. Silver, 1984. Insulin secretion and carbohydrate metabolism during pregnancy in the mare. Equine Vet J. 16(4): 239-246.
Frape, D., 1998. Equine nutrition and feeding, 2nd Edition, Blackwell Science Limited, London.
Freinkel N., N.J. Lewis, R. Johnson and C. Hellerstrom, 1979. Maturation of stimulus recognition and insulin secretion during tissue culture of fetal pancreatic islets. Trans Am Clin Climatol Assoc. 90:86-93
Gentry, L.R., D.L. Thompson Jr., G.T. Gentry, K.A. Davis, R.A. Godke and J.A. Cartmill, 2002. The relationship between body condition, leptin, and reproductive and hormonal characteristics of mares during the seasonal anovulatory period. Journal Anim Sci. 80(10): 2695-2703.
Ghafoorunissa, I.A., 1989. Undernutrition and fertility in male rats. J. Reprod. Fert. 59 (2): 317-320.
Gill, R.J. and G.D. Potter, 1983. Postpartum reproductive performance of mares fed various levels of protein. Texas A&M University, College Station, Texas.

Ginther, O.J. and D.R. Bergfelt, 1993. Growth of small follicles and concentrations of FSH during the equine oestrous cycle. J. Reprod.Fertil. 99(1): 105-111.

Ginther, O.J., 1992. Reproductive biology of the mare: basic and applied aspects. Cross Plains, WI: Equiservices; p. 476–477.

Glade, M.J. and T.H. Belling Jr., 1984. Growth plate cartilage metabolism, morphology and biochemical composition in over- and underfed horses. Growth 48: 473-482.

Guillaume D., B. Bruneau and C. Briant, 2002. Comparison of the effects of two GnRH antagonists on LH and FSH secretion, follicular growth and ovulation in the mare. Reprod. Nutr. Dev. 42(3): 251-264.

Hagenas, L., E.M. Ritzen and H.L. Suginami, 1978. Temperature dependence of Sertoli cell function. Int. J. Androl., Suppl., 2: 449-458.

Henneke, D.R., G.D. Potter and J.L. Kreider, 1981. Rebreeding efficiency in mares fed different levels of energy during late gestation. Proc. Equine Nutr. Phys. Soc. p 101.

Henneke, D.R., G.D. Potter and J.L. Kreider, 1984. Body condition during pregnancy and lactation and reproductive efficiency of mares. Theriogenology 21: 897-909.

Hochereau de Reviers, M.T., C. Monet-Kuntz and M. Courot, 1987. Spermatogenesis and Sertoli cell numbers and function in rams and bulls. J. Reprod. Fertil. Suppl., 34: 101-114.

Hotzel, M.J., A. Caraty and G.B. Martin, 1997. Effects of nutrition on testicular growth in mature Merino rams actively immunized against GnRH. J. Reprod. Fertil. 110 (2): 307-313.

Houseknecht, K.L., C.A. Baile, R.L. Matteri and M.E. Spurlock, 1998. The biology of leptin: a review. J. Anim. Sci. 76(5): 1405-1420.

Huhtaniemi, H. and J. Toppari, 1995. Endocrine, paracrine and autocrine regulation of testicular steroidogenesis. In: Tissue renin-angiotensin system, A.K. Mukhopadhyay and M.K. Raizada (editors), Plenum Press, New York, 33-54.

Hussein, H.S. and J.M. Brasel, 2001. Toxicity, metabolism, and impact of mycotoxins on humans and animals. Toxicology 167 (2): 101-134.

Janosi, S., G. Huszenica, M. Kulcsar and P. Krodi, 1998. Endocrine and reproductive consequences of certain endotoxin-mediated diseases in farm mammals: a review. Acta-Vet-Hung. 46 (1): 71-84.

Jasko, D.J., D.H. Lein and R.H. Foote, 1990. Determination of the relationship between sperm morphologic classifications and fertility in stallions: 66 cases. (1987-1988). J. Amer. Vet. Med. Ass. 197(3): 389-394.

Johnson, L., D.D. Varner and D.L. Thompson Jr., 1991. Effect of age and season on the establishment of spermatogenesis in the horse. J. Reprod. Fertil. Suppl., 44: 87-97.

Johnson, L. and D.L. Thompson Jr., 1983. Age-related and seasonal variation in the Sertoli cell population, daily sperm production and serum concentrations of follicle stimulating hormone, luteinizing hormone and testosterone in stallions. Biol. Reprod. 29: 777-789.

Johnson, L. and D.L. Thompson Jr., 1987. Effect of seasonal changes in Leydig cell number on the volume of smooth endoplasmic reticulum in Leydig cells and intratesticular testosterone content in stallions. J. Reprod. Fertil. 81: 227-232.

Juhler, R.K., S.B. Larsen, O. Meyer, N.D. Jensen, M. Spanò, A. Giwercman and J.P. Bonde, 1999. Human Semen Quality in Relation to Dietary Pesticide Exposure and Organic Diet. Archives of Environmental Contamination and Toxicology. 37 (3): 415-423.

Kilmer, D.N., D.C. Sharp, L.A Berghund, W. Grubaugh, K.J. McDowell and L.S. Peck, 1982. Melatonin rythms in pony mares and foals. J. Reprod. Fert. Suppl. 32: 303.

Klemt, O.W., 1986. The effect of supplementation with synthetic β-carotene on postpartum fertility of thoroughbred mares studied by progesterone estimation in milk. PhD Thesis, Hannover Veterinary School.

Klug, E., R.R. Weiss, L. Ahlswede and G. Schulz, 1976. Effects of beta-carotene and vitamin A on reproductive function in young bulls. Zuchthygiene, 11 (2): 78-79.

Kozink, D.M., M.J. Estienne, A.F. Harper and J.W. Knight, 2004. Effects of dietary l-carnitine supplementation on semen characteristics in boars. Theriogenology 61: 1247–1258

Lewis, L.D., 1996. Feeding and care of the horse. Second Edition. Lippincott Williams & Wilkins, USA.

Lindner, A., M. Haupt, P. von Wittke and H. Sommer, 1993. Effect of Mg supplementation on fertility parameters of mares and vitality of newborn foals. Equine Nutr. Phys. Soc. 305-306.

Liu, C.H., Y.M. Chen, J.Z. Zhang, M.Y. Huang, Q. Su, Z.H. Lu, R.X. Yin, G.Z. Shao, D. Feng and P.L. Zheng, 1982. Preliminary studies on influence of selenium deficiency to the developments of genital organs and spermatogenesis of infancy boars. Acta Vet. Zootech. Sin. 13: 73-77.

Lothammer, K.H. and L. Ahlswede, 1977. Untersuchungen uber eine spezifische, Vitamin- A-unabhangige Wirkung des β-Carotins auf die Fertalitat des Rindes. 3.Mitteillung: Blutserumuntersuchungen, β-Carotin, Vitamin A, SGOT, Gesamtcholesterin, Glukose, anorganischer Phosphor. Deutsche Tierarztl Wochenschr. 84: 220-226.

Magistrini, M., M. Vidament, F. Clement and E. Palmer, 1996. Fertility prediction in stallions. Animal Reprod. Sci. 42: 181-188.

Mantovani, R., P.R. Avezzù and L. Bailoni, 2002. Factors affecting the success of artificial insemination in horse using refrigerated semen. Proc. of 4th Italian Congress "Nuove acquisizioni in materia di ippologia". Campobasso - Italy, 11-13 July, 2003. 211-218.

Marinelli, L. and G. Bono, 1999. Endocrinologia e fisiologia riproduttiva dello stallone. Summa, 16 (1): 7-15.

Marin-Guzman, J., D.C. Mahan, Y.K. Chung, J.L. Pate and W.F. Pope, 1997. Effects of dietary selenium and vitamin e on boar performance and tissue responses, semen quality, and subsequent fertilization rates in mature gilts. J. Anim. Sci. 75: 2994-3003.

Martin, G.B. and S.W. Walkden-Brown, 1995. Nutritional influences on reproduction in mature male sheep and goats. J. Reprod. Fert., Supplement 49: 437-449.

Martin-Rosset, W. and M. Doreau, 1984. Besoins et alimentation de la jument. 355-370. In Le Cheval, R. Jarrige and W. Martin-Rosset Eds, INRA Editions, Versailles, France.

Martin-Rosset, W., Effect of energy intake in late pregnancy on the mare and the foal during the annual reproductive cycle. (unpublished, personal communication).

Martin-Rosset, W., 1990. L'alimentation des chevaux. INRA, Paris.

Matsumoto, A., 1989. Hormonal control of spermatogenesis. In: The testis, Second Edition, H. Burger and D. de Kretser (editors), Raven Press, New York, 181-196.

McCann, J.S., A.B. Caudle, F.N. Thompson, J.A. Stuedemann, G.L. Heusner and D.L. Thompson Jr., 1992. Influence of endophyte-infected tall fescue on serum prolactin and progesterone in gravid mares. J. Anim. Sci. 70(1): 217-230.

McCarthy, M.S., E.M. Convey and H.D. Hafs, 1979. Serum hormonal changes and testicular response to LH during puberty in bulls. Biol. Reprod. 20: 1221-1227.

McDonnell, S.M. and A.L. Hinze, 2005. Aversive conditioning of periodic spontaneous erection adversely affects sexual behaviour and semen in stallions. Animal Reprod. Sci. 89: 77-92.

Meikle, D. and M. Westberg, 2001. Maternal nutrition and reproduction of daughters in wild house mice (Mus musculus). Reproduction, 122: 437-442.

Merkt, H. and A. Günzel, 1979. A survey of early pregnancy losses in West German Thoroughbred mares. Equine Veterinary Journal, 11 (4): 256-258.

Meyer, H., 1995. Pferdefütterung, 3. Auflage, Blackwell Wissenschafts-Verlag, Berlin, Wien

Meyer, H. and B. Stadermann, 1991. Energie- und Nährstoffbedarf hochtragender Stuten. Pferdeheilkunde 7: 11-20.

Miller, K.F., J.A. Wesson and O.J. Ginther, 1981. Interaction of estradiol and a nonsteroidal follicular fluid substance in the regulation of gonadotropin secretion in the mare. Biol. Reprod. 24 (2): 354-358.

Monroe, J.L., D.L. Cross, L.W. Hudson, D.M. Hendricks, S.W. Kennedy and W.C. Bridges Jr., 1988. Effect of selenium and endophyte-contaminated fescue on performance and production in mares. J. Equine Vet. Sci. 8: 148-153.

Morris, R.P., G. Rich, S. Ralston, E. Squires and B.W. Pickett, 1987. Follicular activity in transitional mares as affected by body condition and dietary energy. Proc 10th Equine Nutrition Physiology Symposium, Colorado State University, p 93.

Nadal, M.R., D.L. Thompson Jr. and L.A. Kincaid, 1997. Effect of feeding and feed deprivation on plasma concentrations of prolactin, insulin, growth hormone, and metabolites in horses. J. Anim. Sci. 75: 736-744.

Naden, J., R.P. Amann and E.L. Squires, 1990. Testicular growth, hormone concentrations, seminal characteristics and sexual behaviour in stallions. J. Reprod. Fertil. 88: 167-176.

Nett, T.M., 1993. Reproductive endocrine function testing in stallions. In: Equine Reproduction, A.O. McKinnon and J.L. Voss (editors), Lea & Febiger, Philadelphia, 821-824.

NRC, 1972. Nutrient Requirement for horses, National Research Council, National Academic Press, Washington DC

NRC, 1989. Nutrient Requirement for horses, National Research Council, National Academic Press, Washington DC.

Oster, M. and S. Paufler, 1990. Analysis of reproductive parameters in mare herds of the chief and state stud farms at Marbach and Schwaiganger. Dtsch Tierarztl Wochenschr. 97(3): 107-114.

Ott, E.A. and R.L. Asquith, 1994. Trace mineral supplementation of broodmares. Journal of Equine Veterinary Science, 14: 93-101.

Palmer, E. and A. Fauquenot, 1984. Mesure e prediction de la fertilité des etalons. Etude méthodologique. In: Le Cheval. Reproduction, selection, alimentation exploitation, R Jarrige and W. Martin-Rosset (editors), INRA, Paris, 113-127.

Pickett, B.W., 1993. Factors affecting sperm production and output. In: Equine Reproduction, A.O. McKinnon and J.L. Voss (editors), Lea & Febiger, Philadelphia, 689-704.

Pickett, B.W. and K.A. Shiner, 1994. Recent developments in artificial insemination in horses. Livest. Prod. Sci. 40: 31-36.

Pickett, B.W., L.C. Faulkner and T.M. Sutherland, 1970. Effect of month and stallion on seminal characteristics and sexual behaviour. J. Anim. Sci. 31: 713-728.

Pickett, B.W., L.C. Faulkner, G.E. Seidel Jr., W.E. Berndtson and J.L.Voss, 1976. Reproductive physiology of the stallion. VI. Seminal and behavioural characteristics. J. Anim. Sci. 43: 617-625.

Pitts, W.J., W.J. Millers and O.T. Fosgate, 1966. Effect of zinc deficiencies and restricted feeding from two to five months of age on reproduction of Holstein bulls. J. Dairy Sci. 49: 995-1000.

Pruitt, R.J. and L.R. Corah, 1985. Effect of energy intake after weaning on the sexual development of beef bulls. I. Semen characteristics and serving capacity. J. Anim. Sci. 61 (5): 1186-1193.

Putnam, M.R., D.I. Bransby, J. Schumacher, T.R. Boosinger, L. Bush, R.A. Shelby, J.T. Vaughan, D. Ball and J.P. Brendemuehl, 1991. Effects of the fungal endophyte Acremonium coenophialum in fescue on pregnant mares and foal viability. Am. J. Vet. Res. 52 (12): 2071-2074.

Rae, M.T., S.M. Rhind, P.A. Fowler, D.W. Miller, C.E. Kyle and A.N. Brooks, 2002. Effect of maternal undernutrition on fetal testicular steroidogenesis during the CNS androgen-responsive period in male sheep fetuses. Reproduction, 124: 33-39.

Ralston, S.L., G.A. Rich, S. Jackson and E.L. Squires, 1986. The effect of vitamin A supplementation on seminal characteristics and vitamin A absorption in stallion. J. Equine Vet. Sci. 6 (4): 203-207.

Ralston, S.L., S. Barbacini, E.L. Squires and C.F. Nockels, 1988. Ascorbic acid supplementation in stallion. J. Equine Vet. Sci. 8 (4): 290-293.

Rassu, S.P.G., A. Cannas, R. Cerchi, S. Delogu and G. Enne, 1999. Live yeast use in stallion feeling. In: Recent progress in animal production science. 1, G. Piva, G. Bertoni, F. Masoero, P. Bani and L. Calamari (editors). FrancoAngeli, Milano, Italy, 809-811.

Raymond, S.L., T.K. Smith and H.V.L.N. Swamy, 2003. Effects of feeding a blend of grains naturally contaminated with Fusarium mycotoxins on feed intake, serum chemistry, and hematology of horses, and the efficacy of a polymeric glucomannan mycotoxin adsorbent. J. Anim. Sci. 81: 2123-2130.

Robinson, J.J., 1996. Nutrition and reproduction. Animal Reprod. Sci. 42: 25-34.

Robinson, J.J., C.J. Ashworth, J.A. Rooke, L.M. Mitchell and T.G. McEvoy, 2006. Nutrition and fertility in ruminant livestock, Animal Feed Science and Technology, 126 (3-4): 259-276.

Roser, J.F., 2001. Endocrine and paracrine control of sperm production in stallions. Animal Reprod. Sci., 68: 139:151.

Russel, L.D. and R.N. Peterson, 1984. Determination of the elongate spermatid-Sertoli cell ratio in various mammals. J. Reprod. Fertil. 70: 635-641.

Schams, D., B. Hoffman, K.H. Lotthammer and L. Ahlswede, 1977. Untersuchungen uber eine spezifische Vitamin A unabhangige Wirkung des β-Carotins auf die Fertalitat des Rindes 4. Mittailung: Auswirkung auf hormonale Parameter wahrend des Zyklus. Deutsche Tierarztl Wochenschrift 84: 307-310.

Schöntaler, S., 1998. Intersuchungen zur Selenversorgung von Vollblutstuten und deren Fohlen während Trächtigkeit, Laktation und Aufzucht. J. Insti. Tierernähtung des Fachbereichs Veterinärmedizin der Freien Univ. Berlin, 2170.

Schwarz, A.E., C.G. Felippe, M.M. Bernardi and H.S. Spinosa, 2005. Impaired female sexual behavior of rat offspring exposed to Solanum lycocarpum unripe fruits during gestation and lactation: Lack of hormonal and fertility alterations, Pharmacology, Biochemistry and Behaviour 81: 928–934.

Seitardis, K., 1963. Untersuchungen uber den Vitamin A- und β-Carotin- Gehalt des Blut-plasmas in Rinderherden mit Storung der Fruchtbarkeit unter besondere Berucksichtigung der Carotinversorgung. Dissertation, Tierarztl. Hochschule, Hannover.

Setchell, B.P., 1978. The Mammalian Testis. Cornell University Press, Ithaca, NY.

Setchell, K.D. and A. Cassidy, 1999. Dietary isoflavones: biological effects and relevance to human health. J. Nutr. 129 (3): 758S-767S.

Skinner, M.K., 1991. Cell-cell interaction in the testis. Endocrine Rev., 12: 45-77.

Slob, A.K., J.T.M. Vreeburg and J.J. Van der Werff ten Bosch, 1979. Body growth, puberty and undernutrition in the male guinea-pig. British J. Nutr. 41 (2): 231-237.

Smith, O.B. and O.O. Akinbamijo, 2000. Micronutrients and reproduction in farm animals. Animal Reprod. Sci. 60-61: 549-560.

Sobrinho, L.G., 1993. The psychogenic effects of prolactin. Acta Endocrinol. Copenh. 129 (1): 38-40.

Spiteri-Grech, J. and E. Nieschlag, 1993. Paracrine factrors relevant to the regulation of spermatogenesis: a review. J. Reprod. Fertil. 98: 1-14.

Sticker, L.S., D.L. Thompson Jr., L.D. Bunting, J.M. Fernandez, C.L. DePew and M.R. Nadal, 1995b. Feed deprivation of mares: plasma metabolites and hormonal concentrations and responses to exercise. J. Anim. Sci. 73: 3696-3704.

Stradaioli, G., L. Sylla, R. Zelli, P. Chiodi and M. Monaci, 2004. Effect of l-carnitine administration on the seminal characteristics of oligoasthenospermic stallions. Theriogenology 62: 761–777

Thomas, J.W. and S. Moss, 1951. The effect of orally administered molybdenum on growth, spermatogenesis and testes histology of young dairy bulls. J. Dairy Sci. 34: 929–934.

Thompson Jr., D.L., R.L. St. George, L.S. Jones and F. Garza Jr., 1985. Patterns of secretion of luteinizing hormone, follicle stimulating hormone and testosterone in stallions during the summer and winter. J. Anim. Sci. 60: 741-748.

Thompson Jr., D.L., L. Johnson, R.L. St. George and F. Garza Jr., 1986. Concentrations of prolactin, luteinizing hormone and follicle stimulating hormone in pituitary and serum of horses: effect of sex, season and reproductive state. J. Anim. Sci. 63: 854-860.

Underwood, E.J., 1981. The mineral nutrition of livestock. Commonwealth Agricultural Bureaux, Slough, England.

Van der Holst, W., E.J. Tjalsma and C.I. Wonder, 1984. Experiences with oral administration of β-carotene to pony mares in early spring. In: 35th Annual Meeting of the European Association of Animal Production. pp 2-15.

Van Niekerk, C.H., 1965. Early embryonic resorption in mares. J. S. Afr. Vet. Med. Ass. 36: 61-69.

Van Niekerk, C.H. and J.S. van Heerden, 1972. Nutrition and ovarian activity of mares early in the breeding season. J. S. Afr. Vet. Med. Ass. 43: 351-360.

Van Niekerk, F.E. and C.H. Van Niekerk, 1997. The effect of dietary protein on reproduction in the mare I. The composition and evaluation of digestability of dietary protein from different sources. Jl. S. Afr. Vet. Med. Ass. 68 (3): 78-80.

Van Niekerk, F.E. and C.H. Van Niekerk, 1997c. The effect of dietary protein on reproduction in the mare III. Ovarian and uterine changes during the anovulatory, transitional and ovulatory periods in the non-pregnant mare. Jl. S. Afr. Vet. Med. Ass. 68 (3): 86-92.

Van Niekerk, F.E. and C.H. Van Niekerk, 1997d. The effect of dietary protein on reproduction in the mare IV. Serum progestagen, FSH, LH and melatonin concentrations during the anovulatory, transitional and ovulatory periods in the non-pregnant mare. Jl. S. Afr. Vet. Med. Ass. 68 (4): 114-120.

Van Niekerk, F.E. and C.H. Van Niekerk, 1998a. The effect of dietary protein on reproduction in the mare V. Endocrine changes and conception during the early postpartum period. Jl. S. Afr. Vet. Med. Ass. 69, 3: 81-88

Van Niekerk, F.E. and C.H. Van Niekerk, 1998b. The effect of dietary protein on reproduction in the mare VI. Serum progestagen concentrations during pregnancy. Jl. S. Afr. Vet. Med. Ass. 69 (4): 143-149.

Van Niekerk, F.E. and C.H. Van Niekerk, 1998c. The effect of dietary protein on reproduction in the mare VII. Embryonic development, early embryonic death, foetal losses and their relationship with serum progestagen. Jl. S. Afr. Vet. Med. Ass. 69 (4): 150-155.

Veeramachaneni, D.N.R., J.S. Palmer, R.P. Amann, C.M. Kane, T.T. Higuchi and K-Y.F. Pau, 2006. Disruption of sexual function, FSH secretion, and spermiogenesis in rabbits following developmental exposure to vinclozolin, a fungicide. Reproduction, 131: 805-816.

Voss, J.L. and B.W. Picket, 1974. Effect of a nutritional supplement on pregnancy rate in nonlactating mares. J. Amer. Vet. Med. Assoc. 165: 702.
Walkden-Brown, S.W., B.J. Restall, B.W. Norton, R.J. Scaramuzzi and G.B. Martin, 1994. Effect of nutrition on seasonal patterns of LH, FSH and testosterone concentration, testicular mass, sebaceous gland volume and odour in Australian Cashmere goats. J. Reprod. Fertil. 102 (2): 351-360.
Watson, E.D., D. Cuddeford and I. Burger, 1996. Short communication: Failure of β-carotene absorption negates any potential effect on ovarian function in mares. Equine Veterinary Journal, 28: 233-236.
Weinbauer, G.F. and E. Nieschlag, 1993. Hormonal control of spermatogenesis. In: Molecular biology of the male reproductive system, D. de Kretser (editor), Academic Press, New York, 99-142
Weiss, R.R., 1975 Infleuce of beta-carotene and vitamin A on defined sexual function of young bulls. Tierarztliche Hochschule Hannover, 133.
Williams, J. and P.M. Foster, 1988. The production of lactate and pyruvate as sensitive indices of altered rat Sertoli cell function in vitro following the addition of various testicular toxicants. Toxicol. Appl. Pharmacol. 94: 160-170.

Intrauterine nutrition: Effect on subsequent health

A.H. Tauson[1], P. Harris[2] and M. Coenen[3]
[1]Department of Animal and Veterinary Basic Sciences, The Royal Veterinary and Agricultural University, Grønnegårdsvej 3, DK-1870 Frederiksberg C, Denmark
[2]Equine Studies Group, WALTHAM Centre for Pet Nutrition, Waltham-on-the-wolds, Nr Melton Mowbray, Leics. LE14 4RT, United Kingdom
[3]Institute of Animal Nutrition, Nutrition Diseases and Dietetics, University of Leipzig, Gustav-Kühn-Strasse 8, 04159 Leipzig, Germany

Abstract

Nutrition during foetal life is a significant factor influencing animal and human health as well as lifetime performance. Intrauterine malnutrition may cause metabolic programming of an individual resulting in metabolic and endocrine adaptations that are beneficial for short-term survival, but that are adverse for adult health and longevity. Potential adverse effects include metabolic syndrome, obesity, type 2 diabetes and cardiovascular disease. This paper reviews main rodent and sheep models used in the study of metabolic programming, and reports the significant outcomes of such studies. The importance of glucocorticoids in metabolic programming is briefly described. Furthermore, items of specific relevance for the horse, including considerations regarding the potential effect of intrauterine nutrient supply on adult athletic performance, are reported. It is concluded that the horse, similar to other mammals, is likely to respond to an inadequate maternal nutrient supply by metabolic adaptations. However, substantially more research is needed for all species, but especially regarding the horse.

Keywords: metabolic programming, rodent model, sheep model, glucocorticoids, horse

Introduction

In the past most studies evaluated the growth of the embryo and the foetus in terms of the quantitative aspects and with respect to the accretion of nutrients and energy. This means that currently we have a solid basis of knowledge regarding the intrauterine growth curves of several species (humans, cattle, sheep, dogs) as well as to some extent the equine. The importance of an adequate nutrient supply during foetal and early neonatal life for animal and human lifetime performance and health is increasingly recognised. However, the regulation of growth, the communication between maternal metabolism and the fertilised egg cell as well as the early embryo is incompletely understood. The intrauterine environment is extremely important for the nutrition of the blastocyst, but we do not know the key nutritional drivers. Later on, when the foetus has become an endocrine sensitive individual, the native endocrine system starts to be trained. Obviously this mechanism is triggered by signals coming from the maternal side. Again, we know, to a certain extent, the consequences of disturbances in this communication, such as retardation in mental capacity of humans, – but our knowledge in this area is fragmentary. This situation is well illustrated by glucocorticoids: the foetal side needs to be effectively protected against flooding by glucocorticoids; however, a complete separation of both systems would retard the maturation of the foetal hypothalamic-pituitary –adrenal axis (Arishima et al 1977). One area of particular interest is currently whether the metabolic status of the pregnant dam may cause a metabolic imprinting or programming of the offspring that in turn results in a life-long metabolic adaptation to conditions experienced during foetal or early neonatal life. Many findings suggest that metabolic programming effects are imposed during certain time periods during gestation, critical windows, and that an inadequate nutrient supply in each of these periods may cause a different response. The "foetal origins" hypothesis proposes that alterations in foetal nutrition and endocrine status result in developmental adaptations that permanently change structure, physiology and metabolism, thereby predisposing to cardiovascular, metabolic, and endocrine disease in adult life (cited from Godfrey and Barker, 2000). This long-term metabolic programming effect has been defined as "a permanent change in the structure or function of an organ resulting from a stimulus or an insult acting at a critical period in life" (Lucas, 1991).

This programming effect may cause metabolic adaptations that are beneficial for the short-term survival but might have adverse effect on adult health and longevity. One such example is early programming of glucose - insulin metabolism by foetal undernutrition. The resulting offspring will, if exposed to poor postnatal nutrition have an advantage of the resulting programming, but if exposed to a situation of energy excess will develop obesity and type 2 diabetes in adulthood, i.e. it will express "the thrifty phenotype" (Hales and Barker, 1992).

Given the profound increase in research into the mechanisms underlying metabolic programming during recent years this review will by no means cover this intriguing area of research completely. The main objectives of this paper are to describe and report the main findings from some frequently used rodent and sheep models, known to induce metabolic programming of the offspring, and to convey the current state of knowledge regarding the horse.

Rodent models

Rodents have been abundantly used in metabolic programming studies, and several models have been developed, most of which operate with either protein restricted isoenergetic diets or with global under-nutrition, i.e. restriction of overall dietary allowances hence providing restricted amounts of energy and protein as well as other nutrients.

Isoenergetic low protein diets

A model used in this approach comprises individually housed virgin female Wistar rats with a body weight of 240-260 g. After mating, on day 0 of gestation, they are allocated to either a control (C) diet containing 20% protein or an isoenergetic low protein (LP) diet with 8% protein. These diets are then fed throughout gestation and lactation. After delivery, when pups are 3 days old, large litters are reduced to 8 pups (4 males and 4 females) (Desai *et al.*, 1996). Pups born to LP dams weigh significantly less than those of C dams at birth, and this pattern prevails throughout the pre-weaning period (Desai *et al.*, 1997a). The rat pups born and suckled by C and LP dams were then weaned to a laboratory chow (20% protein) diet at 3 weeks of age, and at 6 weeks of age 2 male and 2 female pups in each litter continued on the laboratory chow diet and the remaining pups were allocated to a highly palatable high fat-high energy diet. The animals were fed the respective diets ad libitum for 6 weeks, and were then, after 48 h food deprivation, killed and studied at 12 weeks of age. Live weights of LP pups remained lower than those of controls throughout the study period, but in both groups pups fed the highly palatable diet gained more weight than those fed the laboratory chow. The activities of key hepatic glycolytic and gluconeogenic enzymes were significantly affected by maternal diet, glucokinase (GK) activity being down-regulated in LP offspring whereas the activity of the gluconeogenic enzyme phosphoenolpuruvate carboxykinase (PEPCK) was increased in LP pups compared with C animals. Post-weaning diet had a clear impact on glycolytic activity, animals on the highly palatable diet having higher GK activity than those on laboratory chow, although this increase was less evident for LP pups. For PEPCK activity feeding of the highly palatable diet tended to decrease activity, but still LP animals fed the highly palatable diet had significantly higher PEPCK than those given laboratory chow. Gender affected the outcome as higher fasting values for plasma insulin suggested that male rats were more insulin resistant than females. Furthermore, in males the highly palatable diet caused significantly higher plasma insulin concentrations than the laboratory chow among both C and LP rats, although the latter had significantly higher concentrations than C animals. Collectively these results demonstrated a permanent change in the activities of key hepatic enzymes of glucose metabolism as an effect of maternal LP feeding, although these enzymes remained responsive to dietary effects in the adult individual. The programming effect seems to have shifted the "set point" for metabolic regulation towards expectation of poor nutrition, because the activity of a glucose utilizing enzyme was decreased whereas that of a glucose producing enzyme was increased (Desai *et al.*, 1997a).

The same maternal protein restriction model has also been used to evaluate if postnatal feeding may modify *in utero* programming effects. In this study half of the pups were cross-fostered so that LP dams nursed C pups (post-natal LP) and vice versa (recuperated), thereby creating 4 treatment groups: C, LP, post-natal LP and recuperated. Pups were weaned onto a standard laboratory chow at 3 weeks of age, and then studied at 21 days and 11 months of age. At weaning LP and post-natal LP pups weighed significantly less than C, and these differences remained until 11 months of age. Maternal protein-restriction influenced the activity of the hepatic insulin-sensitive glycolytic enzyme GK so that its activity was significantly lower in 21 days old offspring to LP dams than in C offspring, and this significant difference still prevailed when the pups were 11 months old. Post-natal nutrition had, however, no influence on GK activity. Both at weaning and when 11 months old post-natal LP rats had similar GK activity as C, and recuperated rats showed the same low GK activity as LP animals. The activity of hepatic PEPCK was higher than in C rats among LP and similarly, among recuperated rats both at 21 days and 11 months of age, and again the post-natal LP group showed the same level of PEPCK activity as the C group. Generally the expression of mRNA for the two enzymes reflected their activities. These findings confirm that maternal protein restriction, permanently throughout life, affects activity and mRNA levels of key enzymes involved in glucose homeostasis in these programmed offspring. The irreversible change of the liver "set point" favours production rather than utilisation of glucose, a direction expected to result in an insulin-resistant liver (Desai *et al.*, 1997b).

The above described studies have pointed out that maternal protein restriction programs the offspring in a manner that is beneficial for survival under poor nutritional conditions, but alters glucose homeostasis in a way that may lead to insulin resistance and type 2 diabetes, especially in a situation of ample food supply. Indeed, young LP offspring have shown an improved glucose tolerance compared with C, but at 15 months of age the situation is reversed, the LP offspring having the worst glucose tolerance (Hales *et al.*, 1996). These effects seem to be related to the response of adipocytes to the action of insulin: in young LP offspring glucose uptake of adipocytes was significantly higher than in C and moreover, insulin stimulated uptake significantly more in LP than in C rats, but in contrast these adipocytes seemed to have a resistance to the antilipolytic action of insulin (Ozanne *et al.*, 1999). Similar studies in 15 months old rats underscored findings of the previous study, and documented that these changes were not related to altered expression of insulin receptors, but they were associated with reduced phosphatidylinositol 3-kinase (PI 3-kinase), a key enzyme in signalling of the metabolic actions of insulin, and activation of protein kinase B (PBK), an enzyme downstream of PI 3-kinase which is thought to stimulate glucose uptake of adipocytes. It was suggested that ineffective PI 3-kinase activation and the consequently reduced PBK activation contribute to explain the insulin resistance of LP adipocytes (Ozanne *et al.*, 2001).

Human studies have indicated that insulin resistance is related to alterations in desaturase activities, and therefore the maternal protein restriction model has been used to evaluate if protein restriction during foetal and early post-natal life may affect the activities of hepatic Δ5 and Δ6 desaturase enzymes in 3 months old rats. It was clearly demonstrated that the activity of Δ5 but not Δ6 desaturase was lower in the LP offspring than in C, and that it was strongly and negatively correlated with insulin concentrations in LP animals. It was suggested that the reduced Δ5 desaturase activity was a key factor in programming the hepatic metabolism in LP offspring and hence, that the following reduced ability to produce certain long chain polyunsaturated fatty acids would lead to insulin resistance (Ozanne *et al.*, 1998).

Metabolic programming effects of maternal protein restriction include, as illustrated above, severe alterations in glucose metabolism, induced insulin resistance and altered important traits of fat metabolism, changes that may predispose for type 2 diabetes and for obesity in later life. Another unfortunate outcome might be that maternal protein restriction programmes young adult rats towards a preference for high fat diets (Bellinger *et al.*, 2004), but in a more recent study this could not be confirmed (Bellinger and Langley-Evans, 2005). The detrimental effects of a poor nutrition during foetal life are furthermore, amplified in LP individuals given a period of rapid catch-up growth: both average longevity and maximum life-span were reduced in mice that were recuperated on a highly palatable cafeteria style diet (Ozanne and Hales, 2004, 2005).

The main focus in most maternal protein restriction studies has been on the metabolic traits of the offspring and less attention has been paid to the metabolism of the pregnant dam, and the alterations that might induce the programming. A study performed according to the maternal LP protocol showed that LP dams had higher food intake than controls in late gestation, were pregnant with a similar number of pups which, as expected, weighed less than those of C. Placenta size was smaller among LP dams than C, but in relation to foetal weight placental weights were the same in the two groups. Rat dams showed some differences in plasma metabolite and hormone concentrations: elevated glucose, insulin and prolactin plus lower progesterone day 14 of gestation in LP dams, whereas triacylglycerol was higher and leptin was lower in LP than in C dams at term. Oestradiol finally, was elevated in LP dams from day 17 of gestation onwards. Despite these differences in dam plasma levels of metabolites and hormones no significant differences regarding the same traits were recorded in pup plasma, the exception being higher foetal glucose day 14 in LP than C foetuses. It was speculated that combined effects of increased prolactin and decreased progesterone might have increased maternal β-cell content and insulin, but that this might have been counteracted later in gestation by increased oestradiol. The fact that leptin did not increase in late gestation among LP dams allowed for a maintained high food intake until term. It was concluded that this study had identified a number of substances that could possibly mediate programming effects for poor glucose tolerance, insulin resistance and the metabolic syndrome (Fernansez-Twinn *et al.*, 2003).

The results reported above mostly have been performed according to the same protocol and produced consistent results, but it has been pointed out that different protein restriction protocols may yield different results, results that are related to differences in the composition of the low protein diets (Langley-Evans, 2000).

Global under-nutrition model

A maternal under-nutrition model that constantly causes intra-uterine growth retardation (IUGR) makes use of virgin Wistar rats, aged about 75 - 100 days. After confirmed mating one group is fed a pelleted rat chow ad libitum throughout pregnancy (AD group). The under-nourished group is fed the same diet at 30% of the intake of the AD group (UN group). After parturition food is freely available for both groups, and litter size is standardized to eight pups. Maternal under-nutrition does not affect litter size but causes a reduction of placental and foetal weights by 25-30%, changes allometric growth patterns and endocrine traits of the somatotrophic axis (Woodall *et al.*, 1996, 1998).

The programming effects caused by this foetal under-nutrition model include several traits that are common with the human metabolic syndrome, and the importance of post-weaning energy supply for the development of hyperphagia, obesity and hypertension have been clearly demonstrated. Vickers *et al.* (2000) used the same general protocol as above, but at birth UN pups were cross-fostered to AD dams to ensure adequate nutrition during the suckling period. After weaning offspring of AD and UN mothers were allocated to post-natal groups to be fed either a standard diet or a hyperenergetic diet. The diets had the same protein energy / total energy ratio. The gestational maternal under-nutrition resulted in foetal growth retardation, and body weights of UN pups remained below those of AD pups until the end of the study. The UN offspring furthermore, were shorter and had more retroperitoneal fat than AD offspring. Offspring of UN dams showed hyperphagia pre-pubertally, post-pubertally and as mature adults. The hyperenergetic diet amplified hyperphagia in post-pubertal and adult UN offspring, interactions between foetal programming and diet being significant. At 100 days of age UN offspring had higher systolic blood pressure and plasma insulin concentrations than AD both on the control and the hyperenergetic diet. Similarly, plasma leptin concentrations were higher in UN than in AD offspring, and here the hyperenergetic diet exacerbated the hyperleptinemia. These findings underline the importance of the post-natal environment for the development of factors that might lead to adult disease. It seems that leptin and insulin resistance, and the resulting hyperleptinemia and hyperinsulinism which were demonstrated among hyper-alimented UN offspring are critical for the development of hyperphagia, obesity and hypertension.

The endocrine system that links the adipose tissue, the brain and the endocrine pancreas and controls feeding behaviour, metabolic regulation and body energy balance is termed the adipoinsular axis (Kieffer and Habener, 2000). This axis has been proposed to be an important link between body fat mass and the function of the pancreatic β-cells. Findings that suggest a permanent dysregulation of the adipoinsular axis in animals treated according to the above model, and demonstrating the same metabolic traits as described, include immunolabeling for leptin in the peripheral cells of the pancreatic islets, and that leptin was co-localised in the pancreatic δ-cells (Vickers *et al.*, 2001a). It was proposed that the phenotype of the UN offspring with hyperleptinemia and hyperinsulinism may be a mechanism enabling animals that have experienced nutrient deprivation during foetal life to store large quantities of triglycerides when food is abundant. In the short term perspective this may be an advantageous strategy, but if the programmed individual constantly is exposed to a plentiful food supply the persisting hyperleptinemia and hyperinsulinism may lead to adipogenic diabetes.

Onset of hyperphagia has been shown to occur before puberty, i.e. before the development of obesity (Vickers *et al.*, 2000). This observation lead to the speculation that, besides the manifold metabolic consequences of maternal under-nutrition, there might be a common biological reason for the association between obesity, the metabolic syndrome, sedentary behaviour and overeating. Indeed, the locomotor activity of 35 days old UN offspring was significantly less than that of AD offspring, and feeding a hyperenergetic diet resulted in a still more sedentary behaviour. Males were more inactive than females, and the diminished locomotor activity among UN offspring was recorded already before the development of obesity. A second study performed with 14 months old AD and UN offspring, which had been fed a healthy diet throughout post-natal life, confirmed that the sedentary behaviour in UN offspring, solely related to prenatal maternal diet, still persisted, and that these individuals were significantly more obese than AD offspring. Hence, these studies suggested that prenatal nutrition may be the origin of the "couch potato" syndrome (Vickers *et al.*, 2003).

The above studies have demonstrated life long detrimental effects of an adverse intra-uterine environment, and the question then arises whether there is a way to reverse these effects. Two studies on adult AD and UN offspring, either fed the control rat chow or the hyperenergetic diet suggest that alleviation of adverse effects might be possible. In the first study a 14 day infusion of IGF-1 by osmotic minipump lead to a pronounced reduction in food intake and body fat mass as well as normalisation of blood pressure in UN offspring. In addition, fasting plasma insulin and leptin concentrations were reduced (Vickers *et al.*, 2001b). In the second study on adult animals the rats were either given saline or growth hormone (GH) injections for 21 days before measurements were performed. As a response to GH treatment systolic blood pressure was markedly decreased in all UN offspring, and GH seemed to have a beneficial effect on cardio-vascular function (Vickers *et al.*, 2002). The altricial neonate may provide a potential target for reversal of intra-uterine programming effects, because of its immaturity at birth. Indeed, neonatal treatment with subcutaneous injections of leptin for 10 days resulted in normalised energy intake, locomotor activity, body weight, body fat mass and fasting plasma glucose, insulin and leptin concentrations in adult UN offspring when compared with saline treated animals. The effect of leptin could be ascribed to a central effect on hypothalamus level, but it might also have modified the postnatal pancreatic organogenesis (Vickers *et al.*, 2005).

The high carbohydrate (HC) rat ("pup in a cup") model

This model is based on the exposure of rat pups to a high carbohydrate diet during the critical window for postnatal pancreatic development, and is therefore founded on the immaturity of the altricial rat neonate. Rat pups are removed from their dams at 4 days of age and artificially reared via ingastric feeding of a HC milk formula with 56% of energy derived from carbohydrate, 24% from protein and 20% from fat. The composition of the formula is quite different from that of rat milk in which 8% of energy is derived from carbohydrate, 24% from protein and 68% from fat. In order to exclude the possibility that programming effects are induced by the artificial rearing *per se*, a control group of pups is artificially reared on a formula with the same energetic composition as rat milk. The HC formula causes an immediate onset of hyperinsulinemia (within 24 h), and despite the HC formula feeding is ended on postnatal day 24, the hyperinsulinemia persists into adulthood. In addition, HC pups show an increased growth rate from day 55 of life, and have developed obesity by an age of approximately 100 days. The pups fed the rat milk like high fat formula (MF) did, in contrast, not develop hyperinsulinemia or adult-onset obesity (Patel and Srinivasan, 2002; Srinivasan *et al.*, 2003; reviews used for this entire section).

Rats reared by this model have mainly been studied in three stages: immediate adaptations, focusing on 12 days old rats during feeding the HC formula, consequences for adult life with focus on changes in 100 days old HC rats and finally, generational effects with focus on changes in the HC rat progeny, i.e. second generation HC rats.

The immediate physiological adaptations include about 6-fold higher plasma insulin concentrations but plasma glucose and body weight not different from those of MF pups. Pancreatic islets isolated from HC pups secreted significantly more insulin in response to glucose stimulation that those from MF pups. Other important changes in HC islets included increased content of GLUT2, and increased activities of enzyme systems that indicated an increased flux through the glycolytic pathway. Furthermore, GLP-1 which promotes insulin secretion by islets via the second messenger cAMP showed increased plasma concentrations as well as islet receptor mRNA in the 12-days-old HC rat. These changes contribute to a lowering of the threshold for insulin secretion, and hence an augmented response to basal glucose.

At the molecular level, insulin biosynthesis and transcription of the preproinsulin gene in islets were enhanced in HC rats, as well as other important factors by which glucose modulates preproinsulin promoter activity, including a phosphorylation cascade involving PI 3-kinase which is a downstream component of the insulin signalling pathway. The increase in gene expression of these factors may suggest that the HC rat maintains its hyperinsulinemic condition by an autocrine effect of insulin. Other changes in the 12 days old HC rat, not related to the pancreatic islets, include increased liver glycogen deposition, increased lipogenic capacity of the liver and precocious induction of GK and malic enzyme.

Artificially reared HC rats are weaned onto laboratory chow on day 24, but they remain hyperinsulinemic in adult life despite being fed a conventional diet. Moreover, they develop obesity after puberty, and are significantly obese by 100 days of age. Metabolic alterations that were recorded for 12-day-old HC rats mainly seem to be programmed to be preserved into adulthood, traits including the increased lipogenic capacity of liver and adipose tissue.

Characteristics of chronic hyperinsulinemia and adult-onset obesity are spontaneously transmitted from HC dams to their progeny, without involvement from the paternal side. Pregnant and lactating HC dams are normoglycemic and hyperinsulinemic, but they produce milk with identical composition to that of MF dams. Moreover, second generation HC pups reared by foster mothers express the hyperinsulinemic phenotype, so the generational effect cannot be explained by the type of milk consumed during rearing. It is believed that the HC phenotype persists into adulthood and is transmitted to the next generation by means of epigenetic mechanisms, triggered by changes in the environment (HC artificial rearing). This early life nutritional challenge may have altered cell-specific DNA methylation patterns, which in turn has caused changes in gene expression patterns in specific tissues, patterns which can be transmitted to daughter cells.

Sheep models

The sheep provides an elegant model of human IUGR: the birth weight of the neonate is in the same order as the human neonate, single or twin births are predominant, and gestation length allows for evaluation of dietary intervention effects during different parts of gestation. The sheep may also provide a valuable model for other domestic animal species. For instance, the size of the conceptus even allows for investigations into foetal ovarian and testicular development from early gestation onwards, investigations that are important in explaining the role of intra-uterine environment for future reproductive capacity of the offspring. Below two models resulting in reduced placental mass, and hence limitation of the supply of glucose, amino acids and oxygen to the foetus will be described and main results outlined.

The adolescent ewe model

Embryos are recovered from superovulated adult ewes, inseminated by a single ram, and transferred in singleton to recipient adolescent ewes aged 6-7 months on day 4 of an induced oestrous cycle. By this procedure the homogeneity of the progeny is maximised and confounding effects of twin or triplet pregnancies excluded. Immediately after transfer, the adolescent ewes are allocated to dietary treatments, either being offered a high (2-2.5 x maintenance) or a moderate (1.25 x maintenance) quantity of a complete diet (10.5 MJ metabolisable energy and 140 g crude protein per kg dry matter). The feeding levels are chosen so as to allow for at weight gain of 50-85 g/day in the moderate intake group and 200-350 g/day in the high intake group during the first two thirds of gestation. The moderate intake group serves as a control, because the intake in this group supports optimum placental and foetal growth for the genotype in question (Wallace *et al.*, 1996).

This model has proved highly robust, and the main results of several studies have been reviewed by Wallace *et al.* (2001, 2004), reviews which this section will be based on if not otherwise stated. Generally, for adolescent ewes delivering live lambs, the high intake has resulted in significantly shorter gestation (about 3 days less), decreased lamb birth weight, decreased placental weight, lower number of foetal cotyledons and higher ratio between foetal and placental weights, as well as lower colostrum yield than for ewes given a moderate intake. Furthermore, the chemical composition of colostrum differed: high intake dams had lower fat and lactose but higher IgG contents than moderate intake dams. However, when related to the lower colostrum yield of the high intake dams the total output of fat, lactose, crude protein and IgG was considerably poorer than in colostrum from moderate intake ewes. Together this results in a lower energy concentration of colostrum from high versus moderate intake dams. Because of its poorer wool cover and relatively larger surface area per unit body mass, as well as its reduced body lipid and lower liver glycogen contents, the IUGR neonate can be expected to have a high energy requirement, and to be susceptible to hypothermia and therefore, colostrum from high intake dams may be inadequate to sustain its needs. The immune status of the neonate may also be compromised because the total intake of IgG may be too small to confer the passive immunity to protect it from infection.

In the growing individual, the hierarchy of nutrient partitioning is promoting the growth of the maternal tissues at the expense of the increasing demands of the conceptus and the mammary gland. High intake dams thus show a considerable weight gain, increasing body condition score, higher body fat content, higher and increasing plasma insulin, leptin and IGF-1 but lower placental lactogen concentrations as gestation progresses compared with moderate intake dams, which have a small increase in body weight, and a stable body condition score throughout gestation. These alterations lead to a lower uterine and umbilical blood flow, and a lower foetal uptake of glucose, amino acids and oxygen in high intake compared with moderate intake dams. When considering that the main placental growth occurs during the first half of pregnancy while the major part of foetal growth occurs during the last third of pregnancy, it is evident that the foetal nutrient requirements are at a maximum in late gestation, and that compromised placental function will result in IUGR. However, when foetal nutrient uptakes are expressed on a weight-specific basis they do not differ between high and moderate intake treatments and the placental mRNA expression of the glucose transporters GLUT-1 and GLUT-3 was similar on the two treatments. These findings show that the growth and vascularisation of the placenta are limiting for nutrient transfer, but that its nutrient metabolism and transfer capacity remain intact. Against this background it is clear that it is important to determine when the placenta is most sensitive to maternal nutrient intake, i.e. establish a critical window. This has been accomplished by nutritional switch-over studies, in which adolescent ewes have been switched from an anabolic to a catabolic state at day 50 of pregnancy and vice versa, thus resulting in treatments HH, MM, HM and MH. Ewes given the high intake from day 50 of pregnancy (HH and MH) showed significantly decreased length of gestation, total placental mass, total foetal cotyledon mass as well as a major decrease in lamb birth weight, whereas the number of caruncles occupied by the conceptus was determined during the first 50 days of gestation only, and therefore was lower in HH and HM dams. These findings point out the profound importance of an adequate maternal nutrition in mid-pregnancy in order to support an optimal placental, and hence foetal, growth trajectory.

It has been considered that factors that influence foetal nutrient uptake and growth may programme persisting changes in the foetal reproductive axis, changes that might limit the programmed individual's life-time reproductive performance. The adolescent ewe model has been used to study effects of maternal nutrition on onset of puberty in offspring. The age at the onset of puberty in IUGR female spring-born lambs was not different from that in normally developed lambs, and there were no differences in the duration of the first cycle, or the number of ewe lambs with normal or aberrant cycles between the two groups of ewe lambs. In male lambs the onset of puberty was indicated by the timing of the increase in plasma testosterone concentrations, and IUGR male lambs showed a 5 weeks delay in this trait compared with normal birth weight male lambs. Although older, the body weights of IUGR male lambs at puberty was the same as for normally developed indicating that body weight was an important determining factor for the onset of puberty (Da Silva *et al.*, 2001).

Although there were no differences in the age at onset of puberty in female lambs between IUGR and normally developed ones, the follicular population and the development of the hypothalamus-pituitary axis may be affected. Pituitary gonadotrophin gene expression and ovarian development of late gestation (day 131) female foetuses have been determined by means of the adolescent ewe model

(Da Silva *et al.*, 2002). Maternal nutritional treatment did not influence FSHβ mRNA expression, but LHβ mRNA in the foetal pituitary gland of IUGR foetuses was significantly higher compared with normally grown, and irrespective of maternal nutrition it was negatively correlated with total placentome mass. This would suggest that the smaller placenta of the IUGR foetuses produced less oestrogen, and hence a smaller feedback signal on the foetal pituitary. The ovarian mass was not different between IUGR and normally grown foetuses, and neither was the cortical layer width. The total number of follicles was, however, strongly negatively influenced in IUGR foetuses. This was mainly caused by a smaller number of primordial follicles. Independent of maternal dietary treatment the number of follicles was positively correlated with foetal weight. The number of follicles available for life-time recruitment is set during foetal life, and therefore it cannot be excluded that the reduced number of follicles present in the ovaries of the IUGR foetuses may negatively influence reproductive performance in adult life.

Maternal undernutrition model

Maternal undernutrition during parts of gestation is another model which has been used to achieve reduced placental growth and IUGR. The protocol for such a model is in brief outlined as follows: Mature ewes are used. They are housed individually at day 28 of gestation and divided into two nutritional groups, one nutrient restricted (NR) which is fed 60% of their calculated ME requirements, and one well-fed (WF) given 225% of their ME requirements, out of which approximately 150% of requirements were consumed. At day 80 the ewes were divided into further two groups, one given 100% (adequately fed; AF) and the other given 150% of their ME requirements (WF). At term therefore, there were four groups namely 1) NR followed by AF, 2) WF followed by AF, 3) NR followed by WF and 4) WF followed by WF. By this approach NR ewes weighed less and had lower body condition scores than WF at day 80 of gestation, but near term these differences had disappeared. At day 80 of gestation placental mass was higher among WF than NR dams, but foetal body weights were similar, and so was the abundance of GLUT-1. Near term NR-AF ewes had higher placental mass than WF-AF and foetal body weight was larger, which was reflected by higher abundance of GLUT-1. For ewes WF in late gestation there were no differences in placental mass, foetal body weight or GLUT-1 abundance, but foetuses weighed more than those of late gestation AF dams. It was concluded that despite NR during the period of rapid placental growth (until mid gestation) did restrict placental growth it had no detrimental effects on the abundance of GLUT-1, and that if nutrient supply was increased to, but not above, the requirement after day 80 of gestation both placental mass and GLUT-1 could be increased (Dandrea *et al.*, 2001).

The same maternal nutrition model was used by Bispham *et al.* (2003), and it was then shown that foetuses sampled near term from dams that were NR until day 80 of gestation had significantly more adipose tissue than those of early gestation WF dams, and the adipose tissue of NR foetuses had increased abundance of IGF-1 and IGF-2 mRNA. Leptin mRNA abundance was reduced in foetuses from dams that were WF in early gestation. NR in early gestation followed by restored maternal nutrition in late gestation was pointed out as a risk factor for later life obesity.

The effects of maternal undernutrition during different critical windows for early foetal ovarian and follicular development (Rae *et al.*, 2001) and foetal testicular steroidogenesis (Rae *et al.*, 2002) have been studied using a model in which mature ewes were fed to support the ME requirement of a pregnant ewe (H) or 50% of that amount (L). Feeding periods applied were mating – day 30 of gestation, and then days 30 – 50 (expt. 1), alternatively mating – day 30 and then days 30 – 65 (expt. 2), giving the treatment groups HH, LH, HL and LL. In expt. 3 finally these treatments were followed by an extra period from day 81 – 110 of gestation, yielding treatments HHH, LHH, HLH, HHL and LLL. Although there was no effect of nutritional treatment on foetal mass at day 50 of gestation, mean foetal ovarian mass was significantly lower in HL and LL animals, and at day 65 of gestation nutrient restriction (LL group) had caused delayed germ cell maturation and onset of meiosis. From Expt. 3 finally, it was concluded that nutrient restriction in each period of gestation delayed ovarian development measured as a significant reduction in the numbers of follicles beyond the primordial stage, a change that might have consequences for later life reproduction performance. A recent study following the same protocol indicates that maternal undernutrition alters proliferation and the expression of apoptosis-regulating genes in the developing foetal ovary (Lea *et al.*, 2006). Also foetal testicular steroidogenesis was responsive to maternal undernutrition: the expression of the key steroidogenically rate-limiting cholesterol transporter was significantly increased as an effect of maternal undernutrition until day 50 of gestation, and plasma testosterone concentrations were generally higher among dams which had undergone a period of undernutrition. However, the absence of differences in plasma mean testosterone concentrations at days 65 and 110 of gestation indicated that the critical window for response to maternal nutrient supply was narrow, and ended before day 65, but still it remains to be determined if the recorded response may have any long-term consequences for male fertility.

Programming by glucocorticoids

It has been proposed that exposure of the foetus to excess glucocorticoids may restrict foetal growth and programme permanent metabolic effects. Evidence that the hypothalamus – pituitary –adrenal (HPA) axis is programmable exists from several species, among them guinea pigs, rats and sheep. Briefly, the foetus can be exposed to glucocorticoids by *de novo* secretion, which increases as the adrenal matures, or in response to foetal stress, or it can be transferred from the mother via the placenta, or finally, it can be locally produced within the chorion trophoblasts and amnion epithelium. During most of gestation glucocorticoid concentrations are low in the foetus and mainly derived from the mother by a materno-foetal concentration gradient which is maintained by 11β-hydroxysteroid dehydrogenase type 2 (11βHSD2) which converts cortisol and corticosterone to their inactive metabolites, and thereby protects the foetus from exposure to maternal corticosteroids. If the foetus is overexposed to glucocorticoids either by maternal administration or by inhibition of 11βHSD2 it has been shown to result in postnatal hypertension, glucose intolerance and abnormalities in HPA function. The mechanisms involved in programming of the HPA axis are described in reviews by Bertram and Hanson (2002) and Fowden and Forhead (2004). Studies with the maternal low protein rat model have shown that both activity and mRNA expression of placental 11βHSD2 is reduced in LP dams, and it has been proposed that down-regulation of 11βHSD2 may be the common pathway by which programming effects are produced (Langley-Evans, 2006).

What can we learn from human studies?

The intense communication between the developing foetus and the maternal metabolism has been shown in human as well as the animal studies illustrated above. Although nutrition during gestation has been intensively investigated in some animals, the emphasis on short term effects – in part by reason of the short life span in farm animals used for food production – reduces the insight available on the more long term effects. Valuable information can perhaps be gained from human studies, although there is considerable dispute over the conclusions that can be drawn. The link between cardiovascular function in the mature individual and foetal exposure by maternal nutrition is such an effect (Langley-Evans, 2001; Huxley and Neil, 2004). Table 1 gives examples of some findings in human studies which it has been suggested show that it is not simply the quantity of a tissue, like bone or liver, in the newborn that can be affected by maternal nutrition but also endocrine and regulatory systems. Some of these may also have some relevance for the horse e.g. blood pressure is of great importance for humans, and considering the equine athlete and the potential role of heart size in performance it seems to be inadvisable to neglect this aspect.

Table 1. Examples of the postulated interactions between conditions for the pregnant woman and effects in the new-born or elderly offspring (Langley -Evans, 2001).

Influencing factor	Area affected
Sucrose intake in early pregnancy, low protein in late pregnancy	Birth weight, placental weight
Link between mother's body stature and foetal growth	Influence on cardiovascular indices
High carbohydrate-low protein in pregnancy	Risk for high blood pressure
Low birth weight	Elevated fasting cortisol levels
Low weight/length-index at birth	Increased excretion of prostaglandin E_2

The impact of nutrient intake during gestation on brain development has been neglected to a large extent in farm animals and humans. It is clearly shown that iodine and selenium play an important role with respect to retardation in brain development (Delange 1998, 2000, 2001, 2002). Delange (2000) concludes that "Iodine deficiency constituents the world's greatest single cause of preventable brain damage and mental retardation". Recently there has been considerable interest in the potential role of EPA and DHA in brain development (Alessandri *et al.*, 2004). In equine nutrition, for both iodine and selenium, there is commonly an oversupply through misuse, but also at the other extreme some animals are given little or no supplementation despite a very low concentration of these nutrients in grass and roughage. In animals retardation in mental development can result in a depressed capacity to respond to critical environmental stressors or conditions demanding adaptive behaviour.

Obviously the interaction between the profile of carbohydrates ingested by the pregnant woman and the conditioning of the foetal as well as of the offspring's regulatory systems is one of the major issues in public health in western countries. In the first instance high glycaemic diets during pregnancy induce an increase in foeto-placental growth (Clapp, 2002). The effect is an increase in birth weight and – as shown above – the induction of insulin resistance in the growing newborn. Abnormal insulin secretion in foals prone to osteochondrosis (OC) (Ralston, 2002; Kronfeld *et al.*, 2005) and the association of laminitis with insulin resistance (Kronfeld *et al.*, 2005a) indicates the need to include nutrition during gestation into the debate on healthy growth and long term health in the horse.

So what do we know about the horse currently?

Wooding and Fowden (2006) recently stated that "equine placentation is characterised by unique features including a secondary blastocyst capsule, endometrial cup formation and the microcotyledenous organisation of the epitheiliochorial structure of the definitive placenta" and they describe key areas where there are similarities and differences between nutrient transfer between the horse and ruminants. These similarities and differences may be reflected in the response of the horse to nutritional imbalances or deficiencies during gestation. However, to date there are no published studies in the horse similar to those described earlier in this paper.

Intrauterine growth retardation (IUGR)

The overall goal for the mare is to have a live foal, which in turn develops into a healthy adult. In the case of a performance horse the goal for the foal is to end up as a sound, healthy and successful athlete whatever the discipline may be. Nutrition of the mare has perhaps in the past been thought much less important than that of the foal. However, in the horse as well as in humans and other species, the important role that nutrition, via the mother, may have in the subsequent health of any offspring is increasingly being recognised (Harris, 2003; Rossdale, 2004; Coenen and Vervuert 2005). Foetal growth and development depends on the intrauterine environment which in turn is responsible for supplying the foetus's metabolic, nutritional and endocrine requirements. The majority of these are provided directly or indirectly from the maternal source.

In the horse by the 7th month of gestation the foetus will be less than 20% of its birth weight. However, by this time significant placental development will have occurred and the greatest increase in crown-rump length occurs in mid-gestation. Foetal growth obviously accelerates markedly during the last three months of gestation. Nearly half the copper (Cu), zinc (Zn), and manganese (Mn) accumulation occurs, for example, in the 10th month. There have been a number of studies in the horse that have manipulated foetal growth by using embryo transfer between thoroughbred and pony mares (e.g. Allen et al 2002, Guissini et al 2003, Ousey et al 2004). These studies confirm the fact that the placental supply of nutrients and oxygen to the foetus depends predominantly on the size of the uterus, and the area of foetomaternal contact (as well as efficacy of nutrient transfer) which in turn is primarily determined by the size of the mare and therefore body size at birth is related primarily to placental area. The result is for any type of horse an optimal foeto-placental contact area in order to ensure nutrient supply from the maternal to the foetal side. However, these cited studies did not look at the effect of nutritional manipulations *per se* on equine foetal growth. Reviewing studies on gestation length in the equine show that under many circumstances of poor nutrition, gestation length increases. This demonstrates the sensitivity of the pregnant individual as well as of the foetus to adverse environmental factors. But it is likely that a prolonged gestation reflects an impaired signalling from the uterus instead of the capacity to compensate for a period of undernutrition.

The relative size of any animal at birth may influence neonatal mortality and morbidity but increasingly, as discussed above, it is being appreciated that, at least in other species, intrauterine effects including more subtle growth retardation may increase the likelihood of developing certain performance limiting conditions in later life. Intrauterine growth retardation (IUGR) covers both a modification of growth potential due to a reduction in growth rate and reduced cellular structure and function. The horse may be particularly vulnerable to IUGR because of its diffuse epitheilochorial placenta which may make areas of the placenta vulnerable to ischaemia etc (Rossdale and Ousey, 1998), and its glucose requirements during pregnancy as discussed below. The equine foetus has a number of significant differences from the rodent and sheep models described previously, which may make it more or less vulnerable to intrauterine disturbances (Rossdale, 2004; Wooding and Fowden, 2006). Growth retardation may occur for a number of non-nutritional reasons but certainly can be induced experimentally by maternal undernutrition, and inappropriate nutrition may impact, for example, on placental development and therefore influence birth weight. It has suggested that there are a number of conditions, based mainly on work in other species, that might "have an IUGR based susceptibility in their aetiology or pathogenesis including hyperlipaemia... and allergic conditions ... osteochondrosis dissecans .. and myopathies" (Rossdale and Ousey, 1998, 2002). As noted by Robinson (1998) for example "does fetal or perinatal growth influence muscle mass and therefore subsequent athletic performance". Austboe and Dolvik (1996) report about the depression in birth weight with reduced calcium supply to the mare, and Meyer (1998) showed that the development of goitre in newborn foals is dependent on the iodine intake of the dam. Growth of organs in turn is a highly complex procedure involving protein synthesis, and obviously amino acids are of outstanding importance (Hoet and Hansen, 1999) but the timing of any nutritional insult seems to be the key. Whilst we may understand the effects of overt amino acid deficiencies on this process we may ask what the effects of more subtle imbalances in amino acids are at certain times of gestation.

Recent work in the pig suggested that maternal nutrition did not affect the proliferation and differentiation of primary myoblasts (Nissen *et al.*, 2003) however, in rats and guinea pigs it does

(Bayol *et al.*, 2004) and it has been stated that the number of muscle fibres that constitute a skeletal muscle can be influenced prenatal by subtle changes in maternal nutrition (Bayol *et al.*, 2004). Work in rats also showed that exposure of the developing foetus to a maternal low protein diet programmed cardiac dysfunction in the offspring in later life (Cheema *et al.*, 2005). As mentioned above, there may be critical "windows of opportunity" when the different organs and tissues can be affected by nutrition (Bayol *et al.*, 2004) and these may differ between species.

It may perhaps be important in the future to differentiate between the premature foal, that is underweight, from the underweight foal, that was born at term - we also need to clearly define immaturity and prematurity. We therefore need to differentiate between the

- Immediate effects of interuterine disturbances on the new born foal and neonate (Rossdale and Ousey, 2002; Rossdale 2004)
- The effects of intrauterine disturbances on subsequent adult health and performance and this in turn may be subdivided into
  1. What is the effect on health and performance as an adult of a foal being born either underweight or showing overt signs of maladjustment. This is obviously influenced by subsequent management.
  2. What is the effect of more subtle influences of nutrition on growth and development in utero.

Thus (1) includes the effect not only of any organ dysfunction or prematurity but also the effect of any catch up growth which may in turn impose its own metabolic stress. In the horse there may be an increased risk of Developmental Orthopaedic Diseases (DOD) for example (Harris *et al.*, 2005) and interestingly some studies have shown in other species that life span is shortened considerably if the period of growth is accelerated to make up for reduced growth *in utero* (Aihie Sayer *et al.*, 2001). Whereas (2) recognises that whilst the overtly small foal or the maladjusted foal may be recognised at birth subtle changes may not be recognised.

Insulin, glucose and carbohydrate metabolism during pregnancy in the mare

The foetal foal apparently deaminates little amino acid and therefore has limited gluconeogenic capacity (Fowden, 1997). It is therefore perhaps more dependent on transplacental supply of glucose than other species studied. This would be in contrast to the foetal calf which needs more amino acids and lactate for energetic purposes than glucose. The foetal foal appears to have a rate of glucose utilisation similar to that of the human foetus *in utero* and in common with other species there are marked changes in the carbohydrate metabolism and pancreatic β cell function of the mare during the pregnancy (Fowden *et al.*, 1984). The changes reported include "hyperinsulinaemia, enhanced ß cell sensitivity to endogenous and exogenous glucose, increased degradation of insulin, enhanced resistance to the action of insulin and exaggerated responses to feeding and fasting". However, unlike other species the high glucose requirement of the foal appears to be met solely by redirecting glucose away from the maternal tissues. As the uptake of glucose by the foetoplacental tissue is dependent primarily on the glucose concentration gradient across the placenta - the enhanced rise in plasma glucose after feeding in the pregnant mare maximises foetal glucose uptake at times when glucose is abundant. There is, however, a change in the insulin sensitivity during pregnancy with an enhanced β cell sensitivity to glucose and a circulating hyperinsulinaemia up to around 270 days of gestation followed by lower insulin concentrations and a reduced β cell sensitivity and a degree of insulin resistance during late gestation (again helping to ensure that more of the available glucose is diverted to the foal). It is thought that maternal glucose utilisation is already near the absolute minimum in the fed state during late gestation and therefore any prolonged hypoglycaemia may have significant effects even precipitating early labour (Fowden *et al.*, 1984). The changes in placental glucose consumption seen in the horse during gestation are not found for example in sheep (Wooding and Fowden, 2006).

What about the effect of diet during this period

Nutrient availability influences the duration of pregnancy (Fowden and Forhead, 2001) and when nutrient availability is limited (for what ever reason) the foetal concentrations of prostaglandins and cortisol rise and those of insulin and thyroxine fall (Fowden. 1985). These are changes which are known from other species to have an impact on cardiovascular functions and also may have a number of consequences on other body systems (Rossdale and Ousey, 2002).

Very little work has been published on the effect of diet during pregnancy, but Hoffman *et al.* (2003) looked at the influence of different supplementary energy sources on glucose metabolism. Metabolic adaptation of the mares to pregnancy was reflected in larger areas under time-concentration curves for plasma glucose and insulin following an oral glucose load, and by slower glucose clearance, during late gestation compared with early lactation (Figure 1).

With respect to the diet, it was evident that mares fed a supplementary concentrate rich in sugar and starch showed a more rapid glucose peak than those fed the fat/fibre supplement, during both late gestation and early lactation perhaps reflecting the adaptation to meals rich in hydrolysable carbohydrate and the feeding-fasting meal cycle. The more sluggish glucose clearance in mares fed the fat and fibre rich supplement more closely mimicked the natural state of horses grazing pasture and not acclimated to feeding-fasting cycles. It was suggested that potentially this more effectively allowed for the adaptation of glucose metabolism required during pregnancy and lactation in order to make energy available to the foetus or suckling foal. A subsequent study evaluated the insulin sensitivity of weanlings whose dams had been fed a starch and sugar rich or a fat and fibre rich diet during the last part of gestation and who themselves had access to their dam's diet pre and post weaning (Treiber *et al.*, 2005). This study showed that adaptation to a high glycaemic diet is associated with increased insulin resistance and a compensatory increase in insulin secretion. Increased insulin secretion maintains glucose homeostasis, but may alter insulin signalling in other systems, such as the somatotropic axis and therefore increase the risk of metabolic diseases (Kronfeld *et al.*, 2005).

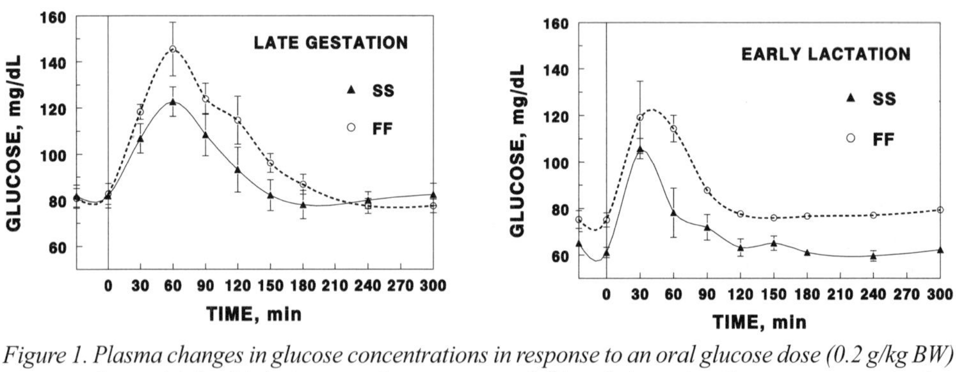

Figure 1. Plasma changes in glucose concentrations in response to an oral glucose dose (0.2 g/kg BW) in mares during (a) the third trimester of pregnancy, and (b) early lactation. Data are summarized as means ± SE. Dietary treatments were forage (grass or hay) plus a supplement rich in either starch and sugar (SS, solid line) or fat and fibre (FF, dashed line).

Other nutrients

Other studies have looked at the effects of supplementing pregnant animals with supra-optimal levels of other nutrients and in particular vitamins and minerals (see Ashworth and Antipatis, 2001). These authors suggest that oxidative stress may be a very important component. A number of studies for example have reported that supplementing pregnant ewes with high levels of vitamin E may improve the vigour of the new born lamb and positively influence growth rate even though neonatal plasma concentrations may be unaffected by such supplementation (Merrell, 1998; Capper et al 2003). It has been shown in sheep and the pig that the formation of surfactant, as well as elastic fibres, in tissues such as the lung is sensitive to vitamin A and fatty acid availability. Similarly, the provision of certain fatty acids has been suggested to be important for the normal development of the neonate - in particular the development of the nervous tissue and brain (Leskanich and Noble, 1999; Allessandri *et al.*, 2004). The results from work on calcium supplementation during pregnancy on birth weight and length in other species, including man, have not been consistent, but there is some evidence to suggest that calcium may have a positive effect on birth weight due to better intrauterine growth and an increased length of pregnancy (Djazayery *et al.*, 2004).

Gambling and McArdle (2004) review the influence of Cu and iron (Fe) on foetal development and emphasise the importance of these elements in growth and development (e.g. long term potential consequences of maternal Cu deficiency include connective tissue abnormalities, cardiac ultrastructural abnormalities, immune suppression and impaired cognitive and behavioural function; and for Zn: increased blood pressure, increased glucose tolerance and impaired cognitive and behavioural function). The authors highlight that effects may be seen even if the offspring have normal dietary intakes from birth.

What about the horse?

Again there is very little work *per se* that looks at this aspect in any detail. Mares have varying reserves, which they can draw on if intakes during pregnancy are inadequate – but at what stage this may influence the foal or future adult horse is currently unknown although one study suggested for example that a low Ca intake of pregnant mares would reduce the intrauterine weight gain of foals (Coenen and Vervuert, 2005). One area where there has been a bit of work undertaken relates to Cu and the possible link with DOD.

A Cu containing enzyme - lysyl oxidase - is involved in the X-linking of protein chains in elastin and collagen of cartilage. Disruption of these X-links due to Cu deficiency may result in biomechanically weakened cartilage and increase the risk of DOD (Hurtig *et al.*, 1993). A number of studies have suggested a relationship between Cu and Zn in the diet and DOD (see Harris et al 2005). However, Cu over supplementation of the foal does not appear to be the answer but recent work supports the suggestion that supplementation during gestation may be of benefit. During gestation the total Cu content of the foetus increases mainly due to storage in the liver and at birth much higher liver Cu concentrations are found than in adult horses (Gee *et al.*, 2000). Foals are born with variable liver Cu stores. Liver Cu concentrations of less than 400 mg/kg DM in new-born foals have been suggested to reflect inadequate absorption or intake of Cu by the dam (Meyer and Tiegs, 1995) although this has been questioned (Gee *et al.*, 2000). Deficits in the suckling foals' Cu needs have been suggested to be met by mobilising hepatic Cu (Cymbaluk and Smart, 1993) which may in part explain the recent studies that have suggested a potential benefit of Cu supplementation during gestation.

In one study (Knight *et al.*, 1990) mares were fed either 13 or 32 mg/kg DM Cu during the last 3 –6months of gestation and first 3 months of lactation and the foals were given creep feed with either 15 or 55 mg/kg DM from an undisclosed time point. Foals remained in the experimental group to which their dam was assigned. Foals from the low Cu group had more articular and physeal cartilage abnormalities at 180 days than those from the supplemented group. Lesions of OC were only seen in the unsupplemented group. However, it was not possible to determine the relative influences of the pre-partum and post-partum feeding from this study. In a large study in New Zealand (see Pearce *et al.*, 1998a-c) Cu supplementation (0.5 mg Cu/kg BW daily; ~ 28mg/kg DM intake) of mares (n=12) in late gestation, significantly decreased the radiographic indices for physitis in the distal third metatarsal bone of their foals at 150 days and the prevalence of articular cartilage lesions in comparison with the control group (n=9). Oral supplementation of the foals (with 0.2 mg/kg BW daily from 3 weeks of age increasing to 0.5 mg/kg BW daily) however, did not affect bone or cartilage compared with untreated cohorts. Supplementing the mares did increase the liver Cu status of foals at birth significantly but had no effect on other tissue Cu concentrations and there was no direct relationship between the radiographic physitis scores and the foal liver Cu contents.

A further study (Van Weeren *et al.*, 2003) correlated the liver Cu status of mares and foals with OC scores – all animals had the same availability of feed but their estimated intakes of Cu ranged from 95 – 153 mg/day and resulted in mean foal liver Cu of 372 mg/kg at birth. No direct link between liver Cu status of mares and foals at birth or radiographical OC development in foals at 5 or 11 months was established. However, foals with higher liver Cu status at birth showed an increased recession of lesions before reaching the threshold age of 8 months. It could be suggested that a slightly better placental supply and greater liver stores at birth helped in the repair process of lesions and that a good Cu supply during gestation may be advantageous. It is therefore possible that a reduced Cu intake/absorption especially during gestation could possibly either be permissive to the development of DOD under certain conditions or may reduce the ability to repair lesions. This conclusion would be supported by the work of Pearce *et al.* (1998a) although further research is needed in this area on a much larger scale.

Conclusions

There is no doubt that the uterus is not just an isolated "bag" which simply enables predetermined growth to occur without any communication with the outside world. Two principles seem to influence the effect of malnutrition on embryonic as well as foetal growth and maturation in case of malnutrition: Firstly, a lack of components for the various processes associated with growth. These induce retardation or damage in the development of specific tissues and the functions associated with those tissues. An affected foal, for example, could show impaired lung defence capacity, muscle failure, bone, cartilage aberrations and an inferior capability to respond onto environmental challenges (cognitive failure). Secondly, a change of foetal endocrine systems may be a result of an "imprint" of the maternal nutritional profile. Possibly the foal like other mammalian foetuses does not perceive for example a high glycaemic response of the mare not as a burden resulting from too much grain feeding but "sees" it as a signal from its environment which needs adaptation and therefore the foal starts to adapt by modifying its own endocrine system.

From interspecies studies it is possible to conclude that changes in cardiovascular and endocrine (possibly the main aspect) functions can result from impaired maternal nutrition without there being, more immediately visible, negative effects on the quantitative aspects of foetal growth. Despite differences between species in specific details it is likely that in the equine, as in other mammals, the foetus will interpret changes in maternal nutrition as a signal from an environment which requires and therefore results in an adapted metabolism at birth. Obviously, much more work is needed in all species, but in particular in the horse, to evaluate these potential connections in more depth.

References

Allen, W.R., S. Wisher, C. Turnbull, F. Stewart, J.C. Ousey, A. Fowden and P.D. Rossdale, 2002. The influence of maternal size on fetal and postnatal development in the horse. 1. Development in utero. Reprod. 123: 445 - 453.

Allessandri, J.-M., P. Guesnet, S. Vancassel, P. Astorg, I. Denis, B. Langelier, S. Aid, C. Poumes-Ballihaut, G. Champeil-Potokar and M. Lavialle, 2004. Polyunsaturated fatty acids in the central nervous system: evolution of concepts and nutritional implications throughout life. Reprod. Nutr. Dev. 44: 509 - 538.

Arishima, K. S., Nakama, Y. Morikawa, Y. Hashimoto and Y. Eguchi,1977. Maternal-foetal interrelations of plasma corticosterone concentrations at the end of gestation in the rat. J. Endocrinol. 72:239-40.

Ashworth, C.J. and C. Antipatis, 2001. Micro-nutrient programming of development throughout gestation. Reprod. 122: 527 - 535.

Austbø, D. and N.J. Dovik, 1996. Different levels of calcium to pregnant mares and growing foals. Proc. 47th meeting EAAP, Lillehammer, Norway.

Bayol, S., D. Jones, G. Golspink and N.C. Stickland, 2004. The influence of undernutrition during gestation on skeletal muscle cellularity and on the expression of genes that control muscle growth. Br. J. Nutr. 91: 331 - 339.

Bellinger, L., C. Lilley and S.C. Langley-Evans, 2004. Prenatal exposure to a maternal low-protein dietprogrammes a preference for high-fat foods in the young adult rat. Br. J. Nutr. 92: 513-520.

Bellinger, L., C. Lilley and S.C. Langley-Evans, 2005. Fetal programming of appetite by exposure to a maternal low protein diet in the rat. Clin. Sci. 109: 413-420.

Bertram, C.E. and M.A. Hanson, 2002. Prenatal programming of postnatal endocrine responses by glucocorticoids. Reprod. 124: 459-467.

Bispham, J., Gopalakrishnan, G.S., Dandrea, J., Wilson, V., Budge, H., Keisler, D.H., Broughton Pipkin, F., Stephenson, T. and Symonds, M.E. 2003. Maternal endocrine adaptation throughout pregnancy to nutritional manipulation: consequences for maternal plasma leptin and cortisol and the programming of fetal adipose tissue development. Endocrinol. 144: 3575-3585.

Capper J.L., R.G. Wilkinson, E. Kasapidou, S.E. Pattinson, A.M. Mackenzie and L.A. Sinclair, 2003. The effect of vitamin E and long- chain polyunsaturated fatty acid supplementation of pregnant and lactating ewes on the transfer of vitamin E to the lamb. In: Proceedings of British Society of Animal Science, p61.

Cheema, K.K., M.R. Dent, H.K. Saini, N. Aroutiounova and P.S. Tappia, 2005. Prenatal exposure to maternal undernutrition induces adult cardiac dysfunction Br J. Nutr. 93: 471 - 477.

Clapp, J.F. 3rd., 2002. Maternal carbohydrate intake and pregnancy outcome. Proc. Nutr Soc. 61: 45-50.

Coenen, M. and I. Vervuert, 2005. The physiological role of minerals and vitamins in the growing horse. In: The growing horse: nutrition and prevention of growth disorders, V. Juliand and W. Martin Rosset (editors), EAAP publication No 114, 173-198.

Cymbaluk, N.F. and M.E. Smart, 1993. A review of possible metabolic relationships of copper to equine bone disease Equine Vet J suppl 16: 19 – 26.

Dandrea, J., V. Wilson, G. Gopalakrishnan, L. Heasman, H. Budge, T. Stephenson and M.E. Symonds, 2001. Maternal nutritional manipulation of placental growth and glucose transporter 1 (GLUT-1) abundance in sheep. Reprod. 122: 793-800.

Da Silva, P., R.P. Aitken, S,M. Rhind, P.A. Racey and J.M. Wallace, 2001. Influence of placentally mediated fetal growth restriction on the onset of puberty in male and female lambs. Reprod. 122: 375-383.

Da Silva, P., R.P. a, P., R.P. Aitken, S.M. Rhind, P.A. Racey and J.M. Wallace, 2002. Impact of maternal nutrition during pregnancy on pituitary gonadotrophin gene expression and ovarian development in growth-restricted and normally grown late gestation sheep fetuses. Reprod. 123: 769-777.

Delange, F. 1998. Screening for congenital hypothyroidism used as an indicator of the degree of iodine deficiency and of its control. Thyroid. 8:1185-92.

Delange, F. 2000. The role of iodine in brain development. Proc. Nutr. Soc. 59:75-9.

Delange, F. 2001. Iodine deficiency as a cause of brain damage. Postgrad. Med. J. 77:217-20.

Delange, F. 2002. Iodine deficiency in Europe and its consequences: an update. Eur J Nucl Med Mol Imaging. 29 Suppl 2: S404-16.

Desai, M., N.J. Crowther, A. Lucas and C.N. Hales, 1996. Organ selective growth in the offspring of protein-restricted mothers. Br. J. Nutr. 76: 591-603.

Desai, M., C.D. Byrne, K., Meeran, N.D. Martenz, S.R. Bloom and C.N. Hales, 1997a. Regulation of hepatic enzymes and insulin levels in offspring of rat dams fed a reduced-protein diet. Am. J. Physiol. 273: G899-G904.

Desai, M., C.D. Byrne, J. Zhang, C.J. Petry, A. Lucas, and C.N. Hales, 1997b. Programming of hepatic-insulin sensitive enzymes in offspring of rat dams fed an isocaloric protein-restricted diet. Am. J. Physiol. 272: G1083-G1090.

Djazayery, M., M. Karandish, F. Moremazi, A. Bherooz, E. Kazerouninejad and M. Mahmoudi, 2004. The effect of calcium supplementation during pregnancy on birth weight and length Proc. Nutr. Soc. 63: 121A.

Fernandez-Twinn, D.S., S.E. Ozanne, S. Ekizoglou, C. Doherty, L. James, B. Gusterson and C.N. Hales, C.N. 2003. The maternal endocrine environment in the low-protein model of intra-uterine growth restriction. Br. J. Nutr. 90: 815-822.

Fowden, A.L. 1997. Comparative aspects of fetal carbohydrate metabolism Equine Vet. J. Suppl. 24: 19 – 25.

Fowden, A.L., R.S. Comline and M. Silver, 1984. Insulin secretion and carbohydrate metabolism during pregnancy in the mare. Equine Vet. J. 16 (4): 239 – 246.

Fowden, A.L. and A.J. Forhead, 2004. Endocrine mechanisms of intrauterine programming. Reprod. 127: 515-526.

Gambling, L. and H.J. McArdle, 2004. Iron Copper and fetal development. Proc. Nutr. Soc. 63: 553 – 562.

Godfrey, K.M. and D.J.P. Barker, 2000. Fetal nutrition and adult disease. Am. J. Clin. Nutr. 71: 1344S-1352S.

Guissani, D.A., A.J. Forhead, D.S. Gardner, A.J. Fletcher, W.R. Allen and A.L. Fowden, 2003. Post- natal cardiovascular function after manipulation of fetal growth by embryo transfer in the horse. J. Physiol. 547: 67 - 76.

Hales, C.N. and D.J.P. Barker, 1992. Type 2 (non-insulin-dependent) diabetes mellitus: the thrifty phenotype hypothesis. Diabetologia 35: 595-601.

Hales, C.N., M. Desai, S.E. Ozanne and Crowther, N.J. 1996. Fishing in the stream of diabetes: from measuring insulin to the control of fetal organogenesis. Biochem. Soc. Trans. 24: 341-350.

Harris, P.A., W. Staniar and A.D. Ellis, 2005. Effect of exercise and diet on the incidence of DOD In: The growing horse: nutrition and prevention of growth disorders. EAAP Publication No 114, V. Julliand and W. Martin-Rosset (editors), 273 – 291.

Hoffman, R.M., D.S. Kronfeld, W.L. Cooper and P.A. Harris, 2003. Glucose clearance in grazing mares is affected by diet, pregnancy, and lactation. J. Anim. Sci. 81: 1764-1771.

Huxley, R.R. and H.A.W. Neil, 2004. Does maternal nutrition in pregnancy and birth weight influence levels of CHD risk factors in adult life? Br. J. Nutr. 91: 459 - 468.

Kieffer, T.J and J.F. Habener, 2000. The adipoinsular axis: effects of leptin on pancreatic beta-cells. Am. J. Physiol. 278: E1-E14.

Kronfeld, D.S., T.M. Hess, B.M. Byrd and R.K. Splan, 2005. Pre-laminitic metabolic syndrome in genetically predisposed ponies involves compensated insulin resistance. J. Anim. Physiol. Anim. Nutr. 89:430-31.

Kronfeld, D. S., K. H. Treiber, T. M. Hess and R. C. Boston, 2005a. Insulin resistance in the horse: definition, detection, and dietetics. J. Anim. Sci. 83 (elec.suppl. 1): E22 - E31.

Langley-Evans, S.C. 2000. Critical differences between two low protein diet protocols in the programming of hypertension in the rat. Int. J. Food Sci. Nutr. 51: 11-17.

Langley-Evans, S.C. 2001. Fetal programming of cardiovascular function through exposure to maternal undernutrition. Proc. Nutr Soc. 60: 505-13.

Langley-Evans, S.C. 2006. Developmental programming of health and disease. Proc. Nutr. Soc. 65: 97-105.

Lea, R.G., L.P. Andrade, M.T. Rae, L.T. Hannah, C.E. Kyle, J.F. Murray, S.M. Rhind and D.W. Miller, 2006. Effects of early maternal undernutrition during early pregnancy on apoptosis regulators in the ovine fetal ovary. Reprod. 131: 113-124.

Lucas, A. 1991. The childhood environment and adult disease: programming by early nutrition in man. Ciba Foundation Symposium 156: 38-55.

Meyer, H. and L. Ahlswede, 1978. The intrauterine growth and body composition of foals and the nutrient requirements of pregnant mares. Anim. Res. Develop. 8: 86 – 112

Nissen, P.M M. Vestergaard and N. Oksbejerg, 2003. Effects of maternal nutrition on serum growth factors in the sow and foetuses and on serum induced proliferation and differentiation of primary myoblasts. Proc. 54th meeting EAAP, Rome, p. 224.

Ousey, J.C., P.D. Rossdale, A.L. Fowden, L. Palmer, C. Turnbull and W.R. Allen, 2004. Effects of manipulating intrauterine growth on post natal adrenocortical development and other parameters of maturity in neonatal foals. Equine Vet. J. 36 (7): 616 - 621.

Ozanne, S.E. and C.N. Hales, 2004. Catch-up growth and obesity in male mice. Nature 427: 411-412.

Ozanne, S.E. and C.N. Hales, 2005. Poor fetal growth followed by rapid postnatal catch-up growth leads to premature death. Mechanisms of Ageing and Development 126: 852-854.

Ozanne, S.E., N.D. Martensz, C.J. Petry, C.L. Loizou and C.N. Hales, 1998. Maternal low protein diet in rats programmes fatty acid desaturase activities in the offspring. Diabetologia 41: 1337-1342.

Ozanne, S.E., C.L. Wang, M.W. Dorling and C.J. Petry. 1999. Dissection of the metabolic actions of insulin in adipocytes from early growth-retarded male rats. J. Endocrinol. 162: 313-319.

Ozanne, S.E., M.W. Dorling, C.L. Wang and Nave, B.T. 2001. Impaired PI 3-kinase activation in adipocytes from early growth-restricted male rats. Am. J. Physiol. 280: 534-539.

Patel, M.S. and M. Srinivasan, 2002. Metabolic programming: causes and consequences. J. Biol. Chem. 277: 1629-1632.

Pearce, S.G., N. D. Grace, J.J. Wichtel, E.C. Firth and P.F. Fennessy, 1998a. Effect of copper supplementation on copper status of pregnant mares and foals. Equine Vet. J. 30: 200 – 203.

Pearce, S.G., N. D. Grace, J.J. Wichtel, E.C. Firth and P.F. Fennessy, 1998b. Effect of copper supplementation on the copper status of pasture fed young Thoroughbreds. Equine Vet. J. 30: 204 – 210.

Pearce, S.G., N. D. Grace, J.J. Wichtel, E.C. Firth and P.F. Fennessy, 1998c. Effect of copper supplementation on the evidence of developmentatl orthopaedic disease in pasture fed New Zealand Thoroughbreds. Equine Vet. J. 30: 211-218.

Rae, M.T., S. Palassio, C.E. Kyle, A.N. Brooks, R.B. Lea, D.W. Miller and S.M. Rhind, 2001. Effect of maternal undernutrition during pregnancy on early ovarian development and subsequent follicular development in sheep fetuses. Reprod. 122: 915-922.

Rae, M.T., S.M. Rhind, P.A. Fowler, D.W. Miller, C.E. Kyle and A.N. Brooks, 2002. Effects of maternal undernutrition on fetal testicular steroidogenesis during the CNS androgen-responsive period in male sheep fetuses. Reprod. 124: 33-39.

Ralston, S.L. 2002. In: Veterinary Clinics of North America Equine Practice:Endocrinology, N.T. Messer and P.J. Johnson (editors). Vet. Clin. Equine 18:295-304.

Robinson, J.S. 1998. Summary of the 3rd international workshop on equine perinatology: comparative aspects. Equine Vet. J. 30: 465 - 466.

Rossdale, P.D. and J.C. Ousey, 1998. Abnormal intrauterine development: potential consequences for survival and athletic performance in the horse. Equine Vet. J. 30: 455 – 456.

Rossdale, P.D. and J.C. Ousey, 2002. Fetal programming for athletic performance in the horse: potential effects of IUGR Equine Vet. Educ. 14 (2): 98 - 112.

Rossdale, P.D. 2004. The maladjusted foal: influences of intrauterine growth retardation and birth trauma. In: Proc. 50th Ann. Conv. Am. Assoc. Equine Practit. Denver, AAEP Lexington.

Srinivasan, M., S.G. Laychock, D.J. Hill and M.S. Patel, 2003. Neonatal nutrition: metabolic programming of pancreatic islets and obesity. Exp. Biol. Med. 228: 15-23.

Treiber, K.H., R.C. Boston, D.S. Kronfeld, P. Harris, 2005. Insulin resistance and compensation in Thoroughbred weanlings adapted to high-glycemic meals. J. Anim. Sci. 83: 2357-2364.

Van Weeren, P.R., J. Knaap and E.C. Firth, 2003. Influence of liver copper status of mare and newborn foal on the development of osteochondrotic lesions. Equine Vet. J. 35: 67-71.

Vickers, M.H., B.H. Breier, W.S. Cutfield, P.L. Hofman and P.D. Gluckman, 2000. Fetal origins of hyperphagia, obesity and hypertension and postnatal amplification by hypercaloric nutrition. Am. J. Physiol. Endocrinol. Metab. 279: E83-E87.

Vickers, M.H., S. Reddy, B.A. Ikenasio and B.H. Breier, 2001a. Dysregulation of the adipoinsular axis – a mechanism for the pathogenesis of hyperleptinemia and adipogenic diabetes induced by fetal programming. J. Endocrinol. 170: 323-332.

Vickers, M-H., B.A. Ikenasio and B.H. Breier, 2001b. IGF-I treatment reduces hyperphagia, obesity, and hypertension in metabolic disorders induced by fetal programming. Endocrinol. 142: 3964-3973.

Vickers, M-H., B.A. Ikenasio and B.H. Breier, 2002. Adult growth hormone treatment reduces hypertension and obesity induced by an adverse prenatal environment. J. Endocrinol. 175: 615-623.
Vickers, M.H., B.H. Breier, D. McCarthy and P.D. Gluckman, 2003. Sedentary behaviour during postnatal life is determined by the prenatal environment and exacerbated by postnatal hypercaloric nutrition. Am. J. Physiol. 285: R271-R273.
Vickers, M.H., P.D. Gluckman, A.H. Coveny, P.L. Hofman, W.S. Cutfield, A. Gertler, B.H. Breier and M. Harris, 2005. Neonatal leptin reverses developmental programming. Endocrinol. 146: 4211-4216.
Wallace, J.M., R.P. Aitken and M.A. Cheyne, 1996. Nutrient partitioning and fetal growth in rapidly growing adolescent ewes. J. Reprod. Fert. 107: 183-190.
Wallace, J.M., D. Bourke, P. Da Silva and R. Aitken, 2001. Nutrient partitioning during adolescent pregnancy. Reprod. 122: 347-357.
Wallace, J.M., R.P. Aitken, J.S. Milne and W.W. Hay, Jr, 2004. Nutritionally mediated placental growth restriction in the growing adolescent: consequences for the fetus. Biol. Reprod. 71: 1055-1062.
Woodall, S.M., B.H. Breier, B.M. Johnston and P.D. Gluckman, 1996. A model of intrauterine growth retardation caused by chronic maternal undernutrition in the rat: effects on the somatotrophic axis and postnatal growth. J. Endocrinol. 150: 231-242.
Woodall, S.M., N.S. Bassett, P.D. Gluckman and B.H. Breier, 1998. Consequences of maternal undernutrition for fetal and postnatal hepatic insulin-like growth factor-I, growth hormone receptor and growth hormone binding protein gene regulation in the rat. J. Molecul. Endocrinol. 20: 313-326.
Wooding, F.B.P. and A.L. Fowden, 2006. Nutrient transfer across the equine placenta: correlation of structure and function. Equine Vet. J. 38 (2): 175 - 183.

Part F - Advances in reproductive biotechnologies

The new biotechnologies of reproduction in horses: recent progresses and applications

F. Camillo[1], C. Galli[2] and E. Palmer[3]
[1]University of Pisa, Veterinari Faculty, 56010 San Piero a Grado, Pisa, Italy
[2]Laboratory of Reproduction Technology, Experimental Italian Institute "Lazzaro Spallanzani", Via Porcellasco 7/f, 26100 Cremona, Italy
[3]Cryozootech S.A., 16 rue André Thome, 78120 Sonchamp, France

Abstract

The biotechnologies of reproduction consist in *in-vitro* manipulations of gametes and /or embryos before reimplantation into a surrogate mother. This allows to use unusual animals for reproduction: immature females as embryo donors, infertile stallions thanks to ICSI technique, infertile or dead mares with the help of in vitro maturation of oocytes and at last castrated males through their clones which will be a replacement stallion for castrated champions. The authors describe the recent progresses obtained in the recent years, the present efficiency of these techniques and their application in the breeding practice.

Keywords: horses, biotechnologies, embryo transfer, cloning

Introduction

This round table presents the new trend in horse technology of reproduction in horses. It does not pretend that all horses are now produced in vitro or by any biotechnology, but, as presented here in the scope of the 3rd European Workshop on Equine Nutrition, this presentation aims at pointing out that new breeding animals should be considered and may receive the attention of nutritionists.

In the old times, the only actors were the barren mare, the foaling mare and the stallion. Then came the new technologies of artificial insemination, embryo transfer, in vitro fertilization and culture and now nuclear transfer. The artificial insemination has allowed a complete separation between the male and female gamete production. Consequently Stallions now have a competition career at the same time as they fertilise hundreds of females. They produce semen all the year round.

The embryo transfer has allowed the reproduction of mares who normally cannot carry pregnancies young mares, performing mares and old mares. As a consequence a mare can produce three or four times more foals than previously. However nobody has really answered the question of the optimal recipient mare.

The in vitro fertilisation by ICSI can overcome subfertility of mares and stallions, allow the use of very small number of sperm cells in storage. However the efficiency of conventional in vitro fertilisation remains insufficient to be used and only ICSI has permitted the first developments.

Dead animals are also used now, either when they are very valuable with the help of post mortem oocyte collection from ovaries,or sperm from epidydimus with the help of CSI. Dead animals are also used to produce recipient ooplasms for nuclear transfer.

Completely sterile animals, such as castrated males are the most recent ones thanks to cloning technology.

All these new breeding animals may have specific requirements and pose specific problems in order to make an efficient production systems. Can we use very young females efficiently without consequences for their future, does intense training influence the gamete production of sport stallions and mares, can we use oocytes of any animal for nuclear transfer?

The most recent scientific developments in embryo transfert and experimental results obtained using these new biotechnologies are reviewed by F. Camillo and C. Galli respectively, while the first commercial application of cloning in domestic animals occurring in the horse is discussed by E Palmer.

Embryo transfer (ET)

This part of the paper will focus on 3 topics: 1) the use of young mares, two and one year old, as embryo donors, 2) studies on embryo transfer in donkeys, 3) commercial applications of ET in Italy

The use of young mares, two and one year old, as embryo donors

lthough mares reach puberty when they are one year old (Wesson and Ginther, 1981; Camillo *et al.*, 2002), usually, they are not bred before the age of three years, or later for sport mares. The use of young mares as embryo donors may allow to anticipate the reproductive life of a valuable animal and to test the reproductive capacity of a sporting mare.

Using two years old fillies as donors has been reported to negatively affect embryo recovery rate: Iuliano and Squires (1985) obtained an embryo recovery rate of 36.3% in two years old Arabian fillies and Steiner and Jordan (1988) found a lower embryo recovery rate in two years old than in mature Hannover mares. In contrast, Savage *et al.* (1989) obtained an embryo recovery rate of 77.7% in two years old Arabian fillies.

Mitchell and Allen (1975) showed that one year old mares were able to conceive but had a high abortion rate. These authors concluded that, although cyclic and fertile, these fillies were not mature enough to carry pregnancy to term.

During different breeding seasons and studies (Camillo et al, 2000 and 2002, Panzani et al, 2004) a total of 84 Haflinger pony mares were employed as embryo donors: 11 maiden from 12 to 16 months of age (one year old mares = 1YM); 57 maiden from 24 to 28 months of age (two years old mares = 2YM); 16 maiden or with a history of normal fertility from 3 to 12 years old (mature mares = MAM) for a total of 44, 101 and 26 oestrus cycles, respectively. Mares of several different breeds, between 2 and 9 years of age, maiden or with a history of normal fertility were employed as recipients.

Oestrous donor mares were naturally bred or artificially inseminated with fresh semen every second day from the detection of a dominant growing follicle until ovulation. Seven to 8 days after ovulation, mares were flushed for embryo recovery. When planned, embryos were transcervically transferred in recipients, which ovulated between one day before to 4 days after the donor. Embryo recovery rate and pregnancy rates in the three groups of mares are reported in Table 1.

No side effects were noticed during the studies following rectal palpation, AI and uterine flushing or hormonal treatment on young mares. The only exceptions were two cases of complete cervical dilatation and expulsion of both uterine flushing catheter and medium during uterine lavage for embryo collection in two 1YM: in these two cases embryo was not recovered.

Table 1. Embryo recovery rate and recipients pregnancy rates at 14 and 25 days in one year old, two years old and mature Haflinger mares.

Age of the donor	Embryo recovery rate	14 days pregnancy rate	25 days pregnancy rate
One year old	21/44 (47.7%)	5/7 (71.4%)	4/7 (57.1%)
Two years old	86/101 (85.1%)	8/16 (50%)	8/16 (50%)
Mature	22/26 (84.6%)	13/20 (65%)	12/20 (60%)

The reproductive performances of 52 former donors (three 1YM and forty-nine 2YM) were controlled in successive breeding seasons: no differences were found comparing the foaling rate of these former donors with the foaling rate of mares of the same breed, age and stud never used before on an embryo transfer program.

The embryo recovery rate of 1YM, although not statistically different, were lower than 2YM and MAM, but similar to per cycle pregnancy rate commonly observed in embryo donors or in mares inseminated with fresh semen. The lower embryo recovery rate in 1YM may be due to a sort of immaturity resulting in a lower quality of oocytes and/or oviductal environment. The pregnancy rate following transfer of embryos recovered from 1YM was similar to the pregnancy rate following transfer of embryos recovered from 2YM and MAM and comparable to the results commonly observed in mature mares (Squires *et al.*, 2004).

In conclusion, the results of this studies demonstrated that young mares can be successfully used as embryos donors without side effects on general or reproductive soundness.

Studies on embryo transfer in donkeys

Many donkey breeds risk the extinction in the Mediterranean area. The Amiata donkey, for example, is present in Tuscany, near the massif of Amiata mountain, in a population of about 500 animals and the Pantesca donkey, that has its roots in the island of Pantelleria, Sicily, considered extinct since 1980, is represented by a population of only 50 animals.

One of the obvious indication of the ET is the conservation of endangered species: in the case of equid ET was employed to try to enlarge the number of Przewalski's Horses *(Equus przewalskii)* (Summers *et al.*, 1987) but data concerning ET in the donkey are still scarce and not encouraging (Allen *et al.*, 1985; Allen *et al.* 1993; Vendramini *et al.* 1997). Allen showed that it was possible to recover embryos from donkeys by non surgical flushing of the uterus and reported a 67% pregnancy rate at 40 days after their transfer in recipient mares by midline laparotomy (Allen *et al.* 1985). However, about 70% of these conceptuses were aborted within day 100 of pregnancy, and half of the remaining foetuses died in the peri partum period (Allen, 1993). Allen's works strongly suggest that mares are not suitable recipients for donkey embryos.

Vendramini *et al.* (1997) transferred donkey embryos to donkeys, both surgically and not surgically, but their rate of success, 5.5%, was much lower than what can be expected after intraspecies embryo transfer in other animal, such horses or cattle.

During 2003 and 2004, in a project of collaboration between University of Pisa and Sicily Region (Azienda Foreste Demaniali della Sicilia and Istituto Incremento Ippico per la Sicilia) 6 Pantesca jennies (2-5 years old), and 15 Ragusana jennies (4-11 years old) were employed as embryo donors and recipients, respectively. Three Pantesca jack stallions known to be fertile were employed to mate the donors. Ovarian activity of animals was evaluated daily during oestrous by transrectal ultrasounds.

From the detection of both a growing follicle ≥ 30 mm in diameter and oestrus behaviour, donors were naturally mated or artificially inseminated with fresh semen every second day until ovulation. Seven to 9 days after ovulation, donors were flushed for embryo recovery using either DPBS (ZE067, I.M.V., L'Aigle Cedeaux, France) or Ringer lactate (Galenica Senese, Siena, Italy) and a "AB Technology Equine Lavage Catether 32 Fr."® (Pullman, WA, USA).

Recovered embryos were evaluated for morphology (McKinnon and Squires, 1989), washed 10 times in DPBS, Ringer lactate or EmCare Holding Solution® (Bio98, Milano) and transcervically transferred (Lagneaux *et al.*, 1988) in recipient ovulating 3-4 days before (non optimal synchronization) or 5-8 days before (optimal synchronization).

The total embryo recovery rate was 62/80 (77,5%) and all embryos but 3 were classified as good or excellent. Overall recipients pregnancy rates at 14 and 50 days were 13/56 (23%) and 10/56 (18%), respectively, with an early embryonic loss of 3/13 (23%). Six embryos were not transferred.

Table 2. Pregnancy rate at 14 and 50 days in recipient at different days following ovulation in donkey to donkey embryo transfer.

Recipient at day	Pregnancies at 14 days (%)	Pregnancies at 50 days (%)	Early embryonic loss
3-4	2/18 (11%)	1/18 (5.5%)	1/2 (50%)
5-8	11/38 (28%)	9/38 (23.7%)	2/11 (18.2%)
Total	13/56 (23.2%)	10/56 (17.8%)	3/13 (23%)

The achieved embryo recovery rate was within the range normally reported for mares, and close to what previously described in donkeys: 53.3% - 63.6% (Allen *et al.*, 1985 and Vendramini *et al.*, 1997). On the other hand, this study confirms that, to date, the limit of ET in donkeys is the very low recipients pregnancy rate. The obtained pregnancy rates were lower than pregnancy rates both after transfer of horse embryos to horses (50-75%, Squires *et al.*, 1999) and surgical transfer of donkey embryos to mares (67%, Allen *et al.*, 1985), but similar to the pregnancy rate previously described after surgical or non-surgical transfer of donkey embryos to donkeys (5.5%, Vendramini *et al.*, 1997). The reasons for these poor results are far to be understood and it is possible than more factors had an effect on the outcome: the synchrony between donor and recipient ovulations was not optimal in about 1/3 of the cases (18/56); donkey embryos may have different requirements in respect to flushing and washing media employed and, finally, it is a common opinion that the difficult catheterisation of the cervix of the jenny, much longer and tortuous than the cervix of the mares, my induce trauma with the consequence of early luteolisys and embryo loss in the recipients. This last hypothesis seems to be negated by the results of a recent preliminary study in which 5/5 recipient jennies were pregnant following transcervical transfer of horse embryos (Camillo et al, unpublished results).

In conclusion, more investigations are needed in this species before embryo transfer can be considered a reliable tool to preserve endangered donkey breeds.

Commercial applications of ET in Italy

The data presented in this part of the paper result from a questionnaire filled by 10 ET groups that correspond approximately to the totality of veterinarians that are involved in commercial ET in horses in Italy and are referred to the breeding seasons between 2001 and 2004.

Technique and media used to recover and to wash the embryos before transfer were changed in the 2004 breeding season: until 2003 most groups employed PBS both for uterine flushing and for embryo holding; publication of papers from France (Moussa et al, 2002) describing the ability of zwitterionic buffers to maintain the viability of equine embryos for at least 24 hours resulted in the use of Emcare for holding the embryos before the transfer by the majority of the Italian groups. In the same time Emcare and mostly ringer lactate replaced PBS for uterine flushing.

In Italy all the contacted veterinarians use now a filter for embryo collection, this due to the shorter time needed, compared to the original French method (Lagneaux et al, 1988). Only three Veterinarians use a laminar flow cabinet and in approximately 50% of the cases the ET group manage his own recipient; up to date, in Italy, there are no centralized groups of recipient; for this reason embryos are not shipped or frozen, but immediately transferred following recovery. All transfers, in Italy, are performed using the transcervical technique.

The following table (Table 3) reports the number of donors, embryo recovery attempts, recovered embryos and recipient pregnant at 14 days in the breeding seasons from 2001 to 2004. The donors were mostly Saddle bred (57%), followed by Trotters (17%), Quarter Horse (18%) and other (8%) breeds.

The high percentage of frozen semen inseminations in Saddle Bred mares is explained by the necessity of importing the best genetic from the countries of North Europe, this due the small number of very important stallion of these breeds in Italy.

Embryo recovery rate was 53%, 55% and 43% for artificial insemination with fresh, chilled and frozen semen, respectively. Total embryo recovery rate and recipient pregnancy rate were similar to data reported by Squires *et al.* (2004) and Carnevale *et al.* (2000), respectively, for commercial ET in USA. Table 4 reports the rate of utilizing fresh, cooled or frozen semen in the different breeds.

In conclusion, in spite of acceptable results generally achieved, the popularity of equine ET is increasing slowly in Italy, probably because of the high costs especially related to the management of the recipients. ET is performed mostly in Saddle Bred mares were in about 50% of cases frozen semen is employed. No data exist about foaling rate of the recipients.

Table 3. Number of donors and cycles, recovered embryos, number and (%), pregnant recipients at 14 days, number and (%), in the commercial embryo transfer activity in Italy.

	Donors	Embryo recovery attempts	Recovered Embryos	Pregnancies at 14 days
2001	67	162	75 (46%)	39 (52%)
2002	73	161	86 (53%)	56 (65%)
2003	103	208	116 (56%)	71 (61%)
2004	115	312	153 (49%)	111 (72%)
Total	358	843	430 (51%)	277 (64%)

Table 4. Type of semen employed in the different breeds in the commercial embryo transfer activity in Italy.

	Fresh semen	Chilled semen	Frozen semen
Saddle Bred	26%	26%	48%
Trotter	36%	56%	8%
Quarter Horse	58%	31%	11%
Others	69%	24%	7%

Experimental results of new biotechnologies in equines

In vitro embryo production

Assisted reproduction techniques are well developed and widely applied in ruminants. The starting material are the immature oocytes recovered from the ovaries of live animals, by ultrasound guided follicular aspiration, or from the ovaries of slaughtered females collected at the abattoir (Galli et al 2003a). Following in vitro maturation, in vitro fertilisation and culture, immature follicular oocytes are converted into viable embryos that are able to establish pregnancies and deliver viable offspring. In domestic species, namely the bovine, several hundred thousands of such embryos are produced each year for breeding purposes. On the contrary, in the horse very little has been achieved so far and the foals derived from embryos produced in vitro may add up only to a dozen world wide.

A major difference with ruminants is the anatomy and physiology of the ovary because of which the mare can be considered a "poor" oocyte donor. Other aspects peculiar to the horse are the recovery of the oocytes that requires the mechanical scraping of the ovarian follicles with a Jacobson curette and the rapid post-mortem degeneration that the ovaries undergo because of their relative large size.

On average 3.76 oocytes per ovary are recovered (see Table 5), of wich 2/3 are of compact morphology and the rest are expanded (i.e. undergoing spontaneous maturation).

With ultrasound guided follicular aspiration of immature follicles from live donors, on average 3.2 oocytes are recovered (see Table 2) with repeated session performed on the same donor. The quality of oocytes matured in vitro can be assessed by transfer to the oviducts of synchronised, inseminated recipients. Zhang et al (1989) showed that high rate of development could be obtained after in vitro maturation and transfer to the oviducts of inseminated recipients.

An alternative option developed by Carnevale *et al.* (2005) involves the puncture of the preovulatory follicle after HCG injection; in this case only one follicle (preovulatory) is aspirated and the oocyte recovered should be fertilised within hours from collection and again is transferred to the oviduct of inseminated recipients.

Table 5. Oocytes recovery from abattoir ovaries.

n of ovaries	240
total number of oocytes	902
n of compacted oocytes	632
n of expanded oocytes	270
average n of oocytes per ovary	3,76

Table 6. Oocyte recovery by ovum pick up.

n of mares	5
n of collections	44
n of follicles	292
average n of follicles per collection	6,6
n of oocytes recovered	141
average n of oocytes per collection	3,2
recovery rate	48%

The second step in order to produce an embryo in vitro is to achieve fertilisation. Very little success has been reported so far with stallion semen. Indeed only one foal has been obtained by Palmer et al (1991) after in vitro fertilisation of an in vivo matured oocyte. Because of these difficulties, the use of intracytoplasmic sperm injection (ICSI) has been attempted in horses to overcome the barrier of in vitro fertilisation. The first report of successful ICSI documented in 1996 by Squires and collaborators was not developed further till Galli and collaborators by using piezo ICSI (a particular type of micromanipulator) consistently and reproducibly generated cleavage stage embryos at high rates (Galli et al 2002) capable to develop into blastocysts suitable for transfer and/or freezing. The same lab showed that using ICSI, the field fertility of the semen is not correlated to embryo development in vitro, providing that, viable sperm could be selected for injection. Under such conditions blastocyst development was similar amongst stallions with different field fertility (Lazzari et al 2002) see Table 7.

This experimental results demonstrate the possibility of using semen available in very small amounts or semen of poor quality (usually after freezing and thawing) whose use would be impossible under conventional breeding.

Cleavage stages embryos must be transferred to the oviduct of the recipient mare requiring endoscopical or surgical procedures that complicates its use in practice. This problem has been overcome by the culture of the ICSI cleaved embryos to the blastocyst stage followed by non-surgical transcervical transfer to the uterus of synchronised recipients. The culture requirements of horse embryos are quite similar to bovine embryos. They grow well in vivo into the surrogate sheep oviducts but also in vitro, albeit at a lower rate in mSOF (synthetic oviductal fluid) see Table 4.

The percentage of embryos developing into the sheep oviduct is comparable to that obatined with the bovine. By contrast, after in vitro culture the rate of embryo development is lower and also the

Table 7. Cleavage and development rate following ICSI with semen of different motility and fertility post-thawing.

group of stallions	N. Met. II injected	N. cleaved	cleavage %	N. comp. morulae/ blastocysts	% comp. morulae/ blastocysts/cleaved
A	117	88	75.2 a	42	47.7 a
B	78	49	62.8 a	21	42.9 a
C	91	72	79.1 a	33	45.8 a
D	46	4	8.7 b	0	0.0 b

Chi square test. Numbers within columns with different letters are significantly different ($p<0.05$). (Lazzari et al 2002)

Table 8. Oocyte recovery by OPU, cleavage and embryo development in the sheep oviduct or in vitro.

N. OPUs	N. oocytes (per OPU)	N. Met. II (% of oocytes) (per OPU)	N. cleaved (% of Met. II) (per OPU)	N. comp. morulae or blastocysts (% of cleaved) (per OPU)
20 (sheep oviduct)	60 (3.0)	46 (76.7) (2.3)	41 (89.1 a) (2.1)	23 (56.1 a) (1.2)
12 (in vitro culture)	49 (4.1)	36 (73.5) 3	25 (69.4 a) (2.1)	5 (20.0 b) (0.4)

Student T test. Numbers with different letters are significantly different ($p<0.05$). (Galli et al 2002)

quality of the embryos measured by cell number is reduced compared to their in vivo counterpart (Tremoleda et al 2003). However, when embryos produced in vitro are given the appropriate time to catch up by transfer to younger recipients (i.e. day 7 IVP embryos transferred to day 5 recipients) then the pregnancy rates are comparable to in vivo produced embryos resulting in the delivery of normal, viable foals, (Galli, unpublished).

Table 9. Diameter and total cell number of Day 7 horse embryos produced either in vivo or ex vivo by culture in SOF or temporary transfer to the oviduct of progesterone treated ewes.

Embryo productionsystem	No.	Diameter (μm)	Number of cells (mean ± SEM)
In vitro (SOF culture)	32*	139.9 ± 1.6a	115.7 ± 15.2a
Semi-in vitro (sheep oviduct)	15	138.1 ± 2.5a	85.8 ± 9.3a
In vivo	10	374 ± 64.1b	1736 ± 567.9b

Within a column, values that differ significantly have different superscripts (^{a,b} $P< 0.001$). **In vitro* produced embryos were derived from both expanded (n=21) and compact (n=11) COCs. (Tremoleda et al 2003)

Nuclear transfer cloning

Somatic cell nuclear transfer has been the subject of much investigation in the last few years and as a result several mammalian species have been cloned (see Galli *et al.*, 2003b as review). In Equids the birth of three mule foals cloned from fetal cells (Woods *et al.* 2003) and one horse foal cloned from adult somatic cells (Galli *et al.* 2003c) have been only recently reported. Remarkably all foals were born alive and survived to adulthood.

Information available in the literature on assisted reproductive techniques in Equids, in particular oocyte maturation and in vitro culture of early pre-implantation embryos. Indeed, the work that led to the cloning of mules (Wood *et al.* 2003) relied on in vivo matured oocytes that were transferred to the oviducts of recipient mares immediately after nuclear transfer and activation, this approach is both very expensive from a financial point of view and also ethically questionable since it involves a lot of surgical procedures on mares. Only the work of Galli *et al.* (2003c) has been carried out completely in vitro up to the blastocyst stage.

Further work carried out by by the same group (Lagutina et al 2005) reported the bitrh of a second foal, genomic copy of a gelded champion, opening the way to the application of cloning in the horse industry to save valuable genes. Much of the factors affecting in vitro production described above are also crucial for nuclear transfer and the success has come from groups that can manage in vitro assisted reproduction. The use of zona free manipulation (Oback et al 2003) has made nuclear transfer more efficient, by increasing fusion rates and cleavage rates (Table 10)

Thus is consistent with the fact that the equine zona pellucida is very etherogeneus and often problematic to manipulate. Horse oocytes are also more difficult to activate. In our preliminary experiments we found that a combination of the most used inhibitors (6-DMAP and Cloheximide) was required to efficiently activate equine oocytes (Galli et al 200?). Several cell types have been used for nuclear transfer from different donors, however like in other species there is no appreciable difference between cell types but there is a huge variation in success rate between different donors (or cell lines) (Table 11)

Table 10. Development of horse NT embryos reconstructed by zona enclosed versus zona free methods.

Donor Cells	Method of NT	N oocytes enucleated	N of couplets Fused (%)	Cleaved N (% of fused)	BL D8	
					N (% of fused)	(% of oocytes)
cumulus	zona-enclos.	113	78 (69)[a]	54 (69.2)[c]	1 (1.3)	(0.9)
	zona-free	104	104 (100)[b]	88 (84.6)[d]	3 (2.9)	(2.9)
adult	zona-enclos.	181	120 (66.3)[a]	82 (68.3)[c]	5 (4.2)	(2.7)
fibroblasts	zona-free	193	187 (97)[b]	159 (85.0)[d]	12 (6.4)	(6.2)

The number of replicates was ≥ 4.
values with different letters within columns differ significantly. Chi square, $P<0.05$.
BL D8 –blastocysts on Day 8. (Lagutina et al 2005)

Table 11. Embryo transfer and pregnancy.

Cell type	Horse	Embryos N	Recipients N	Pregnancy n (%)	35 days n (%)	3 months n (%)	6 months n (%)	Offspring n (%)
Cumulus 22 h IVM	3	3	0 (0)	0 (0)	0 (0)	0 (0)	0 (0)	
fibroblast	C fetal§	33	18	1 (5.6)	1 (5.6)	1 (5.6)	1 (5.6)	0 (0)
fibroblast	A adult	4	2	1 (50)	0 (0)	0 (0)	0 (0)	0 (0)
fibroblast	B adult	71	23	6 (26.1)	4 (17.4)	3 (13)	2 (8.7)	2 (8.7)
fibroblast	C adult	26	12	2 (16.7)	2 (16.7)	1 (8.3)	1 (8.3)	0 (0)
fibroblast	Total adult	101	37	9 (24.3)	6 (16.2)	4 (10.8)	3 (8.1)	2 (5.4)

* - cumulus cells of oocytes from slaughtered mares., § - fetal fibroblasts derived from an aborted cloned fetus of male C., Chi square, $P<0.05$. No statistical differences. (Lagutina et al 2005)

Why are stallions the first clones to reach the breeding practice?

2005 was the year of birth of two clones of famous horses from the cell bank of Cryozootech and we expect them to become stallions. They were obtained in collaboration with Cesare Galli in Italy and with Katrin Hinrichs in USA.

In 2005 these foals have received a passport by an official European stud-book (stud-book Zangersheide), which provides a legal status to these animals and prepares them to be accepted as breeding animals.

Although it is not the first species and not the first success of equine cloning, their birth has a great impact because they are the first that may enter the breeding practice. All problems of clones are not yet completely solved, but I hope to demonstrate here that using a cloned male for breeding is a safe and useful new tool for the breeding industry.

Why do we want to clone an animal?

The first idea when you talk of cloning is that you are making a full photocopy of the donor. Many uses have been imagined: making multiple identical animals for experimental purpose, making the copy of a dead animal to restore endangered genotypes, making multiple bulls with the same genotype for multiplication of high genetic animals, making clones of exceptional carcasses found in slaughterhouses for producing high quality meat etc.

Most of these applications are waiting until one or another unanswered question on cloning has been solved: is the clone absolutely equal to its model for the expected use, will it bring a real progress which is worth the cost and is there any risk for the human health.

Of course the research laboratories and the biotechnology industry work hard on the topic, as scientists find the clones a great model for basic scientific questions and the biotechnologists think of large markets for high value medicines.

What are the differences between a clone and its model, the donor of cells?

First, let us consider clones as perfect identical twins. As performing animals they will differ because of all the environmental factors, other than the true genetic influence. They would be phenotypically equal only if heritabilty was 1. However it is usually somewhere between 0 and 0.50 for most of the traits they are selected for. But we must notice that genetically identical twins will produce exactly the same sperm or oocytes (depending of the sex) and are absolutely equal as vectors of the genetic progress. Fig 1 summarises the different steps where differences can occur between a clone and its model.

The first difference that occurs due to cloning comes from the presence of a recipient ooplasm, which contains mitochondrial DNA. If the mitochondria are involved in any phenotypic differences, then the clone is not equal for performance for two reasons: the heritability and the cytoplasm. For the use as breeding animal, there is a difference between male and female clones. A female clone will produce oocytes with recipient ooplasm and mitochondrial DNA. The difference will be transmitted to its progeny. On the contrary cloned males indeed produce spermatozoa with mitochondria in their mid-piece, but these mitochondria are not transmitted to the next generation as only maternal mitochondria will be maintained. The male clone is still absolutely equal to its model to transmit its nuclear genes. Figure 2 summarises the transmission of DNA from model to clone and from the clone to its offspring.

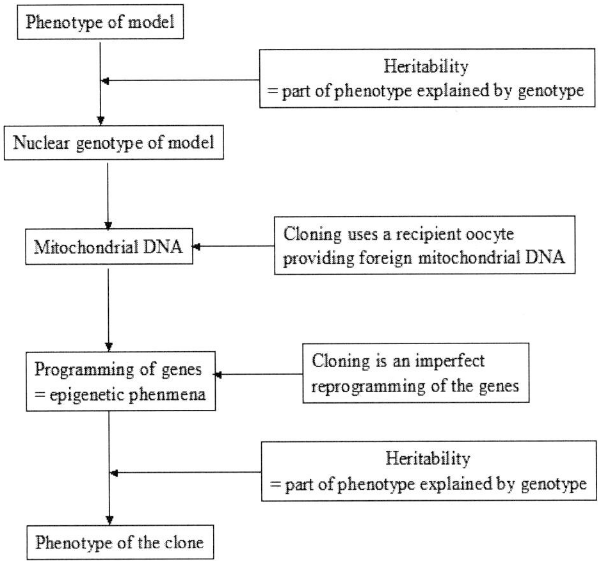

Figure 1. Possible sources of differences between the phenotypes of a a clone and its model.

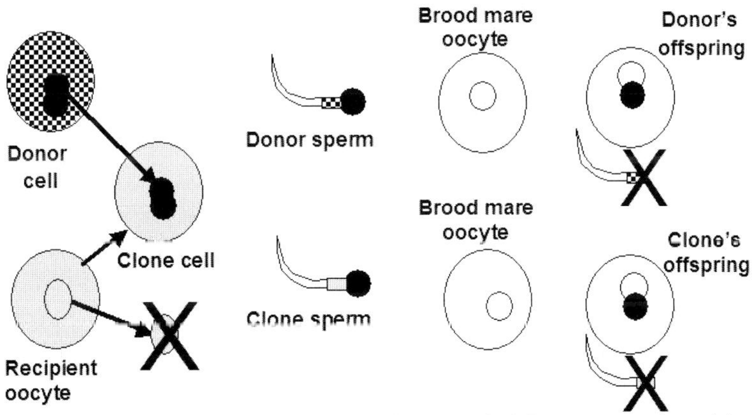

The colour demonstrates the origin of nuclear and mitochondrial DNA: Black for Donor, grey for recipient oocyte and white for brood mare oocyte. The final offspring of the clone is absolutely equal to that of the donor.

Figure 2.Transmission of DNA from the donor to the clone and to the offspring of the clone.

The second difference most often reproached to clones are anomalies which are thought to be epigenetic. This means that the genes are present and normal but that they are not perfectly programmed. Indeed, the operation of cloning is trying to reprogram the genome to the stage following fertilization, but this "trying" is more often hoping. The natural programming of the genome occurs during different phases of the gametogenesis, fertilization and early developpement. The abnormal reprogramming is thought to be responsible for most of the losses that occur during embryonic and foetal development of clones. The animals that survive these stages are thought to be well "reprogrammed". The experts say that after the perinatal period where there is still a high mortality, the clones are more and more equal to control animals and tend to have close to normal survival. However unexpected deaths do occur and a higher than normal mortality occur in cattle. An experiment in mice however did not show any difference in longevity of clones vs control. The possible imperfect programming of the genome increases the possible phenotypic difference between a clone and its model, but it does not increase the difference as breeding animal. The pattern of deprogramming and reprogramming that occurs at each generation (one wave of demethylation followed by methylation of a large part of the genome occur during gametogenesis and a second one occur just after fertilization.) will erase the imperfect programming that occur at the cloning step. No occurrence of large offspring syndrome has been reported in cloned cows or following the use of sperm of cloned bulls.

In conclusion we can say that the clones used as male breeders do not differ from their model as they transmit the same nuclear genes, they do not transmit the mitochondrial DNA of the recipient oocyte and their possible imperfect DNA reprogramming will not be transmitted to their progeny.

As far as genetic progress is concerned, a common objection is that making an equal animal does not provide progress. This is true if all animals are available for breeding as much as necessary. However in some cases, the sport horse is an example, the best animals are not available for breeding because they have been castrated for this use and their high ability has been discovered after the castration. In the case of castrated champions the use of a clone is the only possibility to transmit efficiently his genes into the breeding world.

Another objection is that the cloning process increases the interval between generations as one waits for the test to be completed before cloning is attempted. This is probably the only objection that cannot be ruled out and that can be put on the negative side of the balance. Geneticists have calculated the incidence of using clones of the castrated performers as stallions taking into account the percentage of castrated animals in the population and the increased interval of generations.

Figure 3 shows that, in spite of the increased interval between generations, the yearly genetic progress can be increased by up to 50% in breeds where almost all animals are castrated like endurance or dressage, whereas the benefit is much smaller in breeds where the majority of animals are tested before being castrated, like the race horses.

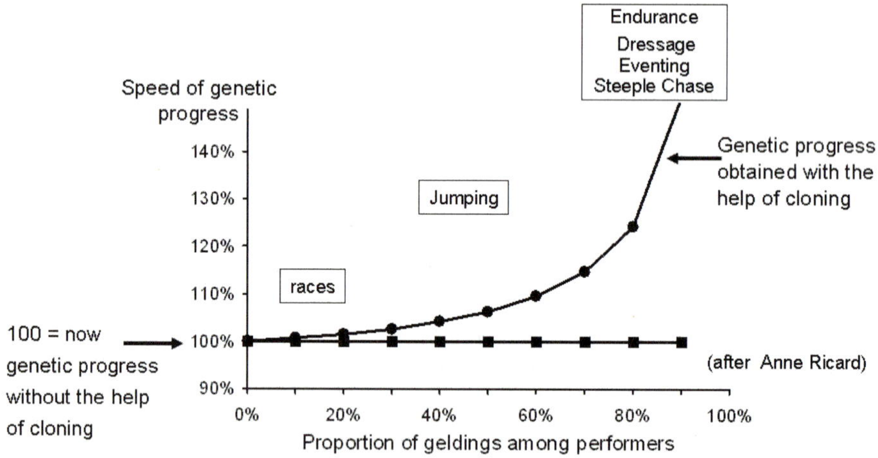

selecting stallions in a wider population of performers will allow a higher selection rate, and consequently more rapid genetic progress

Figure 3. Increase of genetic progress generated by the use of clones of gelded performers as a possible source of stallions in different disciplines, according to the percentage of castrated animals among performers.

European and North American countries are extremely careful about any possible risk for human health of the use of any biotechnology and make no difference in this respect between cloning and any other biotechnology, even if the theoretical risk is hard to imagine. Horse are not considered as food animals in some countries. In other countries they can be legally rejected from slaughter thanks to individual passport inscription by a veterinarian. Consequently this argument has never been objected to cloning horses.

At last, everyone knows that the champion horses have sometimes a big value and that the horse world is used to take financial risks. Another reason why the Horse is probably the first market where cloning is becoming a breeding technique.

In general conclusion, the use of a cloned horse as a stallion find no real objection: it is theoretically absolutely equal to its model for this use, there is no human health involved, there is an economic basis and there is a genetic progress at the end.

Of course we are all looking forward to see the results of this use on the genetic progress in different disciplines. The horse industry is starting to do the real test of a new genetic tool. We are now at the same stage as 60 years ago for Artificial Insemination but changes are much more rapid nowadays.

References

Allen, W.R., J. Kydd, M.S. Boyle and D.F. Antczac, 1985. Between-species transfer of horse and donkey embryos: a valuable research tool. Equine Vet. J. Suppl. 3,53-62.

Camillo, F, I. Vannozzi, A. Rota, D. Panzani, A. Illuzzi and D Guillaume, 2002. Age at puberty, cyclicity, clinical response to PGF2α, hCG and GnRH and recovery rate in yearling mares, Theriogenology; 58:627-630.

Camillo, F, I. Vannozzi, A. Rota, S. Romagnoli and G. Aria, 2000. Comparison of embryo recovery rates from two years old and mature mares, Havemayer Foundation Monograph Series n° 3. Proceedings of the 5th International Symposium on Equine Embryo Transfer, Saari-Helsinki; 86-88.

Carnevale, E.M., R.J. Ramirez, E.L. Squires, M.A. Alvarenga, D.K. Vanderwall and P.M. McCue, 2000. Factors affecting pregnancy rates and early embryonic death after equine embryo transfer. Theriogenology 54, 965:979.

Carnevale, EM, M.A. Coutinho da Silva, D. Panzani, J.E. Stokes and E.L. Squires, 2005. Factors affecting the success of oocyte transfer in a clinical program for subfertile mares. Theriogenology. Aug;64(3):519-27.

Galli, C, G. Crotti, P. Turini, R. Duchi, G. Mari, G. Zavaglia, G. Duchamp, P. Daels and G Lazzari, 2002. Frozen-thawed embryos produced by Ovum Pick Up and ICSI are capable to establish pregnancies in the horse. Theriogenology, 58, 713-715.

Galli, C, R. Duchi, G. Crotti, N. Ponderato, S. Colleoni, I. Lagutina and G. Lazzari, 2003a. Bovine embryo technologies. Theriogenology, 59, 599-616.

Galli, C, I. Lagutina, C. Crotti, S. Colleoni, P. Turini, N. Ponderato, R. Duchi and G. Lazzari, 2003. Pregnancy: a cloned horse born to its dam twin. Nature. Aug 7;424(6949):635.

Galli, C, I. Lagutina and G. Lazzari, 2003b. Introduction to cloning by nuclear transplantation. Cloning & Stem Cells, vol 5 n4, 223-232.

Iuliano, M.F. and E.L. Squires, 1985. Embryo transfer in two-year-old mares. Theriogenology 24, 647-654.

Lagneaux, D., G. Duchamp and E. Palmer, 1988. La transplantation embryonnaire chez la jument, 14eme CEREOPA. 163-181.

Lagutina, I, G. Lazzari, R. Duchi, S. Colleoni, N. Ponderato, P. Turini, G. Crotti and C. Galli, 2005. Somatic cell nuclear transfer in horses: effect of oocyte morphology, embryo reconstruction method and donor cell type. Reproduction. Oct;130(4):559-567.

Lazzari, G, G. Crotti, P. Turini, R. Duchi, G. Mari, G. Zavaglia, S. Barbacini and C. Galli, 2002. Equine embryos at the compacted morula and blastocyst stage can be obtained by intracytoplasmic sperm injection (ICSI) of in vitro matured oocytes with frozen-thawed spermatozoa from semen of different fertilities. Theriogenology, 58, 709-712.

Mitchell, D. and W.R. Allen, 1975. Observations on reproductive performance in the yearling mare, J Reprod Fert Suppl; 23:531-536.

Moussa, M., G. Duchamp, R. Mahla, J.-F. Bruyas and P.F. Daels, 2002. Comparison of pregnancy rates for equine embryos cooled for 24 h in Ham's F-10 and emcare holding solutions. Theriogenology 58 (2-4) 755-757.

Palmer, E, J. Bezard, M. Magistrini and G. Duchamp, 1991. In vitro fertilization in the horse. A retrospective study. J Reprod Fertil Suppl. 44:375-84.

Panzani, D, A. Rota, M. Pacini, I. Vannozzi, G. Aria and F. Camillo, 2004. Transfer of embryos recovered from yearling mares resulted in pregnancies. 15th International Congress on Animal Reproduction, Porto Seguro, Abstracts; 2:409.

Panzani, D., C. Scollo, A. Rota, M. Pacini, I. Vannozzi, S. Balbo and F. Camillo, 2004. Intraspecies embryo transfer in donkeys.

Savage, N.C., L.A. Woodcock and G. Degannes, 1989. Use of two-year-old mares as embryo donors in a commercial embryo transfer programme. Equine Vet J Suppl 8:68-70.

Squires, E.L., E.M. Carnevale, P.M. McCue and J.E. Bruemmer, 2004. Embryo technologies in the horse. Theriogenology 59, 151-170.

Squires, E.L., P.M. McCue and D. Vanderwall, 1999. The current status of equine embryo transfer. Theriogenology 51, 91-104.

Squires, E.L., E.M. Carnevale, P.M. McCue and J.E. Bruemmer, 2004. Embryo technologies in the horse. Theriogenology 59:151-170.

Squires, E.L., J.M. Wilson, H. Kato and A. Blaszczyk, 1996. A pregnancy after intracytoplasmic sperm injection into equine oocytes matured in vitro. Theriogenology, 45, 306.

Steiner, J.V. and M.T. Jordan, 1988. Ovulation rates, embryo collection rates and embryo transfer rates for mature and two-years-old Hanoverian mares. Equine Pract 10:6-8.

Summers, P.M, A.M. Shephard, J.K. Hodges, J. Kydd, M.S. Boyle and W.R. Allen, 1987. Successful transfer of the embryos of Przewalski's Horses (Equus przewalskii) and Grant's Zebra (E. burchelli) to domestic mares (Equus caballus). J. Reprod. Fert. 80,13-20.

Tremoleda, J.L., T.A. Stout, I. Lagutina, G. Lazzari, M.M. Bevers, B. Colenbrander and C. Galli,2003. Effects of in vitro production on horse embryo morphology, cytoskeletal characteristics, and blastocyst capsule formation. Biol Reprod. Dec;69(6):1895-906. Epub 2003 Aug 06.

Vendramini, O.M., J.F. Bruyas, F. Fieni, I. Battut and D. Tainturier, 1997. Embryo transfer in Poitou donkeys, preliminary results. Theriogenology 47, 409.

Wesson, J.A. and O.J. Ginther, 1982. Influence of photoperiod on puberty in the female pony, J Reprod Fertil Suppl 32:269-274.

Woods, G.L., K.L. White, D.K. Vanderwall, G.P. Li, K.I. Aston, T.D. Bunch, L.N. Meerdo and B.J. Pate, 2003. A mule cloned from fetal cells by nuclear transfer. Science. Aug 22;301(5636):1063. Epub 2003 May 29.

Zhang, J.J., M.S. Boyle, W.R. Allen and C. Galli, 1989. Recent studies on in vivo fertilization of in vitro matured horse oocytes. Equine Veterinary Journal, Suppl. 8,101-104.

Management strategy of the broodmare: The case of trotter mares in Italy

A. Falaschini and F. Cappelli
Department of Veterinary Morphophysiology and Animal Production, Alma Mater Studiorum, Via Tolara di Sopra, I40064 Ozzano Emilia/Bologna, Italy

Abstract

Mare, a polyestrous long-day breeder, show maximum reproduction efficiency in spring-early summer, i.e. in April-June in North hemisphere. Trotter mare breeding is influenced by several factors that interfere with their natural reproductive activity. Among these, the need to advance foaling to the early months of the year is directed at obtaining more competitive subjects in terms of morphological development and athletic performance for qualification trials. Among the strategies devised to achieve this goal is the prevention or shortening of the winter anoestrus by means of an artificial photoperiod, diet supplements and hormone treatments. Here we review these strategies and analyse the effects of different management factors in a mare trotter farm; first of all the nutrition of the mare in peripartum in order to meet mare requirements before for foetal growth, than for milk production and allow the new pregnancy. Moreover some aspects of morphological evolution of the foal are discussed.

Key words: mare, management, photoperiod, diet

Introduction

The management of reproduction is extremely important in any species, as it critically affects both technical and economic results. In the main species bred for human consumption (cattle, swine and sheep), such management is directed at optimizing efficiency by minimizing the partum-mating interval. In sows, pregnancy should begin within 4-5 weeks of parturition; in dairy cows within 3 months to allow for a suitable dry period and to exploit the lactation curve; in beef cows the goal is at least one parturition a year. Also in mares a regular foaling cycle is of primary importance, but besides physiological problems other kinds of factors play a role.

Management of the mares

Mares are seasonally polyestrous long-day breeders. In natural conditions, maximum breeding efficiency is achieved in late spring-early summer, when the reproductive apparatus of grazing mares is stimulated by increasing day length, temperature and a qualitatively and quantitatively suitable diet. However, the natural course of trotter mare reproduction is influenced by several management-related factors. Perhaps the most critical of these is that since the age of a horse is calculated from January 1st and trotters begin racing at "two years". Generally running their first race in summer-autumn in Italy, subjects born in June-July will compete with trotters born in January, which thus have a critical advantage in terms of development and athletic performance. This is why breeders try and concentrate births in the first months of the year and may opt against inseminating a mare that has foaled in June-July, since the foal would be born even later (in July-August).

The French mare management scheme described for French Saddle Horse by Micol and Martin-Rosset (1995) adjusted to the conditions prevailing in central Italy is reported in Figure1. The two breeding systems are comparable. In Italy mares are kept out at pasture from spring to the end of December and are then housed in individual box stalls for parturition and mating. However, in Italy only the few breeding farms situated in hill and mountain areas and providing sufficient grazing

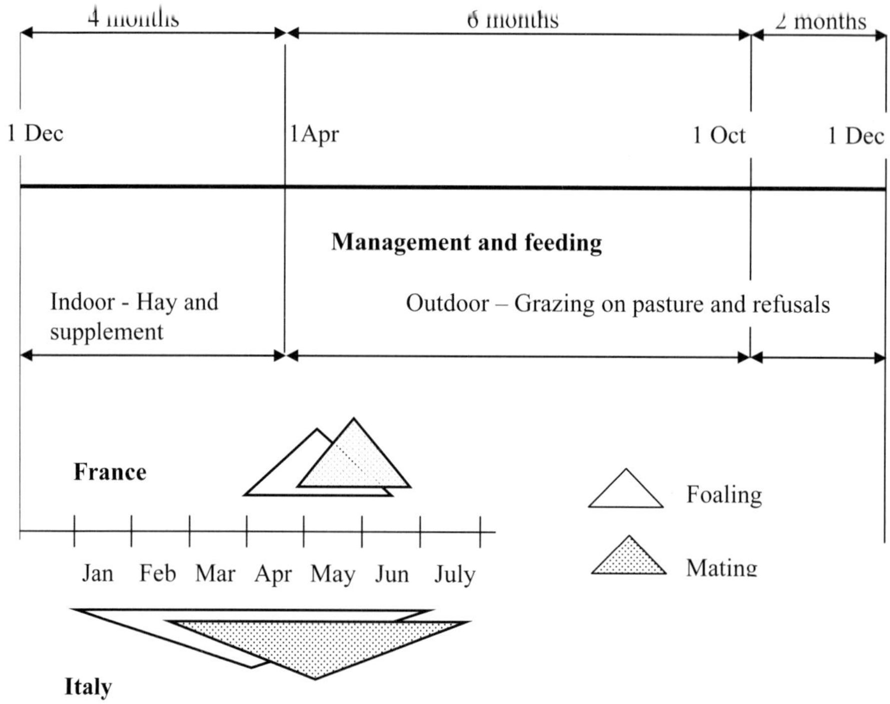

Figure 1. Mare management scheme (modified from Micole and Martin-Rosset, 1995).

levels (>1 ha/mare+foal) can adopt the French management system based exclusively on grazing from spring to late autumn-early winter.

Indeed, the mean yields of Italian pastures from April to November do not allow to offer exclusively fresh feed and grazing of refusals in the last months of the year as in France (see Figure 1). Since in average climatic conditions grazing levels of 0.5-0.7 ha/mare+foal are insufficient, pasture is integrated with hay and energy and protein supplements. On most farms, however, mares are kept in paddocks less for dietary reasons than to allow free movement. The quantity and quality of the supplements vary considerably as a function of pasture composition, phase of production, the mare's physiological state (4-6 kg during lactation; 1-2 kg in the dry period until 2 months before foaling and also in relation to body condition score - BCS), and of course the available type of forage. Corn silage and silage in general is less widely used in indoor dietary regimens in Italy than in France.

Considerable differences between the two countries are found in breeding periods. As shown in Figure 1, whereas the reproductive season of French saddle horses with feeding systems based on high-forage content diets spans 2.5-3 months (including foaling and mating), mainly spring to early summer, in Italy trotter foaling begins with the new year and continues throughout June, while the mating season officially begins on 15 February and, for the reasons stated above, ends by the end of June. Currently, trotters are prevalently inseminated artificially with chilled or frozen semen by a veterinarian, who establishes by ultrasound examination the presence of oestrus and the appearance of the follicle, whose structure directs the decision to perform a single or multiple procedure or postpone it altogether. Artificial insemination (AI) enables a more rational management of the stallion using both chilled and frozen semen which effectively improves its exploitation. Breeders often avoid inseminating the mare during the less fertile foal heat (Loy, 1980; Luxer, 1980), which usually arises 6-10 days post partum, particularly when employing sperm from prize stallions (of which few doses may be available), and await the subsequent oestrus, which presents one month post partum, albeit it obviously extends the foaling-mating interval.

As regards feeding, trotter mares in Italy are usually kept out at pasture in spring through autumn and stabled in winter; however, they receive a forage supplement as well as concentrated feed (usually oats and/or integrated compound feeds), to meet protein and energy requirements, also in the mild season. The compositions of the three rations for pregnant and lactating mares, reported in Table 1, aim at meeting mare requirements, which evolve from the end of gestation to lactation (milk production varies widely among breeds and may exceed 20 l/day). Compound feed supply crude protein and vitamins. Vitamin supplements, too often neglected, meet not only the mare's requirements but also the foal's needs through the colostrum. At the end of gestation the utilisation of vegetable oil allow to supply more energy without increasing dry matter ingestion.

The peripartum is an important phase in which the mare's nutritional needs change. Towards the end of gestation its ingestion ability decreases, especially with regard to forage, while the completion of foetal growth, which is late and exponential as 2/3 of the weight are gained in the last three months, gives rise to further requirements (see the chapter 1 of this issue). The diet in this phase also needs to promote prompt resumption of cycling, and a correct nutrient balance (energy and protein) has been suggested to affect favourably milk production and thus foal growth (Martin-Rosset and Doreau, 1984; Doreau et al, 1988; Salomoni, 1995; Hintz, 1998).

The various aspects discussed above were investigated in a study of the effects of flushing in the trotter mare peripartum that involved two farms (Trombetta *et al.*, 2000). Integration with 25 MJ DE/day (+ 30-35% compared with the control ration) did not induce significant effects on the strictly reproductive parameters (partum to 1st oestrus interval, inseminations/mare and inseminations/ pregnancy), but slightly reduced all of them. The lack of statistical significance may have been due to the already low parturition to conception interval of control mares (11-12 days), which was lower than the one reported by Nagy *et al.* (1998).

A specific problem regarding the vitamins provided in the ration regards β-carotene. Inactivation of grass β-carotene, which begins at harvest and continues throughout storage, involves losses from 150-250 mg/kg of the grass to 10-20 mg/kg DM of the hay in January-February. Various works

Table 1. Rations for pregnant and lactating mares (modified from Salomoni, 1995).

		9th month of gestation	11th month of gestation	1st month of lactation
Meadow hay	kg	6-jul	6-jul	10
Cracked barley + corn	kg	2.5	2.5	4
Compound feed	kg	0.5	0.8-1	0.7
Vegetable oil	g	----	100	150
Dry Matter	kg	8-8.5	8.5-9	13
Digestible Energy	Mj	90	100	150
Crude Protein	g	700	800	1,1
Calcium	g	40	45	60
Phosphorus	g	27	32	45
A Vitamin	IU	30	40	45
D Vitamin	IU	5	5,8	11
E Vitamin	IU	95	95	100

(Ahlswede and Konermann, 1980; van der Holst *et al.*, 1984) have highlighted a positive influence of this provitamin on the reproductive apparatus. In particular, its administration in the peripartum (from 10 days before to 15 days after delivery) promotes the resumption of ovarian activity and significantly affects its blood levels as well as the levels of vitamins A and E (Trombetta *et al.*, 2003), with favourable effects on the metabolism. In fact, until the 15th day post partum the blood parameters merely evidenced higher oestrogen levels; nonetheless, the interval between parturitions was shorter in mares that had received the supplement (369.3 *vs.* 375.1 days). The data for the whole subsequent month evidenced swifter (by ~ 10 days) resumption of ovarian activity (Figure 2). Oestrogen levels also changed, although with different trends in the various subjects. In an another research preformed in the current year (Falaschini, 2006 - unpublished) we have found that β-carotene and artificial photoperiod utilisation allowed to inseminate broodmares in winter anoestrus before February end *vs.* April end for mares with natural photoperiod and without β-carotene.

Several authors have tried to clarify the individual favourable effects of the factors that change in spring: daylight, temperature and diet. Some have investigated mares raised at different latitudes to test the possibility of shortening the winter anoestrus by modifying the photoperiod quantitatively and qualitatively. Camillo *et al.* (1993) used artificial lighting with 200 W bulbs (16 h light/8 h darkness) to supplement natural light in Grosseto (43° degrees N) to assess, among other things, whether the anoestrus could be prevented. Anoestrus took place anyway, but cycling resumed ~ 46 days early. In their 32, predominantly Quarter Horse mares, Hodge *et al.* (1982) noted a reduction in the gestational period (338 *vs.* 348 days) and a non-significant advancement of parturition (1 day). However, this finding is to be attributed to the fact that all mares had foaled in March-April, when the days had already considerably lengthened. In a retrospective study conducted in Australia at 35 degrees S, Guerin and Wang (1994) found a certain influence of temperature, even though it was difficult to distinguish the relative effects of temperature and photoperiod. Oxender *et al.* (1975), in a study performed in Michigan, increased the natural photoperiod by 30 min/day using 250 W bulbs from December until they reached 16 h/day, which were maintained until 21 April. They

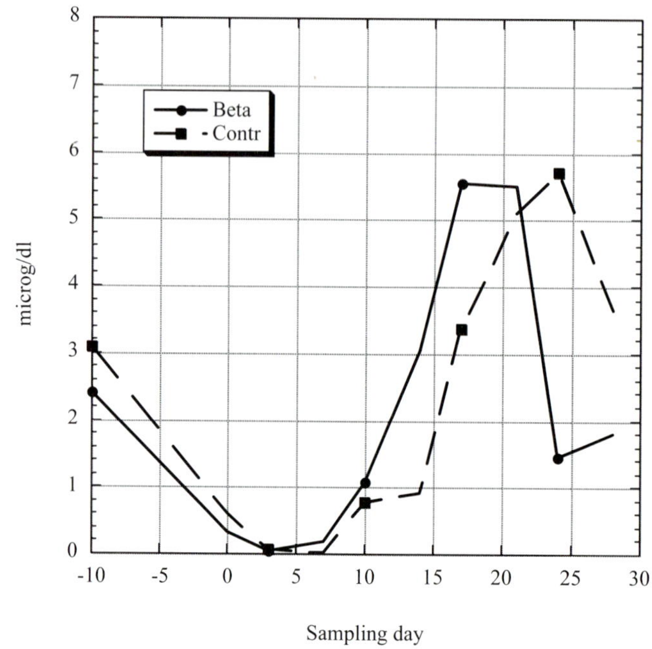

Figure 2. Progesterone levels.

compared these mares with subjects kept outdoors and with an indoor group exposed to natural lighting, and found that in mares exposed to the artificial photoperiod the anoestrus ended 59 days into treatment, i.e. 74 and 50 days earlier, respectively, than in the mares kept outdoors and those stabled in natural light conditions. Another interesting finding was that in the mares exposed to the artificial photoperiod the heat lasted 13 rather than 6-8 days as in controls; this however is not necessarily a positive fact, as it extends the period of observation for the identification of the best time for insemination. In the opinion of Oxender and coworkers, the 24-day advancement in oestrus onset in indoor control mares compared with outdoor subjects could be attributed to temperature, since both groups received the same ration (*ad libitum* hay), and the outdoor mares lost weight (BCS) due to their greater thermoregulation requirements.

In their 10-years study of a group of saddle mares kept in the open all year round with hand breeding, Trillaud-Geyl *et al.* (1990) calculated a mean duration of gestation of 337.7 ± 8.5 days and a mean parturition to conception interval of 29.8 ± 21.7 days. They believe that exploitation of the foal heat would enable foaling to be obtained once a year. However, considering that not all mares conceived each year, that only 59.5% of mares were fertile at the time of the foal heat, and the great variability in time to conception, the interval between parturitions in fact increased from 364.8 ± 19.4 to 396.8 days, or 13 months. When considering a whole herd, a systematic shift of parturitions from spring to summer is thus more realistic.

In the present study, the data of Trillaud-Geyl *et al.* (1990) were used as a reference to assess breeding performances in a large trotter farm based on the records of 293 Italian trotter mares from 1993-2005.

The breeding system on this farm may be considered typical of medium-large trotter mare farms in Italy. About 1-2 months before the expected date of parturition, mares are stabled in individual 3 × 3 m box stalls '(1-2 kg/day according to BCS). The compound feed is raised to 2-3 kg over the last weeks of gestation to meet the requirements of foetal growth, which is especially fast in this period, and prepare the breasts to colostrum and milk production. Parturition in the stable is assisted by farm staff, especially to ensure, and where necessary help, the intake of colostrum by the foal. During lactation the mare receives 4-6 kg/day of concentrated feed. Systematic veterinary checks are then performed to assess oestrus onset and thus the timing of AI in relation to the mare's condition and the availability of semen from the selected stallion. When the weather permits, mares and foals are allowed some hours in the paddock also in winter. Early in March, pregnant mares are turned out to graze in a succession of fenced fields and receive a supplement of hay and concentrated feed and oats (4-6 kg/head/day during lactation). From the third month of life, foal growth is sustained by creep-feeding. At 6-7 months foals are weaned; they are raised outdoors grouped by sex and age and they too receive hay and an energy-protein supplement appropriate to their age.

The numbers of mares present on the farm in the different years is reported in Figure 3, which shows a doubling of figures over the first 8 years, followed by a decline. These changes were the result of management decisions; in particular, mares with reproductive problems and especially those whose foals had not achieved high-level performances were removed from the farm since 2002. The distribution of parturitions by year and month is reported in Figure 4. Statistical analysis ($\chi 2$ test) evidenced highly significant differences ($P<0.001$) among the years. The most interesting finding was the marked reduction in the frequency of January and February parturitions and their shift to April and May and, from 1997, also to June. On average, foaling was "natural", with 64.4% of deliveries taking place in March, April and May in line with Ishii *et al.* (2001). The near-absence of parturitions in July was the result of management choices aimed at reducing the shift of births to the late breeding season. The mean date of birth in the first 3 years fell in the first 10 days of March and then shifted to April until 2002. The exclusion of a large number of mares explains the

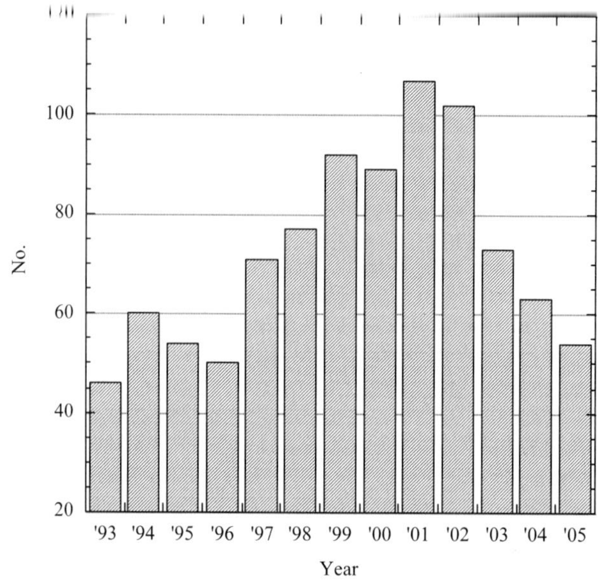

Figure 3. Changes in mares' number.

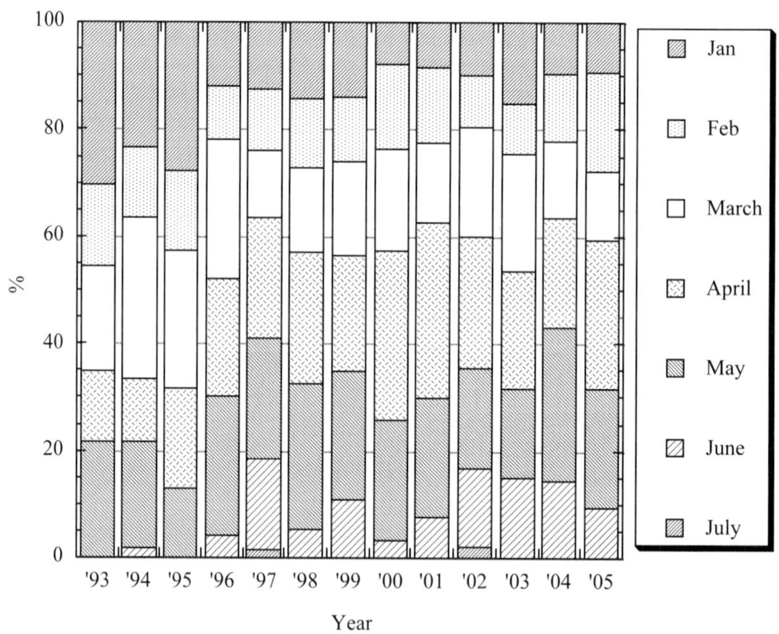

Figure 4. Foaling period in different years.

clear advancement (mid-February) of parturitions in 2003, while in 2004 and 2005 the mean date reverted to late March.

The yearly foaling interval data, reported in Figure 5, show a rising trend, especially in 1994-1999, when the mares were most numerous. The high variability of this interval, especially in 1997, is

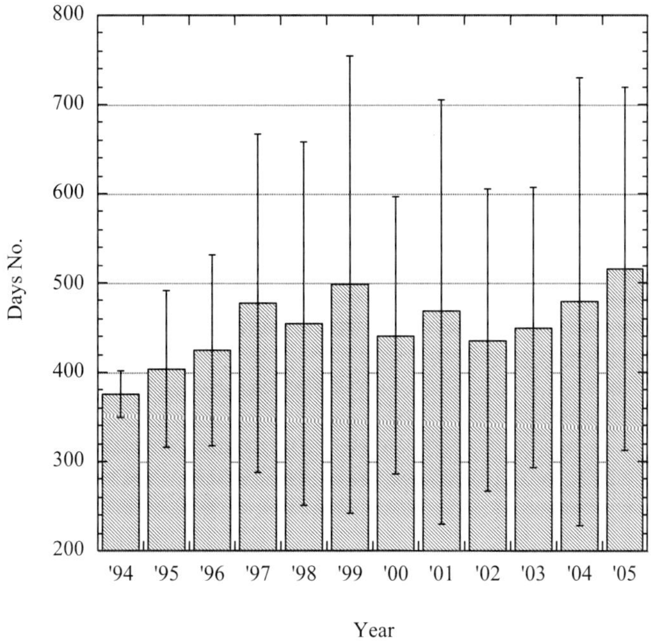

Figure 5. Foaling intervl by year (mean ± SD).

partly attributable to the shift of parturitions mentioned above, which resulted in an increased number of mares that could not be inseminated by July and were thus left unfertilized until the next mating season. This entailed a longer interval between parturitions of at least 6 months; in fact, if the mares that were not pregnant due to management choices are removed from the calculation, the values change considerably, with a mean of 370-390 days vs 516 in 2005 and a maximum standard deviation of 50 days vs 256 days in 1999.

The month-by-month trend of the foaling interval is shown in Figure 6. For parturitions in January to March, this interval is ~ 13 months, in line with the data of Trillaud-Geyl *et al.* (1990), it then declines significantly in April (373 days), to climb steeply again at the end of the season. For the June parturitions (464 ± 153 days), not only is the interval much longer, but the high standard deviation reflects the practice of not attempting a second insemination of the mares that have not conceived with the first, resulting in postponement of the procedure until the next season, at the end of the winter anoestrus. However, barring recourse to artificial interventions (e.g. photoperiod, temperature, hormone courses), the winter anoestrus generally ends in March-April.

Figure 7 summarizes the results of two studies (Trombetta et al., 1997; Falaschini and Trombetta, 1998) of the weight changes of Italian trotter mares monitored from foaling for 7-8 months. Mares were bred in standard conditions, kept in paddocks with the foals and fed hay and 2-3 kg/day oats. Given that all parturitions had taken place in May-June, all mares were inseminated only at the time of the foal heat, and foals were weaned at 5 months. The mares that did conceive at this time (P_1 and $P_{2)}$ were the same that at parturition had weighed more than those that did not subsequently conceive (NP_1 and NP_2).

Although all mares gained weight in the first two months from foaling, only those that had conceived continued to gain weight until the 7th-8th month. This may be ascribed to pregnancy anabolism and subsequently to the weight of the foetus and adnexa and likely to the higher feeding level. By

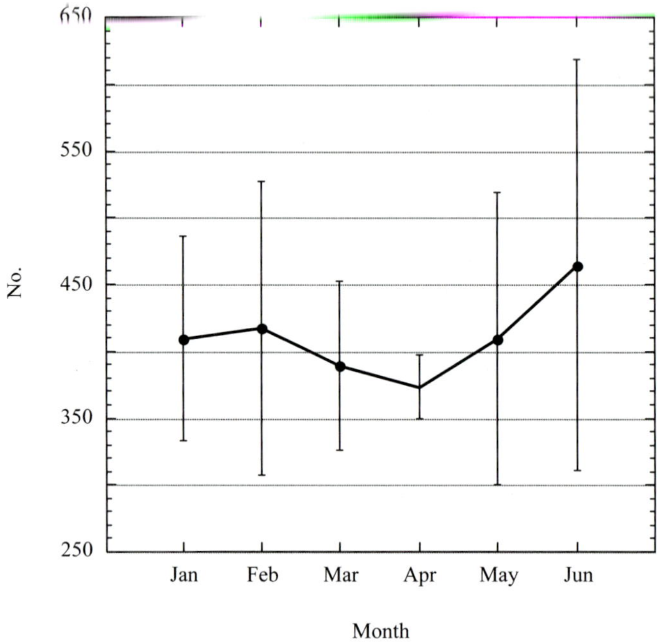

Figure 6. Foaling interval by month (mean ± SD).

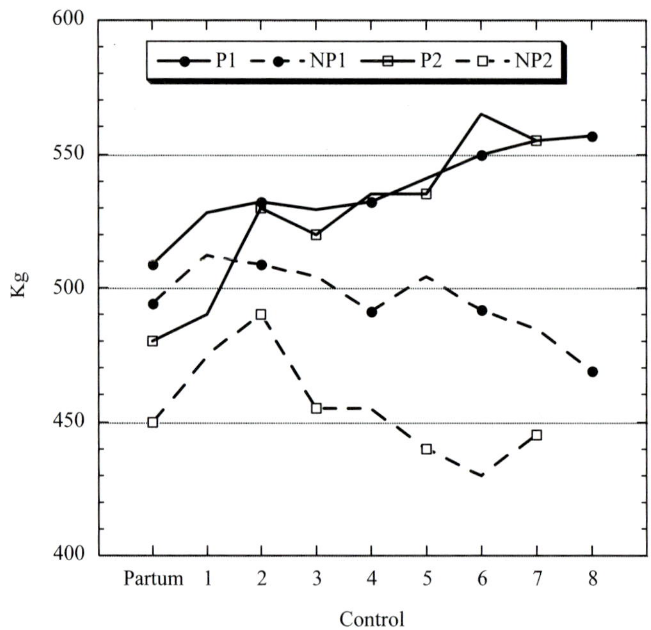

Figure 7. Mare' weight.

contrast, the mares that did not conceive tended to lose weight from the 3rd month post partum, due to a suboptimal dietary nutrient supply. A tendency to neglect the requirements of non-pregnant subjects is fairly common in all species even though, according to Oxender (1975), weight loss has adverse effects such as a greater difficulty to conceive in presence of suboptimal BCS. Indeed, Nagy et al. (1988) reported an increased interval between the first and second ovulation in mares that had lost BCS after the first 60 days from foaling. According to the french evaluation system, the optimum BCS for mares in peripartum can be considered 2.5-3.

Management of the foals

The evolution of some foal morphological parameters from birth to 8 months of age are reported in Figure 8 (Trombetta *et al.*, 1999). These foals were creep fed with 1 kg/head/day while suckling; after weaning at 6 months they received on average 2 kg/head/day until 10 months. It is interesting to note that the curves of height at withers and chest girth were parallel and exhibited a significant correlation ($P<0.0001$; height=51.3 + 0.60 girth). In this study, the increment of height at withers was similar to the one reported by Martin-Rosset (1990) and was ~ 5 cm/month until the 3rd-4th month and then declined to 2.5-3 cm/month until the 12th month.

The mean weight gain of these foals was lower than the one reported by Kohnke (1992), although it should be established for each breed and breeding system. The highly significant correlation found between weight and chest girth ($P<0.0001$; weight = –565.1 + 5.90 × girth) enables calculation of weight even when scales are not available. The regression line should however be recalculated for each genetic type. For foals, the daily growth rate to be pursued is not the maximum possible gain, since it has been shown that an excessively fast growth may have adverse effects and also favour osteochondrosis dissecans (OCD). Foal growth should thus be promoted and sustained with creep feeding using *ad hoc* and highly digestible feeds (flaked barley and corn and extruded soybean) since the earliest months of life, also to compensate for any decline in milk production by the mare.

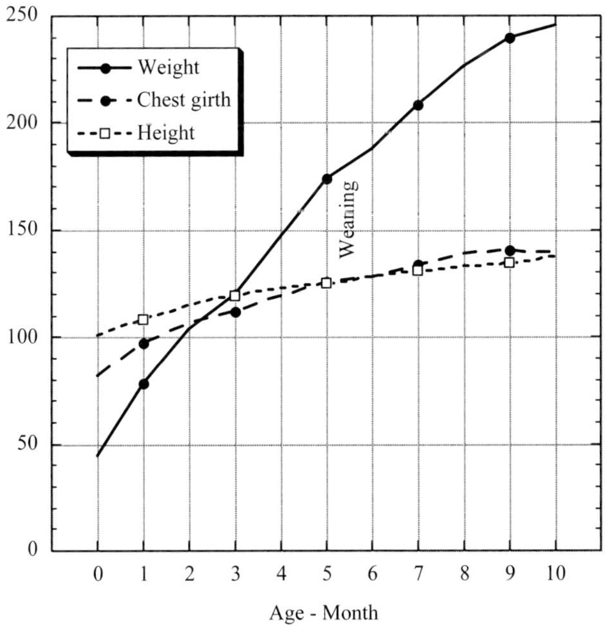

Figure 8. Foals morphological volution.

Discussion

Given that the horse is a free-ranging animal and thus requires to be kept outdoor, one of the main problems of Italian horse breeding is probably the availability of sufficient space for movement as well as for grazing, thus using feed supplements only for short periods.

Such conditions obtain rarely on Italian farms, particularly those situated on the plains, resulting in the need for accurate and balanced dietary supplementation. This is important both for the trotter mare and the suckling foal, until the phase preceding race training. The diet factor thus needs careful attention for the foals in all growth phases, and requirements of the mares can be calculated referring to the BCS.

We have reviewed the main natural factors regulating mare cycling (photoperiod, temperature, and diet). The need for advancing foaling to the first three months of the year entails important management choices, such as postponing the insemination of mares that have foaled late in the season.

Adoption of an artificial photoperiod together with appropriate vitamin supplementation (Falaschini 2006 - unpublished observations) is demonstrating that the winter anoestrus can be shortened and cycling advanced to the end of January.

Finally, indirectly affecting mare management is foal growth from parturition to 12 months of age. In this context, periodic morphological checks (weight, height, chest girth) can provide indications to assess the adequacy of the dietary regimen.
We feel that the several aspects briefly reviewed in this paper can contribute to successful trotter management.

References

Ahlswede, L., H. Konermann, 1980. Experiences with oral and parenteral administration of beta-carotene in the horse. Praktische Tierart. 68: 56-60

Camillo, F., M. Cela, S. Romagnoli, D. Minori, G. Macolino and A. Longo, 1993. Anticipazione dell'attività ovarica della cavalla per mezzo di un fotoperiodo artificiale. Ippologia, Anno 4, n.4: 29-32.

Doreau, M., W. Martin-Rosset and S. Boulot, 1988. Energy requirements and the feeding of mares during lactation: a review. Livest. Prod. Sci., 20: 53-68

Falaschini, A. and M.F. Trombetta, 1998. Variazioni del peso e di alcuni parametri ematici in fattrici di razza trottatore italiano: II anno di monitoraggio. Congresso SISVet. Silvi Marina (TE) 17-19 settembre: 517-518

Falaschini, A., 2006. Effetti della somministrazione di β-carotene a fattrici di razza trottatore: II anno di esperienza. (unpublished)

Ginter, O.J., 1974. Occurrence of anestrus, estrus, diestrus and ovulation over 12-month period in mares. Am J Vet Res, Vol 36. 10:1413-1419.

Guerin, M.V. and X.J. Wang, 1994. Environmental temperature has an influence on timing of the first ovulation of seasonal estrus in the mare. Theriogenology 42: 1053-1060.

Hintz, H.F., 1998. Protein Nutrition of the Mare. Equine Practice. Vol. 20, n 4: 20-21.

Hodge, S.L., J.L. Kreider, G.D. Potter, P.G. Harms and J.L. Fleeger, 1982. Influence of photoperiod on the pregnant and postpartum mare (1982) Am J Vet Res, Vol 43. 10:1752-1755.

Holst, W. van der, E.J. Tjalsma and C.I. Wonder, 1984. Experiences with oral administration of beta-carotene to pony mares in early spring. 35th Annual Meting of the European Association of Animal Production. The Hague, The Netherlands. 6-9 August 1984: 15

Ishii, M., T. Shimamuro, A. Utsumi, T. Jitsukawa, M. Endo, T. Fukuda, T. Yamanoi, 2001. Reproductive performance and factors that decrease pregnancy rate in heavy draft horse bred at the foal heat. J. Equine Vet. Sci. 21(3): 131-136

Konhke, B.V., 1992. Feeding and nutrition, 69 Ed. Birubi Pacific, Australia.

Kooistra, L.H. and O.J., Ginter 1975 Effect of photoperiod on reproductive activity and hai in mares; Am. J. Vet. Res. Vol 36 n. 10: 1413-1419.

Lieux, P., 1980. Comparative results of breeding on the first and second post-foaling heat periods. Proc. Amedr. Assoc, equine Pract.: 129-132

Loy, R.G., 1980. Characteristics of pos-partum reproduction in mares. Vet. Clin, Amer. Large Anim. Pract. 2: 345-348

Martin-Rosset, W. and M. Doreau, 1984 Besoins et alimentation de la jument. 354-370.In « Le cheval » R Jarrige and W Martin-Rosset Eds. INRA Editions 78026 Versailles - France.

Martin-Rosset, W., 1990. L'alimentation des chevaux. 91-93 INRA Paris.

Micol, D. and W. Martin-Rosset, 1995. Feeding systems for horses on high forage diets in the temperate zone. In Journet M., Grenet E., Farce M-H. Thériez M., Demarquilly C. (eds), Recent developments in the Nutrition of Herbivores. Proceedings of the IV International Symposium on the Nutrition of Herbivores: 569-584. INRA Editions, Paris.

Nagy, P., Gy. Huszenicza, M. Juhasz, M. Kulcsar, L. Solti, J. Reiczigel and K. Abary, 1998. Factors influencing ovarian activity and sexual behaviour of postpartum mares under farm conditions. Theriogenology. 50: 1109-1119.

Oxender, W.D., P.A. Noden and H.D. Hafs, 1977. Estrus, ovulation, and serum progesterone, estradiol, and LH concentrations in mares after an increased photoperiod during winter. Am. J. Vet. Res., vol. 38, 2: 203 207.

Salomoni, M., 1995. Alimentazione ed allevamento. Razionamento pratico della fattrice. Rivista di Ippologia. Anno I – N 4: 223-225.

Trombetta, M.F., P.A. Accorsi, P. Pezzi, F. Parmeggiani and A. Falaschini, 2003. Effect of β-carotene integration to Italian trotter mares in peripartum. Ital. J. Anim. Sci. Vol.2 (suppl. 1):589-591.

Trombetta, M.F., S. Mattii and A. Falaschini, 1997. L'allevamento del cavallo da trotto: variazioni del peso e di alcuni parametri metabolici nella fattrice durante l'interparto. Atti XII Congresso Nazionale ASPA. Pisa 23-26 giugno 1997: 335-336.

Trombetta, M.F., S. Mattii, F. Parmeggiani, P. Accorsi and A. Falaschini, 2000. Effetto del flushing sulla ripresa dell'attività riproduttiva e sul quadro metabolico in cavalle di razza trottatore italiano. Atti 2° Convegno "Nuove acquisizioni in materia di alimentazione, allevamento e allenamento del cavallo sportivo". Campobasso 13-14 ottobre 2000: 45-48.

Trombetta, M.F., S. Mattii, M. Pasquini and A. Falaschini, 2000. Morphological evolution of trotter foals in the first year of life: results of a three year study. SISVet Annual Meeting selected abstracts. Anno II, 2000: 166.

Trillaud-Geyl, C., J. Brohier, L. de Baynast, N. Baudoin, E. Rossier and O. Lapierre, 1990. Bilan de productivité sur 10 ans d'un troupeau de juments de selle conduites en plein-air integral. Croissance de produits de 0 a 6 mois. World Review of Animal Production. Val. XXV, n 3: 65-70.

Author index

A
Albenzio, M. 183
Alves, V.C. 253
Austbo, D. 15, 89

B
Bailoni, L. 341
Bergero, D. 263
Boekhoff, M. 341
Brown-Douglas, C.G. 245
Buff, P.R. 155
Burton Staniar, W. 299

C
Caddel, S. 245
Cai, J. 259
Camillo, F. 389
Cappelli, F. 403
Caroprese, M. 183
Casamassima, D. 169, 171
Casini, L. 41
Chiofalo, B. 117, 133, 175, 177, 181
Clément, F. 203
Coenen, M. 89, 367
Colella, G.E. 171
Corazza, M. 41
Curadi, M.C. 257

D
D'Alessandro, A.G. 171
D'Emilio, F. 183
Darien, B.J. 259
Doreau, M. 57, 65, 77
Drogoul, C. 133, 203

E
Ellis, A.D. 341

F
Falaschini, A. 403
Fantuz, F. 167, 179

G
Galli, C. 389
Gambacorta, M. 181
Ganjam, V.K. 155
Gatta, D. 41
Godbee, R.G. 259
Guillaume, D. 315

H
Harris, P. 367

J
Johnson, P.J. 155

K
Keisler, D.H. 155

L
Leitão, L.C. 253
Liesman, J. 163

M
Magistrelli, D. 167
Maglieri, C. 167, 169, 175, 177, 179, 181
Magni, L. 41
Mantovani, R. 341
Marino, R. 183
Martemucci, G. 171
Martin-Rosset, W. 15, 89, 221, 279, 315
Martuzzi, F. 57, 65, 77
Messer IV, N.T. 155
Miraglia, N. 263, 279
Moore, J. 163

N
Nielsen, B.D. 163

O
Orlandi, M. 203, 257
Ousey, J.C. 187

P
Pagan, J.D. 245
Palazzo, M. 169, 171
Palmer, E. 389
Peek, S.F. 259
Pelosi, S. 183
Piccolo, D. 175, 177
Pizzo, R. 171
Polidori, M. 167, 181
Polidori, P. 169, 179

R
Riolo, E.B. 175, 177
Rosi, F. 167

S

Saastamoinen, M. 279
Salazar-Ortiz, J. 315
Salimei, E. 117, 133, 167, 169, 175, 177, 179, 181
Santillo, A. 183
Santos, A.S. 149, 253
Sgorbini, M. 41
Silvestre, A.M. 149
Simone, N. 171
Socci, R. 181
Sousa, B.C. 253
Stamper, T. 163
Starbuck, G.R. 49

T

Tauson, A.H. 367
Trillaud-Geyl, C. 263
Trottier, N.L. 163

V

Valle, E. 263
Varisco, G. 179, 181
Ventorp, M. 203, 263
Vervuert, I. 15, 263
Vincenzetti, S. 179

X

Xu, J. 259

Y

Younge, B. 221